Children's Speech
Sound Disorders

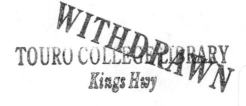

Dedication

Tweets

Caroline Bowen @speech_woman · 14s
Children's Speech Sound Disorders 2e is dedicated to my amazing husband Don Bowen and to #WeSpeechies everywhere!
www.wiley.com/go/bowen/speechlanguagetherapy

Expand   ↰ Reply 🗑 Delete ★ Favorite ••• More

Children's Speech Sound Disorders

SECOND EDITION

Caroline Bowen, PhD CPSP
Speech-Language Pathologist
Honorary Associate in Linguistics, Macquarie University, Sydney, Australia
Honorary Research Fellow, School of Health Sciences, Speech-Language Pathology,
University of KwaZulu-Natal, Durban, South Africa

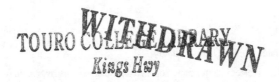
WILEY Blackwell

Library of Congress Cataloging-in-Publication Data

Bowen, Caroline, author.
  Children's speech sound disorders / Caroline Bowen. – Second edition.
    p. ; cm.
  Includes bibliographical references and indexes.
  ISBN 978-1-118-63402-8 (pbk.)
  I. Title.
  [DNLM: 1. Speech Disorders–therapy.   2. Child.   3. Speech-Language Pathology–methods. WL 340.2]
  RJ496.S7
  618.92′855–dc23

                                                                        2014014238

A catalogue record for this book is available from the British Library.

Cover image: Three panel photography by Rachael Moore. Girl with headphones © iStock.

Set in 10/12.5pt Times by Aptara Inc., New Delhi, India

1   2015

Contents

Contributors

Areej Asad, MSc
Speech Language Therapist
Doctoral Candidate
Discipline of Speech Science
School of Psychology
The University of Auckland
Auckland
New Zealand

Elise Baker, PhD
Lecturer
Discipline of Speech Pathology
Faculty of Health Sciences
The University of Sydney
Sydney, New South Wales
Australia

Martin J. Ball, PhD
Professor of Speech and Language Pathology
Linköpings Universitet
Institutionen för Klinisk och Experimentell
    Medicin
Logopedi
Linköping
Sweden

Kirrie Ballard, PhD
Associate Professor
Discipline of Speech Pathology
Faculty of Health Sciences
The University of Sydney
Sydney, New South Wales
Australia

B. May Bernhardt, PhD
Professor
School of Audiology and Speech Sciences
University of British Columbia
Vancouver, British Columbia
Canada

John E. Bernthal, PhD
Professor Emeritus
University of Nebraska-Lincoln
Lincoln, Nebraska
USA

James Robert Bitter, EdD
Professor
Department of Counseling and Human Services
East Tennessee State University
Johnson City, Tennessee
USA

Kenneth M. Bleile, PhD
Professor
Department of Communication Sciences and
    Disorders
University of Northern Iowa
Cedar Falls, Iowa
USA

Barbara Dodd, PhD
Honorary Professorial Fellow
Department Audiology and Speech Pathology
The University of Melbourne
Melbourne, Victoria
Australia

Liz Fairgray, MSc
Speech-Language Therapist
Listening and Language Clinic
Discipline of Speech Science
School of Psychology
The University of Auckland
Auckland
New Zealand

Peter Flipsen Jr., PhD
Professor of Speech Pathology
School of Communication Sciences and
   Disorders
Pacific University
Forest Grove, Oregon
USA

Karen Froud, PhD
Associate Professor of Speech-Language
   Pathology
Director Neurocognition of Language Laboratory
Department of Biobehavioral Sciences
Teachers College
Columbia University
New York
USA

Hilary Gardner, DPhil
Speech and Language Therapist
Senior Lecturer
Department of Human Communication Sciences
The University of Sheffield
Sheffield
UK

Fiona Gibbon, PhD
Professor and Head of Speech and Hearing
   Sciences
Department Speech and Hearing Sciences
University College Cork
Cork
Ireland

Gail T. Gillon, PhD
Professor in Speech-Language Therapy
Pro-Vice-Chancellor, College of Education
University of Canterbury
Christchurch
New Zealand

Karen J. Golding-Kushner, PhD
Golding-Kushner Speech Center, LLC
East Brunswick, New Jersey and
The Virtual Center for Velo-Cardio-Facial
   Syndrome
New York
USA

Brian A. Goldstein, PhD
Dean and Professor, School of Nursing and
   Health Sciences
La Salle University
Philadelphia, Pennsylvania
USA

Sharon Gretz, MEd
Founder and Executive Director
Childhood Apraxia of Speech Association of
   North America
Pittsburgh, Pennsylvania
USA

Anne Hesketh, PhD
Clinical Senior Lecturer in Speech and Language
   Therapy
School of Psychological Sciences
The University of Manchester
Manchester
UK

Chantelle Highman, PhD
Speech Pathologist
Bentley Child Development Service
Department of Health
Perth, Western Australia
Australia

Megan M. Hodge, PhD
Professor Emerita
Director, Children's Speech Intelligibility
    Research and Education Laboratory
Department of Communication Sciences and
    Disorders
University of Alberta
Edmonton, Alberta
Canada

Barbara W. Hodson, PhD
Professor
Communication Sciences and Disorders
Wichita State University
Wichita, Kansas
USA

David Ingram, PhD
Professor in Speech and Hearing
Department of Speech and Hearing Science
Arizona State University
Tempe, Arizona
USA

Deborah G. H. James, PhD
Lecturer, Speech Pathology
School of Health and Human Sciences, Southern
    Cross University
Gold Coast Campus, Bilinga, Queensland
Australia

Victoria Joffe, DPhil
Professor in the Enhancement of Child and
    Adolescent Language and Learning
Associate Dean for Taught Postgraduate Studies
    and Internationalisation
Department of Language and Communication
    Science
School of Health Sciences
City University London
London
UK

Reem Khamis-Dakwar, PhD
Assistant Professor
Director Neurophysiology in Speech Language
    Pathology Lab
Department of Communication Sciences and
    Disorders
Adelphi University
New York
USA

Gwen Lancaster, MSc
Speech and Language Therapist
Language and Learning Team
London Borough of Merton
UK

Suze Leitão, PhD
Senior Lecturer
School of Psychology and Speech Pathology
Curtin University
Perth, Western Australia
Australia

Gregory L. Lof, PhD
Professor and Chair
Department of Communication Sciences and
    Disorders
School of Health and Rehabilitation Sciences
MGH Institute of Health Professions
Boston, Massachusetts
USA

Robert J. Lowe, PhD
Retired
Formerly Professor, Communication Disorders
Bloomsburg University of Pennsylvania
Bloomsburg, Pennsylvania
USA

Patricia McCabe, PhD
Associate Professor
Discipline of Speech Pathology
Faculty of Health Sciences
The University of Sydney
Sydney, New South Wales
Australia

Rebecca J. McCauley, PhD
Professor
Department of Speech and Hearing Science
The Ohio State University
Columbus, Ohio
USA

Karen Leigh McComas, EdD
Professor of Communication Disorders
Assistant Director Center for Teaching and
    Learning
Marshall University
Huntington, West Virginia
USA

Sharynne McLeod, PhD
Professor of Speech and Language Acquisition
Charles Sturt University
Bathurst, New South Wales
Australia

Adele W. Miccio, PhD (1959–2009)
Associate Professor of Communication Sciences
    and Disorders and Applied Linguistics
Co-Director of the Center for Language Science
Pennsylvania State University
University Park, Pennsylvania
USA

Nicole Müller, DPhil
Professor of Speech and Language Pathology
Linköpings Universitet
Institutionen för Klinisk och Experimentell
    Medicin
Logopedi
Linköping
Sweden

Benjamin Munson, PhD
Professor in Speech Language Hearing Sciences
University of Minnesota
Minneapolis, Minnesota
USA

Roslyn Neilson, PhD
Speech-Language Pathologist
Language, Speech and Literacy Services

Jamberoo, New South Wales
Australia

Megan Overby, PhD
Associate Professor
Department of Speech-Language Pathology
Duquesne University
Pittsburgh, Pennsylvania
USA

Michelle Pascoe, PhD
Senior Lecturer in Speech Pathology
Division of Communication Sciences and
    Disorders
University of Cape Town
South Africa

Karen E. Pollock, PhD
Professor and Chair
Department of Communication Sciences and
    Disorders
University of Alberta
Edmonton, Alberta
Canada

Thomas W. Powell, PhD
Professor in Speech-Language Pathology
Department of Rehabilitation Sciences
Louisiana State University Health Sciences
    Center
Shreveport, Louisiana
USA

Suzanne C. Purdy, PhD
Professor and Head
Discipline of Speech Science
School of Psychology
The University of Auckland,
Auckland
New Zealand

Mirla G. Raz, MEd
Speech-Language Pathologist
Communication Skills Center
GerstenWeitz Publishers
Scottsdale, Arizona
USA

Joan B. Rosenthal, MA
Retired
University of Sydney
Sydney, New South Wales
Australia

Susan Roulstone, PhD
Emeritus Professor of Speech and Language
   Therapy
Co-Director Bristol Speech and Language
   Therapy Research Unit
University of the West of England
Bristol
UK

Dennis M. Ruscello, PhD
Professor of Communication Sciences and
   Disorders
Adjunct Professor of Otolaryngology
West Virginia University
Morgantown, West Virginia
USA

Susan Rvachew, PhD
Professor
School of Communication Sciences and
   Disorders
McGill University
Montréal, Québec
Canada

Amy E. Skinder-Meredith, PhD
Clinical Associate Professor
Department of Speech and Hearing Sciences
Washington State University
Spokane, Washington
USA

Hilary Stephens, BSc
Principal Speech and Language Therapist
Nuffield Hearing and Speech Centre
Royal National Throat Nose and Ear Hospital
University College London Hospitals NHS
   Foundation Trust
London
UK

Ruth Stoeckel, PhD
Clinical Speech-Language Pathologist
Mayo Clinic
Rochester, Minnesota
USA

Carol Stoel-Gammon, PhD
Professor Emerita
Department of Speech and Hearing Sciences
University of Washington
Seattle, Washington
USA

Judith Stone-Goldman, PhD
Emeritus Senior Lecturer
Department of Speech and Hearing Sciences
University of Washington
Seattle, Washington
USA

Edythe A. Strand, PhD
Professor of Speech Pathology
Consultant, Department of Neurology
Mayo Clinic
Rochester, Minnesota
USA

Kylie Toynton, BSpPath, MGerontology
Speech Pathologist
Language for Life
Rocky Glen, New South Wales
Australia

Angela Ullrich, PhD
Speech-Language Pathologist
Independent Scholar
Siegen
Germany

Nicole Watts Pappas, PhD
Queensland Health
Children's Developmental Service
Mt Gravatt, Queensland
Australia

A. Lynn Williams, PhD
Professor
Department of Audiology and Speech-Language
    Pathology
Associate Director Center of Excellence in Early
    Childhood Learning and Development
East Tennessee State University
Johnson City, Tennessee
USA

Pamela Williams, MSc
Consultant Speech and Language Therapist/Team
    Manager (Developmental Disorders)
Nuffield Hearing and Speech Centre
Royal National Throat Nose and Ear Hospital

University College London Hospitals NHS
    Foundation Trust
London
UK

Krisztina Zajdó, PhD
Associate Professor
Department of Special
    Education/Speech-Language Pathology
University of West Hungary
Győr
Hungary

Note: See the Contributor Index for the list of
questions answered by each contributor.

About the companion website

This book is accompanied by a companion website:

www.wiley.com/go/bowen/speechlanguagetherapy

The website includes:

- For instructors: Powerpoint and PDF of author's notes for downloading
- For students/readers: Links to the author's personal website (http://www.speech-language-therapy.com/) for web references and resources

Part I

A practical update

Introduction to Part I

Followers of the literature on children's speech sound disorders (SSD) know that much has happened in the 6 years since the first edition of *Children's Speech Sound Disorders* appeared. As with its predecessor, the aim of this work is to provide an accessible, contemporary book on child speech for a readership of clinicians, clinical educators and students in speech–language pathology/speech and language therapy (SLP/SLT).

The uniqueness of this text lies in the inclusion of 54-bite-sized expert essays by 60 internationally respected academicians, clinicians and researchers, representing the fields of audiology, clinical phonology (Grunwell, 1987; Müller & Ball, 2013b), family therapy (Bitter, 2013) and SLP/SLT. The essays, A1–A54 are responses to my questions Q1–Q54, about primary areas in the contributors' own work and how they relate to evidence-based SLP/SLT practice. The questions are not necessarily my own. In fact, most are built on frequently asked questions put to me by colleagues in continuing professional development

or 'training' events, private correspondence and postings to the children's SSD ('phonologicaltherapy') online discussion (Bowen, 2001, 2013). The first two essays are here in the introduction to Part 1. In A1, Sharynne McLeod writes about the international classification of functioning, disability and health – children and youth (ICF-CY) (WHO, 2007), and in A2, taking an international perspective, Michelle Pascoe shares her view of the differences and similarities in child speech practice in different parts of the world.

The contributors

The brief for the contributors has been challenging, as it is a big thing, even for an expert, to condense central aspects of a major body of work into a handful of well thought-out paragraphs, and all of the contributors have delivered brilliantly. Their answers, rarely exceeding 2 000 words, provide quick, readable and sufficiently detailed information for busy colleagues. Attentive readers of the first edition will notice that there are newcomers among the 60 contributors and that their surnames now run from A to Z. They are:

Areej Asad, Elise Baker, Martin Ball, Kirrie Ballard, B. May Bernhardt, John Bernthal, James Bitter, Ken Bleile, Barbara Dodd, Liz Fairgray, Peter Flipsen Jr., Karen Froud, Hilary Gardner, Fiona Gibbon, Gail Gillon, Karen Golding-Kushner, Brian Goldstein, Sharon Gretz, Anne Hesketh, Chantelle Highman, Megan Hodge, Barbara Hodson, David Ingram, Debbie James, Victoria Joffe, Reem Khamis-Dakwar, Gwen Lancaster, Suze Leitão, Gregory Lof, Robert Lowe, Patricia McCabe, Rebecca McCauley, Karen McComas, Sharynne McLeod, Adele Miccio (d), Nicole Müller, Benjamin Munson, Roslyn Neilson, Megan Overby, Michelle Pascoe, Karen Pollock, Tom Powell, Suzanne Purdy, Mirla Raz, Joan Rosenthal, Susan Roulstone, Dennis Ruscello, Susan Rvachew, Amy Skinder-Meredith, Hilary Stephens, Carol Stoel-Gammon, Judith Stone-Goldman, Edythe Strand, Ruth Stoeckel, Kylie Toynton, Angela Ullrich, Nicole Watts Pappas, A. Lynn Williams, Pamela Williams and Krisztina Zajdó.

Having remained current, 8 of the original 49 essays – those authored by Bernhardt and Ullrich, Bleile, Flipsen Jr., Lancaster, Lowe, Rosenthal, Rvachew and Stone-Goldman – appear here unchanged or lightly edited. The essay by the late Adele Miccio is also included unchanged by kind permission of her children Anthony and Claire.

Thirty-two substantially revised and updated contributions come from Baker, Froud, Gardner, Gibbon, Gillon, Golding-Kushner, Gretz, Hesketh, Highman, Hodge, Ingram, James, Joffe, Leitão, Lof, McCauley, McLeod, Munson, Neilson, Pascoe, Pollock, Powell, Raz, Roulstone, Ruscello, Skinder-Meredith, Stoel-Gammon, Stoeckel, Strand, Watts Pappas, Williams, and Williams and Stephens.

Thirteen new contributions are by Bitter; Dodd; Froud and Khamis-Dakwar; Hodson; Goldstein; Ingram; McCabe and Ballard; McComas; Müller and Ball; Overby and Bernthal; Purdy, Asad and Fairgray; Strand; Toynton; and Zajdó.

The questions, which are often multi-part, and about two-thirds of the book, are by me. I write from the perspective of an Australian speech–language pathologist with an international outlook, 40 years of clinical experience, a modest research background, close familiarity with our refereed literature and a commitment to both strong theory and evidence-based practice or E^3BP (Dollaghan, 2004, 2007). As a professional person intent on maintaining work–life balance (Bowen, 2008), I am mindful of the time limitations and conflicting priorities that can make it impossible for clinical practitioners to access the literature relating to child speech as regularly as they would wish; to synthesise, digest and integrate what they have read; and then to apply the knowledge in their work. These constraints mean that clinically applicable information tends to remain in academe, refusing to cross either the theory–therapy gap or the research–practice gap (Duchan, 2001). Speaking clinician-to-clinician, clinician-to-researcher, and researcher-to-clinician once again, this new edition sets out to make critical theory-to-evidence-to-practice connections plain.

The children

The other A to Z of names here comes from the case examples where the reader will meet AJ, Abdi, Adam, Alison, Andrew, Bethany, Bobby, Brett, Brian, Bruno, Ceri, Christopher, Costa, Daniel, David, Dorothy, Emeline, Emma, Fiona, Greg, Harriet, Iain, Jacob, James (and Hannah), Joanna, Jessica, Josie, Kacey, Kenny, Luke, Max, Nadif, Nina, Olaf, Owen, Peter, Philip, Precious, Quentin, Robert, Sam, Sasha, Sebastian, Sigrid, Simon, Sophie, Tad, Tessa, Thomas, Tim, Uzzia, Vaughan, Wesley, William, Xing-Fu, Yoshi and Zach. While the children are real, their names and family members' names are pseudonyms and details relating to some of them have been changed slightly to preserve their anonymity. The exceptions are Gerri, Madison and Shaun whose real names are used by permission.

E³BP

Dollaghan (2007, p. 2) defines E³BP as a dynamic three-way arrangement that combines 'the conscientious, explicit, and judicious integration of best available external evidence from systematic research, best available evidence internal to clinical practice, and best available evidence concerning the preferences of a fully informed patient'. In all discussions of E³BP (e.g., Baker & McLeod, 2011a,b; Powell, A39; Roddam & Skeat, 2010), the important connections between the practitioner's role, good science, academic curiosity and clinical thinking are constantly highlighted. Dollaghan goes on to say, 'E³BP requires honest doubt about a clinical issue, awareness of one's own biases, a respect for other positions, a willingness to let strong evidence alter what is already known, and constant mindfulness of ethical responsibilities to patients'. Pursuing this line of reasoning and emboldening practitioners to reach for balance between total acceptance of their customary practice and an open willingness to explore and accept new ideas, Kamhi (2011, p. 59) argues that, 'the scientific method and evidence-based approaches can provide guidance to practitioners but will not lead to a consensus about best clinical practices'.

Maintaining an E³BP focus, the book is in two parts. Part I concerns theoretical and empirical developments of this decade, and leading earlier work, in the classification, diagnosis and management of children affected by SSD. Against this scientific background, the focus of Part II is the practicalities of day-to-day treatment of children for their SSD and associated issues.

Children with SSD

Children with SSD have gaps and simplifications in their speech sound systems that can make what they say difficult to understand. Nevertheless, most of them persist valiantly in their struggle to communicate intelligibly, despite limited speech sound repertoires, restricted use of syllable structures, incomplete stress pattern inventories and odd pronunciation. They may attempt to accommodate to their difficulties by using speech patterns and structures, or phonological processes (Ingram, 1989), that should not really be present in the utterances of otherwise typically developing children of their ages. For instance, affected English-learning children of 4 or 5, troubled by protracted or problematic speech development, may persist in saying *fin* for *spin*, *twit* for *quit*, or *doom* for *zoom*; and sometimes they simply seem to leave a gap, and the listener hears, for example, *pie* for *pipe*, *up* for *cup*, or *toss* for *Thomas*. They can have poor stimulability, systemic and substitution errors, syllable structure errors, consonant distortions, vowel deviations, atypical prosody, unusual tonality and offbeat timing. Any or all of these intriguing but bothersome speech characteristics can occur singly or in combination; so that the children's speech difficulties can encompass a mixture of phonetic (articulatory), phonemic (phonological or cognitive–linguistic), structural (craniofacial or syndromic), perceptual or neuromotor bases.

Some children have minor speech production difficulties and near perfect intelligibility, likely fitting at the mild end of the conversational Percentage of Consonants Correct (PCC) scale (Shriberg, 1982; Shriberg, Austin, Lewis, McSweeny & Wilson, 1997). But of those referred for·screening or assessments, a large proportion of the children SLPs/SLTs see for *intervention* belongs at the other end of the PCC (or PCC-R) scale displayed in Table i1.1, with moderate-to-severe and severe speech impairments and low intelligibility. As well as making the communication process arduous for the children themselves, their poor speech clarity places extra demands on their parents, siblings, and others close to them. Often, these important individuals have to work overtime, listening super-attentively in order to decipher what the speech-impaired children are saying, regularly finding themselves in the roles of advocate, apologist, code-breaker, go-between and personal interpreter.

Table i1.1 SSD severity scale based on a conversational speech sample (Shriberg, 1982)

Severity interval descriptor[a]	Percentage of consonants correct (PCC)
Mild SSD to normal speech	>85%
Mild to moderate SSD	65–85%
Moderate to severe SSD	50–65%
Severe SSD	<50%

[a]The severity interval descriptors refer to SSD in general and are applicable to children aged 4;1 through 8;6.
The severity interval descriptors apply to SSD and not to specific diagnostic categories under the SSD umbrella. For example, the term 'mild to moderate SSD' can be applied to describe the conversational speech of a child aged 4;1–8;6 with a PCC of 65–85%, using clinical judgement where the percentages overlap. It would be incorrect to refer to that same child as having a 'mild to moderate' articulation disorder/phonological disorder or CAS based on conversational PCC. As well, the descriptors should not be applied to PCCs derived from single-word naming tests.

Under the umbrella heading of either Speech Sound Disorder (American Psychiatric Association, 2013, pp. 44–45) or Speech Sound Disorders (Bernthal, Bankson & Flipsen Jr., 2013; Williams, McLeod & McCauley, 2010), abbreviated SSD either way, the difficulties these young clients face attract labels such as Developmental Phonological Disorder or simply Phonological Disorder, Functional Articulation Disorder or Articulation Disorder, and Childhood Apraxia of Speech (ASHA, 2007) or Developmental Verbal Dyspraxia (DVD) (RCSLT, 2011). All of these diagnoses have a miscellany of perplexing synonyms and acronyms. Irrespective of the classification system used (Waring & Knight, 2013), the diagnostic labels applied, the psycholinguistic profiles generated and the short- and long-term impacts of speech impairment for the children themselves and for their families and society (McCormack, McLeod, Harrison & McAllister, 2010), SLPs/SLTs are charged with the responsibility of dealing effectively with SSD and are uniquely qualified to do so.

Highly unintelligible 3-, 4- and 5-year-old children with moderate-to-severe and severe SSD, as revealed by their PCCs in conversational speech or their performance on single-word-naming (citation naming) tasks, often have complex and difficult-to-analyse speech. Accordingly, they can

pose demanding diagnostic, intervention, reporting and information-sharing challenges for experienced and inexperienced speech and language professionals alike. *Children's Speech Sound Disorders* is about the work clinicians do with such children and their families. It is also about the so-called 'mildly involved' children, many of whom are at school and are older than the moderately and severely affected ones. These older children may have received intervention for brief, through to lengthy periods, continuously or intermittently and have just one or a few persisting and seemingly intractable speech issues, exhibiting insignificant change (Bain & Dollaghan, 1991; Speake, Howard & Vance, 2011). Examples include a stubborn lateral or palatal substitution for /s/ or difficulty producing a particular vowel (Speake, Stackhouse & Pascoe, 2012) so that, for instance, *hat* it sounds like *hut*.

In an individual child, intelligibility concerns may come bundled co-morbidly with other communication impairments (McCauley, A14; Stoeckel, A40), for example, voice disorders, stuttering (Unicomb, Hewat, Spencer & Harrison, 2013), semantic and pragmatic difficulties and language impairment (Tyler, Gillon, Macrae & Johnson, 2011). Some children have other issues of health, development and wellbeing, such as physical or sensory challenges, chemical intolerances and food allergies, intellectual impairment, learning difficulties, and auditory processing and attention deficits. These can be associated with metabolic conditions such as galactosemia (Shriberg, Potter & Strand, 2011) and spectrum disorders such as autism (Shriberg, Paul, Black & van Santen, 2011). In culturally and linguistically diverse clinical settings, numbers of them face the added complication of attempting to acquire more than one language and hence more than one speech sound system (Goldstein, A19; McLeod, Verdon & Bowen, 2013; Yavaş, 2007; Zajdó, A20).

World Health Organization

Whether they are monolingual or multilingual, have an isolated SSD or have an SSD as one of several issues, their lives will be affected in the areas of Body Function, Body Structure, Activity and Participation, Environmental Factors and Personal Factors. These are the headings itemised in the World Health Organization's ICF-CY: the children and youth version of the *International Classification of Functioning, Disability and Health* (WHO, 2001). Question 1 (Q1) is about the ICF-CY, and it goes to speech–language pathologist, Sharynne McLeod.

A tireless worker in speech research and pedagogy, Dr. Sharynne McLeod is Professor of Speech and Language Acquisition at Charles Sturt University, Australia. She is vice president of the International Clinical Linguistics and Phonetics Association (ICPLA), a former editor of the *International Journal of Speech-Language Pathology*, a Fellow of Speech Pathology Australia, and a Fellow of ASHA. Her research has focused on the production of speech sounds in children and adults, and a specific area of inquiry she pursues is the application of the ICF-CY to children with SSD.

Q1. Sharynne McLeod: The ICF-CY and children with speech difficulties

In at least two respects the *International Classification of Functioning, Disability and Health – Children and Youth (ICF-CY)* (WHO, 2007) is far more than a general way of viewing behaviour, ability and health status in children. First, when applied to individual children with SSD it affords an orderly, holistic framework within which to perform an evaluation, select an appropriate therapy, deliver it, and measure and analyse its effects and outcomes, in the process of evidence-based management. Second, it is a vehicle for involving *close* people in a child's life – family, friends, teachers and others – in intervention; and, a means of connecting with the more *distant* people concerned for the child's wellbeing in agencies, funding bodies and policy-making

teams: the ultimate providers and determiners of services.

How does this currently fit together, and what are the interrelationships between the ICF-CY components and clinical practice? As a dynamic work-in-progress, responsive to a changing world environment, the ICF-CY will probably never be quite finished! What would like to see added to or taken from the current schema, and how can therapists working with children and young people with unintelligible speech apply the principles of the ICF-CY and keep up with any changes?

A1. Sharynne McLeod: The contribution of the ICF-CY to working with children with SSD

Children with SSD bring more than their ears and mouths to the clinic. Each of the children on our caseloads brings a unique combination of factors such as relationships with family, friends, teachers and acquaintances; aspects of their lives that are important to them; their personality, learning style and so forth. As SLPs/SLTs we often take these factors into consideration, but rarely do so in an explicit fashion (McLeod, 2004). Instead, our reports and clinic files predominantly contain information about children's speech output such as their ability to produce consonants and vowels correctly.

For over two decades the World Health Organization has been developing an extensive classification system to be used throughout the world to support the health and wellness of all people. This started with the *International Classification of Impairment, Disabilities and Handicaps* (ICIDH) (WHO, 1980) and the most recent version of this is the *International Classification of Functioning, Disability and Health – Children and Youth* (ICF-CY) (WHO, 2007). A description of the history and application of the ICF-CY to children with communication impairments is contained in McLeod and Threats (2008). The five components of the ICF-CY, listed below, have direct relevance to children with SSD (McLeod & McCormack, 2007; also see McLeod, 2006 for a case study).

1. Body structure

   Structures of the ear, nose, mouth, larynx, pharynx and respiration are routinely screened by SLPs/SLTs to determine their potential contribution to SSD. For the majority of children with SSD, body structure is not considered to be a causal factor (Shriberg, Kwiatkowski, Best, Hengst & Terslic-Webser, 1986). In some cases, such as when children have a craniofacial anomaly (e.g., cleft lip and palate), impairment in body structure can impact on children's ability to speak intelligibly and may also impact on their activity and participation in society.

2. Body function

   Articulation, voice, fluency, hearing, respiration, intellectual and specific mental functions such as temperament and personality functions are classified amongst body functions in the ICF-CY. SLPs/SLTs working with children with SSD routinely consider these aspects in their assessment and intervention practices. The majority of SLP/SLT assessment, analysis and intervention tools for children with SSD fall under the category of body function (McLeod & Threats, 2008). Thus, although not specifically stated in the ICF-CY, body function can include measures such as the PCC, the occurrence of cluster reduction and the inventory of consonants phones (McLeod, Harrison, McAllister & McCormack, 2013).

3. Activities and participation

   Learning and applying knowledge; general tasks and demands; communication; interpersonal interactions and relationships; major life areas such as education; and community, social and civic life are all included in the ICF-CY as categories of activities and participation. There are a few tools specifically designed to consider children's activities and participation including: *Focus on the Outcomes of Communication Under Six* (FOCUS©) (Thomas-Stonell, Oddson, Robertson & Rosenbaum, 2010), *Intelligibility in Context Scale* (ICS) (McLeod, Harrison & McCormack, 2012) and the *Speech Participation and Activity Assessment of Children* (SPAA-C) (McLeod, 2004). When we as SLPs/SLTs set goals for children with SSD, it is important that we acknowledge and include these broader aspects of the lives of children with SSD. Thus, communicating intelligibly on the sporting field and in the playground are relevant goals for SLPs/SLTs working in this framework. It is also helpful if we consider the possible mismatch between capacity and performance in these life areas. As children grow older, the impact of SSD on individuals' activities and participation may include an impact on social, educational, occupational, behavioural outcomes as well as on quality of life for these individuals and their families (McCormack, Harrison, McLeod & McAllister, 2011; for a review see McCormack, McLeod, McAllister & Harrison, 2009).

4. Environmental factors

   Products and technology; support and relationships; attitudes; services, systems and policies are all included as environmental factors in ICF-CY. Each of these areas can act as facilitators and/or barriers to children with SSD. In most children's lives, perhaps the most prominent environmental factor is their family. As SLPs/SLTs we need to be aware of facilitating involvement of parents and siblings in assessment and intervention (Barr, McLeod & Daniel, 2008; McLeod, Daniel & Barr, 2013; Watts Pappas, McLeod McAllister & McKinnon, 2008). Another relevant environmental factor is the attitudes of family, friends, acquaintances and people in authority such as teachers as well as health professionals and society (Overby, Carrell & Bernthal, 2007). The attitudes people hold towards children with SSD can either be facilitative or a barrier in these children's lives. Consequently, there may be times when our intervention goals need to be directed towards others, rather than the children with SSD. For example, McCormack, McLeod, McAllister, and Harrison (2010) found that preschool children were concerned that adults had difficulties understanding them so recommended that intervention could focus both on children's 'speech problem' and on the adults' 'listening problem'. Finally, environmental factors include the policies and services that are available for children with SSD. In some nations such as the USA and UK, legislation ensures that children with SSD are provided with relevant services, and these act as an environmental facilitator. In other nations, such as Australia, SLP/SLT services are not legislated, and access to services may be difficult (McLeod, Press & Phelan, 2010) acting as an environmental barrier.

5. Personal factors

Age, gender, race, other health conditions, coping styles, overall behaviour pattern and character style are all included in the ICF-CY as relevant personal factors. Unlike the other components of the ICF-CY, detailed descriptions of personal factors are not included in the manual. However, it is helpful if SLPs/SLTs explore relevant personal factors for each child they engage with.

In conclusion, the ICF-CY is far more than these five discreet components. The interaction between each of these components is essential for visualising the goal of health and wellness. In my view, the advantage of engaging with this comprehensive classification system is that it enables holistic consideration of children with SSD in order to envisage and facilitate fuller participation in society. Recommendations for the enactment of this classification system are found in the *World Report on Disability (WRD)*, WHO and The World Bank (2011) and the nine recommendations from the WRD have been applied to children's communication (McLeod, McAllister, McCormack & Harrison, in press). Increased access to specific services and updated legislation and policies were recommended to support children's ability to communicate.

Evidence, belief and practice

Whether you call it EBP or E^3BP, evidence-based practice is a process and a responsibility. It is located at the juncture between clinicians' engagement with scientific theory and research and their engagement with clients and their worlds. The onus for *adopting* EBP rests with individual clinicians and cannot be imposed by professional associations, workplaces, supervisors, educators, legislators or policy makers. But most clinicians probably only have a small part to play in *constructing* the evidence side of the E^3BP equilateral triangle.

Academic SLPs/SLTs and linguists are largely responsible for developing, evaluating, adapting, synthesising, reporting and teaching about new research, theory, therapy and best practice. They usually do so in laboratory, classroom and CPD/CEU circumstances. Meanwhile, clinicians apply the outcomes of this research endeavour, in anything but laboratory conditions, wherever and with whomever their clients happen to be. So doesn't it seem unreasonable that the burden of converting speech–language pathology into an evidence-based discipline is frequently allocated to practitioners? And that it is done so without providing them with necessary skills, time and resources to keep up with the available evidence and integrate it into practice? Might it not be fairer if the lion's share of the responsibility for the *evidence* aspect of E³BP rested with the individuals who educate SLPs/SLTs, that is, the researchers whose job is to address and answer clinical and educational questions and the policy makers who channel reform?

As well as being unreasonable, it provides an environment in which gaps in communication between researchers, academics, policy makers, employers and practitioners are perpetuated and exacerbated, oftentimes manifesting as uncertainty, antagonism and uncomfortable relationships. Where co-operation, collegiality and sharing would be highly desirable, instead we hear the doubtful voices of academic researchers who are uncertain whether the produce of their hard work is valued or used by clinicians. Then we find conscientious academic teachers whose students complain that they do not teach enough – or indeed *anything* – about the nitty-gritty of practice, as well as exasperated clinicians and CPD/CEU participants criticising messages from the laboratory and the lecture hall as out-of-touch, unrealistic, impractical and impossible to implement. Such criticisms point to the importance of *modelling* and *teaching* principles of E³BP in the academic preparation of new SLPs/SLTs by delivering higher education that is *itself* rooted in and guided by E³BP.

Having put their student days behind them, CPD/CEU participants often clamour for content that is useful and not too theoretical or research focused. Perhaps it was in the context of insistent requests for practical professional development subject matter, almost stripped of theory, that Vicki Lord Larson and the late Nancy McKinley (Larson & McKinley, 2003, p. 26) invoked the famous maxim of gestalt psychologist Kurt Lewin who avowed, 'there is nothing more practical than a good theory to enable you to make choices confidently and consistently, and to explain or defend why you are making the choices you make' (Lewin, 1951, p. 169). Alternatively, their use of the quotation may have been prompted by conversations with students fresh from clinical placements who had been told by experienced SLPs/SLTs that what they had learned in lectures

and from textbooks was 'great in theory' but that in the real world we do it *this* way!

When 'doing it this way' means implementing atheoretical, untested assessment protocols, goal-setting strategies, target-selection approaches or treatment methodologies that have remained essentially unmodified for decades, there may be any number of explanations. It may not necessarily be due to a reluctance to move out of a comfort zone and try something new. Rather, it may relate to a need to rationalise the purchase of particular materials and equipment or to individual clinicians' gaps in knowledge of alternatives. For example, applications of optimality theory in nonlinear phonology (see Rvachew & Brosseau-Lapré, 2012, pp. 282–283 for a brief critique), the psycholinguistic framework (Stackhouse & Pascoe, 2010), core vocabulary therapy (Dodd, Holm, Crosbie & McIntosh, 2010), and the cycles phonological pattern approach (Hodson, 2007, 2010) are not taught in some undergraduate and graduate programs (Hodson, A5), and clinicians may never encounter them in workshops or readings. Furthermore, management pathways within some agencies dictate that the nature of any therapy delivered is determined by personnel concentrations and waiting list management strategies, as opposed to clinical reasoning around the best possible fit between client (and that includes family), therapist and therapy. Or it may be because most of what a particular professional or agency 'does' in SSD management is consultative: working through aides, assistants and teachers (Joffe, A34; McCartney et al., 2005; Pring, Flood, Dodd & Joffe, 2012), rarely seeing clients one-on-one. Or it may even have to do with a mindset that equates 'research findings' with 'impossible to operationalise'.

Controversial, exclusive and untested practices

Our field has a disappointing assortment of commonly implemented, heavily promoted and astonishingly popular controversial practices (Duchan, Calculator, Sonnenmeier, Diehl & Cumley, 2001) such as non-speech oral motor exercises (NS-OME) or non-speech oral motor treatments (NS-OMT) that are currently unsupported by empirical evidence; neither are they theoretically well-grounded (Hodge, A31; Lof, A35; Lof & Ruscello, 2013; McCauley, Strand, Lof, Schooling & Frymark, 2009; Powell, A39) and pointless auditory integration therapies or 'sound therapies' (ASHA, 2004) like the Berard Method (Ears Education and Retraining System), Samonas Sound Therapy, The Listening Program (from Advanced Brain), and Tomatis.

Then there are exclusive therapies such as PROMPT: Prompts for Restructuring Oral Muscular Phonetic Targets. PROMPT is based on muddled theory (Hayden, Eigen, Walker & Olsen, 2010) with an odd interpretation of the DIVA model (for a clear account of DIVA see Callan, Kent, Guenther & Vorperian, 2000). It has flimsy empirical evidence to date (e.g., Dale & Hayden, 2013) alongside copious testimonial support. PROMPT is 'exclusive' in that qualified, certified speech and language professionals must pay to gain additional basic and advanced training and accreditation in order to own 'the knowledge' in the form of special techniques (the prompts), therapy administration manuals, and materials.

Finally, there are popular programs such as the *Entire World of R* series (Ristuccia, 2002; Ristuccia, Gilbert & Ristuccia, 2005; and see Ball, Müller & Granese, 2013 for discussion); the *Kaufman Speech Praxis Kits* for Children (Kaufman, 1998a,b) and the *Kaufman Speech Workout Book* (Kaufman, 2005); and *Easy Does it for Articulation* (Strode Downing & Chamberlain, 1993, 1994) that have weak theoretical credentials and no obvious evidence base.

When clinicians elect to 'do it this way' with 'therapies', kits, manuals and packs that forlornly await scientific evaluation, they may justify their choices in terms of confidence, faith, or resolute *belief* that the treatment in question works. Questioned on their use of a favoured but hotly debated methodology many 'believers' (Gruber, Lowery, Seung & Deal, 2003) will respond that, in their estimation, the intervention approach does not *require* theoretical justification or scientific

evaluation because it is 'known' to be effective! Examples of woolly, occasionally evangelistic, 'it works for me' or 'we don't know how it works but it does' or 'I do it because it has stood the test of time', reasoning abound in mailing lists and SLP/SLT Facebook groups and are inevitably the subject of comment in clinical forums on NS-OME (Lass & Pannbacker, 2008; Lof & Ruscello, 2013).

As well as expressing confidence in the effectiveness of NS-OME, determined proponents also argue the case for them in terms of a weak or absent 'no' case. Taking a moderate stance, Kerridge, Lowe and Henry (1998) have cautioned that we must not confuse the fact of 'currently without substantial evidence' with the idea of 'without substantial value'. Nonetheless, we need to think seriously and critically about the theoretical bases and proposed therapeutic mechanisms (Clark, 2003) of techniques that lack (and in the case of NS-OME, for a *long time* have lacked) empirical support.

Theory–therapy and research–practice gaps

Although there is evidence (Baker & McLeod, 2011a), at a range of levels, supporting many intervention approaches for SSD, there is scant research that provides practitioners with clear clinical guidance. To date there are only a few randomised control trial studies of treatment efficacy for SSD (e.g., Almost & Rosenbaum 1998; Murray, McCabe & Ballard, 2012a,b), few studies have examined rate of change relative to duration and frequency of intervention (Williams, 2012) and most studies have measured accuracy of word production rather than the intelligibility of communicative discourse. Accordingly, it would be difficult – if not impossible – to institute best clinical practice guidelines in SSD based on research findings. This may explain why many practitioners appear to marginalise (Baker & McLeod 2004; Joffe & Pring, 2008; McLeod & Baker, 2004; Pring et al., 2012) and possibly trivialise the relevance of published research as a guide to practice.

Regardless of the reasons some clinicians may have for their reluctance to implement new research or to relinquish theoretically unsupported interventions, the consequence is that the principles of practice are frequently incongruent with the research findings (Duchan, 2001; Ingram, 1998). Musing on Lewin's famous assertion, and conceding that he may have been right about there being nothing more practical than a good theory, Rothman (2004, p. 6) maintains that Lewin's dictum relied on an assumption that 'good' (accurate and applicable) theories are *available* to address practical problems. Arguing the need for a stronger sense of interdependence and collaboration between those engaged in research and those occupied with professional activities, Rothman writes:

If critical advances in health behavior theory depend on an iterative process by which theoreticians and interventionists cooperate in the testing and evaluation of theoretical principles, individuals in both camps need to not only recognize the goals and values of each group, but also trust each other's ability to advance our understanding of both theory and practice.

Positive collaborations

Standing back from accounts of partition between theorists, researchers and practitioners in medicine, education and health sciences, and looking closely at our own SLP/SLT profession, committed as it is to issues of communicative competence and communicative effectiveness, we see encouraging signs of bridge-building, particularly within the doctoral degree process. Conference presentations provide heartening examples of clinicians who have completed, or who are pursuing, clinically oriented doctorates while continuing to work as clinicians during their studies and beyond. Examples of people who, like me, have done so include Highman (A41), Leitão (A53), Neilson (A22), Stoeckel (A40) and Watts Pappas (A30). The connections forged between doctoral candidates, supervisors and advisors, around schol-

arship and the publication process help cement strong collaborative links between laboratory and clinic or classroom.

Two questions

What can a child speech interventionist do when faced with inescapable gaps in the evidence base? Clinical science research and clinical reasoning are not all about incontrovertible evidence and elegant theories. But they have a lot to do with plausibility, healthy scepticism, the questions we ask and how we ask them. According to a highly recommended article by Clark (2003), there are at least two lines of enquiry to adopt in choosing an intervention methodology for a client. First we can ask, 'Is this treatment beneficial?' or '*Does* it work?' To answer this, the therapist examines the evidence base, looking for adequately documented evidence of the effects, effectiveness and efficacy (Olswang, 1998) of the treatment under consideration. If that evidence is unavailable, Clark advises posing a second question: 'Is the treatment approach theoretically sound?' or, '*Should* it work?' This second line of investigation can be successful, according to Clark, only if the practitioner clearly understands (a) the nature of the targeted impairment and (b) the therapeutic mechanism of the proposed treatment – or how the particular approach is *supposed* to work. In this regard, intervention approaches should be based on a solid theory explicating the particular speech behaviour in question. The theory itself should be what Rosen and Davidson (2003) called 'dismantleable' or able to be broken down into components for the purpose of examining them for rationale and effects or (their term) 'empirically supported principles of change', 'explicitly principled therapy' (Crystal, 1972).

Keeping up with the literature

Quality peer-reviewed publications hold a wealth of clinically relevant reports on SSD, but some clinicians do not have easy access to libraries, journals and conference proceedings. The accessibility of research findings is also sometimes reduced because numerous reports are expressed in densely technical and statistical language that is unfathomable for readers who are not researchers. In fact, at times it seems researchers, revelling in their intellectualism, write their reports *only* for their co-authors and a handful of other researchers to read!

Despite bridge building that occurs in doctoral research, discipline-specific electronic mailing lists and social media (Bowen, 2012, 2013), new research-to-practice links and harmonious collegial communication between academe and therapy room are barely perceptible in many clinics. For there, most therapists have little time to integrate new research into day-to-day practice. Neither do they have the chance to *discuss* what they do manage to read, or to *modify* it for their own cultural settings. Enticing new techniques that worked well in one country may need help to travel to another part of the world, or to a different 'world' that may be culturally distant but geographically quite close by. How, for instance, can clinicians working with indigenous populations in remote Australia or Canada or rural New Zealand, or clinical consultants in the UK advising families from the former Soviet Union with English as their second or third language, adapt and apply a powerful clinical insight from a research laboratory in Madison, Wisconsin and make it work for their clients?

Impediments to implementing research findings clinically are not entirely due to time constraints and the propensity for literature reviews, research methods, experimental results, statistical data and discussions to be expressed in impenetrable scientific prose, or unfamiliar language. There is also therapists' inclination to stay with what they know (Dollaghan, 2007; Kamhi, 2011). In terms of treatment approaches, for instance, information has been available for a long time about the advantages for the client, by way of clinical efficiency, of working systemically on error *patterns* (Grunwell, 1975; Hodson, 1982; Ingram, 1974) rather than laboriously targeting individual phonemes one by one (Van Riper,

1978). Similarly, nonlinear phonology, so relevant to phonological assessment and intervention, has been around for at least four decades (Bernhardt, 1992a,b; Bernhardt & Gilbert, 1992; Froud, A38), but it is still generally seen as something new, difficult to incorporate into practice and 'out there' by many practitioners. As well as being conservative in the choice of treatment approach, clinicians have been slow to move on some of the more up-to-date target selection criteria (Bernhardt, 2005; Rvachew & Nowak, 2001, 2003; Williams, 2005) that are now supported by varying degrees of evidence. Tending to follow traditional guidelines by targeting sounds that are, for example, *early developing*, *less complex*, and *stimulable in isolation*, many therapists remain cautious when it comes to embracing new guidelines that would have them work on sounds that are *later developing*, *more complex* and *non-stimulable* (Baker, A13; Baker & Williams, 2010).

Ingram (1998) struck a wise note when he advised against rushing new theory and research into practice as soon as it hits the journals. But the probability of a *widespread* rush to apply new research actually happening is remarkably low. For instance, according to a survey of 270 Australian speech–language pathologists (McLeod & Baker, 2004) it may be that little is adopted from currently available literature, in that just 1.1% of those surveyed said that research influenced their choice of intervention approach. And what an astonishing choice of evidence-based interventions there is!

Cultural and linguistic parochialism

Or is there? Do therapists around the world *know* about the available options? Pascoe (2006), for example, says: 'While there are undoubtedly some issues specific to phonology therapists on different sides of the Atlantic, in general the clients we serve are similar and the theoretical and clinical issues the same', but that, 'it sometimes feels as if there are fewer links between British/European speech and language therapy, and American/Canadian speech and language pathology than there should be'. This redirects attention to another gap: the gradually diminishing tendency for British and European books and important journals in our field to focus on British and European research and North American publications – with notable internationalist exceptions (e.g., Rvachew & Brosseau-Lapré, 2012; Williams et al., 2010) tending to focus on US and Canadian research. From her vantage point in the rainbow nation (Tutu, 1991), Michelle Pascoe reflects on these issues.

Dr. Pascoe qualified as a speech and language therapist/audiologist at the University of Cape Town, South Africa in 1995. She has worked as a speech and language therapist with children with speech, language and literacy difficulties in South Africa and the United Kingdom. Michelle's PhD research focused on intervention for school-age children with speech difficulties and was supervised by Professors Joy Stackhouse and Bill Wells at the University of Sheffield, United Kingdom. She subsequently co-authored books on children's speech and literacy difficulties (Pascoe, Stackhouse & Wells, 2006; Stackhouse, Vance, Pascoe & Wells, 2007) and is the Editor of the *South African Journal of Communication Disorders*. Michelle is currently a Senior Lecturer at the University of Cape Town where she continues to develop her research into intervention for children with speech and literacy difficulties.

Q2.   Michelle Pascoe: Child speech practice: an international view

As a South African speech language therapist who has worked in clinical and academic settings in both the United Kingdom and South Africa and who has co-authored a book (Pascoe et al., 2006) on child speech that reflects an appreciation of theory, research and practice, you have a unique international perspective. What is your take on there being 'fewer links between British/European speech and language therapy and American/Canadian speech and language

pathology than there should be'? And how does child speech practice in your country resemble or differ from what happens – according to both the literature and your own observations – in the United Kingdom, Europe and North America?

A2.   Michelle Pascoe: Going between: intervention for children's speech sound difficulties from an international perspective

British author L.P. Hartley began his brilliant novel with the line: 'The past is a foreign country: they do things differently there' (Hartley, 1953). This reminds me of how our practice as speech and language therapists has changed since the early origins of the profession in the 1950s and 1960s. In our book *Persisting Speech Difficulties in Children* (Pascoe et al., 2006, Chapter 1) we reviewed historical shifts in intervention for children with speech sound difficulties and considered how in some cases the shift from articulation to phonological approaches resulted in 'the baby being thrown out with the bathwater'. But, there are other ways in which we can reflect on differences and similarities in practice – by looking at intervention for children with speech sound difficulties in countries around the globe.

There are many differences in how practitioners around the world assess and manage children's speech difficulties. For a start, terminology gives a clue as to how differently practitioners within the English-speaking world approach speech difficulties. In the US practitioners talk about 'speech pathology', in the UK 'speech and language therapy', and in South Africa... well, sometimes we talk about 'speech–language pathology', sometimes 'speech and language therapy' and sometimes 'speech and hearing therapy'. The latter reflects the way in which

South African speech therapists have, until recently, received a dual training in both speech and language therapy and audiology. There are parts of the world where 'apraxia of speech (AOS)' is preferred over 'DVD' and other places where the term 'childhood apraxia of speech (CAS)' prevails. To a large extent, these differences reflect the different contexts in which we work. Practitioners funded by and working within healthcare may naturally align themselves with medical models of working, more than those working in education contexts. The former may talk more easily of 'speech pathologies' and 'speech disorders' than the latter, who may feel more comfortable with 'delays' and 'difficulties'. The contexts in which we work differ widely and it is inevitable that these will shape our terminology and how we approach our work with children with speech difficulties.

The context in which I carried out my undergraduate training was in South Africa in the first part of the 1990s. On the brink of a new democracy, at the end of the apartheid years, the country was not only geographically isolated but also politically isolated. The effect of this isolation was for those working in the field to look outwards: my training in SLT seemed to involve a carefully integrated perspective on approaches to speech difficulties in the UK at that time (e.g., PACS, Metaphon, Nuffield, Psycholinguistic Approaches) and approaches in the USA and Canada (e.g., Cycles Therapy, Multiple Oppositions, Distinctive Feature approaches). My perspective as a new clinician working with children's speech sound difficulties was thus informed by an amalgamation of some of the most exciting developments happening around the world – making up in breadth what it lacked in depth. My own sense, years later, working in the UK as a clinician and a clinical educator is that it is more easy to be 'spoiled for choice' in a country home to several of the key proponents of particular approaches to children's

speech difficulties. The need to look outwards may be less urgent when you have a wealth of knowledge, research and the associated infrastructure right on your doorstep.

Back in South Africa, things have changed and continue to evolve over time. Although still aware of the bigger picture, the profession is more inward looking as we seek to address the enormous challenges in addressing children's speech and associated literacy difficulties in our own unique context. The country has 11 official languages, yet few resources for the assessment of SSD in languages other than English.

Our knowledge about phonological development in languages other than English is limited, and clinicians who can speak the indigenous languages of the country are few – although this imbalance is slowly changing. isiXhosa, a Nguni language which contains a range of click consonants, ejectives and an implosive is the second most spoken language in South Africa and is widely spoken in Cape Town. Recent research in our department has focused on developing a preliminary set of normative data for the development of isiXhosa speech (Maphalala, 2012; Pascoe & Smouse, 2012) as well as an isiXhosa Speech Assessment ('Masincokoleni' [Let us Chat together!] Maphalala, 2012) that will enable clinicians to more accurately evaluate the speech development of young isiXhosa-speaking children. Work on other languages is happening in similar ways around the country, supporting clinicians as they face the challenges of assessment in our context as well as adding to the linguistic knowledge base for a range of languages. Beyond the borders of our own country, we have strong links with SLPs/SLTs working further north in Africa: in Namibia, Botswana, Tanzania and Ethiopia, for example, A joint project has resulted in the development of preliminary normative data for children acquiring Swahili and a prototype single word assessment for that language (Gangji, 2012).

The challenges in South Africa extend beyond those posed by the rich language diversity of the country: HIV/AIDS and poverty affect a large proportion of the population, for whom speech difficulties are necessarily a low priority. Nevertheless, our work in promoting emergent literacy and the links between phonological awareness and speech processing is vital and should be seen as more than just a luxury. Research is taking place into emergent literacy, speech development and the role of SLT in linguistically diverse classrooms, but a great need for further engagement with these issues.

Although the contexts in which we practice differ, there are surely more similarities than differences when working with children's speech difficulties around the world. South African therapists – and other therapists working in developing countries – need to be careful about chucking out the baby with the bathwater. Instead we should be forging links wherever we can. There is a core of knowledge about linguistics, phonetic transcription, anatomy, target selection, reinforcement and relevance that seems common no matter where we work or in what language. For SLPs/SLTs in South Africa to ignore this core knowledge would be foolish, but we need to adapt ways in which we research and practice so that they are relevant and useful for the population we serve.

The psycholinguistic approach to children's speech and literacy difficulties (Stackhouse & Wells, 1997, 2001) is an approach that exemplifies much of this core knowledge and has been shown to bring about positive changes in children with persisting speech difficulties under ideal (or relatively ideal) circumstances. However, the approach is a flexible one and an important next step, for example, in the South African context is to demonstrate the effectiveness of the approach in different contexts which may include in group settings working through assistants using a variety of languages and with minimal resources. The application of

these concepts in a particular service delivery context will differ – how much therapy can you offer? Do you do it yourself or through co-workers? How involved are parents? For how long to see the child? Will you see them their own or with others? Will you see them at home, in the classroom or clinic? Contextual relevance is key, but examples of good practice and ways of working in a particular context should be shared, trialed and adapted to best suit the population and the place in question.

Happily, in this digital age, communication between practitioners is easier than ever before and websites such as Sharynne McLeod's *Multilingual Children's Speech* (McLeod, 2012) and Caroline Bowen's speech-language-therapy.com (Bowen, 1998) do much to facilitate this exchange. Resources such as the International Guide to Speech Acquisition (McLeod, 2007) and the formation of the International Expert Panel on Multilingual Children's Speech (McLeod et al., 2013) also help develop this global perspective. We can all serve as 'go betweens' making links with others around the world and sharing examples of evidence-based and contextually relevant practice.

A plethora of gaps and questions

Finally, public and private Internet discussions between speech and language professionals have stories to tell. They are noteworthy for demonstrating a plethora of gaps in international communication about SSD. We find experienced therapists in the UK hearing, for the first time, about the cycles phonological pattern approach (Hodson, 2007, 2010; A5), phonotactic therapy (Velleman, 2002, 2003), intervention for developmental dysarthria (Hodge, 2010), or multiple oppositions therapy (Williams, 2006, 2010; A26), and US therapists discovering the psycholinguistic framework (Stackhouse & Wells, 1997; Gardner,

A27), *Metaphon* (Dean, Howell, Waters & Reid, 1995) or PACT (Bowen, 2010; and see Chapter 9) also for first time, many years after they first appeared in the international literature. But how 'international' *is* the literature and who reads it anyway?

So we have it. Questions galore! There are burning questions about clinicians and the evidence base. Where empirically supported intervention guidance exists, will clinicians have time to find it and read it? Will they be able to evaluate it and see it as a professional obligation to do so? Gaps galore! Children with gaps in their speech sound systems and clinicians working to fill those gaps, surrounded by disparities in communication between academe and therapy room; gaps in knowledge, service delivery and evidence; theory–therapy and research–practice gaps; and gaps in international communication. Undoubtedly the list goes on and should include the gaps that can exist between the needs, goals, expectations, roles and responsibilities of therapists and the needs, goals, expectations, roles and responsibilities of individual children, their families and communities. There are even gaps in the way our profession's histories have been recorded (Duchan, 2001, 2010), as Chapter 1 reveals.

References

Almost, D., & Rosenbaum, P. (1998). Effectiveness of speech intervention for phonological disorders: A randomized control trial. *Developmental Medicine and Child Neurology, 40*(5), 319–325.

American Psychiatric Association. (2013). *Diagnostic and statistical manual of mental disorders (DSM-5)* (5th ed., pp. 44–45). Arlington, VA: American Psychiatric Publishing.

ASHA. (2004). Auditory Integration Training [Technical Report]. Retrieved 15 January 2014 from www.asha.org/policy

ASHA. (2007). Childhood Apraxia of Speech [Technical Report]. Retrieved 15 January 2014 from www.asha.org/docs/html/TR2007-00278.html

Bain, B. A., & Dollaghan, C. A. (1991). The notion of clinically significant change. *Language Speech and Hearing Services in Schools, 22*, 264–270.

Baker, E., & McLeod, S. (2004). Evidence-based management of phonological impairment in children. *Child Language Teaching and Therapy, 20*(3), 265–285.

Baker, E., & McLeod, S. (2011a). Evidence-based practice for children with speech sound disorders: Part 1 narrative review. *Language, Speech, and Hearing Services in Schools, 42*(2), 102–139.

Baker, E., & McLeod, S. (2011b). Evidence-based practice for children with speech sound disorders: Part 2 application to clinical practice. *Language, Speech, and Hearing Services in Schools, 42*(2), 140–141.

Baker, E., & Williams, A. L. (2010). Complexity approaches to intervention. In: A. L. Williams, S. McLeod, & R. J. McCauley (Eds.), *Interventions for speech sound disorders in children* (pp. 95–116). Baltimore, MD: Paul H. Brookes Publishing Co.

Ball, M. J., Müller, N., & Granese, A. (2013). Towards an evidence-base for /r/-therapy in English. *Journal of Clinical Speech and Language Studies, 20*, 1–23.

Barr, J., McLeod, S., & Daniel, G. (2008). Siblings of children with speech impairment: Cavalry on the hill. *Language, Speech, and Hearing Services in Schools, 39*(1), 21–32.

Bernhardt, B. (1992a). Developmental implications of nonlinear phonological theory. *Clinical Linguistics and Phonetics, 6*, 259–282.

Bernhardt, B. (1992b). The application of nonlinear phonological theory to intervention with one phonologically disordered child. *Clinical Linguistics and Phonetics, 6*, 283–316.

Bernhardt, B. (2005). Selection of phonological goals and targets: Not just an exercise in phonological analysis. In: A. Kamhi, & K. Pollock (Eds.), *Phonological disorders in children: Clinical decision-making in assessment and intervention* (pp. 109–120). Baltimore, MD: Paul H. Brookes Publishing Co.

Bernhardt, B., & Gilbert, J. (1992). Applying linguistic theory to speech-language pathology: The case for nonlinear phonology. *Clinical Linguistics and Phonetics, 6*, 123–145.

Bitter, J. R. (2013). *Theory and practice of family therapy and counseling* (2nd ed.). Belmont, CA: Brooks Cole: Cengage Learning.

Bowen, C. (1998). *Speech-language-therapy dot com*. Retrieved 15 January 2014 from www.speech-language-therapy.com

Bowen, C. (2001). *Children's Speech Sound Disorders (phonologicaltherapy) Discussion Group*.

Retrieved 15 January 2014 from http://groups.yahoo.com/neo/groups/phonologicaltherapy/info

Bowen C. (2008). Webwords 30: Work-life balance and authentic interests. *Acquiring Knowledge in Speech, Language and Hearing*, *10*(2), 67–68.

Bowen, C. (2010). Parents and children together (PACT) intervention for children with speech sound disorders. In: A. L. Williams, S. McLeod, & R. J. McCauley (Eds.), *Interventions for speech sound disorders in children* (pp. 407–426). Baltimore, MD: Paul H. Brookes Publishing Co.

Bowen C. (2012). Webwords 44: Life online. *Journal of Clinical Practice in Speech-Language Pathology*, *14*(3), 149–152.

Bowen C. (2013). Webwords 46: Social media in clinical education and continuing professional development. *Journal of Clinical Practice in Speech-Language Pathology*, *15*(2), 104–106.

Callan, D. E., Kent, R. D., Guenther, F. H., & Vorperian, H. K. (2000). An auditory-feedback-based neural network model *of* speech production that is robust to developmental changes in the size and shape of the articulatory system. *Journal of Speech, Language & Hearing Research*, *43*(3), 721–736.

Clark, H. M. (2003). Neuromuscular treatments for speech and swallowing: A tutorial. *American Journal of Speech Language Pathology*, *12*(4), 400–415.

Crystal, D. (1972). The case of linguistics: A prognosis. *British Journal of Disorders of Communication*, *7*, 3–16.

Dale, P. D., & Hayden, D. A. (2013). Treating speech subsystems in childhood apraxia of speech with tactual input: The PROMPT approach. *American Journal of Speech-Language Pathology*, *22*(4), 644–661.

Dean, E. C., Howell, J., Waters, D., & Reid, J. (1995). *Metaphon*: A metalinguistic approach to the treatment of phonological disorder in children. *Clinical Linguistics and Phonetics*, *9*, 1–19.

Dodd, B., Holm, A., Crosbie, S., & McIntosh, B. (2010). Core vocabulary intervention. In: A. L. Williams, S. McLeod, & R. J. McCauley (Eds.), *Interventions for speech sound disorders in children* (pp. 117–136). Baltimore, MA: Paul H. Brookes Publishing Co.

Dollaghan, C. A. (2004). Evidence-based practice in communication disorders: what do we know, and when do we know it? *Journal of Communication Disorders*, *37*, 391–400.

Dollaghan, C. A. (2007). *The handbook for evidence-based practice in communication disorders*. Baltimore, MD: Paul H. Brookes Publishing Co.

Duchan, J. F. (2001). *History of Speech-Language Pathology in America*. Retrieved 15 January 2014 from http://www.acsu.buffalo.edu/~duchan/history.html

Duchan, J. F. (2010). The early years of language, speech, and hearing services in U.S. schools. *Language, Speech, and Hearing Services in Schools*, *41*(2), 152–160.

Duchan, J. F., Calculator, S., Sonnenmeier, R., Diehl, S., & Cumley, G. (2001). A framework for managing controversial practices. *Language Speech and Hearing Services in Schools*, *32*, 133–141.

Gangji, N. (2012). Phonological development in Swahili: A descriptive, cross-sectional study of typically developing pre-schoolers in Tanzania. Unpublished Masters Dissertation. University of Cape Town, South Africa.

Gruber, F. A., Lowery, S. D., Seung, H.-K., & Deal, R. (2003). Approaches to speech/language intervention and the true believer. *Journal of Medical Speech-Language Pathology*, *11*(2), 95–104.

Grunwell, P. (1975). The phonological analysis of articulation disorders. *British Journal of Disorders of Communication*, *10*, 31–42.

Grunwell, P. (1987). *Clinical phonology* (2nd ed.). Baltimore, MD: Williams & Wilkins.

Hartley, L. P. (1953). *The Go-Between*. New York: Knopf.

Hayden, D., Eigen, J., Walker, A., & Olsen, L. (2010). PROMPT: A tactually grounded model for the treatment of childhood speech production disorders. In: A. L. Williams, S. McLeod, & R. J. McCauley (Eds.), *Treatment for speech sound disorders in children* (pp. 453–474). Baltimore, MD: Paul H. Brookes Publishing Company.

Hodge, M. (2010). Intervention for developmental dysarthria. In: A. L. Williams, S. McLeod, & R. J. McCauley (Eds.), *Interventions for speech sound disorders in children* (pp. 557–578). Baltimore, MD: Paul H. Brookes Publishing Co.

Hodson, B. (1982). Remediation of speech patterns associated with low levels of phonological performance. In: M. Crary (Ed.): *Phonological intervention, concepts and procedures*. San Diego, CA: College-Hill Press Inc.

Hodson, B. (2007, 2010). *Evaluating and enhancing children's phonological systems: Research and theory to practice*. Wichita, KS: PhonoComp Publishers.

Ingram, D. (1974). Phonological rules in young children. *Journal of Child Language*, *1*, 49–64.

Ingram, D. (1989). *Phonological disability in children* (2nd ed.). London: Whurr Publishers.

Ingram, D. (1998). Research-practice relationships in speech-language pathology. *Topics in Language Disorders*, *18*(2), 1–9.

Joffe, V. L., & Pring, T. (2008). Children with phonological problems: A survey of clinical practice. *International Journal of Language and Communication Disorders*, *43*(2), 154–164.

Kamhi, A. G. (2011). Balancing certainty and uncertainty in clinical practice. *Language, Speech, and Hearing Services in Schools*, *42*(1), 59–64.

Kaufman, N. (1998a). *Kaufman speech praxis treatment kit for children, advanced level.* Gaylord, MI: Northern Speech Services.

Kaufman, N. (1998b). *Kaufman speech praxis treatment kit for children, basic level.* Gaylord, MI: Northern Speech Services.

Kaufman, N. (2005). *Kaufman speech praxis workout book.* Gaylord, MI: Northern Speech Services.

Kerridge, I., Lowe, M., & Henry, D. A. (1998). Ethics and evidence-based medicine, *British Medical Journal*, *316*, 1151–1153.

Larson, V. L., & McKinley, N. L. (2003). *Communication solutions for older students: Assessment and intervention strategies.* Eau Claire, WI: Thinking Publications.

Lass, N. J., & Pannbacker, M. (2008). The application of evidence-based practice to oral motor treatment. *Language, Speech, and Hearing Services in Schools*, *39*(3), 408–421.

Lewin, K. (1951). *Field theory in social science: Selected theoretical papers.* New York: Harper & Row.

Lof, G., & Ruscello, D. (2013, October). Don't blow this therapy session! *SIG 5 Perspectives in Speech Science and Orofacial Disorders*, *23*, 38-48.

Maphalala, Z. (2012). Phonological development of first language isiXhosa-speaking children aged 3;0- 6;0 years: A descriptive cross-sectional study. Unpublished Masters Dissertation. University of Cape Town, South Africa.

McCartney, E., Boyle, J., Bannatyne, S., Jessiman, E., Campbell, C., Kelsey, C., Smith, J., McArthur, J., & O'Hare, A. (2005). 'Thinking for two': A case study of speech and language therapists working through assistants. *International Journal of Language and Communication Disorders*, *40*, 221–235.

McCauley, R. J., Strand, E., Lof, G. L., Schooling, T., & Frymark, T. (2009). Evidence-based systematic review: effects of nonspeech oral motor exercises on speech. *American Journal of Speech-Language Pathology*, *18*, 343–360.

McCormack, J., Harrison, L. J., McLeod, S., & McAllister, L. (2011). A nationally representative study of the association between communication impairment at 4-5 years and children's life activities at 7-9 years. *Journal of Speech, Language and Hearing Research*, *54*(5), 1328–1348.

McCormack J., McLeod S., Harrison L. J., & McAllister L. (2010). The impact of speech impairment in early childhood: Investigating parents' and speech-language pathologists' perspectives using the ICF-CY. *Journal of Communication Disorders*, *43*(5), 378–396.

McCormack, J., McLeod, S., McAllister, L., & Harrison, L. J. (2009). A systematic review of the association between childhood speech impairment and participation across the lifespan. *International Journal of Speech-Language Pathology*, *11*(2), 155–170.

McCormack, J., McLeod, S., McAllister, L., & Harrison, L. J. (2010). My speech problem, your listening problem, and my frustration: The experience of living with childhood speech impairment. *Language, Speech, and Hearing Services in Schools*, *41*(4), 379–392.

McLeod, S. (2004). Speech pathologists' application of the ICF to children with speech impairment *International Journal of Speech-Language Pathology*, *6*(1), 75–81.

McLeod, S. (2006). The holistic view of a child with unintelligible speech: Insights from the ICF and ICF-CY. *International Journal of Speech-Language Pathology*, *8*(3), 293–315.

McLeod, S. (Ed.). (2007). *The international guide to speech acquisition.* Clifton Park, NY: Thomson Delmar Learning.

McLeod, S. (2012). *Multilingual children's speech.* Bathurst: Charles Sturt University. Retrieved 15 January 2014 from http://www.csu.edu.au/research/multilingual-speech

McLeod, S., & Baker, E. (2004). Current clinical practice for children with speech impairment. In: B. E. Murdoch, J. Goozee, B. M. Whelan, & K. Docking (Eds.), *Proceedings of the 26th World Congress of the International Association of Logopedics and Phoniatrics.* Brisbane: University of Queensland.

McLeod, S., Daniel, G., & Barr, J. (2013). "When he's around his brothers . . . he's not so quiet": The private and public worlds of school-aged children with speech sound disorder. *Journal of Communication Disorders*, *46*(1), 70–83.

McLeod, S., Harrison, L. J., McAllister, L., & McCormack. J. (2013). Speech sound disorders in a community study of preschool children. *American Journal of Speech-Language Pathology*, 22, 503–522.

McLeod, S., Harrison, L. J., & McCormack, J. (2012). Intelligibility in context scale: Validity and reliability of a subjective rating measure. *Journal of Speech, Language, and Hearing Research*, 55, 648–656.

McLeod, S., McAllister, L., McCormack, J., & Harrison, L. J. (in press). Applying the World Report on disability to children's communication. *Disability and Rehabilitation*. From http://www.ncbi.nlm.nih.gov/pubmed/24024539

McLeod, S., & McCormack, J. (2007). Application of the ICF and ICF-children and youth in children with speech impairment. *Seminars in Speech and Language*, 28, 254–264.

McLeod, S., Press, F., & Phelan, C. (2010). The (in)visibility of children with communication impairment in Australian health, education, and disability legislation and policies. *Asia Pacific Journal of Speech, Language, and Hearing*, 13(1), 67–75.

McLeod, S., & Threats, T. T. (2008). The ICF-CY and children with communication disabilities. *International Journal of Speech-Language Pathology*, 10(1), 92–109.

McLeod, S., Verdon, S., & Bowen, C. (2013). International aspirations for speech-language pathologists' practice with multilingual children with speech sound disorders: Development of a position paper. *Journal of Communication Disorders*, 46, 375–387.

Müller, N., & Ball, M. J. (2013b). Linguistics, phonetics, and speech-language pathology: Clinical linguistics and phonetics. In: M. Müller & M. J. Ball (Eds.), *Research methods in clinical linguistics and phonetics: A practical guide*. Oxford: Wiley-Blackwell.

Murray, E., McCabe, P., & Ballard, K. J. (2012a). A comparison of two treatments for childhood apraxia of speech: Methods and treatment protocol for a parallel group randomised control trial. *BMC Pediatrics*, 12(3), 1–9.

Murray, E., McCabe, P., & Ballard, K. J. (2012b). The first randomised control trial for treatment of childhood apraxia of speech (ReST vs Nuffield Dyspraxia Program-3). *Communicate: Our natural state. Speech Pathology Australia National Conference*. Hobart, Australia.

Olswang, L. B. (1998). Treatment efficacy research. In: C. M. Frattali (Ed.), *Measuring outcomes in speech-language pathology* (pp. 134–150). New York: Thieme.

Overby, M., Carrell, T., & Bernthal, J. (2007). Teachers' perceptions of students With speech sound disorders: A quantitative and qualitative analysis. *Language, Speech, and Hearing Services in Schools*, 38(4), 327–341.

Pascoe. M. (2006). Review of the book phonological disorders in children: Clinical decision making in assessment and intervention. In: A. G. Kamhi, & K. E. Pollock (Eds.), *Child language teaching and therapy*, 22(2), 243–245.

Pascoe, M., & Smouse, M. (2012). *Masithethe*: Speech and language development and difficulties in isiXhosa. *South African Medical Journal*, 102(6), 469–471.

Pascoe, M., Stackhouse, J., & Wells, B. (2006). *Children's speech and literacy difficulties iii: Persisting speech difficulties in children*. Chichester: John Wiley and Sons.

Pring, T., Flood, E., Dodd, B., & Joffe, V. (2012). The working practices and clinical experiences of paediatric speech and language therapists: A national UK survey. *International Journal of Language and Communication Disorders*, 47(6), 696–708.

RCSLT. (2011). *Royal College of Speech and Language Therapists: Developmental verbal dyspraxia* [Policy Statement], Retrieved 26 April 2014 from http://www.rcslt.org/speech_and_language_therapy/rcslt_position_papers

Ristuccia, C. L. (2002). *The entire world of R instructional workbook*. Carlsbad, CA: Say It Right.

Ristuccia, C. L., Gilbert, D. W., & Ristuccia, J. E. (2005). *The entire world of R book of elicitation techniques*. Tybee Island, GA: Say it Right.

Roddam, H., & Skeat, J. (2010). *Embedding evidence-based practice in speech and language therapy: International examples*. London: Wiley-Blackwell.

Rosen, G. M., & Davidson, G. C. (2003). Psychology should list empirically supported principles of change (ESPs) and not credential trademarked therapies or other treatment packages. *Behavior Modification*, 27(3), 300–312.

Rothman, A. J. (2004). 'Is there nothing more practical than a good theory?': Why innovations and advances in health behavior change will arise if interventions are used to test and refine theory. *International Journal of Behavioral Nutrition and Physical Activity*, 1(11), 1–7.

Rvachew, S., & Brosseau-Lapré, F. (2012). *Developmental phonological disorders: Foundations of clinical practice*. San Diego, CA: Plural Publishing.

Rvachew, S., & Nowak, M. (2001). The effect of target-selection strategy of phonological learning. *Journal of Speech, Language and Hearing Research, 44*, 610–623.

Rvachew, S., & Nowak, M. (2003). Clinical outcomes as a function of target selection strategy: A response to Morrisette and Gierut. *Journal of Speech-Language and Hearing Research, 46*, 386–389.

Shriberg, L. D. (1982). Diagnostic assessment of developmental phonological disorders. In: M. Crary (Ed.): *Phonological intervention, concepts and procedures*. San Diego, CA: College-Hill, Inc.

Shriberg, L. D., Austin, D., Lewis, B. A., McSweeny, J. L., & Wilson, D. L. (1997). The percentage of consonants correct (PCC) metric: extensions and reliability data. *Journal of Speech, Language, and Hearing Research, 40*(4), 708–722.

Shriberg, L. D., Kwiatkowski, J., Best, S., Hengst, J., & Terselic-Weber, B. (1986). Characteristics of children with phonologic disorders of unknown origin. *Journal of Speech and Hearing Disorders, 51*, 140–161.

Shriberg, L. D., Paul, R., Black, L. M., & van Santen, J. P. (2011). The hypothesis of apraxia of speech in children with autism spectrum disorder. *Journal of Autism and Developmental Disorders, 41*, 405–426.

Shriberg, L. D., Potter, N. L., & Strand, E. A. (2011). Prevalence and phenotype of childhood apraxia of speech in youth with galactosemia. *Journal of Speech, Language, and Hearing Research, 54*, 487–519.

Speake, J., Howard, S., & Vance, M. (2011). Intelligibility in children with persisting speech disorders: A case study. *Journal of Interactional Research in Communication Disorders, 2*(1), 131–151.

Speake, J., Stackhouse, J., & Pascoe, M. (2012). Vowel targeted intervention for children with persisting speech difficulties: Impact on intelligibility. *Child Language Teaching and Therapy, 28*(3) 277–295.

Stackhouse, J., & Pascoe, M. (2010). Psycholinguistic intervention. In: Williams, A. L., S. McLeod, & R. J. McCauley (Eds.), *Interventions for speech sound disorders in children* (pp. 219–246). Paul H. Brookes Publishing Co.

Stackhouse, J., Vance, M., Pascoe, M., & Wells, B. (2007). *Children's speech and literacy difficulties IV: Compendium of auditory and speech tasks*. Chichester: John Wiley and Sons.

Stackhouse, J., & Wells, B. (1997). *Children's speech and literacy difficulties I: A psycholinguistic framework*. London: Whurr Publishers.

Stackhouse, J., & Wells, B. (2001). *Children's speech and literacy difficulties II: Identification and intervention*. London: Whurr Publishers.

Strode Downing, R., & Chamberlain, C. (1993). *Easy does it for apraxia school-age*. East Moline, IL: Linguisystems.

Strode Downing, R., & Chamberlain, C. (1994). *Easy does it for apraxia preschool*. East Moline, IL: Linguisystems.

Thomas-Stonell, N., Oddson, B., Robertson, B., & Rosenbaum, P. (2010). Development of the FOCUS© (Focus on the outcomes of communication under six): A communication outcome measure for preschool children. *Developmental Medicine and Child Neurology, 52*(1), 47–53.

Tutu, D. M. (1991, December). *You are the rainbow people of God*. Sermon in Tromsö, Norway.

Tyler, A. A., Gillon, G., Macrae, T., & Johnson, R. L. (2011). Direct and indirect effects of stimulating phoneme awareness vs. other linguistic skills in preschoolers with co-occurring speech and language impairments. *Topics in Language Disorders, 31*(2), 128–144.

Unicomb, R., Hewat, S., Spencer, E., & Harrison, E. (2013). Clinicians' management of young children with co-occurring stuttering and speech sound disorder. *International Journal of Speech-Language Pathology, 4*(15), 441–452.

Van Riper, C. (1978). *Speech correction: Principles and methods* (6th ed.). Englewood Cliffs, NJ: Prentice-Hall.

Velleman, S. (2002). Phonotactic therapy. *Seminars in Speech and Language, 23*, 43–57.

Velleman, S. L. (2003). *Resource guide for childhood apraxia of speech*. Clifton Park, NY: Delmar/Thomson Learning.

Waring, R., & Knight, R. (2013). How should children with speech sound disorders be classified? A review and critical evaluation of current classification systems. *International Journal of Language and Communication Disorders, 48*(1), 25–40.

Watts Pappas, N., McLeod, S., McAllister, L., & McKinnon, D. H. (2008). Parental involvement in speech intervention: A national survey. *Clinical Linguistics and Phonetics, 22*(4), 335–344.

WHO (1980). World Health Organization. *ICIDH: International classification of impairment, disabilities and handicaps.* Geneva: World Health Organization.

WHO (2001). *ICF: International classification of functioning, disability and health.* Geneva: World Health Organization.

WHO (2007). World Health Organization (WHO Workgroup for development of version of ICF for Children. *International classification of functioning, disability and health – Version for children and youth: 2013-CY.* Geneva: World Health Organization.

WHO: World Health Organization and The World Bank. (2011). *World report on disability.* Geneva: World Health Organization.

Williams, A. L. (2005). From developmental norms to distance metrics: Past, present, and future directions for target selection practices. In: A. G. Kamhi, & K. E. Pollock (Eds.), *Phonological disorders in children: Clinical decision making in assessment and intervention* (pp. 101–108). Baltimore, MD: Paul. H. Brookes Publishing.

Williams, A. L. (2006). A systemic perspective for assessment and intervention: A case study. *Advances in Speech-Language Pathology, 8*(3), 245–256.

Williams, A. L. (2010). Multiple oppositions intervention. In: A. L. Williams, S. McLeod, & R. J. McCauley (Eds.), *Interventions for speech sound disorders in children* (pp. 73–94). Baltimore, MD: Paul H. Brookes Publishing Co.

Williams, A. L. (2012). Intensity in phonological intervention: Is there a prescribed amount? *International Journal of Speech-Language Pathology, 14*(5), 456–461.

Williams, A. L., McLeod, S., & McCauley, R. J. (Eds.). (2010). *Interventions for speech sound disorders in children.* Baltimore, MD: Paul H. Brookes Publishing Co.

Yavaş, M. (2007). Multilingual speech acquisition. In: S. McLeod (Ed.) *The international guide to speech acquisition* (pp. 96–110). Thompson Delmar Learning.

Chapter 1

The evolution of current practices

Conceptual frameworks are easy to ignore. Like the air we breathe, their presence is everywhere, once they are looked for. Yet, they are often taken for granted, under-estimated and under-examined. One way to reveal the influence of frameworks today is to study their use in the unfamiliar contexts. For example, an examination of past practices of speech therapists raises questions about what practitioners did then as well as how and why they did it. Such an investigation creates the distance needed for clinicians to apprehend aspects of their own practice that are ordinarily taken for granted.

(Duchan, 2006a)

Judith Felson Duchan, one of our profession's few historians, believes there has been too little work on the evolution of current practices. She observes that most histories of the origins of speech pathology in the United States focus on organisational matters and place the genesis of the profession in about 1925, when workers in the field of speech disorders and speech correction established their own professional association. The chronology by Margaret Eldridge, recording the development of speech therapy in Australia (Eldridge, 1965) and

the Commonwealth of Nations (Eldridge, 1968a, 1968b), has this same institutional focus. By contrast, over a decade Duchan (2001–2011) produced a lively web-based history and several articles (e.g., Duchan, 2009, 2010) broader in scope than their predecessors and distinctive because they include systematic records of the science and ideas underlying practice.

Unlike Duchan's rich histories, the timeline in Table 1.1 provides just a glimpse of the notable SLP/SLT and linguistics influences on contemporary child speech practice, from the 1930s to the beginning of this century. Dodging the trap of presentism (i.e., the practice of evaluating past events, people and motivations by present-day ideas), in the subsequent sections connections are made between our histories of practice and practice today.

Early understandings of 'normal' and 'deviant' speech

The book, *Normal Speech and Speech Deviations* (Travis, 1931) contained just one paragraph on articulation therapy and an appendix containing a

Children's Speech Sound Disorders, Second Edition. Caroline Bowen.
© 2015 John Wiley & Sons, Ltd. Published 2015 by John Wiley & Sons, Ltd.
Companion website: www.wiley.com/go/bowen/speechlanguagetherapy

Table 1.1 Timeline: Milestones in the history of children's speech sound disorders

Pioneers	William Holder (1616–1698) John Thelwall (1764–1834) Alexander Melville Bell (1819–1905)	See Holder (1669) and Duchan (2001) for information about William Holder See Duchan (2006a, 2009) for information about John Thelwall See Duchan (2006b) for information on Alexander Melville Bell
1931	Lee Edward Travis	'The Travis Handbook' contained one paragraph on articulation, and a word list. See also Travis (1957)
1934	Irene Poole	Produced a developmental schedule for 'normal' articulatory proficiency
1937	Robert West	Published *The Rehabilitation of Speech*
1937	Samuel T. Orton	Published *Reading, Writing and Speech Problems in Children*
1938	Sara Stinchfield and Edna Hill-Young	Treated delayed/defective speech with a motor-kinesthetic therapy
1939	Charles Van Riper	Developed a social theory of speech acquisition coupled with an auditory-phonetic therapy
1940	Grant Fairbanks	Published a voice/articulation drill book with listening lists and minimal pairs
1940 -	Theory–Therapy Gap–Research–Practice Gap	The principles of practice were often at odds with theory and research
1941	Roman Jakobson	Developed a linguistics theory of phonological universals
1943	Mildred Berry and Jon Eisenson	Linked a linguistic-mentalist acquisition theory with articulatory-motor therapy
1945	World War II ended	SLP/SLT informed by physiology, psychology and psychiatry (not linguistics)
1948	Kurt Goldstein	Discussed symbol formation and this sort of thinking lead to the novel idea of 'underlying representation' and 'psycholinguistic processing' in phonology
1952	Helmur Myklebust	Used the same term: symbol formation
1957	Charles Osgood	Talked about mediation/ psycho-linguistic processing
1957	Mildred Templin	Published *certain language skills in children*
1959	College of Speech Therapists	Formulated a definition of dyslalia
1959	Margaret Hall Powers	Definition of functional articulation disorder
1968	Noam Chomsky and Morris Halle	Wrote SPE presenting distinctive features theory and generative phonology
1968	Jon Eisenson	Symbol formation
1968	Charles Ferguson	Developed contrastive analysis
1970s	American behaviourism	3-position testing and traditional articulation therapy dominated
1972	Muriel Morley	Implied that 'functional articulation disorder' did not have a neuromotor basis
1973	David Stampe	Explicated natural phonology and phonological processes
1975	Pamela Grunwell	Showed the relevance to SLP/SLT of clinical linguistics
1976	David Ingram	His *Phonological Disability in Children* changed the SLT/SLP view of SSDs
1979	Frederick Weiner	Published *Phonological Process Analysis* (Test)
1980	Lawrence Shriberg and Joan Kwiatkowski	Published *Natural Process Analysis* (Test)
1980	Barbara Hodson	Published *Assessment of Phonological Processes* AAP (Test)
1981	Frederick Weiner	Presented an account of conventional minimal pairs therapy
1982	Stephen E. Blache	Applied distinctive features theory t to phonological assessment and therapy
1983	Barbara Hodson and Elaine Paden	Published *Targeting Intelligible Speech*: Patterns therapy/cycles approach
1984	Dana Monahan	Published (perhaps the first) assessment and therapy package
1985	Pamela Grunwell	Published *Phonological Assessment of Child Speech*: PACS (Test)
1985	Marc Fey	Published the 'Inextricable constructs' article, making everybody think!

Table 1.1 (*Continued*)

Pioneers	William Holder (1616–1698) John Thelwall (1764–1834) Alexander Melville Bell (1819–1905)	See Holder (1669) and Duchan (2001) for information about William Holder See Duchan (2006a, 2009) for information about John Thelwall See Duchan (2006b) for information on Alexander Melville Bell
1985	Carol Stoel-Gammon and Carla Dunn	Published the ground breaking *Normal and Disordered Phonology in Children*
1986	Elizabeth Dean and Janet Howell	Published the developing linguistic awareness article, heralding *Metaphon*
1986	Mary Elbert and Judith Gierut	Published the *Handbook of Clinical Phonology*
1989	Gwen Lancaster and Lesley Pope	Described auditory input therapy for under 3s, and 'difficult' young clients
1990	Elizabeth Dean, Janet Howell, Anne Hill and Daphne Waters	*Metaphon* published as an assessment and therapy resource pack
1992	Marc Fey	Headed up a challenging LSHSS clinical forum
1993	Lawrence Shriberg	Looked at development differently with the early, middle and late 8
1997	Martin Ball and Raymond Kent	Published The new Phonologies – A book for clinicians and linguists
1997	Joy Stackhouse and Bill Wells	Published the first volume of a book series on the psycholinguistic framework
1998-9	B. May Bernhardt and Joseph Stemberger	Developed clinical applications of non-linear phonology
2001	WHO – children and youth classification	International Classification of Functioning, Disability and Health ICF-CY

list of initial–medial–final-sound production practice words. Although 'the Travis Handbook', as it was affectionately or even reverently called, offered a minuscule contribution as far as articulation therapy was concerned, it was highly regarded as a standard text, providing outlines of the neurophysiological bases and clinical subtypes of fluency, articulation and voice problems and aphasia. Uninfluenced by linguistics theory of the day – the Linguistic Society of America was founded in 1924 – Travis presented a view of disorders that had the speech sound (or segment) as the basic unit of speech. There was a hopeful sign in the same year that more was to come when Wellman, Case, Mengert and Bradbury (1931) reported on the development of 'speech sounds' in young children. Publications by other American SLPs soon followed with such revealing titles as: *The Rehabilitation of Speech* (West, Kennedy, & Carr, 1937), *Reading, Writing and Speech Problems in Children* (Orton, 1937), and *Children with Delayed or Defective Speech: Motor-Kinesthetic Factors in Their Training* (Stinchfield & Young, 1938). Robert West (1892–1968) wrote the first section of West, Kennedy and Carr (1937) and

introduced information about articulation difficulties due to oral deformities and hearing impairment. Speech remediation suggestions in the second half of the book included muscle relaxation, non-speech oral motor exercises (NS-OME), phonetic placement strategies and drill.

Another flurry of influential 'child speech' speech pathology publishing activity between 1939 and 1943 started with the first of the nine editions of *Speech Correction: Principles and Methods* (Van Riper, 1939). Charles Van Riper (1905–1994), who had a doctorate in clinical psychology and no formal SLP qualification, emphasised the significance of social context on the day-to-day experience of speech-impaired individuals, with portents of the ICF-CY (McLeod, A1). His social perspective is revealed in his famous definition: 'Speech is defective when it deviates so far from the speech of other people in the group that it calls attention to itself, interferes with communication, or causes its possessor to be maladjusted to his environment' (Van Riper 1939, p. 51). Van Riper's cultural sensitivity and inimitable insight into what he called the 'penalties' of communication impairment may have stemmed from his intrapersonal and interpersonal experiences of stuttering. Discussing what people with communication 'differences' might make of their social situations, and what they might perceive others to read into their symptoms, he wrote, 'The difference in itself was not so important as its interpretation by the speech defective's associates' (p. 66). He reflected sourly on the likely reactions of the said associates, writing: 'Personality is not merely individuality but evaluated individuality' (p. 67). So intensely important was the social level for Van Riper that he recommend trainee speech correctionists undertake assignments, such as lisping for a day, to develop empathy for individuals with speech difficulties and a deeper appreciation of their emotional landscapes. The social aspect was present in his intervention advice, too, when he suggested that correctionists should work with *teachers and parents* in pursuing therapy goals.

Paradoxically, although Van Riper espoused and sustained a sincerely held social view of speech impairment and of disability, his speech intervention approach—classically referred to as 'Traditional Articulation Therapy' or, slightly tongue-in-cheek, 'Van Riper Therapy'—could never have been regarded as communication focused. He incorporated many disparate elements in an atomistic array of peripheral procedures that included stimulus–response routines; sensory training that he called auditory stimulation comprising auditory discrimination, 'ear training' and auditory sequencing; and production drill. These all became part of an auditory–phonetic (or sensory–motor) therapy that is still implemented (Hegde & Peña-Brooks, 2007). In the same productive period, practical manuals, books of exercises, source books and workbooks for the speech correctionist began to appear, replete with word and sentence lists for production practice, listening lists, rhymes, stories, therapy tips, advice and ideas and techniques and activities to be used in speech lessons (Fairbanks 1940; Nemoy & Davis, 1937; Robbins & Robbins, 1937; Twitmeyer & Nathanson, 1932).

Among the techniques that Van Riper did *not* incorporate into his intervention, but which were gaining in popularity, were the motor-kinesthetic (or motokinesthetic) tactile manoeuvres. Van Riper (1939, pp. 198–201) describes them with heavy sarcasm.

We have previously mentioned the Motokinesthetic Method invented by Edna Hill Young as one of the approaches used in teaching a child with delayed speech to talk. It has also been used in the elimination of misarticulations. Essentially, this method is based upon intensive stimulation; however, the stimulation is not confined to sound alone but to tactile and kinesthetic sensations as well. The therapist, by manipulation and stroking and pressing the child's face and body as she utters the stimulus syllable, helps him recognize the place of articulation, the direction of movements, the amount of air pressure, and so on. Watching an expert motokinesthetic therapist at work on a lisper is like attending a show put on by a magician. The case lies on a table with the therapist bending over him. First she presses on his abdomen to initiate breathing as she strongly makes the s sound; then to produce a syllable from the patient, her fingers fly swiftly to close his jaws, spread the lips, and tap a front tooth, thereby signaling a narrow groove of the tongue or the focus of the airstream. Then her magical fingers squeeze together to draw out the sibilant hiss as a continuant.

One therapist, when working with a child, used to "draw out" the s, wind it around the child's head three times then insert it into her ear, thus insuring that it would be prolonged enough to be felt. Each sound has its own unique set of deft manipulations, and considerable skill is required to administer motokinesthetic therapy effectively.

Viewed by the cold eye of the modern speech scientist, many of the motokinesthetic cues seem inappropriate; and a therapist would need sixty fingers and thirty arms to provide sufficient cues to take care of the necessary integration and coarticulation. Moreover, much of our research has indicated that standard sounds are produced in different ways by different people, and that their positioning vary widely with differing phonetic contexts. We suspect that much of the effectiveness of this method is due to its powerful suggestion (the laying on of hands), to its accompanying auditory stimulation, or to the novelty to the situation, which may free the case to try new articulatory patterns. We have used it successfully with some very refractory cases, but we always have felt a bit uncomfortable when doing so, as though we were the Magical Monarch of Mo in the Land of Hocus Pocus.

Disparities between theory, therapy and practice

The release in 1943 of *The Defective in Speech* (Berry & Eisenson, 1942, 1956) provided an alternative interpretation of what might improve children's speech production. They guided a swing away from Van Riperian auditory perceptual and ear training, refocusing on auditory memory span and the motor execution component of speech output, in treatment that saw the therapist administering general bodily relaxation procedures and speech musculature exercises. Today, these are generally referred to synonymously as non-speech oral motor exercises (NS-OME), oral motor therapy, oral motor treatment or oro-motor exercises (the more prominent UK term) sometimes called oro-motor work. Apparently ignoring the social context of and consequences for the client of his or her communication impairment, Berry and Eisenson wrote about the mechanism of first-language learning for the first time in the speech pathology literature. They embraced the associative–imitative model (Allport, 1924) from psychology theory, conceptualising speech in linguistic–mentalist terms. But again, these insights were not reflected in their intervention suggestions. Like Van Riper's, their therapy belied any appreciation of language, and they proceeded from bottom up, starting with tongue, lip and jaw exercises, with stimulation of individual phones, and using phonetic placement techniques and repetitive motor drill.

In her analysis of these inconsistencies, Duchan (2001) highlights the genesis of 'a famil-

iar trait in our professional development, the theory–therapy gap', also commenting that 'a second identifiable gap was between research findings and therapy practices', pointing to an evident interdisciplinary gap that saw speech pathologists failing to take much advantage of the developmental psychology research that flourished from the 1920s to the 1950s.

Dyslalia and functional articulation disorder

SLP/SLT was a young profession when speech sound disorders in children were called 'dyslalia' or 'functional articulation disorders'. In its *Terminology for Speech Pathology*, the College of Speech Therapists (1959) defined dyslalia as: 'Defects of articulation, or slow development of articulatory *patterns*, including: substitutions, distortions, omissions and transpositions of the sounds of speech.' Almost simultaneously in the United States, Powers (1959, p. 711) defined it, with a different name, using the word 'functional' in its medical pathology connotation 'of currently unknown origin' or 'involving functions rather than a physiological or structural cause'. The acronym 'SODA' may have been far from Powers' thoughts when she said, 'the term functional articulation disorder encompasses a wide variety of deviate speech *patterns*. These can be described in terms of four possible types of acoustic deviations in the individual speech sounds: omissions, substitutions, distortions, and additions. An individual may show one or any combination of these deviations.'

How interesting it is to find that as early as 1959 SLPs/SLTs in Britain and the United States had an agreed definition and terminology and included the notion of speech *patterns* when they described speech development and disorders. Nonetheless, it must be remembered that they did so without taking into account speech sounds' organisation and representation, cognitively. The 'phoneme' and constructs like it were the domain of clinical linguistics, and it would not be until 20 years or more after the formulation of the British and

American definitions that the beginnings of a practical assessment and 'therapy connection' (Grunwell, 1975; Ingram, 1976) would be forged between phonological theory and SLP/SLT practice.

In the United Kingdom and Australia, the name 'dyslalia' remained in vogue until the 1960s when the preferred US term, functional articulation disorder, gained currency. The preoccupation of therapists, in the 1960s through to the mid-1970s, with individual sounds in the so-called 'three positions' (initial, medial and final), still constituted a strictly phonetic approach to the problem, somehow isolating the linguistic function of speech from the mechanics or motoric aspects of speech. It is enlightening to return to Grunwell's 1975 critique of contemporary practice and her proposal for a more linguistically principled approach to assessment and remediation than the ones that had evolved from practice in the 1930s.

Functional articulation disorders were graded in severity as mild, moderate or severe. In the severe category were the children with 'multiple dyslalia' or 'multiple misarticulations' whose speech was generally unintelligible to people outside of their immediate families. It was readily acknowledged that children with severe functional articulation disorders could usually imitate or quickly be taught how to produce most speech sounds (Morley, 1972). In other words, the supposed motor execution problem or 'articulation' disorder appeared to reside in the children's difficulty in employing speech sounds for word production, which they *could* produce in isolation. Intervention concentrated on the mechanical aspects of establishing the production of individual phonemes, one at a time, context by context.

By defining the problem in articulatory terms and focussing in therapy on speech and accuracy of production, SLPs/SLTs failed to take into account something that they already knew: that speech serves as the spoken medium of language in a system of contrasts and combinations that signal meaning–differences. That is, when children are acquiring the agreed pronunciation patterns of a language and learning the correspondences between articulatory *movements* and sounds, they are also discovering relationships between *meanings* and sounds.

Linguistic theory and sound patterns

In the 1940s and beyond, linguistics theory blossomed in the hands of scholars like Jakobson (1941/1968), who studied child language, aphasia and phonological universals; Velten (1943), who investigated in the growth of phonemic and lexical patterns in infants; and Leopold (1947), who explored sound learning in the first two years of life. These linguistics developments eventually proved highly relevant to practice, but, in and around the World War II period, the profession tended towards physiology, psychology and psychiatry for elucidation, and not linguistics or education. By the 1950s, however, the literature revealed that thinkers knew something more was going on in speech besides auditory, visual and tactile perception and motor execution of sounds. The idea of an inner process or underlying representation as a clinical construct was imminent. Eisenson (1968) talked about symbol formation; Goldstein (1948) and Myklebust (1952) alluded to inner language; and Osgood (1957) used two terms: mediation and psycholinguistic processing.

The linguistic linkage that enticed speech–language clinicians to consider speech disorders in terms of sound systems or patterns came about when researchers in the area of generative linguistics, Chomsky and Halle (1968), expounded distinctive features theory in *The Sound Patterns of English*, a book so famous and influential in linguistics circles that it is commonly referred to simply as SPE. Contemporaneously, Ferguson (1968) looked at contrastive speech analysis and phonological development (see also Ferguson, 1978; Ferguson & Farwell, 1975; Ferguson, Peizer, & Weeks, 1973). Then, Stampe (1973, 1979) forged another link, but this time in the area of natural phonology, leading most saliently for us to Ingram and his innovative work (Ingram, 1974; 1976) uniquely dedicated to the understanding of disordered speech, and to Grunwell (1975, 1981).

Clinical phonology

In the 1970s, linguists and SLPs/SLTs were talking to each other about language in general and clinical phonology in particular. Finally, what SLPs/SLTs had perceived as multiple individual errors came to be seen as sound class problems, involving multiple members of those classes.

For two phonologists, Pamela Grunwell and David Ingram, there was a clear mission to help the SLP/SLT profession in the practical application of phonological principles to the treatment of children with 'phonological disability'; and many clinicians, myself included, devoured every word they wrote! Clinical phonology, according to Grunwell (1987), a British linguist working in the United Kingdom, was the clinical application of linguistics at the phonological level. Ingram (1989a), an American located in Canada at the time, considered that phonology embraced the study of: (1) the nature of the underlying representations of speech sounds (how they are stored in the mind); (2) the nature of the phonetic representations (how the sounds are articulated); and (3) phonological rules or processes (the mapping rules that connect the two). Around the same period in the United States, Stoel-Gammon and Dunn (1985) provided further theoretically principled guidance in a book about assessment and intervention, as did Elbert and Gierut (1986).

From a therapy point of view, the most radical aspect of the new principles was their focus on changing phonological patterns by stimulating children's underlying systems for phoneme use. There was an apprehensive feeling abroad in the clinical community that, because of the theoretical paradigm shift, therapeutic approaches, intervention goals and therapy procedures and activities should now be different, or at least revamped. Fey (1985, p. 255) answered these concerns and uncertainties in a reassuring article, in which he wrote:

> .... *adopting a phonological approach to dealing with speech sound disorders does not necessitate the rejection of the well-established principles underlying traditional approaches to articulation disorders. To the contrary, artic-ulation must be recognized as a critical aspect of speech sound development under any theory. Consequently phonological principles should be viewed as adding new dimensions and new perspectives to an old problem, not simply as refuting established principles. These new principles have resulted in the development of several procedures that differ in many respects from old procedures, yet are highly similar in others.*

In their response to Q3, Nicole Müller and Martin Ball, both linguists, explore the development of the application of linguistic sciences to speech SLP/SLT practice.

Dr. Nicole Müller received a Master's degree from the University of Bonn, Germany, and a doctorate from the University of Oxford, England. She has taught at the University of Central England, Birmingham, at Cardiff University, Wales, the University of Louisiana at Lafayette and since June 2014 has been a Professor of Speech and Language Pathology at Linköping University, Sweden. Her research combines interests in clinical linguistics (specifically systemic functional linguistics), dementia and bilingualism, with occasional forays into phonetics, speech disorders and aphasia. She co-edits the journal *Clinical Linguistics and Phonetics* and the book series *Communication Disorders across Languages*.

Dr. Martin J. Ball is Professor of Speech and Language Pathology at Linköping University in Sweden. He is co-editor of the journal *Clinical Linguistics and Phonetics* (Taylor & Francis) and the book series *Communication Disorders Across Languages* (Multilingual Matters). His main research interests include sociolinguistics, clinical phonetics and phonology and the linguistics of Welsh. Professor Ball is an honorary Fellow of the Royal College of Speech and Language Therapists and a Fellow of the Royal Society of Arts. Among his recent books are *Research Methods in Clinical Linguistics and Phonetics: A Practical Guide* (co-edited with N. Müller, 2013b) and *Phonology for Communication Disorders* (co-authored with N. Müller and B. Rutter, Psychology Press, 2010).

Q3. Nicole Müller and Martin Ball: Application of linguistic sciences

Crystal (2001) defined clinical linguistics, which had its origins in the 1970s, as 'the application of the linguistic sciences to the study of language disability in all its forms'. It has become an independent discipline in its own right with its own professional association, as well as being a core curriculum subject in the preparation of SLPs/SLTs. On the one hand, it informs SLP/SLT assessment, target selection and intervention practices; and on the other, it provides a tool for critical evaluation of competing linguistic theories and methodologies (Perkins & Howard, 1995). In the process, each discipline impacts the other. How did these two-way influences evolve, what in your estimation are the contributions of clinical linguistics to SLP/SLT practice and vice versa?

A3. Nicole Müller and Martin J. Ball: Clinical linguistics (and phonetics)

On a fairly regular basis, students of speech language pathology/speech and language therapy (SLP/SLT) ask us, 'why do we need to study all that linguistics?' To clinical linguists (and phoneticians), the answer is blindingly obvious: To us, doing SLP/SLT without a solid basis in phonetics and linguistics is like trying to do engineering without physics: One (physics, or linguistics/phonetics) is the enabling science that provides the conceptual basis, and indeed the language, to be able to talk about problems arising in the other (engineering, or SLP/SLT). Having said that, we of course have to add that there are a lot of branches of physics that do not contribute directly to building safer bridges or improving the efficiency of the internal combustion engine. Similarly, there is a lot in linguistics that does not precisely lend itself to clinical applications, such as the development of assessment procedures or of intervention programs. Still, we maintain that speech and language pathologists need a strong grounding in linguistics and phonetics, and we hope to show why in this brief essay.

The term 'clinical linguistics' gained currency in SLP/SLT and linguistics in the wake of David Crystal's publication of a book with that title in 1981. Crystal defined clinical linguistics as the 'application of linguistic science to the study of communication disability, as encountered in clinical situations' (Crystal, 1981, p. 1) and expanded on this definition later: '[C]linical linguistics is the application of the theories, methods, and findings of linguistics (including phonetics) to the study of those situations where language handicaps are diagnosed and treated' (Crystal, 1984, p. 31). For the purposes of this essay, we use the term clinical linguistics in Crystal's sense, that is, as the theoretical backbone providing tools for clinically applied analyses. Other linguists have expanded on Crystal's original definition and include, under the umbrella term of clinical linguistics, research that uses data gathered from participants with a variety of language disorders in order to test hypothesis formed on the basis of linguistic theories. In such studies, clinical data are used to test constructs about language systems, formed on the basis of normal language or, more often, on the basis of native speaker intuition and introspection of how language works (see, for example Ball & Kent, 1987, and for further discussion Müller & Ball, 2013a).

Like other scientists and philosophers, linguists construct taxonomies of categories and build models that aid them in thinking about phenomena they encounter in the real world; in other words, they build theories. The path from linguistic theories to clinical application is essentially a one-way street. The theories and interpretive categories we use to analyse, interpret and hopefully understand language produced by people with a variety of language disorders are by and large, imports, that is, they are frameworks developed with normal language, and typically functioning language users in mind as the models (which are usually taken for granted). There are no linguistic theories (including phonology) of disordered language that do not start out as theories of normal language. However, most modern linguistic frameworks, including phonological theories, have, to a greater or lesser intent, had an impact on clinical linguistics. Some aspiring or practicing clinicians may, on reading this, think, 'but I'm not interested in all this talk about theory. I just want to know what to do in practice'. We need to keep in mind, though, that humans cannot think without theorising, and categorising: Thinking, and talking about, and striving to understand, any phenomenon we encounter is, in essence, an exercise in theorising. And any terminologies and categories that an SLP/SLT uses to describe and understand the phenomena encountered in clinical practice (e.g., speech output impairments) are the product of a set of underlying assumptions about the nature of the phenomena thus categorised. Further, when we use tools provided by linguistic theories to describe, analyse and understand patterns in disordered language, we need to ask ourselves the question whether we take the theoretical model we use as just that, namely a handy hook to hang our thinking on, or whether we assume that the descriptive categories we use are close representations of psychological, or mental, realities.

To illustrate: There is a sizeable body of work that applies Chomskyan generative linguistics, in its various versions, to the study of impaired language. Some key assumptions in generative theory are that language is a 'cognitive system that is represented in a speaker's mind/brain with a grammar as its core element' and the human language faculty is regarded as 'a mod-

ular cognitive system that is said to be autonomous of non-linguistic cognitive systems' (Clahsen, 2008, p. 165–166). The 'mental grammar' is also conceptualised as a modular system with distinct components, that is, lexicon, phonology, morphology and syntax. From such a perspective, language impairments are viewed, and investigated as, 'selective, *within-language* deficits' (Clahsen, 2008, p. 166). The aim of the linguist working within a Chomskyan generative model is to build a generative account of mental categories and operations. Language use, in the generative tradition of clinical linguistics, is of interest only insofar as it can give an insight into the mental representations that give rise to it and is thus not an object of investigation for the generative linguist.

Cognitive linguistic approaches, on the other hand, take different perspectives both with regard to the nature of language and cognition and to language use. In what Langacker (1987, 2000) termed 'cognitive grammar', and in subsequent variants of cognitive approaches to linguistics, such as Bybee and colleagues' cognitive phonology, grammar is considered to emerge from general cognitive abilities; language learning uses the same cognitive abilities as other types of learning, such as 'memory, motor control, categorization and inference making' (Vogel, Sosa & Bybee, 2008, p. 485, following Bybee, 2001). The term 'usage-based' is intended to capture the status of language use as crucial in the shaping of language structure, 'with structure seen as both a generator and a product of language use' (Vogel, Sosa & Bybee, 2008, p. 481). A usage-based account of language acquisition, for instance, gives an important role to language use in a continuous process of modifying and building a child's linguistic system, which in turn is seen as a dynamic, emergent system. This is very different from seeing the role of input as that of a mere trigger for the setting of a finite number of pre-determined parameters in a child's internal grammar, as in the principles and parameters account of generative grammar. Generative and cognitive linguistic approaches are thus diametrically opposed to each other in how they view the relationship between language and cognition on the one hand, and the role of language use in the shaping of language knowledge.

How and why does this matter for clinical practice? And how and why does it matter whether we take theoretical models as 'just models', that is, aids in thinking, or as representing a mental (or psychological) reality? Let us consider the notion of contrastivity in spoken language, which is a fundamental concept in all theories of phonology. Every linguist or SLP/SLT has, at one time or another, learned about the notion of the phoneme as the segment-sized embodiment of contrastivity, more typically defined as the smallest unit of sound in a language that can bring about a change in meaning between two words. There are two ways to think about the *phoneme*: We can treat the phoneme as a *real thing*, something that is psychologically real, a part of language knowledge that is acquired as part of language acquisition (or second language learning), and that in turn, somehow, drives speech production. If we think of phonemes as mental categories in the Chomskyan generative tradition, then we will most likely conceptualise them as made up of distinctive features, and of language use, or input, as a trigger for the setting of feature specifications. Since in Chomskyan generative linguistics phonology and lexicon are thought of as two separate modules within language knowledge, it should, in theory, not matter how rich and varied the language use is that we provide if we target phonemic contrasts in intervention, since, again in theory, any one minimal pair is a representation of a target contrast.

On the other hand, we can use the term *phoneme* as a useful summary that certain minimal differences between otherwise similar sequences of articulator configurations result in acoustic output that is perceived as representing different meanings. Thus, the syllables /tɪp/ and /dɪp/ illustrate that fortis and lenis plosives in English represent different phonemes. Thus, the term *phoneme* embodies a complex of cognitive as well as physical *processes* that link the properties of words as semantic entities with sound production and perception. In other words, /t/ and /d/ are a very economical way of representing that the production of a fortis versus a lenis plosive, in an otherwise identical syllable structure, is 'different enough' to represent different semantic categories, or words. We can further note that this difference is expressed most typically, in English word-initial position, by way of an aspirated voiceless plosive [tʰ] versus a partially devoiced plosive [d̥], and to these latter categories we typically refer to as allophones of their respective phonemes. This way of thinking, in our view, aligns well with cognitive or usage-based models of language: From this perspective, phonology – and with it contrastivity – is considered to be an emergent property of vocabulary learning. In terms of intervention it would therefore make most sense to use many different exemplars to facilitate the emergence of the target contrast.

To summarise: SLPs/SLTs need linguistics (including phonetics) because linguistic frameworks provide tools to discover patterns in communication events involving language (or other) impairments, which in turn can contribute to an explication of communication successes and breakdowns and ideally inform efforts to improve communicative success. We believe that it is most useful to take models just as that, namely, as aids to thinking, rather than as representing the 'mental truth' of language and speech. A further important assumption that we make about a clinically useful linguistics is that it is data driven, in other words: the starting point of our endeavours is always *language use in context*. This means, in turn, that we need to marry theories about discrete phenomena with speech in 'real life': To return to our earlier example, the phoneme neatly captures the notion of contrastivity in terms of a *minimal* contrast: /t/ and /d/ are phonemes of English, represented by IPA symbols for static articulatory configurations. However, speech in real life is about movement, precision and coordination, all of which contribute to 'meaning making', and intervention needs to take this into consideration. With this in mind, we believe that SLPs/SLTs need to critically evaluate the terminologies and categories they encounter and use, which in turn makes it necessary to study the underlying assumptions.

Table 1.2 Developmental schedules for phonetic development

Age of acquisition (Kilminster and Laird, 1978[a])	Order of acquisition (Shriberg, 1993[b])
3;0 p b t d k g m n ŋ w j h	Early 8
3;6 f	m n j b w d p h
4;0 l ʃ tʃ	
4;6 s z dʒ	Middle 8
5;0 ɹ	t ŋ k g v tʃ dʒ
6;0 v	
8;0 ð	Late 8
8;6 θ	ʃ ʒ l ɹ s z ð θ

[a]Data source: single word citation naming.
[b]Data source: monosyllabic words in conversational speech samples.

Articulation development

In work whose impact was far-reaching, Irene Poole, a speech teacher at the University Elementary School in Ann Arbor, MI, pursuing a doctorate, produced a developmental schedule for phonetic development (Poole, 1934). This was consistent with the prevailing, and persisting, view that intervention for speech impairment should be based on typical developmental expectations of 'articulatory proficiency'. Other accounts of phonetic mastery criteria have followed, up to the present day (e.g., Templin, 1957; Sander, 1972; Prather, Hedrick, & Kern, 1975; Arlt & Goodban, 1976; Kilminster & Laird, 1978; Smit, Hand, Freilinger, Bernthal, & Bird, 1990; and so on, through to more contemporary summaries of acquisition by Stoel-Gammon (2010) and McLeod (2013)).

A study of phonetic age-norms by Kilminster and Laird (1978) involved single-word citation-naming by children age 3;0–8;6 in Queensland, Australia, with the aim of determining the ages, in years and months, by which 75% of children had mastered 24 English phones. Most developmental profiles of phonetic acquisition are similarly structured, but Shriberg (1993) took a fresh approach when he produced a clinically useful breakdown of the 'early-8', 'middle-8' and 'late-8' acquired sounds, based on monosyllabic words in conversa-

tional speech samples: reflecting the approximate *order* of acquisition rather than approximate *ages* of acquisition. The norms provided by Kilminster and Laird, and Shriberg's early-, middle- and late-8 are contrasted in Table 1.2.

But, we must remind ourselves that all of this clinically relevant information emerged in the 1970s environment in which practice was still heavily influenced by the medical model and American behaviourism; 'SODA' articulation analysis of errors of (S) substitution, (O) omission, (D) distortion and (A) addition; and 'Traditional Articulation Therapy'. This treatment, or at least close variations of it, is still widely implemented today. For example, Brumbaugh & Smit (2013a, b) surveyed 2084 US clinicians working with 3–6 year olds, gathering 489 usable, fully completed or sufficiently completed responses. They reported that more SLPs indicated that they used traditional intervention than other types of treatment. Of the 489, 49% often or always used traditional therapy, and 33% sometimes did.

Mirla Raz, an experienced licensed speech pathologist certified by the American Speech–Language–Hearing Association, regularly uses the approach in her practice. An SLP in private practice at Communication Skills Center in Scottsdale, Arizona, Ms. Raz has worked extensively with children, remediating speech sound disorders, language disorders and stuttering. She is the author of the *Help Me Talk Right* book series that includes: How to *Teach a Child to Say the "R" Sound in 15 Easy Lessons, How to Teach a Child to Say the "S" Sound in 15 Easy Lessons* and *How to Teach a Child to Say the "L" Sound in 15 Easy Lessons*. In her response to Q4 she describes an intervention for a 4-to-5-year old based on traditional assessment data and combining traditional therapy without the auditory discrimination or ear training step, and with the inclusion of word pairs ('contrastive pairs'). As noted below, the two-word combinations were not necessarily minimal pairs, and this was not minimal pair intervention in the conventional sense (Barlow & Gierut, 2002; Weiner, 1981a, b).

Q4.　Mirla G. Raz: From articulation therapy to Apps

Three of your *Help Me Talk Right* books (Raz, 1993, 1996, 1999) are rooted in the so-called 'Traditional Approach' to the remediation of articulation disorders. Such hierarchical, sound-by-sound interventions still have a place in the speech and language clinician's repertoire, but perhaps not always in a form that would be instantly recognisable to Van Riper (1978). In particular, he would probably be surprised to see oral placement therapy (Rosenfeld-Johnson, 2010) and other non-speech oral motor treatments in such prevalent use alongside his methods (Hodge, A31; Lof, A35). Can you outline and illustrate with a case study both the assessment procedures and the therapy methodology you use and point to evidence in support of the traditional approach? A proliferation of Apps for articulation assessment and intervention is flooding the market (Bowen, 2013; Toynton, A33). Are there certain ones that stand out for you as worthwhile additions to a clinician's toolbox in implementing articulation therapy, is evidence associated with them, and can you speculate on where articulation assessment and intervention Apps might head in the future?

A4.　Mirla G. Raz: One clinician's adaptations of traditional articulation therapy to work with a child with phonological disorder

Among approaches to speech sound disorders in children, traditional therapy has a long history and is widely implemented. However, it is not necessarily the intervention of choice when a client demonstrates numerous phonological errors (Kamhi, 2006). That is because sound-by-sound correction can be time consuming, and there are more efficacious therapy approaches for children with phonological disorder. But, how does an SLP/SLT determine whether or not to use a traditional therapy approach or another approach? The key lies in reviewing assessment data to see if the child's SSD has a predominantly phonemic (phonological) basis, or a predominantly phonetic (articulatory) basis or a combination of these. I avoid approaches such as NS-OME that have little or no empirical support (Lof, A35; McCauley, Strand, Lof, Schooling & Frymark, 2009).

Articulation testing

During my nearly 40 years of evaluating and treating children with SSD, I have steadily relied on the *Goldman-Fristoe Test of Articulation* (Goldman & Fristoe, 1969, 2000) for speech assessment. It is easy to use and offers a clear picture of the child's speech production at the word level. Using the sounds-in-words subtest, one can transcribe and note the child's word productions and speech errors. I transcribe a child's production of a word if more than the targeted sound is in error. If the test indicates the child has, what I regard to be, 'standard substitutions' such as w/l, w/ɹ, f/θ, d/ð, θ/s, ð/z, t/k or d/g, I do not explore further.

If the child is difficult to understand and/or has significant token-to-token variability and I suspect phonological disorder, I then record a sample of the child's conversational speech. The sample can take anywhere from 5 to 15 minutes. I may get a sufficient sample from a talkative child in 5 minutes, whereas with a reticent child may take longer. Doing so is advisable as Eisenberg & Hitchcock (2010) demonstrate. They found that standardised tests did not offer sufficient words to allow an SLP/SLT to draw conclusions about a child's phonetic inventory. The question is what is a sufficient sample? Weston, Shriberg and Miller (1989) were not clear as to how many utterances were required for a sufficient sample but suggested that the number may be as high as 225. It is also important to note that, for some children, obtaining an accurate speech sample is extremely difficult. These are children whose connected speech is so difficult to understand that I have been unable to determine what the child is saying.

Case example

Philip was 4;8 when I began working with him. The Photo Articulation Test (Lippke, Dickey, Selmar & Soder, 1997) had been administered at his school and showed a phonetic repertoire comprising /p/, /b/, /t/, /d/, /j/, /n/, /w/ and /h/. Additionally, he omitted final consonants and only used /w/, /b/ and /n/ intervocalically. Stimulability testing indicated that Philip was able to produce all phonemes, in isolation, with the exception of /k/, /g/, /ɹ/, /w/, /θ/ and /ð/. Just 10% of his speech was intelligible to me, and 5% to the SLP who administered the test.

To rule in or out language impairment I administered the Peabody Picture Vocabulary Test III (Dunn & Dunn, 1997) (Standard Score 113; Percentile Rank 81) and the Preschool Language Scale-3 (Zimmerman, Steiner, & Pond, 1991). His Auditory Comprehension Standard Score was 115 (PR 84);

Expressive Communication Standard Score 108 (PR 70); and his Total Language Score was 113 (PR 81). Clearly this was a child with average language skills. However, his reduced intelligibility made it impossible to accurately assess his conversational language. I felt that any deficits in conversational language would become apparent as I got to know him better and his speech improved.

Philip was scheduled for individual therapy twice weekly for 30 minutes each session. I began Philip's therapy program by targeting /k/ and /g/ using a modified traditional articulation approach. I use the term modified since I have eliminated sound discrimination, comparing and scanning (Van Riper, 1978) from my therapy approach. The first step was to target /k/ and /g/ in isolation. Philip succeeded in producing both sounds the first session, and vowel–consonant (VC) combinations by session 2 and so was challenged to use the velar stops syllable-initial-word-initial (SIWI) and syllable-final-word-final (SFWF) in real words. By the end of the third session, Philip was able to produce the sounds in paired words such as: *come–cow, go–girl, make–bake, hug–bug*). However, a glitch arose when Philip was confronted by a word containing a velar stop and /t/ or /d/. Thus, when he said them, *kite* became *tite*, *goat* became *dote*, *take* became *tate* and *dig* became *did*. To tackle this issue, a 'contrastive pairs' approach was introduced. Philip was shown four different sets of paired pictures comprising initial and final /k/ and /t/ contrasts, and initial and final /g/ and /d/ contrasts. Philip's task was to name the pictures pronouncing both the velar and alveolar stops correctly. In session 6, Philip was asked to use the paired words in short sentences such as *I hug the bug* and *I come to the cow*. During this session, Philip was able to use /k/ and /g/ within words. Initial clusters were introduced in the ninth session. By the 10th session, he was ready to use the targeted sounds in sentence repetition tasks wherein the targeted sounds occurred randomly, as in: *The cat loves catnip* and *The bag is full of chocolate cookies*. He progressed rapidly and by the 12th session he had mastered /k/ and /g/ in elicited conversation. In the elicited conversation condition the therapist manipulates input to encourage the child to use the target conversationally. For instance, playing an airport game, I might ask, 'What do we need to buy to get on the plane?' to elicit 'ticket'. Philip was ready to begin using the targeted sounds in conversation by session 13. As Philip was working on using /k/ and /g/ in conversation, /w/ was introduced. Two sessions later, Philip was able to use /w/ at the sentence level. In session 23, Philip's new goal was to use all sounds, with the exception of /ʃ/, /tʃ/, /dʒ/, /l/, /ɹ/, /θ/ and /ð/ in sentence repetition tasks. Two sessions later, /ʃ/, /tʃ/, /dʒ/ and /l/ were added to the same task. We began working on using all sounds, with the exception of /ɹ/, /θ/ and /ð/, in elicited conversation at session 35 and two sessions later Philip was challenged to begin using the sounds in conversation. At this point, language goals were introduced, because as Philip's speech became more intelligible, grammatical deficits became evident. Soon after, /ɹ/ was targeted and later /θ/ and /ð/. Fourteen months after beginning therapy, Philip, now aged 5:10, had mastered all phonemes and was completely intelligible.

Apps and articulation therapy

It is years since I saw Philip for intervention and he still stands out as one of the most phonologically impaired children on my caseload. Would my therapy program be different today with all the available technology? Would I use Apps to assist me in speech therapy?

When the tablet first came out, I was certain these devices would have a significant effect on clinical practice. I still feel it will. However, at this time Apps for speech therapy have definite limitations. These shortcomings are due to technological limitations. At the time of writing, Apps are not yet able to accurately recognise many individual sounds and their interpretation of sound can be flawed. The technology works best when it recognises the user and when it analyses large communication segments, such as words in phrases. The finer the analysis needed, the less accurate the technology becomes, so that voice recognition technology is highly unreliable when it comes to analysing sounds in words, syllables and in isolation. Let us say that a client is working on /d/ production and the App records the client's production. Let us assume the client produces /b/ instead of /d/. There is a good likelihood that the App will indicate that the sound was produced correctly This is precisely what happened when I tested *Tiga Talk* (Tiga Talk, 2011) by Tactica Interactive, featuring cartoon characters from a Canadian children's television show. Regardless of the sound I produced, the App treated the sound as the correct production. Using such an App, an unsupervised child is rewarded whether he or she says the target sound or another sound. This happened for each of the 23 sounds the App offered.

Another drawback to speech Apps can be the poor sound output quality, making it difficult for the client to hear an accurate model of many sounds. The sound output quality is highly dependent on the quality of the recording device and playback devices. This points to the need for developers to employ a good-quality microphone during the development of any App, because a tablet's speakers will not be able to compensate for substandard recordings. When working with children on articulation, it is essential that all sounds be clearly produced. Apps focusing on minimal pairs are particularly vulnerable to clarity issues when they present contrasts that the child customarily confuses. At the time of writing, it is preferable, in my view, to look for Apps in which the SLP/SLT provides visual feedback, for example by tapping a 'plus' if a child's response is correct or an X if it is incorrect.

Apps and EBP

In the last few years much has been written about evidenced-based practice. SLP/SLT application software technology is so new that there have not yet been studies of the efficacy of using Apps in therapy or for testing. My view is that because Apps are technological versions of the paper materials widely used, the same evidence supporting paper materials may be valid for Apps. SLPs/SLTs must be careful, however, when it comes to taking any statements regarding evidence at face value. For example, SLP and App developer Barbara Fernandes cites work by McGregor, Newman, Reilly and Capone (2002) in support of her 2012 language App *Go-Togethers* (Simms, 2012). Their research does not, in fact, support the claims Fernandes reports for the App's effects.

Apps are becoming increasingly sophisticated with numerous attractive and time-saving features. They currently have the capacity to compute responses for individuals and groups within databases and allow users to record speech and other sounds. As yet, few Apps for speech sound disorders utilise two potentially appealing features: animation and interactivity, and it is hoped that far-sighted developers will move in this direction. Improvements in voice recognition technology have the potential for enhancing our work with children's speech. I anticipate that our devices will one day be able to accurately determine whether or not a sound was said correctly. I envision a client being able to observe how far from the target sound her production was and make the changes according to the device's feedback. But in answer to my own question about whether Apps might have helped in Philip's treatment, the answer at this stage probably has to be a qualified 'no'.

Revolution?

Did the hackneyed term 'paradigm shift' (Kuhn, 1962) overstate what actually happened? *Was* there a phonological revolution? *Did* the new principles change practice? Certainly there were changes in the way assessments were conducted (Grunwell, 1975, 1985a; Hodson, 1980; Hodson & Paden, 1981; Ingram, 1981; Shriberg & Kwiatkowski, 1980; Weiner, 1979), but did the *intervention* work of Elbert, Dunn, Gierut, Grunwell, Hodson, Ingram, Paden, Stoel-Gammon and others alter what happened in therapy? The answer probably has to be, 'not much'. In a US context, Brumbaugh and Smit (2013) report that 33% of their respondents frequently used the cycles phonological patterns approach and suggested the possibility that 'SLPs who treated preschoolers were using hybrid interventions, influenced primarily by traditional intervention, but also by minimal pairs and cycles approaches' (p. 316).

In 2004, when Barbara Williams Hodson, co-developer with Elaine Pagel Paden in the mid-1980s of patterns or cycles therapy (Hodson & Paden 1983, 1991), was asked in an online interview for *Thinking Big News* (Thinking Publications, 2004): 'If you could change one thing in how SLPs work with clients what would it be?' Her response was: 'The one thing I wish most is that SLPs would work on patterns when serving an unintelligible child, rather than to focus on teaching isolated sounds to a criterion'. This resonated with something she wrote some 12 years before (Hodson 1992, p. 247) about the relative lack of application of phonological principles by North American SLPs to either assessment or intervention:

> *My own observation, based on interactions with practising clinicians while giving clinical phonology presentations in some 40 states and 5 Canadian provinces, is that even now in the early 90s, only about 10% of the practising clinicians across the United States and Canada seem to be incorporating any phonological principles in their assessment and/or remediation.*

Dr. Barbara Williams Hodson is a professor in the Department of Communication Sciences and Disorders at Wichita State University. Her research interests include clinical phonology and metaphonology, Spanish phonology, and early literacy. She is a Fellow of ASHA, a recipient of the American Speech and Hearing Foundation Frank Kleffner Lifetime Clinical Achievement Award, and was recognised with ASHA's Honors of the Association in 2009. In A5 she discusses the continuing adherence by many clinicians to sound-by-sound intervention.

Q5.   Barbara Williams Hodson: A phonological patterns focus

In the preface of *Evaluating and Enhancing Children's Phonological Systems: Research and Theory to Practice* (Hodson, 2010 p. xi), there are echoes of the statements you made in 1992 and 2004, mentioning the concerns for severely and profoundly involved clients with highly unintelligible speech, when the focus remained on mastering individual phonemes one at a time (e.g., /f/ singleton) to a pre-selected criterion as contrasted with facilitating phonological patterns (e.g., 'syllableness', final 'consonantness' or /s/ clusters. You go on to write:

> *Most treatment programs are phoneme-oriented. The majority of these focus on mastering each phoneme before progressing to the next target. Some use contrastive techniques (e.g., minimal pairs, maximal oppositions, multiple oppositions). A few target word structures, referred to as 'phonotactic' by Velleman (2002). Our preference for children with severe/profound disordered expressive phonological systems is to target patterns that are deficient, including word structures related to omissions (e.g., /s/ clusters, final consonants) as well as phoneme categories (e.g., velars, stridents). Phonemes are considered to be a means to an end rather than the true targets.*

Given the empirical evidence for cycles (Baker, Carrigg & Linich, 2007; Prezas & Hodson, 2010, p. 144; Rudolph & Wendt, 2014), latterly called the *Cycles Phonological Pattern Approach (CPPA)*, it is really unfathomable that this still needs to be said. Why do not more US clinicians target phonological patterns when they have clients with unintelligible speech?

A5.   Barbara Williams Hodson: Cycles phonological pattern approach

One of our observations in the 1970s was that working on one phoneme-at-a time seemed adequate for a child with a mild speech sound disorder with only a few phonemes in error (e.g., /θ/ and /ɹ/). Children with highly unintelligible speech (i.e., extensive phonological deviations), however, were requiring years of intervention in order to 'master' all of the sounds and word structures. In the mid-1970s, David Ingram's book became available. Ingram (1976) helped us see beyond individual phonemes. As we began experimenting with targeting broad patterns at the University of Illinois clinic, we observed faster intelligibility gains.

One comment I have heard from a rather large number of practicing speech–language pathologists in the United States is that although they learned how to identify the various approaches on exams, they never actually learned how to provide pattern-oriented treatment in their classes or clinical experiences. Often, while watching videos, they seem to be astounded at the huge gains in intelligibility of clients during a period of 2 years or less (contact time 60 minutes per week).

Another consideration is that we do know that everything we do (Ingram, 1983, p.1) leads to improved speech overall. But we also are aware of the critical age hypothesis (Bishop & Adams,

1990) and know that children need to be intelligible by age 5 $\frac{1}{2}$ years or they surely will have greater difficulty acquiring literacy.

The *CPPA* was initiated in 1975 in an experimental clinic for young children with highly unintelligible speech at the University of Illinois (see Hodson, 2011). Rapid changes occurred in our treatment methodology during the late 1970s, as hypotheses were formulated and tested, revised as needed and tested again. For example, singleton /s/ was a common target the first year, which was a mistake. It was observed that when these clients attempted to produce word-initial singleton /s/, they did succeed in producing the /s/, but then they inserted their original substitution /t/; thus *sun* was realised as *stun*. At first the student clinicians taught the child to delete the /t/. Children were then able to say *sun,* but words with /s/ clusters were being produced with /s/ singletons (e.g., *say* for *stay*). It was hypothesised that targeting /s/ clusters before /s/ singletons might be more expedient for children with highly unintelligible speech. Moreover, as children began incorporating /s/ clusters/sequences into their conversational speech, their intelligibility improved dramatically (Gordon-Brannan, Hodson, & Wynne, 1992).

Targeting phonological patterns via *cycles* (time periods varying from 5 to 16 hours depending on each child's needs) was explored at our first experimental phonology clinic, and then this approach was revised numerous times. Typically a phoneme (or consonant cluster) is targeted 1 hour per week (i.e., one 60-minute session, two 30-minute sessions or three 20-minute sessions), with each pattern usually being targeted from 2 to 5 hours per cycle. (Note: the time is doubled [i.e., 120 minutes per target] for children with cognitive delay). Thus, targets for the *CPPA* are Phonological Patterns (e.g., 'syllableness'. final 'consonantness'), with phonemes (e.g., final /p/) serving as a 'means to the end' rather than being the goal.

One other clinical research finding has been learning the importance of incorporating some phonological awareness (PA) activities (e.g., rhyming, syllable segmentation) in treatment sessions. Not only do PA skills help children acquire literacy, the PA tasks also often help children improve aspects of speech (e.g., final 'consonantness' after focusing on rimes in rhyming activities).

Theoretical considerations and underlying concepts

The CPPA is based on developmental phonology theories and cognitive psychology principles as well as on-going clinical phonology research. This approach is aligned most closely with two theories: Gestural Phonology (Browman & Goldstein, 1986, pp. 219–252, 1992) and Dynamic Systems (Thelen & Bates, 2003). Eight underlying concepts (see Table A5.1) serve as the basis for this approach (Hodson, 2010; Hodson & Paden, 1991).

Table A5.1 Underlying concepts

1	Children with 'normal' hearing typically acquire the adult sound system primarily by *listening.*
2	Phonological acquisition is a *gradual* process.
3	*Phonetic environment* in words can facilitate or inhibit correct sound productions.
4	Children associate *auditory* and *kinaesthetic* sensations that enable later *self-monitoring.*
5	Children *generalise* new speech production skills to other targets.
6	An optimal *match* facilitates learning.
7	Children learn best when they are *actively involved/engaged* in phonological remediation.
8	Enhancing a child's *metaphonological* skills facilitates enhances the child's speech improvement and also development of early literacy skills.

Source: Adapted from Hodson (2010)

Targeting phonological patterns

Typically a phoneme (e.g., final /k/) or a word structure (e.g., /s/ clusters in words) is targeted 1 hour per week. At least two exemplars (e.g., /sp/ and /st/) of the current target pattern (e.g., /s/ clusters) are presented before moving on to another target pattern (e.g., velars, liquids) or structure (e.g., final 'consonantness') within the cycle. Most target patterns are recycled one or more times with complexity being increased gradually for each succeeding cycle.

Based on clinical research that is on-going, phonological patterns have been divided into *Primary* (those targeted first and then recycled as needed until they began emerging in conversational speech) and *Secondary* patterns (Figure A5.1).

It is critical that the child be *stimulable* and capable of producing the target sound (assisted by various tactile cues and amplification at first) in order to help the child produce the sound and thus develop a new accurate kinaesthetic image. Amplification is used to help children produce the sound and then to develop a new accurate auditory image. We use a small portable battery-operated amplifier and child-sized headphones. We have been able to elicit sounds with the amplifier that had not been stimulable by any other method. The term 'kinaesthetic image' refers to the sense/awareness in the brain of relative movements/positions of parts of the body (see Servomechanism explanation by Fairbanks, 1954). Sounds that initially are 'nonstimulable' (e.g., /k/) are stimulated/facilitated for a few minutes during each session (i.e., teaching stimulability/appropriate production) and then are targeted as soon as the child can actually produce the sound(s). If sounds are targeted while they are still nonstimulable, the continued production(s) of the incorrect sound(s) can be harmful in that this reinforces the inaccurate kinaesthetic image. Table A5.2 provides information about the typical *CPPA* session structure.

Two-year olds

The *CPPA* session structure has been adapted for toddlers. Most of the children under the age of 3 years who have been referred to the Wichita State University clinic have not been willing to participate in regular production-practice activities. Some are nonverbal; others are unwilling to name pictures or imitate words. These children participate in a cycle (typically 2–3 months of weekly sessions [30–45 minutes in length]) of focused auditory input/stimulation for the primary phonological patterns. The clinician fills the room with objects and activities for a primary pattern phoneme (e.g., *mop top hop up cup tap beep* for final /p/) are incorporated to enhance awareness of final consonants.

The next phonological target is often final /k/, thus facilitating both final 'consonantness' and velars. The child participates in parallel-play activities but is not asked to name words during this cycle. The parents receive a 'listening' list of words (with the week's target pattern) to read to their child each night, but they are instructed not to ask the child to say any particular words at this time (i.e., reduce pressure). These adaptations provide a great foundation.

We have found that the child readily moves to production practice during the ensuing cycle. These children have then progressed rapidly. The new clinicians (students) report that they can tell which patterns were presented during the preceding focused auditory input cycle.

Incorporating complexity

It is important to note that complexity is increased gradually throughout the *CPPA* so that the child is optimally challenged but successful from the beginning of treatment (Hunt, 1961). Most young

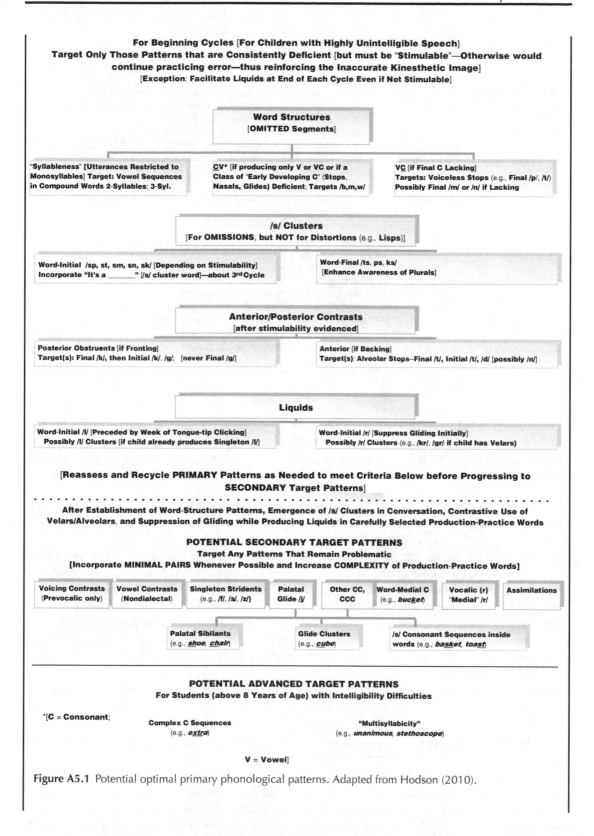

Figure A5.1 Potential optimal primary phonological patterns. Adapted from Hodson (2010).

Table A5.2 Typical clinical session structure

1	Review	Child produces practice words (depicted on large index cards) from the previous treatment session.
2	Listening activity	Clinician reads approximately 20 words using slight amplification (this takes 30 seconds). Child then says new production-practice words for the day while still wearing amplifier headset.
3	Experiential-play motivational production-practice activities	Child says practice word by naming picture or object with correct production of the target pattern for the session before 'taking a turn'. Clinician provides assists (e.g., modelling, tactile cue) as needed so that the child achieves 100% 'correctness' for the target pattern in the practice words.
4	Metaphonological activity	Incorporation of a metaphonological activity: (e.g., rhyming, syllable segmentation).
5	Probing	Probing by clinician to determine optimal target (e.g., singleton phoneme, consonant cluster) for next session's target pattern.
6	Listening activity	Second reading of week's listening list with slight amplification (by parent if possible).
7	Home program	Parents/caregivers are given the following from this day's session to practice with their child 2 minutes every day. (a) week's listening list to read to their child, (b) week's production-practice word (picture) cards for child to name, and (c) metaphonological activity (e.g., folder with 4-line rhyme, syllable segmentation).

Source: Adapted from Hodson (2010)

clients (with initial intelligibility below 20% (Gordon-Brannan, Hodson, & Wynne, 1992) in the university experimental phonology clinics (Wichita State University, San Diego State University, University of Illinois) were judged to be essentially intelligible within 3–4 cycles (i.e., approximately 30–40 contact hours) and simultaneously demonstrated vastly improved phonological systems.

Consonant category deficiencies: Beyond phonological 'processes'

Readers should note that consonant category deficiencies are coded (Hodson, 2003, 2004) if the specified category is lacking because the sound is either being omitted or there is a substitution from a different consonant category. For example, a velar target (/k/) is scored as deficient if it is omitted or if a non-velar sound (e.g., /t/, /j/, /h/) is substituted. This system is necessary because scoring only phonological processes does not always identify what the child needs to target. For example, some children receive a score of zero for fronting, but do not produce any velars because they either omit them or substitute a non-anterior sound (e.g., /h/ or /j/), neither of which is fronting (Hodson 2003, 2004).

Models of phonological acquisition

It has become axiomatic in the literature to say that, because so little is known about normal phonological development, a cohesive, convincing linguistic theory of phonological disorders has yet to be formulated. Ingram (1989a) surveyed various attempts in the field of linguistics to construct a phonological theory that covered both normal and disordered phonological acquisition, indicating that the most likely sources of elucidation of *normal* acquisition might be universalist/structuralist theory (Jakobson, 1941/1968), natural phonology theory (Stampe, 1969), or the Stanford cognitive model (Macken & Ferguson, 1983). Of the three, only that of Stampe was directly tied to a phonological theory.

The behaviourist model

The behaviourist model dominated linguistics from the 1950s to the early 1970s. It applied a psychological theory of learning to explain how children came to distinguish and produce the sound system of the ambient language. Its adherents included Mowrer (1952, 1960), Murai (1963) and Olmstead (1971). They identified the role of contingent reinforcement in gradually 'shaping' a child's babbling to meaningful adult forms through classical conditioning. An important aspect of the model was the emphasis on continuity between babbling and early speech. The behaviourists believed that the infant came to associate the vocalisations of the mother (usually) with primary reinforcements, such as food and nurture, with adults' vocalisations assuming secondary reinforcement status.

Eventually, the infant's vocalisations would become secondary reinforcers (providing self-reinforcement) due to their similarity to adult models. From this point, the caregiver could refine the sound repertoire of the infant through selective reinforcement. The behaviourist framework did not presuppose, or indeed show any interest in, an innate order of speech sound acquisition. The sounds acquired depended on the reinforcement obtained from the linguistic environment.

The structuralist model

The structuralist model (Jakobson, 1941/1968), stemmed from structuralist linguistic theory, and it proposed *discontinuity* between babbling and speech. In addition, the structuralists postulated an innate, universal order of acquisition, with distinctive features emerging hierarchically and predictably. Jakobson regarded babbling as a random activity virtually unrelated to the devel-

opment of the sound system. Evidence of regularities in pre-linguistic vocal patterns (Ferguson & Macken, 1980; Oller, Wieman, Doyle & Ross, 1976) has, however, weakened this position. As well, mid-1970s research challenged Jakobson's hypothesis of a sequence of phonemic oppositions as the basis for the earliest stages of phonological development. Kiparsky and Menn (1977) demonstrated that the child's word count is too small to provide objective evidence of the distinctive features 'unfolding' in the way proposed by Jakobson. Really, the developmental order of phonemic oppositions has proved difficult to ascertain, because analysis has to take into account the adult targets attempted as well as the child's phonetic repertoire. To complicate matters, children seem to selectively *avoid* saying words containing certain consonants that are difficult for them to produce (Ferguson & Farwell, 1975; Schwartz & Leonard, 1982). Studies of evidence of lexical avoidance (or 'lexical selection') lent weight to the theory that, in the first-50-words-stage, children target whole words (Ingram, 1989a, pp. 17–22). The phonetic variability readily observed in children in the 9- to 18-month-age range may also provide evidence against a universal order of phoneme acquisition. Irrespective of such shortcomings, Jakobson's views exerted a tremendous, enduring influence on linguist thought. Ingram (1989a p. 162) counted the structuralist model as one of the 'most likely candidates' for a theory of normal phonological acquisition. He talks about this in A6 and also addresses the topic of whole word measures of correct speech production in A12 in the following chapter.

Dr. David Ingram received his PhD from Stanford University in 1970, where he studied language universals under Professor Joseph Greenberg and phonological acquisition in children under Professor Charles Ferguson. His interest in language disorders was developed during two subsequent years as a Research Associate at the Scottish Rite Institute for Childhood Aphasia. He was a professor at the University of British Columbia from 1972 to 1998 and has been a professor at Arizona State University since 1998. His research is on language acquisition in typically developing children and children with language and phonological disorders. The focus is on both English-speaking children and children acquiring other languages. The language areas of primary interest to him are phonological, morphological and syntactic acquisition. He has published over 100 articles and is particularly known for his seminal work, *Phonological Disability in Children* (1976), and his comprehensive textbook, *First Language Acquisition* (1989b).

Q6.   David Ingram: Theory and speech sound disorders

Can you comment on this quotation from Powell, Elbert, Miccio, Strike-Roussos and Brasseur (1998) who said, 'Perhaps we err in our attempt to find a single theory to support all of our work with children with phonological disorders. When we acknowledge the heterogeneity of this target population, we are logically moving towards acknowledging that different theoretical approaches may have to guide our work with different subgroups. We seem to have moved past the more simplistic "one theory fits all" view'. It is a moot point in SLP/SLT circles whether clinicians spend much time thinking about theories, but most clinicians probably incorporate into their 'theory of intervention' (Fey, 1992b) the idea that you cannot work effectively with children with SSD unless you have a good grasp of normal development. In this context, the notion of 'typical acquisition' is usually around age-of-acquisition and order-of-acquisition schedules that focus on surface forms and not much to do with theories of development and models of phonology. Do you continue to regard the structuralist model as a front-runner in the formulation of a theory of normal phonological acquisition (Ingram, 1989a), and what are the other contenders? How do you see a theory of acquisition informing the development of theories of disorder and intervention, and how can clinicians use this information?

A6.   David Ingram: The role of theory in SSD

This quotation by Powell, Elbert, Miccio, Strike-Roussos and Brasseur (1998) is a well-intended comment on the complexity of determining a theoretical account of children's SSD. The effort to do so has a long history of moving from simpler to more complex explanations. Originally, SLP/SLT began with little if any theory, treating speech sound errors as errors with individual sounds, and with subsequent treatments that were based on the intuitively reasonable assumption that improvement would result from drill and repetition. These early efforts were supported by subsequent acceptance in many circles of behaviourism, a movement clearly described in the present book.

With the demise of behaviourism (Chomsky, 1959), a new era of linguistic explanations emerged, with the result over time being a daunting range of possible theoretical accounts (c.f. summaries in Ball and Kent, 1997). In the 1970s, the field of SLP/SLT was sympathetic to these efforts, and the proposals have constituted major sections of most textbooks since (Stoel-Gammon & Dunn, 1985; Bauman-Waengler, 2004). At least two potential problems arose with these efforts at theoretical explanation. For one, phonological theories became more and more complex and abstract, and de facto harder to assimilate and make clinically relevant. Second, no clear theoretical approach has won out; in the sense of demonstrating it is, without argument, the best and clinically most relevant account. The positive from all this is the impression that a range of intervention approaches 'work' (with some debate whether one or another might be even more effective). The Powell et al. suggestion captures this state of the art. That is, they reflect the impression: (1) that many theories have shown success and (2) that children with a range of speech sound problems respond to different approaches. This leads the authors to the intuitively reasonable conclusion that specific theories, and their subsequent treatment approaches, may work better for some disorders than others.

Like behaviourism, however, this intuitively reasonable assumption is wrong. It errs on both the side of treatment and the side of theory. Concerning treatment, it is certainly good news that a range of treatment approaches work and also good news that SLPs/SLTs know them. There is the implication, however, that a reasonable arsenal of treatment approaches is sufficient to treat SSD. Unfortunately, a range of available treatment approaches is no guarantee of future success without some theoretical grounding. There is no foundation to the prediction that what worked with one child will work with another child, just because the two children appear to be similar based on some assessment. Nor does it make sense simply to run a child through the approaches until one clicks. We need to understand the disorders better than that, and a better understanding can only come from a sound theoretical approach.

Let me try to make this more concrete. Let us say I am a practicing SLP/SLT with excellent skills at two quite different treatment approaches. On the one hand, I am very experienced in using a cycles approach (in a group setting) with target selection based on using developmentally appropriate sounds. At the same time, I am also well trained at using a maximal contrast approach, involving intense one-on-one intervention with target sounds well beyond the child's current developmental level. On Tuesday, I evaluate two children, Barbara and Judy. I conclude from my clinical intuitions that Barbara will benefit from a cycles model, whereas Judy will be best served with the maximal contrast therapy.

At one level, this is evidence-based practice. When I meet with Barbara's parents, I will discuss the cycles approach and refer to Hodson (2004) and other references as needed. When meeting with Judy's parents, however, my justification will be through discussing work by Gierut (2001) and the references therein. I will also be doing exactly what Powell et al. suggest, that is, moving past the simplistic 'one theory fits all' view. I will rely on my clinical experience over many years of practice, an invaluable part of my decision-making process. Given the latitude afforded to me by Powell et al., I also have one additional option. If one or both children do not meet my treatment goals, I can just switch them to the other approach. Or, if I get to attend a national convention in the interim, I can bring home a new approach I might learn at a workshop there. I have also satisfied Powell et al. by not thinking too much about theories throughout the whole process.

Is what I have just described 'best' practice? I do not think so. The bottom line is that knowing a range of treatment approaches and selecting from them as needed for specific subgroups is not sufficient. There needs to be a single theoretical basis for these decisions. In Ingram and Ingram (2001), we discuss a situation similar to the one above. We offer the hypothesis that there may be two subgroups of children with SSD: one with poor whole-word skills and one with good whole-word skills. The former group will be children with poor intelligibility, who are having difficulties matching their speech sounds to the target models. The latter group, on the other hand, are matching the target words relatively well (over 50% of the segments) but are possibly delayed in terms of their speech. We go on to suggest that the former children are candidates for a developmental approach, such as the one described for Barbara. The latter children, however, with good matching skills, may respond well to the maximal contrast approach as mentioned for Judy. Importantly, these decisions follow a single theory, a theory that incorporates whole-word abilities into our account of how children acquire their phonological systems. Within this theory, it makes sense to select the treatments as mentioned, and no sense to do it the opposite way.

Turning to the implications about theories by Powell et al., they make a false assumption about what theories are about. While referring to the 'one approach fits all' view as simplistic, they replace it with a Rodney King 'why can't we all get along' view. Rodney King was an American whose arrest was videotaped and found to include an excessive use of force by the police. This quote was his response to the arrest.

Here is an example of how this point of view could be applied. In Ingram (1989a), I contrast two theories of language acquisition: a maturational approach and a constructionist (Piagetian) approach. These theories make very different claims about how language is acquired. For example, it is known that certain syntactic constructions are acquired late, for example, more complex forms of passive sentences. A maturational account would say that this is because the grammatical principles needed to form passive sentences do not mature until later, say age 6. A constructionist approach would predict that these sentences could be acquired earlier through the right combination of exposure to them and internal developments of the child's language acquisition.

Can these theories co-exist? They can, according to Powell et al. Let us again turn to a concrete example from speech sounds disorders. We know that children acquire certain English sounds late, such as the dental fricatives. On Wednesday, I assess two four-year olds, both referred with problems with these fricatives and a concern that intervention may be appropriate. I reach the following conclusions. One child, Dan, strikes me as very constructionist in his learning, whereas the other child, Tom, appears maturational. My recommendations are as follows. Dan will start an intervention program where we

will use auditory bombardment to stimulate his acquisition of the dental fricatives. We will work on a selective vocabulary with these sounds, which in turn will lead to internal gains in his language knowledge. Poor Tom, however, cannot learn these sounds because his speech development needs to mature. No amount of intervention will help Tom, who will be left alone to acquire these sounds at age six when his maturation is complete. If this makes sense to you, there is some land in Florida I would like to talk to you about.

The Rodney King approach underlies a basic misunderstanding that somehow theories can co-exist. Here is one further demonstration of this misconception. Let us consider a theory of phonological acquisition that proposes children use phonological processes to simplify speech. This theory has many processes, including Fronting (which changes k to t, e.g., 'key' is [ti]) and Backing (which changes t to k, e.g., 'tea' is [ki]). Another theory, NeoJakobson Theory, says that children's productions reflect their underlying distinctive features. This theory allows Fronting, but not Backing, as a natural process. On Thursday, I assess two children: one who shows Fronting (David) and one who is doing Backing (Caroline). My conclusions are that David is using the phonological process theory to acquire his speech sounds, whereas Caroline is using the NeoJakobson theory. Again, this is nonsense. The problem with the phonological process theory (as stated) is that it makes up any process it needs and is therefore too powerful. By explaining everything, it explains nothing. The more restricted theory is to be preferred. How then, can the NeoJakobson Theory account for our data? The theory states that children's first feature distinction is between a labial consonant and a non-labial consonant. The first non-labial consonant can either be a [t] or a [k]. Most children will opt for the [t], a more common sound in early productions, and this choice is the predicted, or unmarked, sound. Some children, however, may select to produce [k] instead, since it still has the same underlying value of the [t], that is, both being non-labial. This becomes, therefore, the less common, or more marked, choice. It is not always easy to evaluate theories and decide that one is more explanatory than the other, but the bottom line is that such evaluations are the way theories are assessed, not by saying they all happily coexist.

If I am to stand by and defend the simplistic (sic) view that one theory fits all, then I should provide some suggestions on what this theory might look like. In Ingram (1997), I outline the basic properties of such a theory. The first point to make is that our theory for SSD has, in the short term, different goals than phonological theory. The latter has as its goal the characterization of the phonological systems of the thousands of languages that exist in the world. Our goal, by no means trivial, is to have a theoretical account of the phonological systems of children's first words, often less than a thousand in number. This goal does not require the extent of theorisation or formalism needed in linguistic theory. As suggested in Ingram (1997), it is possible to isolate the shared assumptions of phonological theory in general to form the basis of our theory of SSD. Here are some of those shared characteristics: the acquisition of an early lexicon involves the acquisition of phonological representations; these early representations, like adult representations, consist of phonological features; the early representations of children are underspecified, that is, they do not contain the full range of features of those for adult speakers; children first acquire a subset of the features underlying all languages; my research leads me to suggest these early features are consonantal, sonorant, labial, dorsal, continuant; voice; the child's productions are speech sounds that have one or more of these features; the first syllables are constructed from a small set, that is, CV, CVC, VC, CVCV, CVCVC; children's productions attempt to

match the adult models, in typical development around 70%.

I will finish with one of my favourite quotes: 'Theory without practice is speculation, practice without theory is dangerous.[1]

---

[1] Source lost in time.

The biological model

Like Jakobson, Locke (1983a, b, c) stressed universality in his proposal of a biological model of phonological development. However, Locke emphasised *biological* constraints rather than linguistic ones. Rejecting Jakobson's idea of discontinuity between babbling and speech, Locke postulated relatively rigid maturational control over the capabilities of the speech production mechanism. For Locke, phonology began before 12 months of age with the pragmatic stage when certain babbled utterances gained communicative intent. At the same time, the phonetic repertoire was essentially 'universal', constrained by the anatomical characteristics of the vocal tract. During the 'cognitive stage' that followed, the biological constraints persisted while the child learned to store and retrieve relatively stable forms of phonemes learned from adult language models. At 18 months, in the 'systemic stage', biologically determined babbling production patterns gave way to more adult-like speech. These speech attempts reflected phonologically the target language. Patterns found *only* in adult speech were acquired and patterns not contained in it were 'lost'.

The natural phonology model

Meanwhile, Stampe (1969) had proposed his natural phonology model of phonological acquisition. He posited that children come innately equipped with a universal repertoire of phonological processes: stopping, fronting, cluster reduction and so on. These processes were 'mental operations' that change or delete phonological units, reflecting the natural limitations and capacities of speech production and perception. In Stampe's view, natural processes amounted to articulatory restrictions, which came into play like reflexes. The effect of these 'reflexes' (which were not reflexes in the physiological 'knee jerk' sense) was one of preventing accurate production of sound differences. This occurred despite the sounds being perceived correctly auditorily and stored as 'correct' adult phonemic contrasts in the linguistic mechanism in the brain. The processes operated to constrain and restrict the speech mechanism *per se*. Stampe held that these universal, innate simplifications of speech output involved children's cognitive, perceptual, and production domains. In essence, he believed that the processes simplified speaking in three possible ways. Given a potential phonological contrast, a process favoured the member of the opposition that was the:

1. least complex to produce;
2. least complex to perceive; or,
3. least complex to produce and perceive.

For instance, given the choice of saying /d/ or /ð/, the assumption was that /d/ was easier, because, in typical development, it was acquired earlier (see Table 1.2); for example, *this* (/ðɪs/) is often realised by young children as /dɪs/ (an example of Stopping).

The child's developmental task was to suppress the natural phonological processes to achieve full productive control of the phonemes of the ambient language. Stampe also believed that, from the time they began using speech meaningfully, children possessed a fully developed, adult-like, phonological perceptual system. Thus, while they exhibited natural processes in output, they already had an underlying representation (a mental image or internal knowledge of the lexical items) of the appropriate adult target form (so 'this' would be /ðɪs/ underlyingly and /dɪs/ on the surface). Stampe relied heavily on a deterministic explanation of phonological change. He maintained that children 'used' processes for the phonological act of simplifying pronunciation.

The progression to adult-like productions (for instance, the use of consonant clusters) repre-

sented mastery of increased constraints (upon output phonology). This development occurred through the suppression of natural processes and consequent revision of the universal system. Change occurred through a passive mechanism of suppression as part of maturation. Stampe did not consider cognitive constraints related to the pragmatics of communication, or of the active learning of a language-specific phonology through problem solving, as in the cognitive model. Possibly the most contentious aspect of Stampe's interpretation of Natural Phonology was his claim that the processes were psychologically real, with Neil Smith (Smith, 1973, 1978) concluding that there was no psychological reality to the child's system because there was no evidence for the 'reflex mechanism' proposed by Stampe in applying, or rather 'using', phonological processes.

The prosodic model

The prosodic model of Waterson (1971, 1981) introduced another novel theoretical construct. It involved a perceptual schema in which 'a child perceives only certain of the features of the adult utterance and reproduces only those he is able to cope with' (Waterson, 1971, p. 181) in the early stages of word production. Waterson (1971), Braine (1974), Macken (1980) and Maxwell (1984) asserted that, in infants, both perception and production are incomplete at first. Both developed and changed before they could become adult like. Unlike the more generally applied phonological process-based (segmental) description, Waterson's schema provided a gestalt of child production rather than a segment-by-segment comparison with the adult target. Waterson's approach is useful in describing the word productions of toddlers and may explain those that are not obvious reductions of adult forms.

The cognitive/Stanford model

The Stanford or cognitive model of phonological development (Ferguson, 1968; Kiparsky &

Menn, 1977; Macken & Ferguson, 1983), and also Menn's (1976) 'interactionist discovery model', construed the child as *Little Linguist*, a captivating idea that dates back at least as far as Comenius (1659). Comenius insisted that, for a child, language learning was never an end in itself but rather a means of finding out about the world and forming new concepts and associations. In problem-solving mode, the child met successions of challenges and mastered them, thereby gradually acquiring the adult sound system.

Because the child was considered to be involved actively and 'cognitively' in the construction of his/her phonology, the term cognitive model was used. Phonological development was an individual, gradual, and creative process (Ferguson, 1978). The Stanford team proposed that the strategies engaged in the active construction of phonology were individual for each child and influenced by internal factors: the characteristics and predispositions of the child, and external factors: the characteristics of the environment. The external factors might include the child's ordinal position in the family, family size, child-rearing practices and interactional style of the adults close to the child.

Levels of representation

Both David Stampe and Neil Smith recognised only two levels of representation. Stampe saw phonological processes as mapping from the underlying representation to the surface phonetic representation, whereas Smith (1973) saw realisation rules assuming this function. Stampe and Smith insisted that the child's phonological rules or processes were innate or learned extremely early. Then, Ingram (1974) coined the term 'organisational level' to connote a third, intervening component, related to, but distinct from, the perceptual representation of the adult word. A similar three-level arrangement, implicit in Jakobson's distinctive features theory, was central to cognitive or Stanford theory.

Smith rejected the hypothesis that each child has a unique system and assumed full, accurate perception and storage of adult speech targets. He proposed a set of ordered and universal phonological tendencies and realisation rules. Realisation rules were physical expressions of abstract linguistic units. Any underlying form had a corresponding realisation in substance. In this instance, phonemes were 'realised' or manifested in 'phonic substance' as phones (whereby meanings were transmitted). Smith's understanding was that the processes acted as a filter between the correctly stored adult word and the set of sounds produced by the child. Again, the problem arose of the child being perceived as passively allowing the realisation rules to 'apply' in reflecting the adult word.

Theories of development, theories of disorder, and theories of intervention

The theoretical assumptions upon which any speech-intervention approach is based are derived first from a theory or theories of normal phonological development, or how children normally learn the speech sound system through a combination of maturation and learning. Exploring this idea, Stoel-Gammon and Dunn (1985) posited four basic interacting components necessary for the formulation of a model of phonological development:

1. An auditory–perceptual component, encompassing the ability to attend to and perceive linguistic input.
2. A cognitive component, encompassing the ability to recognise, store and retrieve input and to compare input with output.
3. A phonological component, encompassing the ability to use sounds contrastively and to match the phonological distinctions of the adult language.
4. A neuromotor component, encompassing the ability to plan and execute the articulatory movements underlying speech.

From the practitioner's beliefs and assumptions about *normal* development comes a theory of *abnormal* phonological development: that is, a theory of disorders that explains why some children do not acquire their phonology along typical lines. Then, from the theories of normal and abnormal acquisition, and their formalisms, a theory of *intervention* can evolve. The nature of a theory of intervention (or theory of therapy) depends on how the individual clinician understands, interprets, incorporates, adapts, and modifies knowledge of normal and abnormal acquisition, and what theoretical assumptions are made in the process. Michie and Abraham (2004) suggested that intervening without a theory of therapy could lead to 'reinventing the wheel rather than re-applying it'. Expanding on this point, they explained that, if we can isolate which parts of a treatment are doing the work (the 'active ingredients', so to speak) of facilitating desired goals, it is possible to 'fine-tune' therapy to maximise those effective components while reducing components that do not seem to exert much effect on the outcome.

A theory of therapy, that is, how best to improve the speech of a child with SSD beyond the progress expected with age must logically rely on *assessment procedures* that are congruent with the interventionist's theories of development, disorders and intervention (Fey, 1992a, b; Ingram, A6). In this regard, our timeline should record the development, mainly in the 1980s, of new speech assessments based around Natural Phonology theory and emphasising phonological process analysis. These included, in order of publication: Weiner (1979), Shriberg and Kwiatkowski (1980), Hodson (1980), Ingram (1981), Grunwell (1985a), and Dean, Howell, Hill and Waters (1990). Phonological process analysis introduced the concept of an abstract level of knowledge. This was revolutionary in its time and was the phonological version of syntactic deep structure.

The first minimal pair therapy, inspired by Natural Phonology, appeared in the literature when Frederick Weiner had a novel idea. Calling it 'the method of meaningful contrast' (Weiner, 1981a), he described what we now know as 'conventional' (Barlow & Gierut, 2002) minimal pair therapy. More therapy ideas based on linguistic principles followed rapidly. For example, a year later, Blache (1982) presented a systematic approach to minimal pairs and distinctive feature training in a book chapter; Hodson and Paden (1983) produced the first edition of *Targeting Intelligible Speech*, which described their 'patterns' approach, popu-

larly called 'cycles therapy', and since rebadged as the *Cycles Phonological Pattern Approach: CPPA* (Hodson, A5); Monahan (1984, 1986) devised a minimal pairs therapy kit called *Remediation of Common Phonological Processes*; and Elbert and Gierut (1986) wrote the *Handbook of Clinical Phonology*. In the same period that all this action was happening in the United States, in the United Kingdom, Grunwell (1983, 1985b) provided intervention guidance in peer-reviewed journal articles; Dean and Howell (1986) wrote an inspiring article about the metalinguistic aspect of therapy for child speech that heralded the development of the *Metaphon Resource Pack* (Dean, Howell, Hill & Waters, 1990); and Lancaster and Pope (1989) developed a therapy manual, *Working with Children's Phonology*, that focused on an auditory input therapy (thematic play or naturalistic approach) approach suitable for very young children and older children with cognitive and attention-span challenges (Lancaster, A24). Still in the United Kingdom, the first of a series of books (Stackhouse & Wells, 1997) devoted to an influential psycholinguistic framework appeared (Gardner, A27).

A clinical forum on phonological assessment and treatment, edited by Marc Fey, was published in 1992 in one of the ASHA journals, *Language, Speech, and Hearing Services in Schools (LSHSS)*. Other such forums followed in 2001, 2002, 2004 and 2006, but this particular one, with articles by Edwards (1992), Elbert (1992), Fey (1985, 1992a, b), Hodson (1992), Hoffman (1992), Kamhi (1992) and Schwartz (1992), remain extraordinarily helpful as a comprehensive introduction. In one of the articles, Fey (1992b) captured the clear distinction between intervention approaches, intervention procedures and intervention activities when he described and applied a structural plan for analysing the form of language interventions, such as phonological therapies. This hierarchical plan (displayed in Table 1.3) was adapted by Bowen (1996) and discussed in Bowen and Cupples (1999a).

For clinicians, one good reason for knowing the theoretical underpinnings of the 'therapies' or 'interventions' in his/her repertoire is that it enables them to pick and choose among them, or

Table 1.3 Theory to intervention hierarchy

1. PHONOLOGICAL THEORY

CLINICIAN'S <u>OWN</u> THEORY OF DEVELOPMENT ~ THEORY OF DISORDERS ~ THEORY OF INTERVENTION
CONGRUENT WITH

↓↑

2. PHONOLOGICAL ASSESSMENT APPROACHES

↓↑

CONGRUENT WITH

↓↑

3. PHONOLOGICAL INTERVENTION APPROACHES
INCORPORATING GOAL SELECTION AND GOAL ATTACK VIA 3 LEVELS OF INTERVENTION GOALS

<u>LEVEL 1</u>
BASIC INTERVENTION GOALS
(1) To facilitate cognitive reorganisation of the child's phonological system, and phonologically oriented processing
strategies;
(2) to improve the child's intelligibility.

<u>LEVEL 2</u>
INTERMEDIATE INTERVENTION GOALS
To target *groups* of sounds related by an organising principle
(e.g., phonological processes / patterns / rules; or phoneme collapses)

<u>LEVEL 3</u>
SPECIFIC INTERVENTION GOALS
To target a sound, sounds or structure, using <u>vertical strategies</u>, e.g., working on it until a criterion is reached, then
moving to a new goal; or <u>horizontal strategies</u>, e.g., targeting several sounds within a process, and/or targeting more
than one process simultaneously, and/or targeting syllable structures, metrical stress, etc. simultaneously with another
target; or <u>cyclical strategies</u>, e.g., addressing several goals cyclically, focusing on only one goal per treatment session.

↓

4. INTERVENTION PROCEDURES
e.g., stimulability training, or phonetic production

↓

5. INTERVENTION ACTIVITIES
Contexts and events, such as games and tasks

Source: Available from: www.speech-language-therapy.com/images/14.png

even to combine aspects of them, based on client need. In suggesting that we should be more aware of theories, it should not be assumed that theories are only incorporated into intervention if we, as clinicians, are conscious of them. As Duchan (personal correspondence 2008) points out, 'I feel that we can look at any intervention and deduce its theoretical underpinnings or at least the assumptions it is based on, even if the clinician cannot articulate them. For example, drill is based on an assumption or theory that learning is like exercise, the more you practice saying a sound or word, the better you "know" or can say it next time'.

Fey's useful hierarchy covered the steps involved in modifying and adapting theoretical principles into a practicable intervention approach. It shows the progression from (1) a given phonological theory (e.g., Natural Phonol-

ogy) to (2) a phonological analysis that is congruent with that theory of phonological development (e.g., Independent Analysis and Relational Analysis) to (3) the phonological therapy approach under consideration (e.g., Conventional Minimal Pairs Therapy), informed by (1) and (2). It then allows description of three levels of intervention goal—basic goals, intermediate goals and specific goals—with goal-selection and goal-attack as critical components. From these arise (4) the intervention procedures of choice within the selected therapy model or a coherent combination of models and (5) workable intervention activities that are both consistent with the preceding four levels and suitable for a particular client.

The 'other' clinical forums, so useful to clinicians, referred to above include one in *LSHSS* edited by Barlow (2001, 2002); one in the

American Journal of Speech-Language Pathology edited by Williams (2002a, b); another in *Child Language Teaching and Therapy*, guest edited by Bernhardt (2004); and, one in *Advances in Speech-Language Pathology* (now renamed the *International Journal of Speech-Language Pathology*) edited by McLeod (2006). More specific clinical forums dealing with particular therapy approaches are also available to guide the clinician. For example, there is one on Metaphon (Dean, Howell, Waters & Reid, 1995) in *Clinical Linguistics and Phonetics*, and one on Parents and Children Together: PACT (Bowen & Cupples, 1999a, 1999b) in the *International Journal of Language and Communication Disorders*.

Looking back at Table 1.1 and the 70-year period from the Travis articulation paragraph in 1931 to the impact of phonology in the 1970s, via the information explosion of the Internet era, to the ICF-CY view of speech impairment post 2001, we see the dominant influence of linguistics on child speech practice. Bleile (personal correspondence 2005) sees the effects of linguistics, and particularly the impact of phonology, on our practice as being less than we thought it would be. He uses the analogy of waves on a beach and a 'wave height' metaphor from surfing. The first wave, distinctive features theory, was 'over head' and went way, way up the beach; then came natural phonology theory and phonological processes, 'head high' and not so far up the beach; following that, nothing was quite 'shoulder high' or even 'waist high', with metrical phonology, auto-segmental phonology and other nonlinear approaches creating small ripples, barely wetting the sand. Can it be that linguistic theory is now exhausted as a source of ideas and insights about phonological disorders, like behavioural psychology that ran out of puff in the 1970s? Perhaps information-processing models like the psycholinguistic model of speech processing and production (Stackhouse & Wells, 1997, 2001) hold promise of enticing waves on the intervention side in the future. Maybe it is time for big new insights to come from biology, particularly developmental neurology and genetics. This notwithstanding, there are aspects of linguistic and psycholinguistic theory that we clinicians should

be well acquainted with, because certain linguistic principles can help in devising evidence-based therapies that are conducive to treatment efficacy.

Communication and advocacy

Our recent history has unfolded alongside the creation and expansion of the Internet, comprising the World Wide Web (Berners-Lee, 2002) and e-mail, and the growing use of information and communication technology (ICT), including social media by academics in general and speech and language professionals in particular (Bowen, 2003, 2012), and consumers of SLP/SLT services. E-mail, electronic mailing lists, message boards and other web-based discussion and sharing including Facebook, Pinterest and Twitter have facilitated quick, easy and enjoyable international communication and collaboration among academics and specialist clinicians who have the time to devote to it and have provided novel opportunities for professionals and consumers to engage with each other. Part of this Internet expansion has included the growth of child speech-related advocacy websites, the most prominent of which is the Apraxia-KIDS website (www.apraxia-kids.org), the online face of the Childhood Apraxia of Speech Association of North America (CASANA).

Ms. Sharon Gretz, M.Ed. is the founder and executive director of CASANA. She has been recognized and awarded in the United States for her work in advocating for children with apraxia of speech and their families. Sharon brings many perspectives to the field as both parent and professional, having completed extensive graduate course work in Communication Sciences and Disorders at the University of Pittsburgh while also being the parent of a child with CAS. Frustrated in 1997 by the lack of information on CAS, she worked with local and international SLP academics and clinicians to develop training programs for SLPs and accessible web-based information for families new to diagnosis, those seeking on going support and individuals interested in the research side. She talks about this in A7.

Q7.   Sharon Gretz: Consumer advocacy and childhood apraxia of speech

As the parent of a young adult who had severe CAS at the age of three, founder and Executive Director of Apraxia-KIDS and the Childhood Apraxia of Speech Association of North America (CASANA) and a doctoral student in communication sciences and disorders, you have made an extraordinary contribution to our field and have a unique perspective on SLP/SLT child speech practice. Impressively, CASANA has become the only national non-profit organization in the United States and internationally with the sole focus of CAS. Can you provide a little of the history of what inspired you to follow this path and share your thoughts on the mutual needs, goals, expectations, roles, responsibilities and costs for the child (or adolescent or young adult), family and therapist in the assessment, therapy and management of CAS? Where do consumer advocacy and web-based communication fit, and what is your vision for the future of organisations like CASANA and smaller, more local 'CAS associations' that currently need to raise funds in order to operate?

A7.   Sharon Gretz: Apraxia-KIDS^{SM} and the childhood apraxia of speech association of North America (CASANA)

Beginning in 1994 and for a span of several years, from my seat behind a one-way mirror, I witnessed my child's emergence as a speaker and communicator. I witnessed his incredible struggle, effort, resolve and ultimate success. Eventually, after over 200 individual speech therapy sessions, my son who had been diagnosed with severe childhood apraxia of speech (CAS) and dysarthria was a 'talker', his speech intelligible. To say that observing the painstaking, persistent work of both clinician and child was inspiring is an understatement. Fuelled by an appreciation for the good outcomes possible with proper diagnosis, treatment and clinician–parent partnerships, I turned my thoughts to what I could do to help others in similar circumstance. In the mid- to late 1990s little information on CAS existed that was comprehensible to families, and training opportunities on the topic for practicing professionals were infrequent. The Apraxia-KIDS^{SM} listserv, followed by the website, were early efforts to address gaps in information and to create an international community of concern regarding children affected by this disorder. These developments highlighted at least three critical needs for parents and caregivers to

- gain support for the emotional and practical aspects of raising children with CAS;
- develop advocacy skills to benefit children with CAS; and
- learn how to help their children with speech and communication practice at home.

The Childhood Apraxia of Speech Association of North America (CASANA) was founded in 2000 to address those needs, and more. Since 2000, CASANA has served as a catalyst and a galvanizing force for heightened professional interest, education, research and caregiver support, worldwide, for children with CAS and their families. High-quality websites and online communities such as the Apraxia-KIDS^{SM} website and email LISTSERV, Facebook groups and Twitter; and face-to-face events, such as the Walk for Children with Apraxia®, appear to play a vital role providing reliable information and emotional and practical support. For example, Boh, Csiacsek, Duginske, Meath and Carpenter (2006) found that 93% of surveyed parents of children diagnosed with CAS used Internet sites as information sources regarding their child's disability. Overwhelmingly, parents report that the *most* helpful information they receive comes from the Apraxia-KIDS[SM] listserv (Lohman, 2000) and not from treating SLPs/SLTs. Furthermore, Farinelli, Allen and Babin (2013) found that network support alone, and no other variable, appeared to predict levels of depression and health in parents of children with CAS. They reasoned that given the relative rarity of CAS, parents of affected children might have a heighted need for a sense of belonging and connectedness than parents dealing with more common disabilities. Farinelli et al. suggested that professionals be aware of this dynamic and support families in connecting with others with similar experiences. Finally, many SLPs/SLTs report that they routinely visit specific consumer group websites, such as Apraxia-KIDS.org, to gain information about clinical cases (Nail-Chiwetalu & Bernstein Ratner, 2007).

In the years since CASANA formed, it has been a privilege to watch young people who had been affected by the disorder reach young adulthood. They, too, inspire our movement to bring awareness, information, support, education and research to CAS. Several of them serve as important ambassadors and role models for the importance of early intervention, specialised help and opportunity.

Apraxia-KIDS[SM] and CASANA at work

To illustrate the impact that Apraxia-KIDS and CASANA resources have on families and children, consider the story of a mother named 'Jenna' and her son 'Jacob'. Jenna subscribed to the Apraxia-KIDS listserv in a panic. Jacob 5;0 had received private and school-based speech therapy for nearly 3 years. Although identified through public early intervention as having CAS at about three, and treated by three SLPs, he had

just a handful of intelligible words. Jenna realised, through reading the Apraxia-KIDS[SM] listserv and website, and by asking specific questions relating to Jacob's situation, that several factors might account for his poor progress and considered potential solutions. First, his school speech therapy, delivered in a group with five other children, was not the recommended service delivery model for a child with severe CAS. Jenna learned that by law (Individuals with Disabilities Education Improvement Act [IDEA], 2004) she was considered a team member in her son's individual education planning (IEP) and that there were rules governing the process that might help her advocate for improved services for Jacob, including individual speech therapy. Additionally, Jenna came to understand that bubble and horn blowing activities that occupied most of Jacob's private speech therapy time were also not likely to make significant differences in his speech production skills (Hodge, A31; Lof, A35). Finally, Jenna came to understand that working at home with Jacob in specific ways would benefit generalization of his developing speech skills.

With help from local parents involved with CASANA's groups, Jenna located a new private SLP. She now felt prepared to interview the SLP to ensure that the professional understood the nature of CAS, its appropriate treatment and the need to actively involve Jenna. When she attended a national conference on CAS in a nearby state, she learned more about CAS itself, and about associated problems that Jacob faced and that might persist.

Soon, Jenna was able to ecstatically report to her online community that Jacob had made significant progress in speech and communication. He now had friends at school; his handwriting was improving; and his reading difficulties were being addressed. Jenna had hope for Jacob's future and felt more competent and confident as his chief advocate. She was delighted when Jacob's new school SLP attended a CASANA workshop to learn more about appropriate assessment and treatment for CAS. Several years down the track, Jenna now *answered* questions posed by new parents to the listserv, sharing the information she had learned with others in similar circumstances.

The story of Sara and her daughter Kacey illustrates how CASANA and its support for families evolved in recent years. Sara learned about CASANA's annual conference on its Apraxia-KIDS[SM] Facebook group. Kacey was 4;6, and despite having a lot of speech therapy had few intelligible words. Sara was looking for new information and a better understanding of her daughter's condition so that Kacey could become a fully verbal communicator. She applied for, and was granted a CASANA parent scholarship to attend the conference, where she was delighted to finally meet other parents who had children with CAS. Sara gained hope by observing and speaking to youth and young adults – volunteers at the event – who had a history of CAS. Among the numerous conference sessions she attended, covering therapy approaches, advocacy and related conditions, was one about genetic conditions that may be accompanied by CAS. The talk prompted Sara to consider locating a geneticist to test her daughter. Several months later, Sara contacted CASANA staff to report that Kasey's genetic testing yielded a positive finding. Kasey had a rare copy number variant (CNV), with several cases discussed in the professional literature as having an association with CAS. Thinking this new information might provide answers as to why her daughter's speech progress was slower and more limited than expected, Sara was anxious to contact parents who might have children with the same genetic condition. CASANA staff told Sara about the online Apraxia Research Registry. The online registry is a CASANA project in which families assist researchers in a 'bottom up' approach by entering extensive and detailed data regarding their child's history.

Because of life situations like those of Jenna, Jacob, Sara and Kacey, CASANA's board of directors believes that its work is of an urgent nature. CAS, as a severe speech disorder, has serious ramifications on the quality of life (including activities and participation, McLeod, A1) for affected children and youth. Beyond the complicated and challenging speech disorder and its co-morbidities, issues around the children's inclusion, relationships, education, emotional functioning, social wellbeing and independence are also at stake (Markham & Dean, 2006).

Accomplishments and challenges for the future

CASANA has experienced success in bringing worldwide attention to the challenges of CAS. In a dozen years, CASANA has grown from hosting and growing online information and support to also providing a variety of educational events, funding and supporting research, and providing more in the way of individual support to children and families.

In terms of education, each year CASANA provides CAS workshops, seminars and an annual summer conference. CASANA's webinars alone have provided training to thousands of parents and professionals in over 30 countries, including remote locations where training on CAS is limited. Additionally, a strategy to boost regional CAS expertise was devised through the development of an Apraxia Intensive Training Institute, in which selected clinicians with moderate levels of experience are taught and mentored by 'master clinicians' with CAS expertise. Trainees complete over 40 hours of CAS education and submit and pass an extensive case study presentation, demonstrating knowledge gained. To date, CASANA has graduated 40 geographically dispersed clinicians from the institute.

In recent years, CASANA has funded pilot treatment research grants, leading to increased journal publications on intervention and treatments for CAS. The CASANA Apraxia Research Registry (see above) allows parents to contribute to new understandings and research into CAS by entering comprehensive data on all aspects of their child's prenatal, birth and post-natal history, speech and language history, intervention history, medical and family history. Moreover, in 2013 CASANA hosted the 2013 Childhood Apraxia of Speech Research Symposium in which international researchers presented on the 'state of the art' in CAS research, including genomic, neuroimaging, diagnostic marker, and neurocognitive behavioural areas. CASANA will use this information to plan and implement its research funding direction, and plans to disseminate it to a worldwide audience via online video sharing.

In an effort to assist low- to moderate-income families financially, CASANA has initiated two programs. First, 'iPads for Apraxia' provides tablet computers and protective cases to a number of children with apraxia each year, aiding them in speech practice and communication. Priority is given to children who are older and those that are severely impacted by CAS. Responding to the growing financial impact families experience in trying to provide appropriate levels of intensity and frequency of speech therapy for their children, CASANA has partnered with another organization, to fund a program to provide small speech therapy grants for children.

CASANA's events serve to increase community awareness, offer support, and raise funds for its programs and research. For example, what started as a local event in one community has led to the Walk for Children with Apraxia® movement. In 2013, for example, 80 communities in the United States and Canada and over 16 000 individuals directly participated. The walks and the donations generated at the community level are CASANA's largest funding source and allowed for the vital expansion of programs and research. Of equal importance, the events serve to bring together affected children and families with a community and web of support. CASANA's 2013 inaugural Apraxia Awareness Day was highly successful with thousands of participants distributing worthwhile information about CAS and its serious impact, and about the resilience, gifts and talents of the many affected children and youth who deserve an opportunity to be heard.

As more research is conducted and published about best assessment and treatment practices; genetic, biophysical and behavioural markers of CAS; and its long-term ramifications, consumer groups will continue to have a role in the widespread dissemination of important lifespan information regarding toddlers, children and youth with this disorder. A continued challenge will be to educate professionals and parents to evaluate readily available Internet and social media information and to critically judge its authority, reliability and credibility. A likely additional challenge is maintaining adequate funding for consumer non-profit groups like CASANA. In some ways, the organization is a victim of its own success. Through its work, there is increased interest in and attention to CAS. This interest and attention leads to increased demand for assistance and education, requiring additional funding. Diversified financial resources to support and sustain existing operations and new programs into the future are essential.

Terminology

Gretz (A7) includes, among the motivational factors driving the development of CASANA, the paucity of information on CAS that could be interpreted by families. Her observation accords with the view of McNeilly, Fotheringham and Walsh (2007) that terminology in communication sciences and disorders 'presents a significant barrier to the profession's advancement in research, clinical effectiveness, public image and political profile'. Insisting that change is imperative, McNeilly et al. are clear that, 'influencing attitudes and understanding about something as fundamental and closely tied to one's professional identity as terminology is no small task'. They also underscore the need for sufficient will, resources, and cooperation, as well as a realistic timeframe within which to effect such change. Against the historical backdrop provided here in Chapter 1, the following chapter covers a range of currently applied systems of terminology and the issues that surround them, as well as accounts of the classification, description and assessment of children's speech.

References

Allport, G. (1924). *Social psychology.* Boston: Houghton-Mifflin Co.

Arlt, P. B. & Goodban, M. J. (1976). A comparative study of articulation acquisition as based on a study of 240 normals, aged three to six. *Language, Speech, and Hearing Services in Schools, 7,* 173–180.

Baker, E., Carrigg, B. & Linich, A. (2007). What's the evidence for . . . the cycles approach to phonological intervention? *ACQuiring Knowledge in Speech, Language and Hearing, 9*(1), 29–31.

Ball, M. J. & Kent, R. D. (1987). Editorial. *Clinical Linguistics and Phonetics, 1,* 1–5.

Ball, M. J. & Kent, R. D. (Eds). (1997). *The new phonologies: Developments in clinical linguistics.* San Diego, CA: Singular.

Barlow, J. A. (2001). Recent advances in phonological theory and treatment. [Special Issue]. *Language, Speech, and Hearing Services in Schools, 32,* 225–298.

Barlow, J. A. (2002). Recent advances in phonological theory and treatment, Part II. [Special issue]. *Language, Speech, and Hearing Services in Schools, 33,* 4–69.

Barlow, J. A. & Gierut, J. A. (2002). Minimal pair approaches to phonological remediation. *Seminars in Speech and Language, 2*(1), 57–67.

Bauman-Waengler, J. (2004). *Articulatory and phonological impairments: A clinical focus* (2nd ed.). Boston: Allyn and Bacon.

Berners-Lee, T. (2002). The World Wide Web - Past Present and Future: Exploring universality. *Japan Prize Commemorative Lecture.* Retrieved 15 January 2014 from www.w3.org/2002/04/Japan/Lecture.html.

Bernhardt, B. (2004). Introduction to the Issue: Maximizing success in phonological intervention. *Child Language Teaching and Therapy, 20,* 195–198.

Berry, M. D. & Eisenson, J. (1942). *The defective in speech.* New York: Appleton-Century-Crofts.

Berry, M. D. & Eisenson, J. (1956). *Speech disorders: Principals and practices of therapy.* New York: Appleton Century Crofts.

Bishop, D. V. M. & Adams, C. (1990). A prospective study of the relationship between specific language impairment, phonological disorders and reading retardation, *The Journal of Child Psychology and Psychiatry, 31*(7), 1027–1050.

Blache, S. E. (1982). Minimal word pairs and distinctive feature training. In: M. Crary (Ed.), *Phonological intervention: Concepts and procedures.* San Diego: College-Hill Press Inc.

Boh, A., Csiacsek, E., Duginske, R., Meath, T. & Carpenter, L. (2006). *Counseling parents of children with CAS.* American Speech-Language-Hearing Association, Boston, MA.

Bowen, C. (1996). *Evaluation of a phonological therapy with treated and untreated groups of young children.* Unpublished doctoral dissertation. Macquarie University.

Bowen, C. (2003). Harnessing the net: A challenge for Speech Language Pathologists. The 2003 Elizabeth Usher Memorial Lecture. In: C. Williams & S. Leitão (Eds), *Nature, nurture, knowledge, proceedings of the speech pathology Australia National Conference* (pp. 9–20). Hobart. Available from www.speech-language-therapy.com/pdf/papers/2003usher.pdf.

Bowen, C. (2012). Webwords 44: Life online. *Journal of Clinical Practice in Speech-Language Pathology, 14*(3), 149–152.

Bowen, C. (2013). Webwords 45: Apps for speech-language pathology intervention. *Journal of Clinical Practice in Speech-Language Pathology, 15*(1), 36–37.

Bowen, C. & Cupples, L. (1999a). Parents and children together (PACT): A collaborative approach to phonological therapy. *International Journal of Language and Communication Disorders, 34*(1), 35–55.

Bowen, C. & Cupples, L. (1999b). A phonological therapy in depth: a reply to commentaries.

International Journal of Language and Communication Disorders, 34(1), 65–83.

Braine, M. D. S. (1974). On what might constitute a learnable phonology. *Language, 50,* 270–299.

Browman, C. P. & Goldstein, L. (1986). Towards an articulatory phonology. In: C. Ewen & J. Anderson (Eds), *Phonology yearbook 3* (pp. 219–252). Cambridge: Cambridge University Press.

Browman, C. P. & Goldstein, L. (1992). Articulatory phonology: An overview. *Phonetica, 49,* 155–180.

Brumbaugh, K. M. & Smit, A. B. (2013a). Treating children ages 3–6 who have speech sound disorder: A survey. *Language Speech, and Hearing Services in Schools, 44*(3), 306–319.

Brumbaugh, K. M. & Smit, A. B. (2013b). Supplementary material for treating children ages 3–6 who have speech sound disorder: A survey. *Language Speech, and Hearing Services in Schools, 44*(3), 306–319. Downloaded Nov 2, 2013 from http://lshss.asha.org/cgi/content/full/44/3/306/DC1.

Bybee, J. L. (2001). *Phonology and language use.* Cambridge: Cambridge University Press.

Chomsky, N. (1959). A review of B. F. Skinner's *Verbal Behavior. Language, 35,* 26–58.

Chomsky, N. & Halle, M. (1968). *The sound pattern of English.* New York, NY: Harper and Row.

Clahsen, H. (2008). Chomskyan syntactic theory and language disorders. In: M. J. Ball, M. R. Perkins, N. Müller & S. Howard (Eds), *The handbook of clinical linguistics* (pp. 165–183). Oxford: Blackwell.

College of Speech Therapists. (1959). *Terminology for speech pathology.* London: College of Speech Therapists.

Comenius, J. A. (1659). *Orbis sensualium pictus.* (Facsimile of first English edition of 1659): Adelaide: Sydney University Press.

Crystal, D. (1981). *Clinical linguistics.* Vienna & New York: Springer.

Crystal, D. (1984). *Linguistic encounters with language handicap.* Oxford: Blackwell.

Crystal, D. (2001). Clinical linguistics. In: M. Aronoff & J. Rees-Miller (Eds), *The handbook of linguistics* (pp. 673–682). Oxford: Blackwell.

Dean, E. & Howell, J. (1986). Developing linguistic awareness: A theoretically based approach to phonological disorders. *British Journal of Disorders of Communication, 21,* 223–238.

Dean, E., Howell, J., Hill, A. & Waters, D. (1990). *Metaphon resource pack.* Windsor, Berks: NFER Nelson.

Dean, E. C., Howell, J., Waters, D. & Reid, J. (1995). *Metaphon*: A metalinguistic approach to the treatment of phonological disorder in children. *Clinical Linguistics and Phonetics, 9,* 1–19.

Duchan, J. F. (2001). *History of Speech-Language Pathology in America.* Retrieved 15Jan, 2014 from: http://www.acsu.buffalo.edu/~duchan/history.html.

Duchan, J. F. (2006a). How conceptual frameworks influence clinical practice: Evidence from the writings of John Thelwall, a 19th-century speech therapist. *International Journal of Language and Communication Disorders, 41,* 735–744.

Duchan, J. F. (2006b). The phonetic notation system of Melville Bell and its role in the history of phonetics. *Journal of Speech Language Pathology and Audiology, 30,* 14–17.

Duchan, J. F. (2009). The conceptual underpinnings of John Thelwall's elocutionary practices. In: S. Poole (Ed.), *John Thelwall: Radical romantic and acquitted felon* (pp. 139–145). London: Pickering & Chatto.

Duchan, J. F. (2010). The early years of language, speech, and hearing services in U.S. schools. *Language, Speech, and Hearing Services in Schools, 41*(2), 152–160.

Dunn, L. M. & Dunn, L. M. (1997). *Peabody picture vocabulary test III.* Circle Pines, MN: American Guidance Service.

Edwards, M. L. (1992). In support of phonological processes. *Language, Speech, and Hearing Services inSchools, 23,* 233–240.

Eisenberg, S. L. & Hitchcock, E. R. (2010). Using standardized tests to inventory consonant and vowel production: A comparison of 11 tests of articulation and phonology, *Language, Speech, and Hearing Services in Schools, 41*(4): 488–503.

Eisenson, J. (1968). Developmental aphasia: A speculative view with therapeutic implications. *Journal of Speech and Hearing Disorders, 33,* 3–13.

Elbert, M. (1992). Consideration of error types: A response to Fey's 'Articulation and phonology: Inextricable constructs in speech pathology.' *Language, Speech, and Hearing Services in Schools, 23,* 241–246.

Elbert, M. & Gierut, J. (1986). *Handbook of clinical phonology: Approaches to assessment and treatment.* San Diego College-Hill Press.

Eldridge, M. (1965). *A history of the Australian college of speech therapists.* Melbourne, Melbourne University Press.

Eldridge, M. (1968a). *A history of the treatment of speech disorders*. Edinburgh & London: E. & S. Livingstone.

Eldridge, M. (1968b). *A history of the treatment of speech disorders*. Melbourne: F.W. Cheshire.

Fairbanks, G. (1940). *Voice and articulation drillbook*. NY: Harper.

Fairbanks, G. (1954). Systematic research in experimental phonetics: A theory of the speech mechanism as a servosystem. *Journal of Speech and Hearing Disorders, 19*, 133–139.

Farinelli Allan, L. & Babin, E. (2013). Associations between caregiving, social support, and well-being among parents of children with childhood apraxia of speech. *Health Communications, 28*(6), 568–576.

Ferguson, C. A. (1968). Contrastive analysis and language development. *Monograph Series on Language and Linguistics, 21*, 101–112. Georgetown University.

Ferguson, C. A. (1978). Learning to pronounce: The earliest stages of phonological development in the child. In: F. D. Minifie & L. L. Lloyd (Eds), *Communicative and cognitive abilities - early behavioural assessment* (pp. 273–297). Baltimore: University Park Press.

Ferguson, C. & Farwell, C. (1975). Words and sounds in early language acquisition. *Language, 51*, 419–439.

Ferguson, C. A. & Macken, M. (1980). Phonological development in children: Play and cognition. *Papers and Reports on Child Language Development, 18*, 138–177.

Ferguson, C. A., Peizer, D. B. & Weeks, T. A. (1973). Model-and-replica phonological grammar of a child's first words. *Lingua, 3*, 35–65.

Fey, M. E. (1985). Clinical forum: Phonological assessment and treatment. Articulation and phonology: Inextricable constructs in speech pathology. *Human Communication Canada*. Reprinted (1992) *Language, Speech, and Hearing Services in Schools, 23*, 225–232.

Fey, M. E. (1992a). Phonological assessment and treatment. Articulation and phonology: An introduction. *Language Speech and Hearing Services in Schools, 23*, 224.

Fey, M. E. (1992b). Phonological assessment and treatment. Articulation and phonology: An addendum. *Language Speech and Hearing Services in Schools, 23*, 277–282.

Gierut, J. (2001). Complexity in phonological treatment: Clinical factors. *Language, Speech, and Hearing in Schools, 32*, 229–241.

Goldman, R. & Fristoe, M. (1969). *Goldman-fristoe test of articulation*. Circle Pines, MN: AGS.

Goldman, R. & Fristoe, M. (2000). *Goldman-fristoe test of articulation* (2nd ed.). Circle Pines, MN: American Guidance Service.

Goldstein, K. (1948). *Language and language disturbances*. NY: Grune and Stratton.

Gordon-Brannan, M., Hodson, B. & Wynne, M. (1992). Remediating unintelligible utterances of a child with a mild hearing loss. *American Journal of Speech-Language Pathology, 1*, 28–38.

Grunwell, P. (1975). The phonological analysis of articulation disorders. *British Journal of Disorders of Communication, 10*, 31–42.

Grunwell, P. (1981). *The nature of phonological disability in children*. New York: Academic.

Grunwell, P. (1983). Phonological development in phonological disability. *Topics in Language Disorders, 3*, 62–76.

Grunwell, P. (1985a). Developing phonological skills. *Child Language Teaching and Therapy, 1*, 65–72. 1985a is in Chapter 1.

Grunwell, P. (1985b). *Phonological assessment of child speech (PACS)*. Windsor: NFER-Nelson.

Grunwell, P. (1987). *Clinical phonology* (2nd ed.). Baltimore: Williams & Wilkins.

Hegde, M. N. & Peña-Brooks, A. (2007). *Treatment protocols for articulation disorders*. San Diego, CA; Plural Publishing.

Hodson, B. (1980). *The assessment of phonological processes*. Danville, Illinois: Interstate.

Hodson, B. (1992). Clinical forum: Phonological assessment and treatment. Applied phonology: Constructs, contributions and issues. *Language, Speech, and Hearing Services in Schools, 23*, 247–253.

Hodson, B. (2003). *Hodson computerized analysis of phonological patterns*. Wichita, KS: PhonoComp Publishers.

Hodson, B. (2004). *Hodson assessment of phonological patterns* (3rd ed.). Austin, TX: Pro-Ed.

Hodson, B. (2007, 2010). *Evaluating and enhancing children's phonological systems: Research and theory to practice*. Wichita, KS: PhonoComp Publishers.

Hodson, B. (2011, April 05). Enhancing phonological patterns of young children with highly unintelligible speech. *The ASHA Leader*, 16–19.

Hodson, B. W. & Paden, E. P. (1981). Phonological processes which characterize unintelligible and unintelligible speech in early childhood. *Journal of Speech and Hearing Disorders, 46,* 369–373.

Hodson, B. W. & Paden, E. P. (1983). *Targeting intelligible speech: A phonological approach to remediation.* San Diego: College-Hill Press.

Hodson, B. W. & Paden, E. P. (1991). *Targeting intelligible speech: A phonological approach to remediation* (2nd ed.). Austin, TX: Pro-Ed.

Hoffman, P. R. (1992). Synergistic development of phonetic skill. *Language, Speech, and Hearing Services in Schools, 23,* 254–260.

Holder, W. (1669). *The elements of speech, an essay of inquiry into the natural production of letters: with an appendix concerning persons deaf and dumb.* London: John Martyn.

Hunt, J. (1961). *Intelligence and experience.* New York: Rowland Press.

Individuals with Disabilities Education Improvement Act [IDEA] (2004). Public Law 108–446. 20 USC 1400. 108th Congress.

Ingram, D. (1974). Phonological rules in young children. *Journal of Child Language, 1,* 49–64.

Ingram, D. (1976). *Phonological disability in children.* London: Edward Arnold.

Ingram, D. (1981). *Procedures for the phonological analysis of children's language.* Baltimore: University Park Press.

Ingram, D. (1983). Case studies of phonological disability. *Topics in Language Disorders, 3*(2), 1.

Ingram, D. (1989a). *First language acquisition: Method, description and explanation.* Cambridge: Cambridge University Press.

Ingram, D. (1989b). *Phonological disability in children* (2nd ed.). London: Cole & Whurr Publishers.

Ingram, D. (1997). Generative phonology. In: R. D. Kent & M. J. Ball (Eds), *The new phonologies: Developments in clinical linguistics* (pp. 7–33). San Diego, CA: Singular Press.

Ingram, D. & Ingram, K. (2001). A whole word approach to phonological intervention. *Language, Speech and Hearing Services in Schools, 32,* 271–283.

Jakobson, R. (1941/1968). *Child language, aphasia and phonological universals.* The Hague: Mouton.

Kamhi, A. G. (1992). The need for a broad-based model of phonological disorders. *Language, Speech, and Hearing Services in Schools, 23,* 261–268.

Kamhi, A. G. (2006). Treatment decisions for children with speech-sound disorders. *Language, Speech, and Hearing Services in Schools, 37*(4), 271–279.

Kilminster, M. G. E. & Laird, E. M. (1978). Articulation development in children aged three to nine years. *Australian Journal of Human Communication Disorders, 6*(1), 23–30.

Kiparsky, P. & Menn, L. (1977). On the acquisition of phonology. In: J. Macnamara (Ed.), *Language learning and thought.* New York: Academic Press.

Kuhn, T. S. (1962). *The structure of scientific revolutions.* Chicago: The University of Chicago Press.

Lancaster, G. & Pope, L. (1989). *Working with children's phonology.* Oxon: Winslow Press.

Langacker, R. (1987). Foundations of cognitive grammar. Volume *I: Theoretical prerequisites.* Stanford: Stanford University Press.

Langacker, R. (2000). A dynamic usage-based model. In: M. Barlow & S. Kemmer (Eds), *Usage-based models of language* (pp. 1–63). Stanford: CSLI Publications.

Leopold, W. F., (1947). *Speech development of a bilingual child, Vol. 2. Sound learning in the first two years.* Evanston: Northwestern University Press.

Lippke, B. A., Dickey, S. E., Selmar, J. W. & Soder, A. L. (1997). Photo-articulation test (3rd ed.). Austin, TX: Pro-Ed.

Locke, J. L. (1983a). Clinical phonology: The explanation and treatment of speech sound disorders. *Journal of Speech and Hearing Disorders, 48,* 339–341.

Locke, J. L. (1983b). *Phonological acquisition and change.* New York: Academic.

Locke, J. L. (1993c). *The child's path to spoken language.* Cambridge, MA: Harvard University.

Lohman, P. (2000). Results of summer 2000 apraxia-kids parental survey. Retrieved 10 Sept, 2013, from http://www.apraxia-kids.org/library/results-of-summer-2000-apraxia-kids-parental-survey/.

Macken, M. A. (1980). The child's lexical representations: the 'puzzle - puddle - pickle' evidence. *Journal of Linguistics, 16,* 1–17.

Macken, M. A. & Ferguson, C. A. (1983). Cognitive aspects of phonological development: Model, evidence and issues. In: K. E. Nelson (Ed.), *Children's language, 4.* Hillsdale N.J.: Lawrence Erlbaum.

Markham, C. & Dean, T. (2006). Parents' and professionals' perceptions of quality of life in children with speech and language difficulty. *International Journal of Language and Communication Disorders, 41*(2), 189–212.

Maxwell, E. M. (1984). On determining underlying representations of children: A critique of the current theories. In: M. Elbert, D. A. Dinnsen & G. Weismer (Eds), Phonological theory and the misarticulating child. *Asha Monographs. 22.* Rockville MD: ASHA.

McCauley, R. J., Strand, E., Lof, G. L., Schooling, T. & Frymark, T. (2009). Evidence-based systematic review: Effects of nonspeech oral motor exercises on speech. *American Journal of Speech-Language Pathology, 18,* 343–360.

McGregor, K. K., Newman, R. M., Reilly, R. M. & Capone, N. (2002). Semantic representation and naming in children with specific language impairment. *Journal of Speech, Language, and Hearing Research, 45,* 998–1014.

McLeod, S. (2006). The holistic view of a child with unintelligible speech: Insights from the ICF and ICF-CY. *International Journal of Speech-Language Pathology, 8*(3), 293–315.

McLeod, S. (2013). Speech sound acquisition. In: J. E. Bernthal, N. W. Bankson & P. Flipsen Jnr (Eds), *Articulation and phonological disorders: Speech sound disorders in children* (7th ed., pp. 58–113). Boston, MA: Pearson Education.

McNeilly, L., Fotheringham, S. & Walsh, R. (2007). *Future directions in terminology.* Symposium: Terminology in communication sciences and disorders: a new approach. Copenhagen: 27th World Congress of the International Association of Logopedics and Phoniatrics.

Menn, L. (1976). Evidence for an interactionist discovery theory of child phonology. *Papers and reports on language development, 12,* 169–177. Stanford: Stanford University.

Michie, S. & Abraham, C. (2004). Identifying techniques that promote health behaviour change: Evidence based or evidence inspired? *Psychology and Health, 19,* 29–49.

Monahan, D. (1984). Remediation of common phonological processes. Tigard, Oregon: CC Publications.

Monahan, D. (1986). Remediation of common phonological processes. Four case studies. *Language Speech and Hearing Services in Schools, 17,* 187–198.

Morley, M. (1972). *The development and disorders of speech in children* (3rd ed.). Edinburgh: Churchill Livingstone.

Mowrer, O. (1952). Speech development in the young child: The autism theory of speech development and some clinical applications. *Journal of Speech and Hearing Disorders, 17,* 263–268.

Mowrer, O. (1960). *Learning theory and symbolic processes.* New York: John Wiley and Sons.

Müller, N. & Ball, M. J. (2013a). *Research methods in clinical linguistics and phonetics.* Chichester, UK: Wiley-Blackwell.

Müller, N. & Ball, M. J. (2013b). Linguistics, phonetics, and speech-language pathology: Clinical linguistics and phonetics. In: M. Müller & M. J. Ball (Eds), *Research methods in clinical linguistics and phonetics: A practical guide.* Oxford: Wiley-Blackwell.

Murai, J. (1963). The sounds of infants, their phonemicization and symbolization. *Studia Phonologica, 3,* 18–34.

Myklebust, H. (1952). Aphasia in childhood. *J. Exceptional Children, 19,* 9–14.

Nail-Chiwetalu, B. & Bernstein Ratner, N. (2007). An assessment of the information-seeking abilities and needs of practicing speech-language pathologists. *Journal of the Medical Library Association, 95*(2), 56–57.

Nemoy, E. & Davis, S. (1937). *The correction of defective consonant sounds.* Boston: Expression Company.

Oller, D. K., Wieman, L. A., Doyle, W. J. & Ross, C. (1976). Infant babbling and speech. *Journal of Child Language, 3,* 1–11.

Olmstead, D. (1971). *Out of the mouths of babes.* The Hague: Mouton.

Orton, S. T. (1937). *Reading, writing and speech problems in children: A presentation of certain types of disorders in the development of the language faculty.* NY: W. W. Norton.

Osgood, C. (1957). *A behavioristic analysis of perception and language as cognitive phenomena, contemporary approaches to cognition.* Cambridge: Harvard University Press.

Perkins, M. & Howard, S. (1995). Principles of clinical linguistics. In: M. Perkins & S. Howard (Eds), *Case studies in clinical linguistics.* London: Whurr Publishers.

Poole, I. (1934). Genetic development of articulation of consonant sounds in speech. *Elementary English Review, 11,* 159–161.

Powell, T. W., Elbert, M., Miccio, A. W., Strike-Roussos, C. & Brasseur, J. (1998). Facilitating [s] production in young children: an experimental evaluation of motoric and conceptual treatment approaches. *Clinical Linguistics and Phonetics*, *12*, 127–146.

Powers, M. H. (1959). Functional disorders of articulation. In: L. E. Travis (Ed.), *Handbook of speech pathology and audiology*. London: Peter Owen.

Prather, E. M., Hedrick, D. L. & Kern, C. A. (1975). Articulation development in children aged two to four years. *Journal of Speech and Hearing Disorders*, *40*, 179–191.

Prezas, R. F. & Hodson, B. W. (2010). The cycles phonological remediation approach. In: A. L. Williams, S. McLeod & R. J. McCauley (Eds), *Interventions for speech sound disorders in children* (pp. 137–157). Baltimore, MD: Paul H. Brookes Publishing Co.

Raz, M. G. (1993). *How to teach a child to say the "S" sound in 15 easy lessons*. Scottsdale, AZ: Gersten Weitz Publishers.

Raz, M. G. (1996). *How to teach a child to say the "R" sound in 15 easy lessons*. Scottsdale, AZ: Gersten Weitz Publishers.

Raz, M. G. (1999). *How to teach a child to say the "L" sound in 15 easy lessons*. Scottsdale, AZ: Gersten Weitz Publishers.

Robbins, S. D. & Robbins, R. (1937). *Corrections of speech defects of early childhood*. Boston: Expression Co.

Rosenfeld-Johnson, S. (2010, May). Muscle placement and movement patterns for speech clarity and feeding safety. *Workshop presented at the Annual Conference of the Canadian Association of Speech-Language Pathologists and Audiologists, Whitehorse*, Canada.

Rudolph, J. M. & Wendt, O. (2014). The efficacy of the cycles approach: A multiple baseline design. *Journal of Communication Disorders*. http://dx.doi.org/10.1016/j.jcomdis.2013.12.003

Sander, E. (1972). When are speech sounds learned? *Journal of Speech and Hearing Disorders*, *37*, 55–63.

Schwartz, R. G. (1992). Advances in phonological theory as a clinical framework. *Language, Speech, and Hearing Services in Schools*, *23*, 269–276.

Schwartz, R. G. & Leonard, L. (1982). Do children pick and choose? *Journal of Child Language*. *9*, 319–336.

Shriberg, L. D., (1993). Four new speech and prosody-voice measures for genetics research and other studies in developmental phonological disorders. *Journal of Speech and Hearing Research*, *36*, 105–140.

Shriberg, L. D. & Kwiatkowski, J. (1980). *Natural Process Analysis*. New York: Academic Press.

Simms, R. (2012). *Go togethers*. Desoto TX: Smarty Ears.

Smit, A. B., Hand, L., Freilinger, J. J., Bernthal, J. E. & Bird, A. (1990). The Iowa articulation norms project and its Nebraska replication. *Journal of Speech and Hearing Disorders*, *55*, 779–798.

Smith, N. V. (1973). *The acquisition of phonology: A case study*. Cambridge: Cambridge University Press.

Smith, N. V. (1978). Lexical representation and the acquisition of phonology. Paper given as a forum lecture, Linguistic Institute, *Linguistic Society of America*.

Stackhouse, J. & Wells, B. (1997). *Children's speech and literacy difficulties I: A psycholinguistic framework*. London: Whurr Publishers.

Stackhouse, J. & Wells, B. (2001). *Children's speech and literacy difficulties II: Identification and intervention*. London: Whurr Publishers.

Stampe, D. (1969). The acquisition of phonetic representation. *Papers from the 5th regional meeting of the Chicago Linguistic Society*. 443–454.

Stampe, D. (1973). *A dissertation on natural phonology*. Unpublished doctoral dissertation, University of Chicago.

Stampe, D. (1979). *A dissertation on natural phonology*. New York; Academic Press.

Stinchfield, S. & Young, E. H. (1938). *Children with delayed or defective speech: Motor-kinesthetic factors in their training*. Stanford, CA: Stanford University Press.

Stoel-Gammon, C. (2010). Relationships between lexical and phonological development in young children. *Journal of Child Language*, *38*(1), 1–34.

Stoel-Gammon, C. & Dunn, C. (1985). *Normal and disordered phonology in children*. Baltimore: University Park Press.

Templin, M. C. (1957). Certain language skills in children. *Monograph Series No. 26*. Minneapolis: The Institute of Child Welfare, University of Minnesota.

Thelen, E. & Bates, E. (2003). Connectionism and dynamic systems: Are they really different? *Developmental Science*, *6*, 378–391.

Thinking Publications (2004). *Barbara Hodson: Phonological Intervention Guru*. Thinking Big News, Issue 22, December.

Tiga Talk (2011). *Tiga Talk speech therapy games V1.3*. Winnipeg, Canada: Tactica Interactive.

Travis, L. E. (1931). *Speech pathology: A dynamic neurological treatment of normal speech and speech deviations*. NY: D. Appleton Co.

Travis, L. E. (1957). *Handbook of speech pathology*. NY: Appleton-Century-Crofts.

Twitmeyer, E. B. & Nathanson, Y. S. (1932). *Correction of defective speech*. Philadelphia, PA: P. Blakiston's Son and Co.

Van Riper, C. (1939). *Speech correction: Principles and methods*. New York: Prentice-Hall.

Van Riper, C. (1978). *Speech correction: Principles and methods* (6th ed.). Englewood Cliffs, N.J.: Prentice-Hall.

Velleman, S. (2002). Phonotactic therapy. *Seminars in Speech and Language, 23*, 43–57.

Velten, H. (1943). The growth of phonemic and lexical patterns in infant language. *Language, 19*, 281–292.

Vogel Sosa, A. & Bybee, J. L. (2008). A cognitive approach to clinical phonology. In: M. J. Ball, M. R. Perkins, N. Müller & S. Howard (Eds), *The handbook of clinical linguistics* (pp. 480–490). Oxford: Blackwell.

Waterson, N. (1971). Child phonology: A prosodic view. *Journal of Linguistics, 7*, 170–221.

Waterson, N. (1981). A tentative development model of phonological representation. In: T. Myers, J. Laver & J. Anderson (Eds), *The cognitive representation of speech*. Amsterdam: North Holland.

Weiner, F. (1979). *Phonological process analysis*. Baltimore: University Park Press.

Weiner, F. (1981a). Treatment of phonological disability using the method of meaningful contrast: Two case studies. *Journal of Speech and Hearing Disorders, 46*, 97–103.

Weiner, F. (1981b). Systematic sound preference as a characteristic of phonological disability. *Journal of Speech and Hearing Disorders, 46*, 281–286.

Wellman, B. L., Case, I. M., Mengert, I. G. & Bradbury, D. E. (1931). Speech sounds of young children. *University of Iowa Studies in Child Welfare*, 5(2). Iowa City: The Iowa Child Welfare Research Station: University of Iowa.

West, R., Kennedy, L. & Carr, A. (1937). *The rehabilitation of speech*. NY: Harper and Bros.

Weston, A. D., Shriberg, L. D. & Miller, J. J. (1989). Analysis of speech samples with SALT and PEPPER. *Journal of Speech and Hearing Research, 32*, 755–766.

Williams, A. L. (2002a). Prologue: Perspectives in the phonological assessment of child speech. *American Journal of Speech-Language Pathology, 11*, 211–212.

Williams, A. L. (2002b). Epilogue: Perspectives in the phonological assessment of child speech. *American Journal of Speech-Language Pathology, 11*, 259–263.

Zimmerman, I. L., Steiner, V. G. & Pond, R. E. (1991). *Preschool language scale-3*. San Antonio, TX: The Psychological Corporation.

Chapter 2

Terminology, classification, description, measurement, assessment and targets

In the area of speech sound disorders (SSD), considerable barriers are engendered by difficult nomenclature. Picture new students, individuals re-entering the profession or clinicians switching from adult to child caseloads, facing the task of reading the SSD literature from the 1970s onwards, encountering a morass of conceptual, classificatory and descriptive terms. These terms come primarily from medicine, linguistics and psychology, only to be enveloped in a mystifying array of like-sounding terms, drawn from the study of literacy in the fields of education and psychology. Within and across disciplines, the *same* words are often used to denote *different* concepts and phenomena: 'phonological processes' being a case in point (Scarborough & Brady, 2002). Among the first things to strike the reader will be the impact of the medical model and symptomatological and aetiological frameworks, adopted singly or in tandem. Quickly realising the need for a medical or nursing dictionary and a glossary of key genetics terms (as in Table 2.1), the reader will discover broad, trichotomous symptomatic distinctions between *articulation disorder*, *phonological disorder* and *childhood apraxia*

of speech (CAS). Historically, this was not the case. For example, Grunwell (1975), who really understood the difference, wrote an article with the paradoxical title: 'The phonological analysis of articulation disorders' that reflected the jumbled state of the terminology at the dawn of the phonological revolution.

Waring and Knight (2013) critically reviewed current classification systems for SSD, concluding that, 'There is a need for a universally agreed-upon classification system that is useful to clinicians and researchers. The resulting classification system needs to be robust, reliable and valid. A universal classification system would allow for improved tailoring of treatments to subgroups of SSD which may, in turn, lead to improved treatment efficacy' (p. 25).

The most commonly used classification system in clinical settings is based around three *aetiological* distinctions: *unknown* cause, *putative* or supposed cause and *known* cause. SSD is usually considered to be idiopathic, with 'no identifiable causal factor', and is often given the designation 'functional speech disorder'. Here, 'functional' implies 'unknown cause'. Children

Children's Speech Sound Disorders, Second Edition. Caroline Bowen.
© 2015 John Wiley & Sons, Ltd. Published 2015 by John Wiley & Sons, Ltd.
Companion website: www.wiley.com/go/bowen/speechlanguagetherapy

Table 2.1 Glossary of genetic terms

Aetiology	The study of causes or origins.
Alleles	Humans carry two sets of chromosomes, one from each parent. Equivalent genes in the two sets might be different, for example because of single nucleotide polymorphisms. An allele is one of the two (or more) forms of a particular gene.
DNA (deoxyribonucleic acid)	The molecule that encodes genetic information and is capable of self-replication and synthesis of *RNA*. DNA consists of two long chains of nucleotides twisted into a double helix and joined by hydrogen bonds between the complementary bases adenine and thymine or cytosine and guanine. The sequence of nucleotides determines individual *Hereditary* characteristics.
Environment	All circumstances surrounding an organism or group of organisms, especially: (a) The combination of external physical conditions that affect and influence the growth, development and survival of organisms. (b) The complex of social and cultural conditions affecting the nature of an individual or community.
Gene	A *Hereditary* unit consisting of a sequence of *DNA* that occupies a specific location on a chromosome and determines a particular characteristic in an organism.
Gene expression	The process by which a gene's coded information is converted into the structures present and operating in the cell.
Genome	The complete DNA sequence of an organism.
Genotype	The genotype is the genetic makeup, rather than the physical appearance (*Phenotype*), of an organism or group of organisms. It involves the combination of *Alleles* located on *Homologous Chromosomes* determining a specific characteristic or trait.
Hereditary	(a) Transmitted or capable of being transmitted genetically from parent to offspring. (b) Appearing in or characteristic of successive generations. (c) Of or relating to heredity or inheritance.
Homologous chromosomes	A pair of chromosomes containing the same linear gene sequences each derived from one parent.
Incidence	The number of new cases of a disorder or disease during a given time interval, usually per annum, expressed as *Incidence Proportion (Risk)* or as *Incidence Rate*.
Incidence proportion	The number of new cases divided by the size of the population at risk. For example, if a stable population contains 1000 pre-schoolers and 2 develop a condition over two years of observation, the incidence proportion is 2 cases per 1000 pre-schoolers.
Incidence rate	The number of new cases per unit of person-time at risk. Using the previous example, the incidence rate is 1 case per 1000 person-years, because the incidence proportion (2 per 1000) is divided by the number of years (2). Using person-time rather than just time covers circumstances in which participants exit studies before they are completed.
Inheritance	(a) The process of genetic transmission of characteristics from parents to offspring. (b) A characteristic so inherited. (c) The sum of characteristics genetically transmitted from parents to offspring.
Locus	Locus (pl. loci): The position on a chromosome of a gene or other chromosome marker; also, the DNA at that position. The use of locus is sometimes restricted to mean regions of DNA that are expressed. See *Gene Expression*.
Monogenic disorder	A disorder caused by a mutant allele of a single gene.
Oligogenic disorder	A phenotypic trait produced by two or more genes working together.
Phenotype	The phenotype comprises the observable physical or biochemical characteristics (*Phenotypic Traits*) of an organism, as determined by both genetic makeup (*Genotype*) and environmental influences. It is the expression of a specific trait, such as stature or blood type, based on genetic and environmental influences.
Polygenic disorder	Genetic disorder resulting from the combined action of alleles of more than one gene (e.g., heart disease, diabetes and some cancers). Although such disorders are inherited, they depend on the simultaneous presence of several alleles; thus the hereditary patterns usually are more complex than those of single-gene disorders.
Prevalence	The total number of cases of a disease or condition in a given population at one time.

(continued)

Table 2.1 (*Continued*)

RNA (ribonucleic acid)	A polymeric constituent of all living cells and many viruses, comprising a long, usually single-stranded chain of alternating phosphate and ribose units with the bases adenine, guanine, cytosine and uracil bonded to the ribose. The structure and base sequence of RNA are determinants of protein synthesis and *Transmission* of genetic information.
Symptom	A symptom is a sign or an indication of disorder or disease, especially when experienced by an individual as a change from normal function, sensation or appearance. Symptomatic classifications of SSDs are based on speech characteristics or 'symptoms' such as limited phonetic repertoire, or persistence of normal phonological patterns.
Transmission	Genetic transmission is the transfer of genetic information from genes to another generation or from one location in a cell to another location in a cell.

with functional SSD comprise the largest subgroup within child speech impairment, whereas children who have SSD of *known* (or 'organic') aetiology fall into several, much smaller subgroupings. In a survey, Broomfield and Dodd (2004b) established that functional SSD affects 6.4% of *all* children in the United Kingdom; an interesting finding in relation to Shriberg and Kwiatkowski (1994) in the United States, who proposed that 7.5% of *all* children age 3–11 experienced SSD (of known and unknown aetiology).

Where does 'functional' fit?

For some researchers (e.g., Gierut, 1998 in an important 'state-of-the-art' article), the large 'functional' component includes children with CAS, children with articulation disorders and children with phonological disorders, all included in the same category. Other scholars (e.g., Ruscello, 2008), who also make the known-versus-unknown aetiological distinction, place children with phonetic (articulatory) and phonemic (phonological) difficulties in the populous 'unknown origin' group, followed by small subgroups of children who have at least one observable explanation for their speech difficulties. From Ruscello's perspective, children in these subgroups may exhibit a range of organic issues: *craniofacial anomalies*, such as cleft lip and palate or dental malocclusion; *sensory impairments*, such as hearing loss; and *motor speech disorders*, such as a dysarthria (Hodge, 2010), apraxia due to a known cause,

or idiopathic CAS, affecting speech–motor planning and/or speech–motor execution, in varying combinations. Ruscello uses the overarching term 'sound system disorder(s)' (SSD) to embrace all possibilities as opposed to my preferred term, 'speech sound disorder(s)' (*also* SSD). A noteworthy aspect of the 'functional' speech disorders is that there are now suggested subgroups that *are* linked to causes (Flipsen, Jr., 2002).

Subtypes

Drawing on data from several hundred case studies, Shriberg (2006) summarised seven putative subtypes of SSD (listed below) in a Speech Disorders Classification System (SDCS) based on genetic (inherited) and environmental risk factors. Furthermore, he suggested clinical prevalence percentages for the first four of these seven, coding them with 'working terms' and abbreviations as subtypes of *speech delay*. Prevalence was not estimated for a fifth speech delay subtype, Speech Delay-Dysarthria (SD-DYS), but potentially it would amount to less than 2% of the SSD speech delay population. In a separate SSD category of *speech errors*, Shriberg included Speech Errors-Sibilants (SE-/s/) and Speech Errors-Rhotics (SE-/r/). He added two additional (unnumbered) categories of SSD, also based on genetic and environmental risk factors whose working terms and abbreviations were Undifferentiated Speech Delay (USD) and Undifferentiated Speech Sound Disorder (USSD). An additional category, Motor

Speech Disorder Not Otherwise Specified (MSD-NOS) was added in 2009 (Shriberg et al., 2010).

1. Speech Delay-Genetic (SD-GEN), 56% of referrals
2. Speech Delay-Otitis media with Effusion (SD-OME), 30% of referrals
3. Speech Delay-Developmental Psychosocial Involvement (SD-DPI), 12% of referrals
4. Speech Delay-Apraxia of Speech (SD-AOS), <1% of referrals
5. Speech Delay-Dysarthria (SD-DYS)
6. Motor Speech Disorder Not Otherwise Specified (MSD-NOS)
7. Speech Errors-Sibilants (SE-/s/)
8. Speech Errors-Rhotics (SE-/r/)

Undifferentiated Speech Delay (USD)
Undifferentiated Speech Sound Disorder (USSD)

Shriberg classified the *primary origin* or probable aetiology of the putative subtypes as

1. SD-GEN: Polygenic/Environmental
2. SD-OME: Polygenic/Environmental
3. SD-DPI: Polygenic/Environmental
4. SD-AOS: Monogenic? Oligogenic?
5. SD-DYS: Monogenic? Oligogenic?
6. SE-/s/: Environmental
7. SE-/r/: Environmental
    USD: Any of 1–5
    USSD: Any of 1–7

With regard to the *processes affected*, Shriberg's breakdown was

1. SD-GEN: Cognitive–Linguistic
2. SD-OME: Auditory–Perceptual
3. SD-DPI: Affective–Temperamental
4. SD-AOS: Speech–Motor Control
5. SD-DYS: Speech–Motor Control
6. SE-/s/: Phonological Attunement
7. SE-/r/: Phonological Attunement
    USD Processes Affected: Any of 1–5
    USSD Processes Affected: Any of 1–7

Waring & Knight (2013, p. 12) comment, 'The SDCS is still primarily a research tool driven by a search for genetic factors associated with speech disorders. The value of the theoretical underpin-

nings of the SDCS may not be fully apparent until the repercussions of genetic research impact upon speech pathology, sometime in the future. If researchers are able to identify specific markers that can be readily employed by clinicians to classify children with SSD of unknown origin into the eight putative SDCS subgroups, the classification system would become clinically useful. Further validation is required before the SDCS is used as a clinical tool'.

When classification systems based around aetiological distinctions with causal subgroups are applied, clinicians attempting differential diagnosis discover that the speech of some children is impossible to pigeonhole because it seems to 'belong' in more than one category. Broomfield and Dodd (2004a) discuss the unsurprising elusiveness of neat clinical categorisation, pointing out that it has caused several authors (Fox, Dodd & Howard, 2002; Stackhouse & Wells, 1997) to question the clinical utility of the aetiological approach. Commenting on Shriberg's (1997) SDCS aetiological system, Broomfield and Dodd note three difficulties: (1) children do not fall easily into one subgroup or another; (2) it bears doubtful universality since it has not been trialled with non-English-speaking children; and (3) it provides no mechanism to account for developmental change. They go on to suggest that one alternative to the medical model approach is the theoretically strong psycholinguistic profiling approach proposed by Stackhouse and Wells (1997). But again, Broomfield and Dodd (2004a) are unconvinced, querying its utility on three points: one, its having little regard to surface phonology; two the lengthy diagnostic process involved in applying the framework; and three, the uncertainty of its universal applicability.

By contrast, Dodd (1995, 2005) proposed a differential diagnosis model with psycholinguistic foundations that is based primarily on linguistic profiling and speech subtypes. In it, specific speech subtypes are matched to discrete areas of psycholinguistic difficulty or breakdown that are 'testable' or 'differentially diagnosable'. Dodd's model enjoys some support for its universal applicability (Goldstein, 1996; So & Dodd, 1994). It embraces four subtypes that can occur at any age or stage of speech development, plus a fifth category for CAS. They are

- **Phonological delay:** in which children have a phonemic difficulty and all phonological rules or processes evident in a child's speech output are attested in typical development, but are characteristic of children chronologically younger than the child in question (this large group accounts for 57.5% of referrals).
- **Consistent deviant phonological disorder/ also known as consistent atypical phonological disorder:** in which children have a phonemic difficulty with co-occurring non-developmental or unusual errors and developmental rules or processes, with the presence of unusual processes signalling that the child has impaired understanding of the target phonological system (this group comprises 20.6% of referrals).
- **Inconsistent deviant phonological disorder/ also known as inconsistent phonological disorder:** in which children have a phonemic difficulty and exhibit delayed and non-developmental error types and variability of production of single-word tokens equal to or greater than 40% (this group covers 9.4% of referrals).

- **Articulation disorder:** in which children had a difficulty at the phonetic level and are unable to produce particular perceptually acceptable phones. They exhibit substitutions or distortions of the same sound in isolation, words and sentences, during imitation, elicitation and spontaneous speech tasks (this group amounts to 12.5% of referrals).
- **Childhood apraxia of speech:** in which children have difficulty at the motor planning, programming and execution levels, exhibiting multiple deficits involving phonological planning, phonetic programming and motor programming implementation (less than 1% of children with SSD have CAS).

Broomfield and Dodd (2004a) stress that children with CAS, as described by Ozanne (1995, 2005), have 'deviant' surface speech production patterns that may sound *similar* to those of children with inconsistent deviant phonological disorder. They point to key differences between the two, in terms of *proposed level of breakdown* and in terms of *symptomatology*. These differences are contrasted in Table 2.2 and the reader is referred to Dodd (2005) for interesting discussion.

Commenting on the model, Waring and Knight (2005, p. 12) say, 'Dodd's differential diagnosis is a clinically feasible, inclusive classification

Table 2.2 A comparison of CAS and inconsistent deviant phonological disorder

Childhood apraxia of speech (CAS) (Ozanne, 1995, 2005)	Inconsistent deviant phonological disorder (Dodd, 1995, 2005)
Level of breakdown Children's speech processing breaks down at the phonetic programme assembly level, with associated phonological planning and motor speech program implementation difficulties	*Level of breakdown* Children's speech processing difficulties are primarily at the phonological planning level
Spontaneous vs. imitated speech Spontaneous speech is closer to their intended target than imitated speech	*Spontaneous vs. imitated speech* Imitated speech is closer to their intended target than spontaneous speech
Phonological awareness (PA) skills Children tend to have intact PA skills	*PA skills* Children are likely to have an associated deficit in PA
Oromotor or feeding difficulties Children often have oromotor or feeding difficulties	*Oromotor or feeding difficulties* Children do not often have oromotor or feeding difficulties
Clarity and precision Children have an overall lack of clarity and precision	*Clarity and precision* Children are likely to be more precise
Suprasegmental characteristics Children's voice, prosody and fluency may be affected	*Suprasegmental characteristics* Children's voice, prosody and fluency are usually intact

system that divides children with SSD of unknown origin into discrete subgroups. More research is needed to profile the cognitive–linguistic difference between the subgroups. The validity of Dodd's classification system would be strengthened by replication studies, conducted by different research groups'.

Clinicians' use of classification terms

Faced with a range of approaches to classification, clinicians and researchers tend to use cover terms differently from each other, and there is variation from clinician to clinician and from researcher to researcher, sometimes relative to 'what they grew up with'.

'Articulation disorder' as a cover term

Clarity is achieved when 'articulation disorder' is taken to mean phonetic-level difficulties and 'phonological disorder' implies phonemic or cognitive–linguistic difficulties with organisation of the speech sound system. Nevertheless, in clinical settings, some speech-language pathologists and speech and language therapists (SLPs/SLTs) use the term 'articulation disorder' loosely and inaccurately. This is noticeable, and reasonable, when they opt for 'articulation disorder' to refer to *any* SSD, in explaining a child's speech difficulties in what they perceive to be simple language, to people who do not have a background SSD. Less excusably, they also do it when using professional patois to communicate with SLP/SLT colleagues, referring to *all* speech disorders as 'articulation disorders' (or 'artic' disorders).

'Phonological disorder' as a cover term

Some authorities use 'phonological disorder' as an overarching heading that embraces phonological disorder, articulation disorder and other SSDs. For example, Gierut (1998) uses 'functional phonological disorder' synonymously with 'phonological disorder' and under that heading includes five groupings. The first two are *phonetic disorders* and *phonemic disorders*, and she is careful to note that these two are not mutually exclusive. The third is *motor speech disorders*, including 'childhood apraxia'. Gierut's fourth category encompasses *functional phonological disorders associated with more global involvement of multiple aspects of the linguistic system*, for example in children with specific language impairment (p. S86). The fifth is *phonological disorders with organic bases*, such as hearing impairment, craniofacial anomalies, 'mental retardation' (intellectual disability) and 'childhood apraxia' (again). She also mentions a sixth group of children: those with 'phonological differences' or 'phonological difficulties' who are culturally and linguistically diverse, pointing out that these children with 'dialect differences, or native language differences' may not have a phonological disorder as such.

Rvachew and Brosseau-Lapré (2012) use 'developmental phonological disorders' (cf. Bowen, 1998a) in the title of a magnificent book that covers the range of developmental SSD across three subcategories: Speech delay, apraxia and residual errors; and excludes non-developmental speech disorders and speech differences. Rvachew and Brosseau-Lapré follow the Shriberg, Austin, Lewis, McSweeny and Wilson (1997) version of the SDCS. In it, 'Developmental Phonological Disorder' refers to children with speech delay (persisting substitution and deletion errors in children under 9) or Developmental Apraxia of Speech (DAS) or Residual Speech Errors. As indicated above, this classification system was updated in Shriberg, Fourakis et al. (2010) and DAS was replaced by SD-AOS (or CAS). Rvachew and Brosseau-Lapré emphasise that 'a majority across all three subcategories have specific underlying problems with phonological processing'. Rvachew who is 'profoundly uninterested in any arguments about what to call this particular population of children' discusses terminology at www.developmentalphonological disorders.wordpress.com in a July 14, 2012 blog post. This scholarly blog is a noteworthy and valuable resource for clinical SLPs/SLTs. Moreover, Rvachew invites instructors to comment and engage with her 'on the topic of teaching students about phonological (or speech sound) disorders'.

'Sound system disorders' as a cover term

Ruscello (2008) achieves simplicity and clarity with Shelton's (1993) classificatory term 'sound system disorders' (SSD), but he does not indicate the percentages of occurrence for his four subtypes. The expression 'sound system disorders' denotes, one: children with clinically significant sound production errors of unknown aetiology who have an SSD of unknown origin that includes phonetic (articulatory) production errors or phonemic (phonological) production errors or both (this is the largest category according to Ruscello); two: children with craniofacial anomalies termed 'oral structure deficits'; three: children with sensory deficits (i.e., hearing loss); and four: children with motor speech disorders whose sound system disorders have known aetiology in the form of a neurological deficit. Interestingly, my colleagues at the University of KwaZulu-Natal in Durban, South Africa, have expanded this particular cover term, calling it Speech Sound System Disorders (SSSD), so making it sound less like something is wrong with your hi-fi.

'Speech sound disorder' as a cover term

In its policy and clinical guideline documents and practice portal, ASHA uses the rather consumer friendly cover term 'speech sound disorder', with the articulation/phonology dichotomy, noting that, 'Intervention in speech sound disorders addresses articulatory and phonological impairments, associated activity and participation limitations and context barriers and facilitators by optimizing speech discrimination, speech sound production

and intelligibility in multiple communication contexts' (ASHA, 2004b).

It is adopted in the title of McLeod, Williams and McCauley (2010) and in the current work. Speech sound disorder is also the preferred term of Bernthal, Bankson and Flipsen, Jr. (2013) and within the influential Phonology Project, at the Waisman Center at the University of Wisconsin-Madison. An interpretation of Shriberg's (2006) conceptualisation of how 'speech sound disorder' evolved from 'articulation disorder' is displayed in Table 2.3.

Speech sound disorder is the term used in the DSM-V (American Psychiatric Association, 2013, pp. 44–45) too, though their description in 315:39 (F80.0) under 'Neurodevelopmental disorders' is confusing. Despite extensive collaboration with ASHA staff and members (Paul, 2013; and see www.asha.org/slp/dsm-5), it includes statements such as, 'verbal dyspraxia is a term also used for speech production problems' and excludes hearing loss from aetiology (cf. Purdy, Fairgray & Asad, A52 and see Schonweiler, Ptok & Radu, 1998) with no qualifying comment. The DSM-V diagnostic criteria are

A. Persistent difficulty with speech sound production that interferes with speech intelligibility or prevents verbal communication of messages.

B. The disturbance causes limitations in effective communication that interfere with social participation, academic achievement or occupational performance, individually or in any combination.

C. Onset of symptoms is in the early developmental period.

D. The difficulties are not attributable to congenital or acquired conditions such as cerebral palsy, cleft palate, deafness or hearing loss, traumatic brain injury or other medical or neurological conditions.

In the *Multilingual children with speech sound disorders: Position paper* (International Expert Panel on Multilingual Children's Speech, 2012; McLeod, Verdon & Bowen, 2013) Speech Sound Disorders is used as an 'umbrella term for the full

Table 2.3 From articulation disorder to childhood SSD: 1920–2005

Articulation One cover term	Two cover terms	No preferred cover term	→ Overlapping cover terms	One cover term	One cover term	Speech One cover term
'Articulation disorder' covered the UK term 'dyslalia' and later 'functional articulation/ speech disorder' in the United States	Children had an articulation or a phonological difficulty. Phonology impacted error description and assessment, but intervention was 'articulatory'	Articulation disorder and phonological disorder were used confusingly and almost synonymously in the literature and by clinicians	Children had a phonological difficulty or an articulation difficulty, with the emphasis on phonology, and frequently observed overlap between the two	'Phonological disorder' incorporated delayed or disordered phonology, with phonetic and phonemic levels and mapping rules	'Phonological disorder' now incorporated PA and phonological memory acknowledging the speech– literacy link	SSD was preferred in the literature, but clinicians still referred to children's articulation or phonology difficulties
Articulation	Articulation and phonology	Articulation or phonology	Articulation– phonology	Phonology	Phonology	Speech sound disorders
1920–1970	1971–1980		1981–1990		1991–2004	2005–

range of speech sound difficulties of both known (e.g., Down syndrome, cleft lip and palate) and presently unknown origin.' Including difficulties with speech perception, phonological representation and prosody in their description, they say that:

> *Children with speech sound disorders can have any combination of difficulties with perception, articulation/motor production, and/or phonological representation of speech segments (consonants and vowels), phonotactics (syllable and word shapes), and prosody (lexical and grammatical tones, rhythm, stress, and intonation) that may impact speech intelligibility and acceptability.*

Terms related to intervention

The intra- and interprofessional miscommunications that arise from having several approaches to the classification and description of SSD, and the tendency for professionals to mix-n-match them with abandon, spill over into intervention-related terminology and nomenclature. Gierut (1998), for example, talks about four 'phonolog-

ical treatments': traditional sensory-motor articulation therapy, cycles therapy, the *Metaphon* approach and conventional minimal pair therapy. Summarising the traditional sensory-motor articulation approach, Gierut cites Van Riper and Emerick (1984) and Winitz (1969, 1975), whose work in speech intervention well and truly predated any explicitly motivated *phonological* intervention, and likely predated the term 'phonological therapy'. She then provides an account of cycles (Hodson & Paden, 1991), with its traditional and metaphonological flavour (Kamhi, 2006, p. 275), about which Fey (1992) famously remarked, 'there is nothing inherently phonological about the use of cycles' (p. 279). At the same time, he added that because the approach aims to encourage gradual system-wide change, it is highly consistent with the goal common to all phonological approaches of facilitating reorganisation of the child's system. The third account Gierut provides is of conventional minimal pair therapy (Weiner, 1981), the only one on her list of four to meet all of Fey's (1985, reprinted 1992) exacting criteria for a 'phonological' therapy following the three 'phonological principles' outlined below.

In Weiner's approach, the therapist works at real-word (meaning) level, confronting children with their own homonymy, providing a semantic motivation to change production, thereby facilitating phonological reorganisation. The fourth 'phonological treatment' Gierut outlines is *Metaphon* (Dean, Howell, Waters & Reid, 1995), in which the SLP/SLT aims to eliminate persisting phonological processes via metalinguistic awareness tasks (Howell & Dean, 1994) involving imagery, minimal contrast activities, feigned listener confusion and guided discussion to promote self-monitoring of output.

Three phonological principles

Like Grunwell (1975) and Ingram (1976), Fey (1992) observed three basic principles underlying what he called phonology-based approaches to treatment such as conventional minimal pairs therapy (Weiner, 1981).

1. Modifying groups of sounds, or syllable structures

    The first principle concerned the modification of *groups* of sounds attacked according to an organising feature or systematic rule (of the child's), rather than focusing on the 'correction' of individual phonemes. Targeting groups of sounds indicates acknowledgement of the systematic nature of phonology and the prospect of promoting generalisation of new learning across the child's speech sound system. The speech production errors that the systemic rules represented fell into two main categories: *substitution errors* (also called *systemic errors*) where one sound or sound class is substituted for another (as in stopping, fronting, gliding, backing and assimilation); and *structural errors*, where the structure of the syllable or word changes (as in cluster reduction, diminutisation, schwa insertion or epenthesis, final consonant deletion, initial consonant deletion and weak syllable deletion). For example, if a child who was 'stopping' treated all fricatives as voiced stops, producing, system-

atically, *fun* as /bʌn/, *sum* as /dʌm/ and *shoe* as /du/, and so on, the therapist would target fricatives as a sound class, or frication as a feature, rather than treating, say, /f/ then /s/, then /ʃ/, and so on, position by position in word-initial, within-word and word-final contexts. Similarly, if a child's speech were characterised by prevalent final consonant deletion, with many open syllables and productions like /kɒ/ for *cough*, /bʌ/ for *bus*, /pɛ/ for *pet* and /ɛ/ for *edge*, the therapist would encourage final consonant inclusion across his or her system, in preference to treating word-final /t/, /f/, /s/ and /dʒ/ individually and serially as word-final singleton omissions.

2. Establishing feature contrasts

    The second principle was around establishing feature contrasts as opposed to perfecting articulatory execution sound by sound and word position by word position. Phonetic placement techniques, such as *hunting* (Van Riper & Irwin, 1958), the 'trail blazing' (*sic*) *progressive approximations* method (Van Riper, 1963), the *successive approximation* procedure (Kaufman 2005; McCurry & Irwin, 1953), and *shaping* (Bernthal & Bankson, 2004; Shriberg, 1975) are all goal attack strategies used as intermediary steps towards adult-like phonetic execution of a therapy target. In the process of fostering such articulatory precision, clinicians may verbally encourage children to produce 'a good crisp /s/', 'a clear /tʃ/', 'a perfect /k/', 'a sharp /t/', 'a beautiful /ŋ/', or 'a lovely /l/'. But in phonological therapy, the child is rewarded for creating *contrast* by using a sound in the target sound class, or a reasonable approximation of the target. For instance, with a child working at the systemic (substitution process) level to eliminate stopping of fricatives, a production like /ʃʌn/ for *sun* rather than /dʌn/ for *sun* would be rewarded, because /ʃ/ and /s/ are in the same (fricative) sound class, and both are voiceless. With a child working at the structural level, trying to learn final consonant inclusion, a production such as /biːm/ for *bean* rather than /biː/ for *bean* would be rewarded, because a final consonant was included, and furthermore the /m/ is a nasal consonant (like /n/). The clinician's acceptance of phonemic contrast and the lack of emphasis on fine tuning of phonetic form, particularly in the early stages of therapy, can be difficult to explain or 'sell' to parents and caregivers (and even some SLPs/SLTs), especially if they are anxious and eager to see progress. Their expectation of a clinician's role may be that we are 'supposed to be' encouraging perfection, and they can find it hard to understand that, if a goal in therapy is to eliminate stopping of fricatives, then /fɪp/ for *ship* is 'more correct' than /dɪp/ for *ship* and /sɪp/ for *ship* is even better!

3. Working at word level and making meaning

The third principle had to do with the goal of making *meaning*, with the implication that the therapy itself must perforce be constructed around listening to, discriminating between, decoding and saying 'real' words. Indeed, it is a truism that phonological therapy *must* be at word level or above (i.e., word, phrase, sentence or conversational level) in order to signal to the child that the purpose of having a system of sound contrasts, or a phonological system, is to communicate (or to make meaning). The child discovers that homophony must be avoided and appropriate contrast established. If *come*, *crumb*, *drum*, *gum*, *plum*, *some* and *thumb* are all collapsed and realised homonymously as [dʌm], they come to appreciate that something (phonological) *has* to change.

Characteristics of phonological disorder

Stoel-Gammon and Dunn (1985) reviewed the small (at the time) literature on the relationship between normal and disordered child phonology, finding a general view that, while there were many similarities between normal and disordered speech sound systems, there were also substantial differences between them. Their useful list of the most frequently described characteristics of developmental phonological disorders (as distinct from

'phonetic' or 'articulation' disorders) included the presence of

1. Static speech sound systems that had plateaued at an early level of development.
2. Extreme variability in production, without gradual improvement.
3. Persistence of phonological processes beyond typically expected ages.
4. 'Chronological Mismatch' (Grunwell, 1981) with mastery of 'later', 'difficult' sounds and structures and errors with sounds usually acquired early in development.
5. Idiosyncratic rules or processes that rarely occur in normal phonology.
6. Restricted use of contrast.

Misuse of terms

There is a regrettable tendency among SLPs/SLTs to 'improve on' the term phonological disorder, replacing it with: *'phonological processing disorder'*, *'phonological process disorder'*, or *'phonological processes disorder'*. Although they have crept into the vernacular, achieving prominence in the workplace, on the Web, in e-mail discussion, and on professional association websites, none of these three inappropriate terms is an acceptable synonym for either 'phonological disorder' or 'developmental phonological disorder'.

Four easily confused 'phonological terms'

Phonological disorder in the area of speech (Grunwell, 1987; Ingram, 1989a), phonological processes in the area of speech (Stampe, 1969), phonological processes in the area of literacy (Scarborough & Brady, 2002) and phonological processing in the area of literacy (Snowling, Bishop & Stothard, 2000) are four different things.

1. **Phonological disorder (speech)**

Phonological disorder, also known as developmental phonological disorder, is an SSD at the cognitive–linguistic level, manifested in (surface) speech error patterns. In clinical settings, it is unusual to hear phonological disorder called 'phonological speech disorder' (Gillon, 1998) or 'expressive phonology disorder' (Bird, Bishop & Freeman, 1995). We obviously do not need *more* terms, but if we *did*, these would be good, explanatory ones to use because they help to distinguish (a) phonological impairment in terms of speech error patterns, from (b) phonological impairment in terms of literacy, specifically in relation to Phonological Awareness and phonological processing (Gillon, 2004, pp. 89–90).

2. **Phonological processes (speech)**

Stampe's (1969) natural phonology theory introduced the concept of phonological processes. A phonological process was a *descriptive rule or statement* (*not* a 'process' in the sense of a series of actions or steps taken in order to achieve a particular end) that accounted for structural or segmental speech errors of substitution, omission or addition. As explained in Chapter 1, Natural Phonology theory stressed the importance of natural phonological processes as a set of universal, obligatory rules governing a particular phonology. These innate processes represented the *constraints* a child modifies or suppresses in order to learn more *advanced forms* in the process of mastering spoken language. The constraints, according to Stampe, disallowed the production of all but the simplest pronunciation patterns in the early stages of phonological development. 'Advanced forms' really implied the correct 'adult' realisation of the sound.

Recall from Chapter 1 that Stampe saw the processes as being universal, innate and psychologically real, operating to constrain and restrict the speech mechanism, and that he believed children actively 'used' processes for the phonological act of simplifying pronunciation via a 'reflex mechanism'. In this sense, because he considered the processes to be real 'mental operations', Stampe believed that the processes provided an *explanation* of children's speech sound errors.

Stampe's legacy includes a range of useful descriptors for the speech characteristics of

typically developing children and children with SSD, such as 'stopping of fricatives', 'velar fronting', 'deaffrication', and 'cluster reduction', that are widely utilised by SLPs/SLTs. But descriptions they *are*, and explanations they are *not*. Table 2.4 displays a selection of the common phonological processes (or phonological deviations or phonological rules or phonological patterns in some literature) that can be used to describe error patterns in phonologies that are developing *normally*, phonologies that are *delayed* and phonologies that are *disordered*. The cut-off ages for the elimination of the deviations displayed in the table in simplified form to share with families are those suggested by Grunwell (1987). For Grunwell, the term 'deviation' implied that the child's production deviated from the adult target production.

3. **Phonological processing (literacy)**
4. **Phonological processes (literacy)**

Scarborough and Brady (2002) provide an essential glossary (for the literacy enthusiast or phonology tragic) of what they call the 'phon words', carefully distinguishing between the many phonological concepts and terms that are found in contemporary literacy theory, research, practice and pedagogy. In such contexts, 'phonological processing' is used collectively to refer to the phonological information-using abilities and codes (or 'phonological processes') that are fundamental to learning to read and write. These are 'abilities', or 'mental operations', that cannot be directly measured. They include phonological *representations* (Sosa & Stoel-Gammon, 2010), phonological *memory*, phonological *knowledge*, phonological *awareness*, and phonological *naming*.

Scarborough and Brady define phonological processing as: 'The formation, retention, and/or use of phonological codes or speech while performing some cognitive or linguistic task or operation such as speaking, listening, remembering, learning, naming, thinking, reading, or writing' (p. 318). They note that these phonological processes do *not* require conscious awareness, asserting that PA

Table 2.4 Common phonological processes and their *approximate* ages of elimination in typical acquisition (Grunwell, 1987)

Phonological process (phonological deviation)	Adult target vs. child's realisations		Description	Approximate age of elimination
	Adult	Child		
Context sensitive voicing	PIG: pɪg KISS: kɪs	bɪg gɪs	A voiceless sound is replaced by a voiced sound. In these examples, /p/ is replaced by /b/, and /k/ is replaced by /g/. Other examples might include /t/ being replaced by /d/, or /f/ being replaced by /v/	3;0
Word-final devoicing	RED: ɹɛd BAG: bæg	ɹɛt bæk	A final voiced consonant in a word is replaced by a voiceless consonant. Here, /d/ has been replaced by /t/, and /g/ has been replaced by /k/	3;0
Final consonant deletion	HOME: houm ROUGH: rʌf	hou ɹʌ	The final consonant in the word is omitted. In these examples, /m/ is omitted (or deleted) from 'home' and /f/ is omitted from 'rough'	3;3
Velar fronting	KISS: kɪs GIVE: gɪv WING: wɪŋ	tɪs dɪv wɪn	A velar stop or nasal is replaced by an alveolar stop or nasal respectively. Here, /k/ in 'kiss' is replaced by /t/, /g/ in 'give' is replaced by /d/ and /ŋ/ in 'wing' is replaced by /n/	3;6
Palatal fronting	SHIP: ʃɪp TAJ: tɑʒ	sɪp tɑʒ	The palato-alveolar fricatives /ʃ/ and /ʒ/ are replaced by alveolar fricatives /s/ and /z/	3;9
Consonant harmony	CUPBOARD: kʌbəd DOG: dɒg	pʌbəd gɒg	Pronunciation of the whole word is influenced by the presence of a particular sound in the word. Here, /b/ in 'cupboard' causes the /k/ to be replaced /p/, which is the voiceless cognate of /b/, and /g/ in 'dog' causes /d/ to be replaced by /g/	4;0
Weak syllable deletion	AGAIN: əgɛn TIDYING: taɪdiɪŋ	gɛn taɪɪŋ	Syllables are either stressed or unstressed. Here the weak syllables in 'again' and 'tidying' are omitted	4;0
Cluster reduction	BLUE: blu ANT: ænt	bu æt	Consonant clusters occur when two or three consonants occur in a sequence in a word. In cluster reduction part of the cluster is omitted. Here, /l/ has been deleted from 'blue' and /n/ from 'ant'	4;0
Gliding of liquids	REAL: ɹiəl LEG: lɛg	wiəl jɛg	The liquid consonants /l/ and /ɹ/ are replaced by the glides /w/ or /j/. In these examples, /ɹ/ in 'real' is replaced by /w/, and /l/ in 'leg' is replaced by /j/	5;0
Stopping	FUNNY: fʌni JUMP: dʒʌmp	pʌni dʌmp	A fricative consonant or an affricate consonant is replaced by a stop. Here, /f/ in 'funny' is replaced by /p/, and /dʒ/ in 'jump' is replaced by /d/	See below

Approximate ages of elimination for stopping of fricatives and affricates

/f/, /s/	FUNNY: fʌni→pʌni SIP: sɪp→ tɪp	3;0
/v/, /z/	VAN: væn → bæn ZOO: zu → du	3;6
/ʃ/, /dʒ/, /tʃ/	SHIP ʃɪp → dɪp JUMP: dʒʌmp → dʌmp CHIP: tʃɪp → tɪp	4;6
/θ/, /ð/	THING: θɪŋ → tɪŋ THEM: ðɛm → dɛm	5;0

is sometimes treated as a separate category because it deals with tasks and constructs that *do* require conscious reflection on the phonological structure of words (Hesketh, A28; Neilson, A22).

Scarborough and Brady believe the term 'phonological processing' in literacy contexts obscures important distinctions between *constructs* (underlying mental operations that *cannot* be directly observed or measured) and *tasks* (that *can* be directly observed or measured), and between 'the various tasks themselves, with regard to their requirements for other sorts of processing'.

Web questions

It its first 15 years, my website (Bowen, 1998b) attracted approximately 14 000 emails containing questions and/or requests for advice from among over 1 000 000 unique site visitors from around the world at the rate of between 10 and 20 emails a week. About half of the email came from SLP/SLT professionals and students and the other half from parents, adults with communication disorders and interested members of the general public.

A large number of the questions received relate to classification and terminology. For example, the parent of an unintelligible 4 year old asked, 'Can you please tell me the difference between an articulation disorder and a phonological disorder; how can you tell them apart; and are they treated differently?' Another wrote, 'My five year old was diagnosed by one therapist who said he had a phonological disorder, but the therapist who is actually treating him says he has "a phonological processing disorder" and that we need to work on "his artic". I am so, so confused by this: help!' And this came from a colleague: 'Although I have been an ASHA-certified school-based SLP for over 20 years, and most of my caseload is "artic", I have to say I am confused about the difference between phonetic speech sound disorders, and phonemic speech sound disorders. In simple terms, what exactly is the difference, and can they exist concurrently in the same child?'

Such questions prompted the development of a plain English response on the website, a variation of which is shown in Box 2.1. Predictably, in light of the prevalence of SSD, it is one of the most-retrieved pages there and much used by students, clinical educators, and practitioners, including those preparing talks for consumer groups.

Box 2.1 How do articulation disorder and phonological disorder differ?

A PLAIN-ENGLISH EXPLANATION FOR CONSUMERS

How do articulation disorder and phonological disorder differ?

In order to understand the difference, it is important to know that SLPs/SLTs make a distinction between *speech* and *language*. Human language is partly innate and partly learned from our interactions with the people in our world. The 'learned' part is like a code, or sets of systematic rules that enable us to communicate ideas and express wants and needs. Reading, writing, gesturing and speaking are all forms of language. For convenience, we can think of language as having two divisions: *receptive language*, or understanding what is said, read or signed; and *expressive language*, or speaking, writing or signing. Our overall grasp of what linguistics, neurology, psychology and related disciplines reveal about the nature of typical speech and language development, and what can go wrong with them, is critical to understanding an individual child's speech and or language difficulty.

When we think about speech as the spoken medium of language, we find, among other things, that speech has a phonetic level and a phonemic level. The phonetic level takes care of articulation: the motor act of producing vowels and consonants, so that we have a repertoire of all the sounds we need in order to speak our language(s). The phonemic level is in charge of phonology: the 'brain-work' that goes into organising the sounds from the phonetic level into patterns of sound contrasts that enable us to make sense when we talk.

An articulation disorder is a *speech* disorder that adversely affects the phonetic level so that the child has difficulty saying particular consonants and vowels. The reason for this may be *unknown* or poorly understood as is the case for children who do *not* have serious problems with muscle function; or the reason may be *known* and well understood as is the case for children with dysarthria who do have serious problems with nerve and muscle function (like children with cerebral palsy), or children with craniofacial differences, such as *some* children with cleft lip and palate. By contrast, a phonological disorder is a *language* disorder that affects the phonemic organisation level. The child has difficulty organising his or her speech sounds into a system of contrasts, often referred to as phonemic contrasts. One way of understanding this is to think of the phonetic level as happening 'in the mouth' or even 'on the lips' and the phonemic level as happening 'in the mind' (Grunwell, 1989). The phonemic level is sometimes referred to as the linguistic level or the cognitive level.

Can phonetic and phonemic difficulties co-occur?

Yes, they can: the same child can have both. Some of their intelligibility challenges can have an articulatory basis and others of their challenges can have phonological bases.

Can they occur with other speech or language disorders?

Again, the answer is 'yes'. For example, the same child may have co-occurring difficulties at the phonetic level, the phonemic level, the motor planning level and perceptual level.

Can individuals with CAS have some combination of all these other issues too?

Yes, they can. In addition to having difficulties with planning the movements required for speech, children with CAS can have phonetic and/or phonemic issues. Because of their knowledge base, SLPs/SLTs are able to distinguish between the many speech and language disorders they have to assess (or 'differentially diagnose') in the course of their work, and they can also recognise these co-occurrences.

Where can I find out more?

There is further information, written for a general readership, about children's SSD on the author's website: www.speech-language-therapy.com.

Two major sub-groups

Within the overall SSD client population, there are two major sub-groups of children: (1) poorly unintelligible preschoolers with low percentages of consonants correct (PCCs) and multiple errors; and (2) acceptably intelligible school-aged students with high PCCs and 'residual errors'. In practice, clinicians often reserve the terms 'articulation disorder' and 'functional articulation disorder' for the reasonably intelligible children of all ages, with one or just a few speech production difficulties, characteristically involving /s/, /z/, /l/ and /ɹ/ and, in some settings, /θ/ and /ð/ also.

A high proportion, but we do not know precisely *how* high, of the unintelligible pre-schoolers have a phonological impairment entailing linguistic difficulties with organising speech sounds into patterns of sound contrasts. A small proportion (<1% of the paediatric SLP/SLT SSD caseload) has CAS, thought to be due to a deficit in speech motor control (ASHA, 2007; Shriberg, 2004, 2006; Shriberg, Campbell, Karlsson, McSweeney & Nadler, 2003). Each and every SSD can co-occur (e.g., phonetic and phonemic issues in the same child), and each can occur with other communication disorders (e.g., CAS and stuttering in the same child) or with other conditions (e.g., phonological disorder and ADHD in the same child).

Speech assessment: Screening

Speech assessment involves careful, informed observations and hypothesis testing. The process typically begins with the referral followed by a preliminary, informal *screening* procedure in which the SLP/SLT listens to and watches the child speak. Usually without discussion or collaboration, the SLP/SLT develops, independently, a tentative explanation, or hypothesis, about the nature of any apparent difficulties with a view to conducting further investigations if needed. This initial screening may be as simple as making observations of the child in conversation, either with the therapist or with a parent, sibling or peer, or it may involve a short screening test. Appropriate screening reflects sensitivity to cultural and linguistic diversity (Goldstein, A19). In family-centred practice (Watts Pappas, A30), which is by no means universal, there is collaboration around the nature and conduct of further assessment. The SLP/SLT provides pertinent information, but it is a family's decision whether to proceed, who should be present in assessment sessions, and so on.

A person who is not an SLP/SLT may be called upon to conduct initial screening and it may involve the use of computer software. For example, the 66-picture computerised *Phoneme Factory Phonology Screener* developed in the United Kingdom is designed for teachers to administer to children whom they suspect have speech sound difficulties, before referring them to SLP/SLT services for assessment. The teacher listens as the student names the pictures, writing down alphabetically or phonetically the child's production of one particular sound per word.

The software has the capability of generating a report, based on what the teacher records, specifying the errors and patterns revealed, with normative comparisons and an indication of whether the child's speech difficulties are 'developmental' or 'disordered'. Any recommendation to refer to speech therapy is based on this report. The report also guides the teacher to appropriate activities to use in an associated software title in the series, the *Phoneme Factory Sound Sorter* program.

In testing the software, 408 children were assessed on the screener by a teacher–researcher and by an SLT using the phonology subtest of the *DEAP* (Dodd, Zhu, Crosbie, Holm & Ozanne, 2002). These two measures of the children's speech were used to determine the screener's sensitivity (71%), specificity (99%) and positive predictive values (81%). The order of testing was randomised (i.e., sometimes the children were assessed first by the teacher and sometimes first by the SLT) so as to control for order effects.

The first author of the *Phoneme Factory* software packages, Dr. Sue Roulstone, is Emeritus Professor of Speech and Language Therapy, University of the West of England, Bristol and a co-director of the Bristol Speech & Language Therapy Research Unit. She is a Fellow of the Royal College of Speech & Language Therapists and was Chair from 2004 to 2006. She received an Honorary Doctor of Health degree from Manchester Metropolitan University in 2013. Her research interests include evaluation of SLT service delivery, child and family perspectives on speech and language impairment, epidemiology of speech and language impairment and professional judgement and decision-making, and her response to Q8 reflects these interrelated topics.

Q8.   Sue Roulstone: Child speech screening and 'phoneme factory'

Screening and assessment practices vary widely. In its preamble to preferred practice patterns (ASHA, 2004b), it states that the document provides 'an informational base to promote delivery of quality patient/client care. They are sufficiently flexible to permit both innovation and acceptable practice variation, yet sufficiently definitive to guide practitioners in decision making for appropriate client outcomes'. The document goes on the say, 'Pediatric speech-language screening is conducted by appropriately credentialed and trained speech–language pathologists, possibly supported by speech–language pathology assistants under appropriate supervision'. How do screening practices in the United Kingdom differ from those specified in the ASHA guidelines? Has the *Phoneme Factory* been a successful innovation as a referral tool, and can you clarify teachers' use of the screener in relation to the *Phoneme Factory Sound Sorter* intervention component? Is this work children do while waiting for SLT intervention?

A8.   Sue Roulstone: Screening for speech impairments

I would first like to highlight different uses of the word 'screening' within the profession and more widely in health and education services. Generally, screening is used to suggest a level of assessment that provides a pass/fail outcome, indicating whether or not a child has a speech and language difficulty that requires more in-depth, confirmatory assessment. However, there are several stages along the diagnostic pathway at which 'screening' might be used, and for the purposes of this discussion, I would like to identify three.

1. Early identification screening of at-risk populations

    First, screening is used to describe a public health process in which children within a defined population are tested, in order to identify those at risk for speech and language problems so as to refer them for further diagnostic testing; the aim of such screening is to provide early identification, preferably in a pre-symptomatic stage, and provide treatment at the earliest appropriate opportunity (Hall & Elliman, 2003, p. 135).

2. Informal SLP/SLT triage screening

    A second use of screening describes part of the initial assessment process carried out by an SLP/SLT. In Q8, Caroline described an 'informal screening procedure' carried out by SLPs/SLTs at the first assessment of child following referral. Pickstone (2007) called this a 'triage' process whereby the experienced SLP/SLT makes judgements about the priority status of the newly referred child to make best use of resources and monitor the urgency and needs of those being referred.

3. Formal screening assessment

    Third, screening assessments might be used to gather a quick overview of speech output that indicate whether further investigation is warranted. The screeners of the *DEAP* (Dodd et al., 2002) and *HAPP-3* (Hodson, 2004) might be used for this purpose.

These different types of screening represent a gradual focusing of the identifica-

tion and diagnostic process and in order to decide who could or should carry out screening, it can be helpful to determine which stage in the diagnostic process is being described and the purpose of screening at that point. Within the United Kingdom, the first type of screening is regarded as a public health role, performed by health and education professionals. These personnel might be health visitors, teachers and nursery (daycare and pre-school) staff, who work in primary care and paraprofessionals in some community settings, trained for a particular procedure (Pickstone, Hannon & Fox, 2002). A health visitor is a registered nurse or midwife who has undertaken post-registration training to qualify as a member of the primary healthcare team. The promotion of health and the prevention of illness across the lifespan are central to the role of the health visitor.

The *Royal College of Speech and Language Therapists* (Gascoigne, 2006) sees SLTs' role in the public health arena as strategic in nature – advising on the types of procedures to be used, training the other professionals involved. Indeed, SLTs in the United Kingdom rarely conduct this kind of screening directly themselves. Occasionally, where SLTs are establishing the needs in a particular population, for example, setting up a new service in a school or a preschool setting, SLTs might be directly involved in population screening. However, following this, the screening and referral process would be handed back to the people in regular contact with the child; the SLT's role would be to provide materials and training. On the other hand, the second and third types of screening for speech and language impairment would be regarded as the role of the state-registered SLT, perhaps supported by an SLT assistant within some constrained contexts. Furthermore, Pickstone (2007) reports the use of more experienced therapists in the triage process in order to utilise their expertise in decision making.

Population screening

In the rest of the discussion, screening is used in the first sense, where the testing is part of a public health process aiming to identify which children should be referred for further confirmatory or diagnostic assessment. According to the UK National Screening Committee (n.d.) online resource:

Screening is a public health service in which members of a defined population, who do not necessarily perceive they are at risk of, or are already affected by a disease or its complications, are asked a question or offered a test, to identify those individuals who are more likely to be helped than harmed by further tests or treatment to reduce the risk of a disease or its complications.

Systematic reviews of screening for speech and language impairments (Law, Boyle, Harris, Harkness & Nye, 1998; Nelson, Nygren, Walker & Panoscha, 2006) conclude that although there several assessments with adequate sensitivity and specificity (i.e., they identify a reasonable proportion of cases [sensitivity] and a reasonable proportion of children who were not cases [specificity]), no comparisons have been made of the different procedures. The lack of consensus regarding which children *should* be identified for treatment and the uncertainty that those identified by screening procedures would be the ones who would most benefit from intervention was also noted. The impact of screening assessments on actual referral and identification practices is rarely evaluated; neither is the use of risk factors to assist screening decisions. In the absence of a clear evidence base, there has been no nationally recommended process for screening for speech and language impairment in the United Kingdom and the emphasis has been on primary prevention and providing universal access to advice for parents (Hall & Elliman, 2003, p. 262; Pickstone et al., 2002). Nonetheless, most SLT departments,

in collaboration with local primary care and education agencies, have developed and publicised local criteria to guide referrals. However recent UK government initiatives (DfE, 2012), responding to evidence that shows the negative outcomes for children with early speech and language delay, have introduced a new progress check between the ages of 2 and 3 years that includes an evaluation of communication and language. Health visitors or nursery staff working with a child of this age are required to provide parents with a developmental profile with the aim of identifying any aspects of their development that are of concern. The profiling process does not focus particularly on speech but on indicators of communication and language development more generally.

Phoneme factory

Thus, the original UK policy context around the development of *The Phoneme Factory* did not support the introduction of screening assessments targeting the population as a whole. So it was not our original intention to develop a screening assessment when we initiated the *Phoneme Factory* (a software suite comprising the *Phoneme Factory Sound Sorter* (Wren & Roulstone, 2006) and the *Phoneme Factory Phonology Screener* (Wren, Hughes & Roulstone, 2006)) project.

In the United Kingdom, where therapists are working with children of school age (4;0 and upwards), therapy is typically school based and curriculum focused (Gascoigne, 2006, p. 224). The original aim of the *Phoneme Factory* project was therefore to develop a therapy tool that could be set up by therapists for use by teachers in class that had credence for teachers as useful to the speaking and listening and pre-literacy curriculum. We reasoned that therapists frequently left poor quality picture and paper-based activities for teachers (e.g., photocopied sheets). As these got lost, or crumpled and separated from instructions, they were either not implemented or incorrectly implemented in terms the SLTs' goals. We felt that computer software had much to offer in providing fun, interactive materials that maintained their quality. Furthermore because the activities need little adult input, they were less prone to unintentional and unhelpful modifications by the teacher or assistant working with the child.

Conscious that the software once left in the classroom would inevitably be used more widely by education staff, we developed seven software games that were primarily PA activities and unlikely to cause children harm even if they were used indiscriminately for children not under the care of the SLT. The games could be configured to fit with the individual child's speech targets. As we predicted, once piloted in the classroom, teachers were keen to have greater access to the software games. Our advisory therapist group too felt that they had potential general applicability to children beyond the SLT remit, who perhaps had minimal speech output immaturities or literacy problems. Our position is that engagement of teachers with the work of SLTs is crucial to the success of intervention for children of school age and therefore we should make the software accessible to teachers. So our challenge became how to make *Phoneme Factory* therapy software (i.e., the Sound Sorter component (Wren & Roulstone, 2006)) more accessible without the risk of teachers perceiving that they now had a tool that obviated the need for therapy referral. This was the dilemma that precipitated the development of the screener (Wren et al., 2006).

The aim was to produce a reliable screener that allowed teachers to identify children with expressive phonological systems that were below age expectations, in order to refer for further investigation by an SLT. Further, we aimed to produce a screener that would provide teachers with feedback about the child's phonology, encompassing

suggestions for activities that could be carried out by the teacher using the therapy software. The original therapy software was designed to allow therapists to configure the games to suit individual children's phonological system, target sounds and contrasts. So we developed the therapy software further to include specific teacher settings that did not require detailed analysis of a child's system, but that would nonetheless provide appropriate activities (or games). These teacher settings, in the current software, include a random selection of PA games as well as pre-set games for developing PA related to developmental the substitution processes of stopping, fronting, context sensitive voicing, gliding and deaffrication and the structural process of final consonant deletion. An Australian version of the Phoneme Factory Sound Sorter Software is under development as part of a research program to evaluate its effectiveness for children with SSD (McLeod, Baker, McCormack, Wren & Roulstone, 2013–2015). The games aim to fulfil four purposes, namely:

- to provide interim activities whilst a child is awaiting an SLT appointment;
- to provide relevant activities should the therapist not be able to visit the school to program the software themselves or to provide a teacher with support activities;
- to provide activities for children whose articulation or phonology is perhaps a little immature but does not warrant further referral; and
- to provide general PA activities that might be of use to any child as pre-reading activities.

Having developed the screener, the next stage of the research program will be to assess the impact of the use of both the screener and the sound sorter software on referral processes and on the development of children's phonology – using a wider sample of SLT and teacher views of the software. So there is still research to be done on how the software works in practice. However, here is an illustrative example of how things might work out.

Case illustration

Christopher is a newcomer to Year 1. Aged 5;3, he has moved home during the summer. No information is available to his teacher, Amala, at the start of term and she immediately notices that Christopher is very difficult to understand. Amala allows Christopher a little while to settle into class, before completing the *Phoneme Factory* screener with him. The screener report indicates that Christopher has developmental and non-developmental errors and the need for referral to an SLT for assessment. Amala discusses a printout of the report with Christopher's parents and with their permission refers him to the SLT service. The screener report has also suggested sound sorter activities appropriate to his needs: namely, the pre set teacher settings for 'fronting', 'final consonant deletion' and 'general PA'. He waits two months to see the SLT who uses his screener information as a baseline against which Christopher's progress over the two months is measured. The therapist's in-depth assessment of Christopher's phonology shows he consistently replaces /k/ and /g/ with /d/ and all word initial fricatives with /h/; and omits all final consonants. On her next visit to the school, the therapist configures the *Phoneme Factory* sound sorter to target Christopher's systematic sound preference for /h/ SIWI. Already familiar with the games, Christopher can use the software independently and Amala allows him time each day to enjoy the PA activities. Therapy continues using a combination of the individually configured software games and individual sessions with the therapist, Christopher and Christopher's mother working on a combination of PA/input tasks using the sound sorter and activities to remediate his production errors.

Diagnostic evaluation

Child speech assessments for the purpose of diagnosis are prompted by: (1) referral, including referral by a child's family; (2) a child's medical, sensory or developmental status, for example, the speech of children with cleft palate is routinely assessed in most of the industrialised world (Golding-Kushner, A17); or (3) failing a speech–language screening (see ASHA, 2004c, for further information). They are conducted by appropriately credentialed SLPs/SLTs, working individually or as members of collaborative teams that may include the child, family and others (Watts Pappas, A30).

Speech assessments are administered to children as needed, requested or mandated or where there are indications that individuals have articulation and/or phonology impairments associated with their body structure/function and/or communication activities/participation (McLeod, A1).

Depending on the presenting picture, the SLP/SLT typically examines the phonetic, phonological, perceptual, phonotactic, prosodic, speech motor and intelligibility aspects of the child's speech. In evidence-based practice (E³BP), the particular tests chosen depend on the child's presentation, the educated preferences and theoretical orientation of the clinician, and client/patient values and wishes.

The case history interview and 'red flags'

The case history interview and/or a history questionnaire provide helpful information about the child and the family that may assist the therapist to manage the assessment and intervention process sensitively and appropriately. Ideally, information gathering is conducted with an eye to the potential 'red flags' for speech impairment (summarised in Box 2.2), including family history (Stein et al., 2011) or the risk and protective factors (Harrison & McLeod, 2010) that alert the clinician to a range of important risk factors and 'leads' to pursue.

Box 2.2 Red flags for speech impairment to consider in case history taking

Failure to babble or late onset of canonical babbling Overby and Caspari (2013) are conducting research into early vocalisations relative to CAS (see below)	Infants start to produce canonical (speech-like) CV and VC strings of babble at around 0;7 and all infants should be producing canonical babble, at least some of the time, before their first birthday. Canonical babbling may go hand-in-hand with all sorts of other perfectly normal baby noises including strange vocalisations, squeals and gurgles. Babble and real speech overlap for months, with the baby producing both. Failing to babble, and late-onset of canonical babble, are both associated with (1) hearing impairment and (2) motor speech disorder (MSD). Also, late canonical babbling is predictive of delayed language development. www.vocaldevelopment.com
Otitis media with effusion (OME)	OME between 12 and 18 months is associated with speech delay. Query this in children with grommets (PE tubes), especially if inserted at 1–3 years of age.
Glottal replacement	Glottal replacement, when it is not dialectal, alerts clinicians to the possibility of SSD.
Initial consonant deletion	ICD is not attested in first language learners of English, alerting us to the possibility of moderate and severe SSD. It is found in typical development in some languages, for example, French, Finnish, Maltese, Spanish and Thai.
Small phonetic inventory	Small repertoires of consonants and/or vowels may signal moderate and severe SSD (moderate/severe phonological disorder and/or CAS).
Inventory constraints	Six missing consonants (inventory constraints) or six sounds in error, across three manner categories signal severe SSD. For example, two stops, two fricatives, two glides.
Backing of obstruents stops fricatives affricates	Backing of obstruents is a diagnostic marker for speech delay associated with otitis media with effusion (Shriberg et al., 2003). Article: www.waisman.wisc.edu/phonology/pubs/PUB15.pdf
Vowel errors Do vowels 'wander'?	Prevalent or inconsistent vowel errors are a diagnostic marker for CAS. Children with CAS and those with moderate/severe phonological disorder frequently experience difficulties producing vowels (Gibbon, 2013). Vowel errors may occur in as many as 50% of children with these diagnoses (Eisenson & Ogilvie, 1963; Pollock & Berni, 2003). 24–65% typically developing children below 35 months have a high incidence of vowel errors. By 35 months errors are far less prevalent (0–4%). (Pollock, 2013).
Persisting FCD	Final consonant deletion coming up to the third birthday alerts the clinician to the possibility of SSD. Typically, FCD is eliminated by about age 2;10–3;3.
Beginning readers' conversational PCC <50%	PCC below 50% when formal reading instruction starts (at about the age of 5;6) is associated with literacy acquisition difficulties. *Conversational PCC* – Based on a sample of at least 200 Utterances (Shriberg, 1982).

PCC	Severity scale for children 4;1–8;6
>85%	Mild SSD
65–85%	Mild–moderate SSD
50–64%	Moderate–severe SSD
<50%	Severe SSD

Critical age hypothesis	The critical age hypothesis is that literacy acquisition is likely to be compromised if children are not intelligible by the age of 5;6, especially if they also have semantic and syntactic difficulties (Bishop & Adams, 1990).
Mild speech difficulties >6;9	Persistent, mild speech production difficulties beyond the age of 6;9 are associated with literacy acquisition difficulties (Nathan, Stackhouse, Goulandris & Snowling, 2004).
'Losing words'	If parents say their child 'loses words', it may be significant, but it is not a 'CAS indicator'/'SSD indicator'. The 'losing words' phenomenon occurs in early typical development. However, it may indicate language regression due to epilepsy (e.g., Landau–Kleffner syndrome), tumours, etc.
Intellectual disability	1. Persons with cognitive impairment are likely to have speech sound errors. 2. The most frequent error type is likely to be deletion of consonants. 3. Errors are likely to be inconsistent. 4. The pattern of errors is likely to be similar to that of very young children or children with SSD of unknown origin (Shriberg & Widder, 1990).

Video observations of early characteristics of CAS

Overby and Caspari (2013) note that SLPs/SLTs are hesitant to diagnose CAS in children younger than 2 years of age because of the paucity of information about early (birth – toddler) characteristics of the disorder, low volubility (little talking (DeThorne, Deater-Deckard, Mahurin-Smith, Coletto & Petrill, 2011)) in children with suspected CAS, and phonological overlap between CAS and other SSDs. Using home videos provided by children's parents, Overby and Caspari (2013) compared the early sounds made by four children diagnosed with CAS between the ages of 3 and 5 years old to those of two typically developing children. Sounds examined in this study were organized into the following groups: *vegetative sounds* (burps, hiccoughs, sneezes, gulps, reflexive grunting, etc.); *fixed signals* (recurring motor sequences such as laughs, cries and moans that do not vary across individuals); *protophones* (quasivowels that are speech-like but not transcribable); and *fully resonant productions* that were transcribable (marginal babbling and canonical babbling for variable purposes). Because they were interested in tracking children's development of perceptually accurate motor productions (an assessment consideration in the identification of CAS), they included fully resonant vowels and *speech* (meaningful speech or made up words) as fully resonant productions.

Emphasising the preliminary nature of this work, the individual variation among children with CAS, the current small sample size and the need to expand their comparison group to infants and toddlers with non-CAS severe SSDs, they found that children later diagnosed with CAS demonstrated, as infants and toddlers, a lack of diversity in place, manner and voicing compared to typically developing children. Children with CAS had a 'place' preference for bilabials and alveolars; a 'manner' preference for stops and nasals; limited babbling defined by reduced syllable shapes (dominated by vowels and CVs); and consonants that disappeared.

Confirming anecdotal reports by parents that infants and toddlers with CAS are 'silent babies', Overby and Caspari (2013) found the average volubility (number of utterances per unit of time) for children with CAS to be one-fifth to one-third that of the typically developing children. The authors preliminarily suggested the following with regard to intervention between 6 and 20 months.

1. If a child is at high risk for CAS, focus on babbling (CVCV, VCVC, etc.) at 6–12 months.
2. After 14–16 months, consider increasing the child's use of velar and glottal phonemes.
3. After 14–16 months, consider increasing the child's use of fricatives and glides.
4. By 19–20 months, voiceless sounds should be evident and more than 20% of the child's productions.
5. Target phonemes should include: /h/, /k/, /w/, /j/, fricatives.

Independent and relational analysis

Stoel-Gammon (1988) considered that an analysis of a child's phonology should involve an independent analysis and a relational analysis. As a *mnemonic we* can conceptualise the *independent analysis* as a handful of inventories and the *relational analysis* as a handful of percentages. The analyses are based on data from a single-word (SW) and conversational speech (CS) sample, of around 200 words if possible. In recording results, it is important to differentiate between what was found in the SW sample on the one hand, and what was in the CS sample on the other.

For Stoel-Gammon, a completed independent and relational analysis includes:

1. What the child attempted to produce (an independent analysis of adult forms).
2. What the child actually produced (an independent analysis of child's corpus).
3. What was produced correctly by the child (a relational analysis).
4. What was produced incorrectly by the child (a relational analysis).

5. The nature of the child's incorrect productions (a phonological process analysis and other errors).
6. The extent (percentage of occurrence) of phonological processes and other errors.

Independent analysis: The independent analysis is a view of the child's unique system without reference to the target (adult) phonology. It consists of a consonant inventory; vowel inventory; syllable-word shapes or phonotactic inventory; and a syllable–stress patterns inventory.

By ascertaining what is *not* present in the sample, the examiner develops an account of vowel and consonant inventory constraints (absent phones and phonemes); positional constraints (e.g., a sound such as /k/ might not occur word initially in CVC words like *cap*, although it occurs word finally in CVC words like *pack*); sequential or phonotactic constraints (the C and V combinations that the child does not use); and syllable stress pattern inventory constraints (e.g., the child might use strong–weak word stress (as in *dolly*) but not weak–strong (as in *mistake*). Note that in tonal languages an independent analysis of the tones present and absent would also be conducted.

Relational analysis: The relational analysis is a normative comparison that looks at the child's system relative to an idealised version of the target (adult) phonology, as it would be with each sound said 'perfectly' and comprises:

- PCC in SW and CS;
- percentage of vowels correct (PVC) in SW and CS; and
- phonological processes in SW and CS expressed as percentages of occurrence.

Combining elements of SODA analysis (described in Chapter 1) and place-voice-manner (PVM) analysis (Hanson, 1983; Table 2.5), production errors or mismatches between the child's realisations and the adult target (or 'standard sound') are identified by sound class and position within words.

Errors are described in terms of patterns (e.g., using the HAPP-3, Hodson, 2004), phonological processes (e.g., via the ALPHA-R, Lowe, 2000), DEAP (Dodd et al., 2002), KLPA-2 (Khan & Lewis, 2002), GFTA-2 (Goldman & Fristoe, 2000), or PACS (Grunwell, 1985), or phoneme collapses (via the SPACS, Williams, 2003), depending on the clinicians' theoretical orientation and the assessment needs of the child, and, in the clinical reality also, depending on the test instruments available. In tonal languages a relational analysis of tones would be included as required.

Table 2.5 Place–voice–manner (PVM) chart for PVM analysis

	Manner	Voicing	Bilabial	Labiodental	Interdental	Alveolar	Palato-alveolar	Palatal	Velar	Glottal
			Labial			**Coronal**			**Dorsal**	
Obstruents	Stop	Voiceless	p			t			k	ʔ
		Voiced	b			d			g	
	Fricative	Voiceless		f	θ	s	ʃ			h
		Voiced		v	ð	z	ʒ			
	Affricate	Voiceless					tʃ			
		Voiced					dʒ			
Sonorants / Liquid	Nasal	Voiced	m			n			ŋ	
	Lateral	Voiced						l		
	Rhotic	Voiced						ɹ		
	Glide	Voiced	w					j	w	

Source: Available from www.speech-language-therapy.com/images/pvmchart.png
Obstruent: A consonant formed by obstructing outward airflow, causing increased air pressure in the vocal tract.
Sonorant: A vowel or a consonant produced without turbulent airflow in the vocal tract. A sound is sonorant if it can be voiced continuously at the same pitch.

Dr. Carol Stoel-Gammon joined the Speech and Hearing Sciences faculty at the University of Washington in 1984 and has a PhD in Linguistics from Stanford University; she became an ASHA Fellow in 2005 and is currently a Professor Emerita at the University of Washington. Her many research interests include linguistic and early linguistic development, cross-linguistic studies of phonological acquisition, early identification of speech and language disorders, phonological acquisition in children with speech and language disorders, relationships between phonological and lexical acquisition, effects of hearing loss on phonological development and phonological development of children with Down syndrome. In her reply to Q9, she considers the practical realities for the SLP/SLT in administering an appropriate, effective and efficient speech assessment when time is limited.

Q9. Carol Stoel-Gammon: Speech data collection and analysis

As Masterson, Bernhardt and Hofheinz (2005) wrote, 'efficient treatment depends on many factors, one being a valid and reliable assessment from which to derive a treatment plan. Conversational data are potentially representative of a client's everyday speech and in that regard are an ecologically valid basis for planning effective and efficient treatment. A clinician-controlled single-word sample, in comparison, may not elicit a client's typical speech production patterns'. Taking into account the unavoidable trade-off between the available time and choosing an appropriate sampling and analysis methodology, how would you guide a clinician with just 1 hour in which to administer a speech assessment for an unintelligible preschooler and 1 more hour to complete the analysis? How can the 2 hours be best spent?

A9. Carol Stoel-Gammon: Assessment of the speech of an unintelligible preschool child

Meet 'Brett', 4;9, referred by his preschool teacher, who is concerned because she has rated his intelligibility at just 50%. His parents, 'John' and 'Vicki', have little difficulty understanding his speech, but are anxious to act on the teacher's concerns because even close relatives often need them, or Brett's sister 'Dorothy', 3;6, to interpret for them. Brett has received no previous SLP/SLT assessment or intervention when he becomes acquainted with 'Eric', the new graduate SLP/SLT who has just 1 hour to gather speech assessment data and related information. Sensibly, Eric has assigned Brett an early morning appointment, hoping that he will be fresh enough to perform well. Dorothy is at preschool and Brett is reassured to have both parents in the unfamiliar clinic room during the assessment, observing, participating and responding to Eric's questions and clarification requests when Brett is difficult for *him* to understand.

Eric has already viewed Brett's normal audiogram and tympanogram, read the teacher's brief report and reviewed the family's responses to a case history questionnaire mailed to them 3 weeks previously and returned a few days ago. He knows that Brett: (a) is reserved at preschool, seldom talking with peers; (b) shows frustration on the rare occasions that family members ask him to repeat himself, usually responding crossly with 'never mind'; (c) is sometimes teased by older neighbourhood children because he says *bwett* for *Brett*; (d) relies on Dorothy to interpret his wishes at times; (e) is a happy, confident boy in general, with good athletic skills and is eager to speak more clearly.

The first 30 minutes of the consultation comprised the case history interview, an unremarkable (but nonetheless essential) oral muscular examination and conversing with

Brett to establish rapport and gain an initial impression of his communication skills. The history uncovers nothing of note. Language development is age appropriate and there are no indications of CAS or dysarthria. Rather, everything points to phonological impairment with the possibility of both phonemic and phonetic issues.

Like many SLPs/SLTs, Eric is equipped with a good-quality audio recorder, but does not have video. He has assembled a suitable standardised articulation and phonology assessment (such as the *HAPP-3*, the *GFTA-2* or *DEAP*) and books, games and toys to tempt Brett to talk, so that Eric can gather SW and spontaneous CS samples, imitated utterances and intelligibility and stimulability data. It is important to note that a CS sample is essential in speech assessment, providing information that is unavailable from an SW articulation test. Analyses of aspects of these data will occur within the assessment hour, and, if required, Eric will do additional analyses later.

In my view, the most important parts of the assessment are twofold: first, the data collected should reveal the general nature of Brett's speech production patterns; second, the analyses should provide a basis for a treatment plan. Although the clinician may not be able to determine the precise substitution and deletion patterns for each phoneme of English, the data should show Brett's phonetic inventory in terms of sounds and syllable/word structures; voice quality; prosodic features; consistency of productions at the segmental and word levels; and his stimulability for absent sounds and syllable and word structures.

CS sample

Potentially, the spontaneous speech sample, gathered and recorded over 10–15 minutes, will bring to light Brett's: (1) 'everyday' language abilities in terms of mean length of utterance (MLU) and vocabulary; (2) production patterns in terms of speech rate, phrasal intonation and fluency; (3) ability to perform revisions and repairs; and (4) overuse, if any, of a particular phoneme in running speech, a phenomenon referred to 'systematic sound preference' (Grunwell, 1985). Eric will obtain a sample of Brett's conversation with his parents and with Eric himself. John and Vicki will be asked to repeat any words Eric does not understand to facilitate later analysis. Using the clinician as a conversational partner in sampling should demonstrate how Brett responds when his (relatively unfamiliar) conversational partner does not understand him. Does he simply repeat the utterance, modify it, refuse to respond or pretend not to hear?

SW sample

In SLP/SLT contexts, the SW sample is typically drawn from a phonology or articulation test, such as the three mentioned above. The SW information it provides complements that gained from the CS sample. Because Eric knows what the intended targets are in his chosen test, he will be able to perform a relational analysis that displays which aspects of word productions do and do not match the target. Relational analysis is impossible with poorly intelligible CS samples with a high proportion of unknown target words.

Stimulability assessment

The term stimulability assessment refers to a dynamic evaluation (Strand, A45) wherein a clinician provides verbal, visual, tactile or auditory cues to determine whether the child is able to adequately produce a sound or syllable structure with clinician support and scaffolding (Glaspey & Stoel-Gammon, 2007; Miccio, A23). Having first ascertained from his SW and CS data Brett's sound and syllable structure constraints (absent phonemes and phonotactic combinations), Eric will determine whether Brett can produce, with support, his missing consonants and vowels in isolation, and consonant phonemes in at least two syllable positions (e.g., initially and finally).

Consistency assessment

Consistency of production refers to the degree to which the pronunciation of a word (or sometimes a phoneme) remains the same across various productions (Stoel-Gammon, 2007). To assess variability, Eric will have Brett repeat five or six words, produced in error in the SW sample, several times. Then, to determine any effects of utterance length on consistency of production, he will elicit words (both those in error and those produced accurately) in increasingly complex environments. (e.g., by having Brett imitate *ball, basketball, basketball player*, and *big basketball player*).

Analysing these data

The time needed for analysis rests on several factors, including Eric's transcription skills, his familiarity with the analysis measures, and the intelligibility of the sample, but it should be 'doable' within an hour if the SLP/SLT is experienced. Following steps 1–5 below can streamline the procedure.

1. **SW relational analysis**

    Let us assume that Eric has gathered and transcribed, online, using broad transcription and a few helpful diacritics, 45 known words. He will check his online transcriptions against his audiotape and make necessary corrections and additions and then compare Brett's productions with idealised adult targets, in *relational* analyses that will provide numerical measures of accuracy. The quantitative measures of Brett's produc-

tions thus gained will be: (a) PCC, (b) PVC and (c) percentage CV structure correct. The latter measure allows Eric to quantify the degree to which segment and syllable deletions occur in Brett's speech. In addition, Eric examines the *nature* of Brett's errors in terms of error patterns (often referred to as phonological processes). The error analysis allows Eric to see whether Brett's errors resemble those of younger, typically developing children or are disordered or idiosyncratic. Taken together, these relational measures will give Eric an idea of Brett's accuracy levels in elicited SW productions and of his error types. He will also examine the accuracy of polysyllabic words, including stress placement, using the words and phrases from the consistency assessment.

2. **SW independent analysis**

    Now Eric will focus exclusively on Brett's productions without reference to the adult target. Using a checklist, he simply notes the presence or absence of certain sound classes and syllable structures. The checklist is based on responses to the following seven questions, and they relate to Brett's word productions regardless of accuracy of pronunciation. Does the single-word sample include: (1) Stops at three places of articulation? Voiced and voiceless stops? (2) Nasals at three places of articulation? (3) Voiceless and voiceless fricatives and/or affricates, and how many of each? (4) Liquids? (5) Closed syllables? (6) Consonant clusters? (7) Three-syllable words? From this analysis, Eric will be able to determine the number and diversity of consonants and word structures Brett produces in SW productions.

3. **CS analysis**

    Now Eric listens to the CS sample, glossing (i.e., writing down the words) 50–70 fully or partially intelligible utterances, half from the Brett–parent conversation and half from the Brett–Eric one. He will also record the number of unintelligible (to him) utterances. By dividing the intelligible utterances by the total utterances and multiplying by 100, Eric gains an idea of Brett's percentage of intelligible utterances in CS. If Brett produces full sentences, yielding a relatively high MLU, a sample of 50 partially or fully intelligible utterances will suffice. One-word responses such as 'yes' and 'no' should not be included in the utterance count, as they provide little information about Brett's phonological system.

After glossing, Eric listens once again to portions of the CS (about 100–120 utterances in all) and uses the checklist above to determine presence/absence of the sound classes and word structure forms in Brett's spontaneous speech. This independent analysis will be based on both intelligible and unintelligible utterances, and accuracy of production is not considered. In addition, Eric rates the 'normalcy' of Brett's voice quality, speech rate, lexical stress patterns, sentence rhythm and prosody (Skinder-Meredith, A43), noting any systematic sound preferences.

4. **Comparing the SW and CS analyses**
    The final step in Eric's analysis (and this should be considered a 'first pass' or 'overview') is to determine how Brett's SW and CS production patterns compare. In many cases, particularly for children who have received SLP/SLT intervention for their speech, SW phonetic inventories are relatively large, word structures are fairly complex and accuracy of pronunciation may be quite good. In contrast, CS may be characterised by simple CV syllable structures and limited consonant and vowel inventories.

5. **Looking further**
    The procedures outlined above can provide a broad, rather than deep, understanding of Brett's speech. If, for example, the assessment indicated that Brett had particular problems with vowels and multisyllabic words, Eric would later use relevant, more in-depth instruments to gain a more fine-grained analysis. It must be acknowledged that many published SW articulation tests do not assess all the vowels of English (discussed in Stoel-Gammon & Pollock, 2008) and even fewer assess words of more than two syllables; therefore, a full understanding of difficulties in these areas is only possible via additional assessments.

Interpreting the analyses

Now Eric must interpret his findings carefully in order to plan an effective and efficacious program of treatment. Speculatively, possible outcomes of the analysis and potential treatment approaches are summarised in the following three scenarios.

Scenario 1

Brett exhibits small SW and CS consonant and syllable structure inventories, and consequently a low PCC, low percentage of word structures correct, and of course, limited intelligibility. Accordingly, Eric thinks fast and considers treatment that focuses on phonetic inventory expansion, across place and manner classes and across syllable structures.

Scenario 2

SW and CS comparisons indicate high PCC scores for Brett's SW productions but a low PCC for spontaneous speech. Eric decides that the focus of intervention must be on transferring Brett's abilities in single words to running speech, and he talks to John and Vicky about how they can help with this generalisation.

Scenario 3

Brett's SW and CS phonetic inventories are large, and he has a good range of word structures, but he has low accuracy in terms of segments and word structures and is highly inconsistent. So Eric sets about developing an intervention program to stabilise Brett's productions and encourage segmental and structural accuracy.

Summary

The key points of this assessment are as follows:

1. Assessment data gathering should be broad based, examining productions in a variety of imitated, elicited and spontaneous contexts: single words, spontaneous speech, word repetitions and words/phrases produced with and without clinician support.
2. The analysis should involve both relational and independent approaches and focus on a variety of parameters: segmental accuracy; nature and consistency of segmental errors and word structure errors; vowel inventory and vowel accuracy; presence/absence of sound classes and word structures; stress at the word and sentence levels; and rate, rhythm and intonation patterns of spontaneous sentence productions.
3. The assessment procedures identified will provide a broad overview of Brett's speech. The time needed for analysis is reduced by the use of a checklist approach. Once preliminary analyses are completed and areas of concern are identified, additional assessments should be performed, as needed.

Summarising these assessment data

The sheer volume of analysed data collected from more talkative children can be overwhelming, but there is a range of ways to organise them to pro-

vide a quick but detailed overview of a child's speech. For example, Baker (2004) offers a practical four-page phonological analysis summary and management plan, and in the same volume there is a user-friendly assessment of vowels summary (Watts, 2004).

Intervening early

The question of 'how young is too young?' for speech assessment and intervention, or to put it more positively, 'how old is "old enough"?' frequently arises. Who better to explore this issue than the co-author of the *Toddler Phonology Test* (McIntosh & Dodd, 2011)?

Dr. Barbara Dodd is honorary research professor at four Australian universities and continues to be involved in student clinical supervision, teaching and research. Her interests include children's changing speech and language abilities in the areas of listening, speaking and thinking; the need for differential diagnosis of different types of SSD and the links between diagnosis and intervention approach; the evaluation of the types of research evidence available on intervention approaches; and issues in service delivery. The author of a key reference book (Dodd, 2005) and a classification system for phonological disorder, she is widely published in the peer-reviewed literature and is lead author of the *Diagnostic Evaluation of Articulation and Phonology (DEAP)* (Dodd et al., 2002).

Q10. Barbara Dodd: Management of toddlers with phonological disorder

The literature indicates that early intervention to expand lexical development and improve expressive language can enhance the intelligibility of 2-year-old children. These findings suggest that early intervention for phonological disorders might prevent a child's atypical speech output from becoming entrenched, avoiding its negative consequences for children and families. This possibility raises important clinical issues. Should individual children's speech development be measured in the context of their general language acquisition? At what age can a toddler be diagnosed as phonologically disordered? What steps can parents and clinicians take in order to identify toddlers who are at risk for phonological disorder? How can provision of clinical services for 2 year olds be justified to budget holders? What interventions might be appropriate for 2- and 3 year olds?

A10.   Barbara Dodd: Assessment and intervention for 2 year olds at risk for phonological disorder

Children utter their first word at around 12 months of age. Six months later, toddlers usually have a vocabulary of at least 50 words and by 24 months they are constructing sentences (Cattell, 2000). Nevertheless, SLP/SLT services rarely provide intervention for 2 year olds with communication disorders, except for cases of craniofacial anomaly, and sensory, neurological or cognitive deficits. Referral and intervention for most children with SSD occurs after 3 years (Broomfield & Dodd, 2005a). This conventional age of referral reflects assumptions that early assessment of speech and language is not valid or reliable and that intervention with 2 year olds is unlikely to be cost-effective (Hodson, 2011; Reilly et al., 2010). These assumptions are evaluated in the light of language acquisition research about the onset of speech disorder; the clinical evidence base concerning the benefits of early intervention; and the negative consequences of unintelligible speech for children and families. The essay is framed by the specific questions posed in Q10.

Should children's speech development be measured in terms of their general language acquisition?

The interaction between different language domains during early, typical development is poorly understood. Research usually focuses on one aspect of communication rather than delineating linguistic relationships during development. One way of exploring the issue is to consider the co-occurrence of linguistic impairments. Few of the 19% of all children who are late talkers have long-term difficulties (Whitehouse, Robinson & Zubrick, 2011). Those who do have syntactic rather than lexical or phonological difficulties (Rice, Taylor & Zubrick, 2008), and this suggests that there are different developmental trajectories for specific domains of language. In contrast, an incidence survey indicated that around 20% of 320 children with speech impairment also performed poorly on measures of syntax, vocabulary or pragmatics (Broomfield & Dodd, 2004b). Co-occurrence of speech and language disorders might affect natural history of phonological impairment and response to therapy (Wren, Roulstone & Miller, 2012).

The nature of the interaction between speech and language can be explained in at least two ways. One causal factor might affect more than one aspect of language (e.g., deprived language learning environment, fluctuating hearing loss). Alternatively, a domain-specific deficit might affect other aspects of language. For phonology, children who delete word final consonants fail to mark tense, plurality and possession, and this can result in misdiagnosis of specific language impairment (SLI). Children with highly unintelligible speech adopt strategies to enhance communication such as use of generic words (e.g., man) rather than specific terms (e.g., judge) and short MLU (Dodd, 1995). Until research describes the developmental relationship between phonology and other aspects of language, the issue might be considered from a clinical perspective. One randomised control trial (Broomfield & Dodd, 2005b) indicated that children with dual speech and language diagnoses did as well in intervention targeting their specific subtype of speech difficulty as children with isolated speech impairments. Current understanding, then, supports a focus on speech development, rather than general language acquisition. If verbal language is being produced, the question is whether parents and clinicians are able to identify children with difficulties.

At what age can a toddler be diagnosed as phonologically disordered?

Few studies provide reliable predictive data identifying early clinical markers for emerging language disorders (Paul & Roth, 2011). Nevertheless, toddlers identified as typically developing have been shown to maintain those skills, implicating the following measures as possible risk indicators: receptive language, joint attention and consonant inventory (Watt, Wetherby & Shumaway, 2006). While speech characteristics (e.g., limited word imitation, restricted phoneme repertoire) are significant markers for early identification of language learning difficulties, speech disorder is not considered in recent reviews (Crais, 2011; Paul & Roth, 2011).

This is surprising given previous research. One case study (Leahy & Dodd, 1987) charted the development of phonological disorder from 21 months, when AJ's mother started regularly tape-recording her speech. AJ's phonological system was characterised by bizarre error patterns (e.g., bilabial fricatives marked many consonant clusters) that were apparent at 21 months and persisted unchanged until initial clinical assessment at 3;8. Thirteen fortnightly phonological con-

trast intervention sessions resulted in AJ's phonology being age appropriate by 4;2.

Further, 2 year olds' typical phonological development is well described (e.g., McIntosh & Dodd, 2008) with Baker and Munro (2011) reviewing procedures for identification of 2 year olds with phonological difficulties. There are also standardised assessments. The Goldman-Fristoe Test of Articulation (Goldman & Fristoe, 2000), a 34-item picture-naming test, has norms for 2 year olds' PCC. In contrast, the Toddler Phonology Test (McIntosh & Dodd, 2011) relies on a qualitative measure to identify 2 year olds at risk of phonological disorder at 3 years.

What steps can parents and clinicians take in order to identify toddlers who are at risk for phonological disorder?

The early language in Victoria study evaluated parental descriptions of their children's speech sound production (Ttofari Eecen, 2011). The results indicated that neither parental description nor clinical assessment of speech sound production at 8 or 12 months predicted SSD 4 years later. While parents could identify 2- and 3-year-old children as typically developing (i.e., few false positive identifications of SSD), they were unable to identify children whose development was atypical (i.e., many false negative judgements). Perhaps parents are unwilling to recognise speech difficulties in very young children. Early intervention, however, is dependent upon valid and reliable early identification of speech disorder, indicating a need for a formal assessment that identifies toddlers at risk for speech disorder.

Most studies describing 2 year old's phonology include few subjects, focus on narrow age bands and assess a limited range of speech behaviour (McLeod & Bleile, 2003). While individual differences in toddlers' developmental trajectories might account for variation in word shapes, phonetic repertoires and error patterns observed, the wide range of data sampling methods contributed to the discrepancies reported. Nevertheless, there was consensus that 2 year olds produce multisyllabic words, predominantly using a CVC syllable shape although 30% of clusters are realised. PCC findings for 2 year olds ranged from 69.2 to 86.2 with phonemes identified as absent from their phonetic repertoires being: /v tʃ dʒ θ ð ŋ ɹ ʒ z ʃ l/. The predominant error patterns reported were cluster reduction, weak syllable deletion, assimilation, stopping, fronting of velars and palatals, gliding and consonant deletion. These data suggest that standardised assessment of 2-year-old speech might have predictive power.

Toddler phonology test

The *Toddler Phonology Test – TPT* (McIntosh & Dodd, 2011) consists of 37 target words derived from 31 pictures of the *Diagnostic Evaluation of Articulation & Phonology* (*DEAP*, Dodd et al., 2002). The target words, selected from age of acquisition norms (Morrison, Chappell & Ellis, 1997), include both mono- and multi-syllable words, test a range of syllable structures, most English phonemes and 17 two-element consonant clusters. The *TPT* was standardised in the United Kingdom and Australia on representative populations of children (*N*=364), including a group of 30 toddlers exposed to English as an additional language. Each child's picture naming was transcribed online using the International Phonetic Alphabet, allowing both quantitative (PCC and PVC) and qualitative measures (number and type of atypical errors, phoneme repertoire). Atypical errors are those not produced by more than 10% of the normative samples (e.g., initial consonant deletion: [u] *shoe*; backing: [hæk] *hat*).

Any assessment for the early identification of speech difficulty needs to be sensitive and has strong predictive validity. Toddlers may be unintelligible because of developmental speech errors, but this does not mean that they are at risk for speech disorder (McIntosh & Dodd, 2008). The Australian standardisation of the *TPT* indicated that its quantitative data had poor predictive validity. All five children performing below the normal range on the *TPT*'s *quantitative* measures at first assessment performed within normal limits on the *DEAP* (Dodd et al., 2002) when they were three. The *TPT*'s *qualitative* data, however, was predictive. Children making a high number of atypical errors at age two, also made many atypical errors at age three, and had PCC scores below typical expectations. The predictive validity for the UK standardisation (McIntosh & Dodd, 2011) reassessed 22 randomly selected children 12 months after initial testing on the *TPT* on the *DEAP*, when they were aged between 38 and 48 months. There was no correlation between the two assessments on quantitative measures (PCC, PVC), suggesting that severity measures at 2 years of age do not predict emerging speech difficulties. Of the 22 children in the longitudinal sample, seven made five or more atypical errors. Those seven children performed significantly less well on PCC 1 year later than the 15 children who had made fewer than five atypical errors. To confirm that finding, four children who had made 10, 12, 27 and 47 atypical errors at their first assessment, and could be contacted, were reassessed on the *DEAP*. All four were identified as having disordered phonology. One had an inconsistency score of 70%; the other three used atypical error patterns consistently.

In summary, 2-year-old children can be reliably identified as at high risk for speech disorder. The measure that predicted phonological disorder was the number of atypical phonological errors made. Severity measures, like PCC and PVC, were *not* useful predictive indicators of phonological impairment. It is, however, not yet possible to detect phonological delay at age 2;0 (i.e., using error patterns typical of a younger toddler) as there are no normative data for less than 2 years.

How can the provision of clinical services for 2 year olds be justified?

Law, Reilly and Snow (2013) argue that services for paediatric communication disorder should focus on primary prevention, through public health programs responding to whole populations' social needs. Head Start (US) and Sure Start (UK) are cited as early intervention public health programs that successfully addressed communication, preventing disorder from becoming established and its negative sequelae developing. If this model were adopted, clinicians might identify toddlers who would benefit from intensive intervention. Early focus on phonology might avert the social, behavioural and academic (especially written language) disadvantage associated with persisting unintelligible speech (McCormack, McLeod, Harrison & McAllister, 2010). For example, a meta-analysis indicated that early intervention improved educational (school completion) and social (lower arrest rates for juvenile crime) outcomes at 20 years for people from low SES backgrounds (Reynolds, Temple, Robertson & Mann, 2001). The cost of unintelligible speech to individuals, families and society is a persuasive argument.

What type of intervention is appropriate for 2;0–3;0-year-old children?

Several intervention strategies are documented for toddlers with communication impairments.

Lexical intervention

Girolametto, Steig Pearce and Weitzman (1997) examined the effect of lexical intervention on the phonological development of 25 toddlers, aged between 23 and 33 months who were at the single-word stage and diagnosed as late talkers. Half the participants were randomly assigned to an intervention group and half to a non-treated control group. Parents of toddlers in the intervention group were 'trained to employ frequent, highly concentrated presentations of target words without requiring responses' (p. 338). Toddlers receiving intervention acquired a greater variety of complex syllable shapes, expanded their speech sound inventories and marked more word initial and final consonants. As expected, these qualitative changes were not reflected by PCC, given toddlers' developmental errors.

Parent administered language intervention program

A randomised controlled trial (Buschmann et al., 2009) evaluated a parent-based language intervention group program for 25 month olds with expressive SLI. The participants, who had no receptive language or non-verbal cognitive deficits, were randomly assigned to an intervention ($n = 29$) or a no-treatment ($n = 29$) group. Mothers of toddlers in the intervention group attended the Heidelberg Parent-based Language Intervention. Seven-two-hour sessions over three months, plus one three-hour session six months later, focused on enhancing interaction by following the child's lead, language modelling and shared picture book reading. Re-assessment was blind to group membership. At 3 years, 75% of the intervention group showed age-appropriate expressive language compared to 44% of the no-treatment group. Only 8% of the intervention group versus 26% of the control group met criteria for SLI, indicating that the program significantly reduced need for later treatment.

Targeting executive function: Cognitive linguistic therapy

None of the approaches described were developed to specifically target the ability to acquire understanding of a phonological system: its contrasts and phonotactics. Yet it is this knowledge, reflected by number of consistently used atypical errors, which best predicts phonological development (Dodd & McIntosh, 2010). Phonological contrast therapy explicitly teaches contrasts to eliminate error patterns such as 'backing' and to establish legal syllable structure phonotactics (e.g., in English /ŋ/ and /ts/ cannot occur word initially). Most young children spontaneously derive these phonological rules, rarely producing illegal sound combinations. Perhaps the best intervention for toddlers making atypical errors would be to target the ability to derive phonological rules.

Holm and Dodd (2011) compared two groups of 4–5-year-old children exposed for eight weeks to 45-minute, twice weekly, intervention sessions at school, with daily follow-up activities. The 'phonological contrast' group (N = 10) received minimal pairs therapy targeting consistently used atypical error patterns. The 'rule group' (N=10) received the same amount of therapy, delivered identically, targeting the ability to abstract non-verbal and verbal rules and to apply those rules in untaught activities. Each session was split into three 15-minute segments where the rule-governed nature of the activities was made explicit, stressing 'rules' and 'patterns' and links between activities.

Planning, sequencing, sorting, pattern-focused play and activities: Patterns were initially demonstrated and explained, followed by activities requiring children to detect and describe the rules or patterns. Complexity increased over time in activities like sorting

(category, colour, size), sequencing puzzles and planning.

Language rules and word patterns: Activities focused on syntax (e.g., sequencing by tense marking), story sequencing (e.g., sequencing cards to retell a story), PA activities (e.g., finding the phonological feature that matched a picture set, such as number of syllables, initial or final sounds/clusters, rhymes).

Phonological output: Minimal pair contrasts were used to target each child's disordered processes and then dominant developmental processes.

Both groups made statistically significant improvement ($F_{1,18}$ = 95.13, $p < 0.001$) following intervention. There was no difference between the intervention groups despite the 'rule group' spending significantly less time targeting speech output. Standardised assessments showed that the 'rule group's' PA and rules abstraction abilities also improved significantly, perhaps indicating a better prognosis for literacy. Although this trial's participants were aged around 5 years, the methods might be adapted for younger children to target the suspected deficit underlying emerging speech disorder.

Summary and conclusions

Phonological disorder is apparent from speech onset. Standardised assessment allows valid and reliable identification between 24 and 36 months. Different therapy approaches have been clinically trialled, or are being developed, for toddlers with impaired speech. Consequently, it seems time to re-evaluate current practice. The current referral system fails to identify toddlers at risk; severity measures are poor markers for later speech disorder; targeting speech errors directly may not be effective; and type of intervention activities would need to change to engage toddlers. The prospect is challenging but worthwhile. It is time to reconsider the age at which speech pathologists should implement assessment and intervention for phonological disorder.

Severity measures

Having analysed and organised a child's speech data, the clinician may want to quantify severity for his or her own information; to inform parents, as part of the process of ensuring appropriate services for the child; or for insurance purposes. The issue of determining and reporting severity of involvement has exercised the research skills of Peter Flipsen, Jr. So, he seemed the ideal person to answer the question posed in Q11.

Dr. Peter Flipsen, Jr. is a Professor of Speech Pathology in the School of Communication Sciences and Disorders at Pacific University, in Forest Grove, Oregon. Widely published, he has the distinction of being third author of the seventh edition of the highly respected classic text *Articulation and Phonological Disorders* (Bernthal et al., 2013). A portion of Dr. Flipsen's current research program is devoted to examining atypical acquisition of speech sound production skills in children.

Q11. Peter Flipsen, Jr.: Measuring the severity of SSD

There appears to be considerable uncertainty about the best way to rate severity of involvement in child speech disorders, and it is also difficult to get a sense of how it is attempted in current clinical practice, and why clinicians want or even need these ratings. The findings of Flipsen, Hammer and Yost (2005) indicate that the use of impressionistic rating scales for determining severity of involvement in children with speech delay is problematic. What alternative procedures and measures have better clinical utility, and what do you see as the best 'next step' in further investigation of severity measures?

A11. Peter Flipsen, Jr.: Severity and SSD: a continuing puzzle

When we begin discussing severity of involvement, one question my students often ask is 'why do we even need to assess severity? Isn't it enough to just say that the child qualifies for services?' In some instances, it is not necessary, but sometimes it is. In an era of manpower shortages and expanding demands for SLP services, we often need to prioritize our time. Where the law permits (not in the United States), children with milder problems may be placed on waiting lists, while those with greater degrees of involvement are given higher priority for services. Severity ratings may also be of value for clinicians who try to improve their efficiency by working with children in groups with group membership often being determined by level of severity (I have not seen much evidence for the effectiveness of group interventions however). Finally, I have even heard that some insurance companies determine the amount of service they will pay for based on severity ratings (i.e., children with milder problems would be entitled to fewer treatment sessions).

When the situation demands it, my sense is that most clinicians typically rely on impressionistic severity rating scales. But as indicated in the question, such scales are problematic. In our study (Flipsen et al., 2005) we looked at ratings from a group of 10 very experienced clinicians (with at least 10 years of clinical experience working with children) and even they did not agree very well on their ratings of severity for a group of 17 children with speech delay of unknown origin. Admittedly the scale we gave the clinicians was just a set of numbers on a line with 1 being 'normal' and 7 being 'severe'. And we did not tell them what to think about – we just said 'tell us how severe you think the problem is'. Some clinicians and some of my students have since suggested that we should tell clinicians what specifically to focus on when they make their ratings. Some existing rating scales do that, but I cannot honestly say I know whether clinicians agree any more than usual with such scales. In any event, ratings obtained from rating scales may not be reliable because clinicians may simply be considering different things in their ratings. Assuming we need to focus the clinician's attention on specific things, we then have to decide what to tell them what to focus on. That was a major goal of our study. We started by identifying the clinicians who agreed the most with each other (we found six who did) and we looked at what those clinicians were considering. We looked at how their ratings correlated with a whole long list of possible severity measures. It appeared that they were considering number, type and consistency of errors at both the single sound and whole word levels. But we based our analysis on the ratings of only six clinicians, so we do not know if we cannot generalise these findings to all clinicians. Perhaps more importantly, we did not have enough data in our study to allow us to figure out whether any of the things they considered were more important than any of the others. Clearly a much larger study is needed.

Percentage consonants correct

So what is a busy clinician to do? There is not yet a definitive answer, but one measure that continues to show up in the research literature is PCC. Back in 1982, Shriberg and Kwiatkowski developed this measure and showed that it correlated very nicely with severity ratings of CS samples obtained from a much larger group of clinicians (who used the same scale as in Flipsen et al., 2005). Shriberg and Kwiatkowski (1982) showed that if PCC is less than 50%, clinicians rated the sample as severe; if it was 50–65%, they rated the sample as moderate to severe; if it was 65–85%, they rated it as mild to moder-

ate; and if it was greater than 85%, they rated it as mild. It should be noted that the samples used for the ratings were obtained from children age 4;1–8;6 (mean = 5;9), so it is not clear if these severity categories are valid for children outside this age range.

The calculation of PCC requires recording a CS sample that includes at least 200 intelligible words. It should be a conversation; it is not clear whether similar severity ratings would be obtained with narrative samples. The sample should then be transcribed using narrow phonetic transcription; it is important to use narrow transcription because the severity categories determined by Shriberg and Kwiatkowski (1982) were based on a definition of PCC which assumes that omissions, substitutions and distortions (indicated by the presence of diacritics) are all errors. If broad transcription were to be used, distortions are being ignored, and the resulting measure is actually called PCC-R (Percentage Consonants Correct – Revised). See Shriberg et al. (1997) for a discussion of different variations on PCC including measures that consider vowels. In any event, once the narrow transcription of the sample is completed, all of the consonants that were attempted should be examined and a tally made of those which are correct and those that are not (any omissions, substitutions or distortions). Here is the formula for calculating PCC:

$$PCC = (\text{# of correct consonants}/ \text{total # of consonants attempted}) \times 100$$

PCC limitations

PCC is not perfect however. One practical problem with using it clinically is that age differences are not accounted for. If two children both have a PCC score of 75%, would it really mean the same thing if one child was 3 years old and the other was 8 years old? Probably not. In addition, error types may not be the same at different ages. That 3 year old may be producing mostly omission and substitution errors, while that 8 year old may be producing mostly residual distortion errors (Gruber, 1999).

One way to get around the age question (though it does not directly address the error-type issue) would be to know how PCC normally changes with age. Normative studies do not yet exist and clearly need to be developed, but Austin and Shriberg (1996) have developed 'reference data' based on several hundred children with normal or normalized speech (who happened to have been part of various research projects). That report provides means and standard deviations for PCC over a wide range of ages. These PCC data can be freely downloaded from www.waisman.wisc.edu/phonology/bib/tech.htm and could be used by American clinicians (since the children all spoke dialects of American English) to estimate how many standard deviations the child is from their age peers. For clinicians in other countries, such reference data could be developed.

A related 'concern' with PCC is the fact that it is only valid to translate the scores into severity categories if your PCC values come from CS. I refer to this as a concern (and not a problem) only, because many clinicians still fail to assess CS. Several studies over the years (e.g., Andrews & Fey, 1986; DuBois & Bernthal, 1978; Healy & Madison, 1987; Morrison & Shriberg, 1992; Wolk & Meisler, 1998) have shown that performance in single words is usually different from performance in conversation and thus CS should probably be evaluated directly. On the other hand, Masterson et al. (2005) showed that PCC values derived from one particular single-word task were not significantly different from PCC values derived from conversational samples.

Imitative PCC

Arguments from clinicians against evaluating CS are twofold. They say they do not

have the time, and they say they are not sure they will get a good sample of all the speech sounds. In response to these concerns, Johnson, Weston and Bain (2004) developed a sentence repetition task that includes a representative sample of the consonants of English, and they showed that PCC scores on their task are not significantly different from PCC scores obtained from CS samples. Administering and scoring the sentence-repetition task is much faster than recording and transcribing CS. The task itself is shown in an appendix of their publication and includes a phonetic transcription and a formula for calculating PCC. Each sentence is read aloud to the child and as the child repeats it, the clinician simply crosses out any consonant phoneme that was not produced correctly (again any omission, substitution or distortion). Johnson and colleagues did not however, directly examine whether severity ratings would be the same on the two tasks. This probably does need to be done as the link from PCC scores on their task to PCC scores from conversation to severity rating from conversation is an indirect one at best. But if you really cannot do CS analysis, it may be a place to start.

Parents' concerns and questions

If parental involvement in SLT is a requirement, there should be a greater focus on their perceptions, needs and concerns, particularly during the early phase of their involvement... Where recognition of the parental perspective could influence future decision making and negotiation of treatment... it emerged from the parents' accounts that even where they became involved in their child's therapy, this did not lessen, in their eyes, the need for the therapist to be involved. The therapist was perceived by parents as the provider of the direction and means for therapy (Glogowska and Campbell, 2000, p. 403).

Questions parents ask

Providing satisfactory answers to questions from parents is a key responsibility for SLPs/SLTs working with children with SSD. Some of their questions are posed prior to and during the referral process. For example, the SLP/SLT may receive a call from a parent wanting to know if speech assessment is possible with a 2 year old – or 'how young is too young?' (Dodd, A10 provides guidance). Or, a parent of an adolescent or young adult might call to ask whether they have left it too late for assessment and intervention for a previously untreated speech difficulty – or 'how old is too old?' In both of these instances, the clinician would encourage the parents (or their 'older' child) to pursue speech assessment.

No matter the child's age, once the speech assessment has been carried out, parents, caregivers or the client in the case of an adolescent or young adult are provided with a report. This may be a verbal report in some cases, but often it is a written report; and in various settings, reports in writing are mandatory. The initial questions parents ask their SLP/SLT, and often *keep* asking, arising from such reports, are usually related to *severity* ('How serious is my child's problem?'), *prevalence* ('Do many children have this problem?'), *aetiology* ('What caused this problem?'), *classification* ('Is it a delay or a disorder?'), *prognosis* ('Can the problem be corrected?'), *intervention* ('What are you, or we, going to do about the problem?') and *target selection* and *goal setting* ('Where do we start working on the problem?'). Severity, prevalence and aetiology are discussed above and will be addressed briefly again here, relative to the kinds of answers clinicians can provide to families.

Questions families ask: Severity

Other than presenting them with impressionistic estimates based on experience with similar chil-

dren, there are three simple-to-use aids available to help in answering questions about severity, each of which is based on objective measures. The three: PCC, percentage of occurrence of processes or patterns and normative data can be used in combination with each other, alongside informal intelligibility ratings.

Percentage of consonants correct

While it has limitations (Flipsen, A11), PCC can be useful in providing an impression of 'severity of involvement' to parents. It is important to explain to them that not everything to do with speech impairment can be neatly classified in terms of severity, and that the severity increments (Mild–Normal, Mild–Moderate, Moderate–Severe and Severe) suggested by Shriberg (1982) for PCCs of >85%, 65–85%, 50–65% and <50% respectively, as displayed in Box 2.2, cannot be applied with children younger than 4;1 or older than 8;6.

Note also that the severity increment descriptors relate to children with SSD in general, not to specific diagnoses that fall under the SSD umbrella heading. This means that a child with a PCC below 50 can *only* be said to have a 'severe SSD'. If that same child had a diagnosis of phonological disorder, for example, it would be *incorrect* to say that the child had a 'severe phonological disorder'. Similarly, if the child had a PCC below 50 and a diagnosis of CAS it would be incorrect to say that he of she had 'severe CAS' solely on the basis of the PCC.

An advantage of using this simple scale is that it can be the basis for demonstrating progress (or lack of progress) over time, to families. As well, some children, from the age of about 4;0, particularly those who are entranced by numbers or who like to see progress represented graphically, enjoy seeing their PCCs rise and find it encouraging. Simple imagery using a drawing of a ladder, mountain, flight path or train journey (with a PCC of 50 shown at the half-way mark and 100 or thereabouts at the summit or destination and gradations between) can provide pleasure and motivation.

Percentage of occurrence of processes, or patterns

Likewise, when the occurrence of phonological patterns or phonological processes is expressed in percentage terms (e.g., Cluster Reduction 100%) in initial reporting to parents, it provides a straightforward way for them to appreciate their child's therapy gains as the percentages drop. Again, this can be conveyed to those children who are spurred on by performance feedback and extrinsic reinforcers (Lowe, A49).

Normative data

Age norms for the phonetic acquisition (Table 1.2) and typical ages of elimination of processes (Table 2.4) may be helpful for parents and can allay anxiety in those who are inclined to expect too much too soon, like the many parents who worry unnecessarily about gliding of liquids and interdental /s/ and /z/ in 3 year olds!

Informal intelligibility ratings

The speech and language therapist who by definition is an 'expert' listener may not be the best judge of a child's intelligibility overall. The views of others, including parents/carers, teachers/assistants and peers, need to be sought in order to establish a child's functional intelligibility (Speake, Stackhouse & Pascoe, 2012, p. 294).

Intelligibility ratings are notoriously unreliable, but they have considerable clinical utility. As well as being informative for parents, it can be quite a useful exercise for clinicians to ask for impressionistic ratings of intelligibility on a five-point scale from parent(s) or a significant other, such as a grandparent or preschool teacher, and

compare these with the therapist's own rating. Those doing the rating are asked, 'How intelligible is [the child's name] in day-to-day conversation. How much of what he [or she] says do *you* understand?' They then select a point on the following scale. Sometimes they will qualify their ratings, for example, by observing that the child is less intelligible when tired, unwell, or rushed, or that intelligibility often seems better when the child speaks on the telephone, and this is useful information for the clinician to have.

1. Completely intelligible
2. Mostly intelligible
3. Somewhat intelligible
4. Mostly unintelligible
5. Completely unintelligible

Reviewing the original intelligibility ratings for the child and comparing them with current ratings, once intervention is underway and progress is evident, can provide encouragement to parents, which they may convey to their child receiving therapy. Occasionally, it is enlightening to ask children how intelligible they believe they are by getting them to rate a familiar adult as a listener ('How well does dad understand your words?' and 'How well does he understand—'s [naming another child or adult] words?').

Questions families ask: Prevalence

In the United States, children with SSD comprise the largest proportion of the caseloads of school-based SLPs (Katz, Maag, Fallon, Blenkarn & Smith, 2010). Indeed, around 93% of SLPs in US schools serve children with SSD (ASHA, 2012), while 3–6 year olds who have SSD constitute 75% of the population served in preschools and other settings (Mullen & Schooling, 2010).

According to surveys conducted in the United Kingdom, some 6.5% of all children have SSD (Broomfield & Dodd, 2004) and in a 2012 study (Pring, Flood, Dodd & Joffe, 2012), 82% of surveyed paediatric SLTs served children with speech difficulties. Broomfield and Dodd reported that of 1100 children referred to a mainstream paediatric speech and language therapy service over a period of 15 months, 57.5% had phonological delay, 20.6% consistently made non-developmental errors, 9.4% made inconsistent errors on the same lexical item and 12.5% had articulation disorder; and no child was diagnosed with DVD (CAS).

Researchers who conducted a community (non-clinical) study of 1097 Australian 4–5-year-old children, McLeod, Harrison, McAllister and McCormack (2013) found that 143 of the children had parent/teacher reported speech concerns. When tested, 86.7% of the 143 had standard scores below the normal range for the PCC on the DEAP, and their consonants errors involved the late-8 acquired consonant phonemes (Shriberg, 1993b), displayed in Table 1.2.

Questions families ask: Aetiology

As discussed above, we still do not know in *precise* terms the causes of the so-called SSDs of unknown origin, but their aetiology is no longer such a mystery (Flipsen, 2002; Shriberg, 2006). In view of this, perhaps we could relinquish 'functional' in clinical settings, as it has become something of a misnomer. We can now provide parents with suggestions as to *likely* causes relative to putative aetiological subtypes (Shriberg, 2006; Shriberg et al., 2010). This is surely preferable to unsatisfactory (to parents) responses like 'We don't really know'. Current research suggests that 'functional' SSD may be due to genetic transmission of a linguistic processing deficit, middle ear disease or genetic transmission of a speech motor control deficit. Each can occur co-morbidly, in varying degrees, in the same child.

Genetic transmission of a linguistic processing deficit (60%)

The first putative cause, accounting for about 60% of referrals, is the genetic transmission of a linguistic processing deficit, expressed as a problem with speech production. There are findings to support the theory of aetiology for this group

in the form of large family studies, particularly the K.E. family study of a rare genetic disorder in the United Kingdom (Vargha-Khadem, Watkins, Alcock, Fletcher & Passingham, 1995). Exploration of the risk factors for childhood speech disorder by Fox et al. (2002) led to a finding that between 28% and 60% of children with a speech and language deficit have a similarly affected sibling or parent, or both. Family history is also commonly revealed in the day-to-day experience and informal 'genotype research' (Table 2.1) of clinicians, not only in case history taking, but also in the frequent appearance on our speech caseloads of siblings, cousins or otherwise closely related children.

Middle ear disease (30%)

In the second group, covering about 30% of referrals, are the children who have experienced or who are experiencing fluctuating ('fluctuant') conductive hearing loss, typically associated with episodic otitis media with effusion (OME), or middle ear disease (Casby, 2001). Otitis media is the most frequently diagnosed disease in infants and young children (Dhooge, 2003). Findings that have arisen from structural equation modelling techniques (Shriberg, Flipsen, Kwiatkowski & McSweeny, 2003) suggest that speech effects are most closely tied to hearing loss associated with frequent OME occurring in the 12–18 months age range (for further discussion, see Purdy, Fairgray & Asad, A52).

Genetic transmission of a speech motor control deficit (10%)

The remaining 10% are understood to have a genetically transmitted deficit in speech motor control, and in this grouping are the children with CAS. There are several on-going collaborative genetic projects around CAS aimed at developing the phenotype for this disorder. Perceptual and acoustic techniques are being used to gather, analyse and quantify affected children's and family members' speech, speech motor control and prosody.

In fact, all three putative subtypes are under active investigation by teams of researchers. The goals of this research are to understand the origins of the disorders and to support the development of assessment and treatment methods that enable consumers and SLPs/SLTs to make optimal clinical decisions for affected children. Data collection and data analysis are centred around epidemiologic, molecular genetic and speech–language data on each of the three, in the contexts of both genotype and phenotype research.

Questions families ask: Delay or disorder

Information about children's SSD is readily available online to many, but certainly not all, consumers of SLP/SLT services. Parents of children with communication difficulties are probably in a better position to 'educate' themselves about the nature and treatment of SSD than ever before. These educated consumers may present with questions not only about the terminology they encounter (see Box 2.1), but also about classification. One aspect of classification that often provokes anxiety is the question of whether their child's speech difficulty is classified as being delayed or disordered (Dodd, 2011), and this is another of David Ingram's areas of interest.

Dr. David Ingram, a professor in the Department of Speech and Hearing Science at Arizona, was introduced in the previous chapter in the preamble to A6. Here, in A12 he compares whole word measures with measures of consonant correctness and explains how these measures can be used to identify speech delay and speech disorder.

Q12.   David Ingram: Whole word measures

As measures of correct production of whole words, percentage of correct consonants (pCC) and Proportion of Whole-word Prox-

imity (PWP) differ. PCC is a measure for consonant correctness only, while PWP covers consonant correctness, consonant substitutions and vowel usage. How do the data these measures represent intersect to allow the clinician to distinguish speech delay from speech disorder?

A12.   David Ingram: Whole-word measures: using the pCC–PWP intersect to distinguish speech delay from speech disorder

Overview

Determining the severity of phonological impairment in children can be pursued across a continuum from a simple assessment of the percentage of correct consonants (pCC) to much more complex (and time consuming) analyses of phonological patterns, an enterprise requiring a background in linguistics in general and phonological analysis in particular. I have been a proponent over the years of the latter (Ingram, 1976, 1981). In more recent years, however, I have also examined ways to do insightful assessment of a much simpler nature referred to as whole word assessment (Ingram, 2002). The present discussion will be a comparison of whole word measures with the assessment of consonant correctness.

Whole word assessment involves measures that consider three aspects of the child's speech productions, that is consonant correctness, consonant substitutions and vowel usage. Notice that whole word assessment includes the consideration of *consonant correctness*, so it values the importance of this aspect of speech, but is at the same time more inclusive. When only consonant correctness is measured, differences between children regarding incorrect consonants are missed. It is possible for children to have similar rates of consonant correctness, but differ in their rate of consonant deletion versus *consonant substitution* for non-acquired consonants. In whole word assessment, children who have high rates of consonant deletions receive lower scores than children who predominantly use consonant substitutions. A similar difference can be found when *vowel usage* is considered. Children may have similar rates of consonant correctness, but differ in their use of vowels. It has been known for a long time (e.g., Ingram, 1981) that some children prefer monosyllabic words, e.g., *cat*, *dog*, while either avoiding or deleting syllables in longer words. Other children, however, do well at the production of longer words, and in some cases at the expense of consonant correctness.

These differences can be shown by taking a very simple example of four hypothetical children's productions of the word 'banana' as follows: Child 1 [nan], Child 2 [nana], Child 3 [mana] and Child 4 [bamama]. If only consonant correctness were considered, Children 1 and 2 do best with two correct consonants (67%), followed by Children 3 and 4 who have a single correct consonant (33%). When substitutions are considered, Child 4 does better than Child 3 because he or she produces three consonants rather than just two consonants. When vowels are considered, Child 2 does better than Child 1 because the former child produces two syllables rather than just one.

In summary, I have identified three aspects of a child's productions that are simple to identify and measure: consonant correctness, consonant substitutions and vowel usage. Only one of these, consonant correctness, has been commonly used in speech assessment, both in articulation tests and in the assessment of conversational samples (Shriberg, 1982). It may be that in some instances, this aspect is sufficient to gain an initial impression of speech severity. That said it takes relatively little further effort to include an assessment of consonant substitutions (versus deletions) and vowel usage. Further, these may help the SLP/SLT to identify speech patterns missed by consonant correctness alone. As will be discussed shortly, their inclusion also leads to complexity measures for both the child's productions and their target words that are lacking in assessments examining just consonant correctness. They further allow a measure of proximity between the child's words and their targets that allows for a distinction of two kinds of children with phonological disorders, a topic to be discussed after a more explicit description of the whole word measures.

PCC versus pCC

As mentioned, whole word assessment includes a measure that considers the rate of consonant correctness, using the acronym 'pCC'. This measure needs to be distinguished from the popular measure of consonant correctness referred to as PCC (or PCC-R), displayed in Table i1.1, and described in A11 by Peter Flipsen, Jr. PCC differs from pCC in at least two ways. First, PCC has been developed for use in conversational samples, not single-word assessment. The whole word measurement of pCC has not restricted its use in this manner. Second, PCC has been recommended for usage with all the tokens in a conversational sample. By contrast, my colleagues and I have used whole word assessment, for sampling lexical types and not tokens. If a lexical type (word) is used several times, the child's most typical production is used. This is an important point for it means that a comparison of studies using PCC versus pCC may show different rates of consonant correctness. No comparison of the difference, to my knowledge, has been conducted. It should be noted that these decisions to use the measures on consonant correctness in this manner are not inherent in the measures, but in the decisions on how they have been applied. Both PCC and pCC can be calculated by the same formula, described by Flipsen, Jr. (A11):

pCC/pCC
= number of consonants/total number of consonants attempted × 100

Phonological mean length of utterance (pMLU)

The central point of whole word measurement is that the assessment considers word complexity, both in terms of the complexity of the *target words* and the *child's productions*. Words are considered simple when they have a small number of consonants and vowels, and more complex when these numbers increase. The measure of word complexity begins with the target words. The complexity of an individual word is determined by the simple calculation of scoring 2 points for each consonant, and 1 point for each vowel. Since this is a measure that has the same intent for speech assessment as the calculation of MLU has for language assessment, I refer to it as the *phonological mean length of utterance* (pMLU). The formula is as follows:

$$\text{Target pMLU} = C(2) + V/W$$

(where C = number of consonants, V = number of consonants and W = number of words)

Simple words like 'cat' (two consonants and one vowel) will receive a score of 5, while a longer word such as 'banana' (three consonants, three vowels) receives a score of 9. Children using very simple words at the early stages of lexical development have Target pMLUs in the range of 3–5. These scores increase as the lexicon increases in size though no normative data are yet available.

The next step in whole word assessment is to determine the pMLU of the child's pro-

ductions. This is done similarly as in the Target pMLU by assigning points to the child's productions, in this instance using the three aspects of children's speech productions discussed earlier. Correct consonants receive two points each, while consonant substitutions and vowels receive one point each. These are then tallied and an average score is determined as done for the Target pMLU by dividing the sum of these counts by the total number of words. The formula is as follows:

$$\text{Child pMLU} = CC(2) + CS + V/W$$

(where CC = number of correct consonants, CS = number of consonant substitutions)

The Child pMLU values will be higher when rates on consonant correctness, consonant substitutions and vowel usage increase, and they will be lower when these values decrease. An example of this for a simple word would be the following productions of 'cat', [kat], [tat], [ta], which would have Child pMLU scores of 5, 3 and 2 respectively. Another example for a longer word is the four productions for 'banana' given earlier, [nan], [nana], [mana], [bamama], which would receive Child pMLU scores of 5, 6, 5, 7. Notice the discrepancy between these scores and the pCC values, where the fourth form has the highest Child pMLU score, but the lowest pCC score. It is due to examples such as these that I have recommended that whole word assessment be used in conjunction with pCC (Ingram, 2012). The target pMLU and child pMLU scores provide an idea of whether the child is both producing and/or attempting words with either high or low complexity. Along the way, a score of consonant correctness is also determined.

Whole word proximity (PWP)

Once the pMLU scores have been calculated, there is one further measure to be applied, this being the *Proportion of Whole Word*

Proximity (PWP), or more simply *Proximity*. This proportion is obtained by dividing the target pMLU into the child pMLU, measuring the closeness of child's productions to their targets. The formula is as follows:

$$PWP = Child\ pMLU/pMLU$$

The assessment of proximity for typically developing 2-year-old English speaking children has found values usually around 65% or above. Single-word examples would be 0.67 (or 67%) for 'banana' [nana] (6/9), and 0.80 (or 80%) for 'cat' [tat] (4/5). We have found these values to be somewhat higher for similarly aged Spanish-speaking children (Hase, Ingram & Bunta, 2010). Conversely, we have found Proximity score for children assessed with SSD to be lower, often at 50% or below. In Ingram and Ingram (2001), we provide a discussion of how these measures can be utilised in the planning for phonological intervention.

PCC, PWP intersect

More recently, I have been involved in two further developments in the elaboration of these measures for whole word assessment and consonant correctness. One of these improvements is the consolidation of the proximity measure and the pCC measure into a single measure referred to as the pCC, PWP Intersect. This development was the result of research conducted by Elena Babatsouli and Dimitrios Sotirpoulos in Greece who have demonstrated mathematically that pCC and PWP are in a linear relationship. A child's PCC score will predict the range of possible PWP scores. When children show high rates of consonant deletion and low vowel usage, pCC scores and PWP scores are relatively close together, though PWP will always be higher since it scores more than consonant correctness. Conversely, when children show low rates of consonant correctness, but high rates of consonant substitutions and vowel usage, the scores are much further apart.

The second development occurred when we began using the intersect measure to assess phonological samples from both typically developing children and children with SSD. It turned out (not surprisingly!) that the intersect measure was being influenced by word complexity, particularly by word length, and syllable complexity, particularly in words with consonant clusters. After much trial and error, the decision was made to divide children's words for assessment into the following four categories along two dimensions of monosyllables versus multi-syllables, and words with clusters versus words without clusters:

Monosyllabic words with only singleton Cs, e.g., 'go', 'eat', 'cat'
Monosyllabic words with at least one consonant cluster, e.g., 'grape', 'lamp' 'cramp'
Multisyllabic words with only singleton Cs, e.g., 'mama', 'ticket', 'banana', 'telephone'
Multisyllabic words with at least one consonant cluster, e.g., 'spigot', 'Aardvark'

Two patterns of acquisition based on word complexity

The following preliminary results have been found to date. First, with typically developing 2-year-old children, these categories fall into a linear relation, where words with mono-syllables tend to have higher pCC and PWP scores than words with multi-syllables, and words without clusters have higher scores than words with clusters. That is, consonant correctness correlates with word complexity, the simpler the word, the higher the rate of consonant correctness.

Second, the results obtained from analyses of children with SSD have identified two distinct patterns. For one set of children, the results are similar to those just described for young typically developing children. That is, these children show a correlation between word complexity and consonant correctness, and in this sense look like younger typically developing children. I have identified this pattern as one of *speech delay*. The second group of children, however, does not show this correlation. For this group, consonant correctness does not noticeably increase across the four categories of word complexity. For these children, their difficulty in producing non-acquired speech sounds is stable and not impacted by word complexity. I have used the term *speech disorder* for this group, since it is not the pattern found in typically developing children. Their PWP scores are influenced by the complexity of the words they produce, however, since longer words with more vowels and substitution increase PWP values. Values can also increase if cluster errors involve substitutions rather than deletions.

Concluding remarks

The results just discussed indicate the pCC assessments are good predictors of phonological acquisition for typically developing children and children with SSD who show the pattern of speech delay. The pCC assessment alone, however, is not as helpful for the children with the pattern of speech disorder, where pCC values vary little across categories of word complexity. For these children, the more inclusive whole word measure of proximity, more explicitly the impact of consonant substitutions and vowel usage within the categories.

The identification of the two kinds of speech disorders through the pCC, PWP Intersect measure also consequently has important implications for treatment assessment and intervention. For assessment, it has implications for the usage of articula-

tion tests, since such tests vary in the number of words they use across these four categories discussed. For treatment, it suggests that different goals may be necessary for the two types of children. One possibility is that children with speech delay may be more responsive to interventions based on maximal contrasts (Baker, A13; Williams, A26), while children with speech disorder may be less so. Treatment studies will be needed to examine this and other possible differences in treatment options for these two kinds of children.

The questions families ask: Prognosis

Questions about the anticipated duration of intervention (see Dodd, 2009 and Williams, 2012 on dosage and intensity of service delivery) and the eventual prognosis may be couched in a variety of ways, from 'How much treatment does my child need?' (This may sound like an enquiry about the probable cost in money and time) to a more direct, 'Will my child's speech be normal by the time he/she starts school?' and even 'Will my child's speech improve to the point that no one would know there was ever a speech difficulty?' Such questions are commonly asked early in the therapeutic engagement, often before any assessment or therapy has taken place. For most children with SSD, the outlook is optimistic (Gierut, 1998; Kamhi, 2006; Shriberg, 1997). Shriberg reported that approximately 75% of children with speech delay had normal range speech performance by the age of six (with or without SLP/SLT intervention), and that the balance (25%) normalised by nine, with just a few showing residual errors, typically involving /s/, /ɹ/ and /l/. Because we do not have robust intervention outcome data for the small CAS subgroup quite yet, statements to parents must be more guarded, but we can say that therapy for CAS has been shown to be effective even in severe cases (Jakielski, Kostner & Webb, 2006; McCabe & Ballard, A47; Strand, Stoeckel & Baas 2006).

The questions families ask: Which method do you use?

It is quite usual for parents to ask their new therapist, 'Which method do you use?' especially if they have been advised – perhaps by a non-SLP/SLT – that a particular method is desirable or even '*the* method' of choice. There is, of course, a range of evidence-based treatment approaches for SSD (Baker & McLeod, 2011) including CAS (McCabe & Ballard, A47; Strand, A45; Williams & Stephens, A46), and many commercially available resources, which range from having *ample* to *low* to *no* empirical support. These resources, including a proliferation of application software (Apps), are on the open market, and some parents buy them with a view to 'going it alone' or augmenting what an SLP/SLT puts in place (Toynton, A33).

When parents ask about the method the clinician uses, it may be an indication that they believe a 'best method' exists, a favoured 'therapy package' can be accessed or that there is a certain 'therapy kit' or manualised intervention tool that they should be seek out. For example, they may ask, 'Are you a PROMPT therapist? (Mentioning a widely practiced technique whose effects remain equivocal (Hayden, Eigen, Walker & Olsen, 2010)); or 'Do you do TalkTools?' (Naming a popularly applied but non-evidence based oral motor therapy product range); or 'Do you do auditory integration training?' (Referring to a range of controversial therapies such as *Tomatis*, *Samonas Sound Therapy*, and *The Listening Program*, that have no scientific basis, and about which ASHA (2004a) declared, in a Technical Report, 'AIT has not met scientific standards for efficacy that would justify its practice by audiologists and speech–language pathologists'); or 'Should we buy Speech Buddies?' (A currently non-evidence-based tool associated with many unsubstantiated efficacy claims, marketed to both consumers and professionals).

Some families hear about interventions that lack empirical support via the Internet, and their questions may be fuelled by statements like, 'If you feel one of your family members may benefit from PROMPT, the first thing you should do is find a PROMPT therapist' (source: www.promptinstitute.com). Similarly, 'Our resources are the best in the industry, and our products cater to every age and learning style, enabling effective treatment that parents can encourage outside of traditional speech therapy' and 'It's important that parents and children alike learn as much as they can about oral motor and speech therapy, so that together, they can experience the development and personal growth that comes with our products and resources (source: www.talktools.com/parents/). And, 'Speech Buddies are so effective that the findings were presented at the 2012 American Speech-Language-Hearing Association's conference showing that kids learn 2 to 4 times faster' (source: www.speechbuddy.com/parents/how-it-works).

Such statements lend themselves to questions like, 'Are you a PROMPT therapist?' or 'Are you a *TalkTools® therapist*?' and 'Do you use Speech Buddies?' Other parents will come armed with samples such as homeopathic tinctures, dietary supplements, or therapeutic listening CDs. Some will bring pamphlets and articles promoting various 'cure all' interventions such as craniosacral therapy (bodywork), astrological, or alternative medicine solutions, as a sure fire treatment for SSD. In general they wish to ascertain whether the clinician will cooperate with, or at least not actively oppose, their 'alternative practitioners'.

When parents ask about controversial or 'experimental' interventions a short talk by the clinician on E^3BP is rarely appropriate. My strategy has been to reframe their question as, 'What you are asking me is, "is this treatment scientific?"' and then inform clients that I am unaware of 'scientific evidence' in support of the intervention concerned, but that I will take another look to see if I am up-to-date with the available literature. If I find nothing, when I see the parent again I will tell them that, and follow up by saying 'I want ___'s speech therapy to be based in the best science', explaining in straightforward terms that SLP/SLT is a science-based profession (see Leitão, A53; Powell, A39; Stoeckel, A40 and Chapter 7, page 376 for further discussion).

Question families seldom ask: Target selection, goal setting and generalisation

Although parents commonly ask about the overall therapy approach a clinician uses, it is fairly rare for them to ask about target selection, goal setting and generalisation, except perhaps to suggest working on a particular sound or word that worries or irritates them. For example, some parents are eager to work on interdental substitutions for /s/ and /z/ or difficulties with /ɹ/ and /l/ because of issues of stereotyping and social indexing (Munson, A51). Phonological generalisation is something clinicians think about all the time—carefully choosing targets with an eye to maximal impact. The minority of parents that *do* ask may be reassured if we convey, in accessible language, that we:

- exercise clinical judgement in selecting targets (breaking 'the rules' advisedly at times);
- select targets using linguistic criteria while taking into account motivational factors;
- take into consideration attributes of the child and the parents;
- are flexible in choosing targets and feature contrasts; and
- are mindful of, and refer periodically to, the growing evidence base for explicitly principled target selection criteria (listed in Table 8.1).

One person who is interested in the impact of target selection upon phonological generalisation is Dr. Elise Baker. Elise is a speech–language pathologist and academic with The University of Sydney. She has particular interests in phonological intervention research, the conduct of evidence-based practice and the relationship between phonological and lexical learning. She also enjoys thinking about how theory informs practice and how practice can inform theory.

Q13.   Elise Baker: Complex treatment targets

The term 'phonological generalisation' refers to a change in a child's phonological system that goes beyond the treatment words or treatment (sound or structure) targets used during therapy. How can a clinician set about using theoretical concepts in phonology, such as markedness, implicational relationships, sonority and complexity to prioritise intervention targets in order to facilitate widespread change in children's phonological systems for less SLP/SLT time?

A13.   Elise Baker: The why and how of prioritising complex targets for intervention

SLPs/SLTs have a tradition of prioritising early developing and stimulable speech sounds when working with children who have a phonological impairment. Such targets are considered easier and less frustrating for children to learn. Other time-honoured criteria influencing target selection include speech sounds that are in the child's name, important to the child or family or prominent in the ambient language; and production patterns that attract teasing are unusual, highly variable or greatly affecting intelligibility. Such factors may be relevant, but the logic and principles they reflect are not necessarily grounded in an understanding of the nature of the problem or phonological theory. Consider the child who says Sue /su/ as [ɬu], shoe /ʃu/ as [ʃu] and two /tu/ as [tu]. Phonemic contrasts are preserved. The obvious target for this child is /s/. What about the child who says Sue /su/, shoe /ʃu/ and two /tu/ all as [tu]? Phonemic contrasts are lost. In this case, the child needs to learn the phonological *system* rather than an individual sound. Empirical research guided by phonological theory suggests that complex (rather than simple) targets can be an efficient means of facilitating change in children's *systems* (Gierut, 2007; Gierut & Hulse, 2010). What are *complex* targets? An appreciation of the answer to this question requires an understanding of several theoretical concepts. These definitions are cumulative. An understanding of one definition assumes you have understanding of prior definitions.

Linguistic universals

These are phonological characteristics or traits across (nearly) all languages. Universals may be *absolute* in nature, such as all languages have stops or they may be *tendencies* across many languages, such as most languages have at least one nasal phoneme (O'Grady, Archibald, Aronoff & Ree-Miller, 2005).

Markedness

Phonological characteristics that are uncommon across languages such as /θ/ are termed marked (Velleman, 1998). Universal characteristics such as stops are unmarked. Marked traits are usually more complex and later developing, like /θ/ in English. Ordinarily, a marked trait occurs in a language if its unmarked (implied) counterpart also occurs (O'Grady et al., 2005).

Implicational relationships/universals

The existence of a marked trait in a language implies the existence of the unmarked counterpart. For instance, stops and fricatives are related by implication because the existence of fricatives in a language implies the existence of stops. This next point is important because of its relevance to target selection. If a child has stops they will not, by implication, have fricatives. If a child has frica-

tives however, by implication they will have stops. What does this have to do with target selection? If a 4 year old with unintelligible speech has few stops (e.g., only /t, d, b/) and is taught the more marked trait of fricatives, then by implication this child might acquire the targeted fricatives *and* the previously absent stops. A comparable situation exists with clusters implying affricates. Clinical illustrations provided by Gierut (2007) tell of child '154' (3;2), and child '147' (3;1). Pre-treatment neither used affricates phonemically, nor produced clusters. Child 154's treatment target was /tw/. Post-treatment, this child had learned /tw/ both affricates /tʃ, dʒ/ and other clusters. Child '147's treatment target was /tʃ/ and only /tʃ/ was learned. Post-treatment child 147 'showed little to no further generalization, either to other affricates (i.e., use of /dʒ/) or clusters' (Gierut, 2007, p. 10) indicating that clusters may be the targets of choice. Which clusters? Are some clusters better targets than others? This question is difficult to answer if we use a traditional typological classification (e.g., /l, ɹ, w, s/ clusters). For instance, if we compare /pl/ and /sn/ – which cluster is more marked? While the /s/ in /sn/ is more marked than /p/ in /pl/, the /n/ in /sn/ is less marked than the /l/ in /pl/. A more helpful classification system uses sonority.

Sonority

This is a useful concept for capturing a property of a speech sound 'determined by features such as its loudness in relation to other sounds, the extent to which it can be prolonged, and the degree of stricture in the vocal tract' (Davenport & Hannahs, 2010, p. 245). Speech sounds vary in sonority – some are more sonorous than others. Consider the word *help*. If you need to say this word loudly, you would prolong the speech sound in the word that carries the most sound and has the least degree of stricture in the vocal tract – the vowel. It would not be /h/ or /p/ because they contain very little sound and cannot be drawn out or prolonged. Steriade (1990) proposed a numerical *sonority hierarchy* to capture this varying sonority in speech sounds. Most sonorous are vowels (=0), then glides (=1), liquids (=2), nasals (=3), voiced fricatives (=4), voiceless fricatives (=5), voiced stops (plosives) (=6), and finally voiceless stops (=7). When we talk, we prefer to articulate words with a rise and fall in sonority. For instance, in a word like *print* we start with the least sonorous segment (voiceless plosive) followed by liquid with the vowel at the peak, then the less sonorous nasal, finally falling to the least sonorous voiceless stop. It would be unnatural to say [rpɪtn]. This rise-then-fall tendency is called the *sonority sequencing principle*. Consonant clusters varying according to their degree of rise towards the vowel (for syllable-initial clusters) or fall away from the vowel (for syllable-final clusters). For instance, /tw/ has a large rise from plosive to glide (i.e., /t/ → /w/) while /sl/ has a small rise from voiceless fricative to liquid (e.g., /s/→ /l/). Using the numerical values from the sonority hierarchy, consonant clusters can therefore be grouped according to their *sonority difference scores* (Ohala, 1999). Onset clusters with a small score have a small rise while onset clusters with a larger score have a larger rise. For example, /kw/ (7–1) has a sonority difference score of 6, while /fl/ (5–2) scores 3. Gierut (1999) predicted that consonant clusters with small sonority difference scores would be more marked than clusters with larger sonority difference scores, because of the natural tendency to start syllables with a bang and end with a whimper (Gussenhoven & Jacobs, 2011). Classifying clusters according to sonority difference, Gierut (1999) confirmed that those with small sonority difference scores (e.g., /fl/, scoring 3) were indeed more marked than consonant clusters with larger sonority difference scores (e.g., /tw/ scoring 6). For example, Child 6

(3;8) detailed in Gierut (2007) produced no clusters prior to intervention for /bl/. Following intervention the child acquired /tw, kw, pl, bl, sw, fl, sm, sn, sp, st/ in addition to varying but improved production of: /f, v, θ, ð, s, z, tʃ, h, l, ɹ/. Child 2 (4;2) in the same study was taught the relatively less marked /kw/ with its larger sonority difference score. This child did not acquire clusters in response to intervention, but showed generalisation to two untreated singletons /ʃ, dʒ/. Baker (2007) reported that targeting /s/+C, specifically /sp, st, sn/, saw some children learning /s/ clusters *and* other untreated clusters (e.g., pre-treatment David used /kw/ only, while post-treatment he acquired /sp, st, sk, sm, sn, pɹ, bɹ, kɹ, bl, stɹ/). Not all of Baker's participants had such far-reaching changes, with some only learning initial /s/ clusters. Further, it was noted that the participants' pre-treatment productive phonological knowledge influenced what they learned about the phonological system. Morrisette, Farris and Gierut (2006) postulate that initial /s/+ stop 'clusters' are adjuncts, not true clusters because they violate the sonority sequencing principle. For example, /sp/ in *speak* /spik/ begins with a more sonorous sound followed by a less sonorous sound before rising to the vowel. Such adjuncts are therefore not subject to the implicational relationships among true clusters with respect to sonority. It seems that clusters with a small sonority difference of 3 like /sl, fl/ or 4 like /bl/ may better promote generalised change to singletons and clusters. Gierut (1999), Gierut and Champion (2001), and Morrisette et al. (2006) provide case evidence and target selection guidelines.

Complexity

Here we have a useful abstract concept for studying systems, the constituents of systems and how they inter-relate in organised hierarchies. The reader is referred to Rescher

(1998) for a philosophical overview of complexity. Consider a speech sound. It is part of a child's phonological system, abiding by laws (or rules) determining its relationship with the other sounds and structures (e.g., syllables, word shapes and stress patterns). It has a relative complexity status being either more or less complex than other system constituents. Furthermore, the phonological system interacts with other linguistic and cognitive systems. A metaphor illustrates what this means for selecting intervention targets. Elbert (1989) suggested that the phonological system is a puzzle children solve as they learn to talk. Imagine a jigsaw puzzle depicting an elephant on bare, dry ground. Some puzzle-pieces are 'complex', containing more information about the bigger picture. They also have more spaces where other pieces can attach. A child with a severe phonological impairment characterised by a limited phonetic inventory may have a few puzzle-pieces depicting dry ground, though they are unhelpful in informing the bigger picture. Upon receiving an informative or 'complex' puzzle-piece: the elephant's head and trunk, say, the child possesses important bigger picture information, enabling quicker, more efficient completion of more parts of the puzzle than would be possible had they received another less informative puzzle-piece. Using the basic tenets of learnability theory, Gierut (2007) argues that to learn the system efficiently, children with phonological impairment must be taught complex parts of the system (i.e., informative puzzle-pieces) beyond what they have already learned. This idea is not limited to child phonology.

The benefit of preferring complex targets rather than simpler targets is apparent in other language domains including syntax (Thompson & Shapiro, 2007) and semantics (Kiran, 2007). In a clinical forum on the complexity account of treatment efficacy (CATE), Thompson (2007, p. 3) noted that 'while challenging the longstanding clinical notion that treatment should begin with simple structures, mounting evidence points toward the facilitative effects of using more complex structures as a starting point for treatment'. In a discussion on complex targets in the context of phonological intervention, Gierut (2001) proposed four general, evidence-based categories. A brief summary with examples follows.

1. *Complex linguistic structures:* Marked properties or structures of the phonological system are complex and have been shown to imply unmarked properties. For example, consonants imply vowels (Robb, Bleile & Yee, 1999); fricatives imply stops (Elbert, Dinnsen & Powell, 1984); affricates imply fricatives (Schmidt & Meyers, 1995); clusters (except for /sp st sk/) imply affricates (Gierut & O'Connor, 2002); and true clusters with small sonority differences imply true clusters with larger sonority differences (Gierut, 1999). See Gierut (2001, 2007) and Gierut and Hulse (2010) for helpful reviews.

2. *Complex psycholinguistic structures:* The phonological and lexical systems interact (Storkel & Morrisette, 2002). Just as the type of speech sound prioritised for intervention influences the extent and efficiency with which children's phonological systems change, so too it seems does the type of word. Characteristics of words studied to date include: word frequency, neighbourhood density, age of acquisition and lexicality (i.e., real versus non-words) (e.g., Bellon-Harn, Credeur-Pampolina & LeBoeuf, 2013; Cummings & Barlow, 2011; Gierut & Morrisette, 2010, 2012a,b; Gierut, Morrisette & Champion, 1999; Gierut, Morrisette & Ziemer, 2010; Morrisette & Gierut, 2002). Clear interpretation and clinical recommendation from this literature is currently difficult, given the diversity (and sometimes conflicting) findings. For instance, Morrisette and Gierut (2002, p. 153) suggested that 'if the ultimate goal is

to promote system-wide change in the phonology, then the best targets are likely to be high-frequency words'. This implies that sounds taught in real words may be better than sounds taught in non-words, because non-words (by nature) are low frequency (Cummings & Barlow, 2011). However, sounds taught in non-words have been associated with more widespread change relative to real words (Cummings & Barlow, 2011; Gierut & Morrisette, 2010; Gierut et al., 2010). Sounds taught in later (rather than earlier) acquired words have also been associated with greater system-wide change, regardless of word frequency status (Gierut & Morrisette, 2012a). These findings suggest that perhaps the age-of-acquisition status of a word may be 'the higher order word-level property, with word frequency being its derivative' (Gierut & Morrisette, 2012a, p. 124). Regarding neighbourhood density, sounds taught in words from low-density neighbourhoods (i.e., words with relative few phonetically similar counterparts or neighbouring words) have been associated with greater accuracy in the *treated* sounds relative to sounds taught in words from dense neighbourhoods (Morrisette & Gierut, 2002). In light of this finding, Morrisette and Gierut (2002, p. 153) suggest that 'if a desired goal of treatment is to promote change in only the treated sound, then low-density words with few phonetically similar counterparts might be the most appropriate forms to present.' What about high-density words? Can they have a positive therapeutic effect on children's phonological systems? In a study involving 10 children with phonological impairment, Gierut and Morrisette (2012b) reported that the children 'made the greatest gains in expressive phonology following treatment of frequent words from dense neighbourhoods' (p. 830). Clearly, the characteristics of words influence and interact with children's phono-

logical systems. Research is needed to disentangle and clarify the effect of the frequency, age of acquisition, lexicality and neighbourhood density characteristics of words in phonological intervention. There is also a need to discover the combined effect of such characteristics (Gierut & Morrisette, 2012a). Based on current knowledge, it would seem that if sounds in real words are to be targeted, it may be more efficient to select later developing high-frequency words, from a combination of low- and high-density neighbourhoods – to capitalize on the desire for improvement in both treated sound(s) and the wider system.

3. *Complex articulatory phonetic factors:* Stimulability reflects an individual's capacity for articulatory complexity. According to Powell (2003), as non-stimulable sounds are more complex, they should take priority over stimulable sounds to facilitate generalization to both stimulable and non-stimulable sounds. Powell, Elbert and Dinnsen (1991) provide supporting evidence. Rvachew and Nowak's (2001) research supports an alternative view: selection of stimulable sounds. Rvachew and Brosseau-Lapré (2012) also discuss the importance of phonemic perception training alongside phonetic place procedures for improving stimulability.

4. *Conventional clinical factors:* Developmentally later acquired sounds are more complex and are thought to facilitate to greater system-wide changes than earlier acquired sounds (Gierut, Morrisette, Hughes & Rowland, 1996). Sounds consistently in error, underpinned by least productive phonological knowledge, are considered more complex (Gierut, Elbert & Dinnsen, 1987). Simultaneous selection and pairing of two or more sounds that differ by major class and have maximal feature differences is more complex, facilitating greater system-wide

changes compared with targeting one sound (Gierut, 1992). For a differing view based on dynamic systems theory, readers are referred to Rvachew and Bernhardt (2010). Briefly, Rvachew and Bernhardt (2010, p. 48) found that 'children who received treatment for complex targets experienced very little gain in phonological knowledge, even for those phonemes that were directly targeted', suggesting that 'new phonological structures be introduced in such a way as to build on the child's pre-existing strengths, stabilize emerging forms, and prepare the child to actively learn from the ambient language input'.

So, how do you identify complex targets?

What follows is a brief overview of the selection of complex targets, grounded in Gierut and colleague's research. First, discover what the child knows about the phonological system they are learning through an independent and relational phonological analysis (Stoel-Gammon, A9). List any singleton consonants and clusters not used by the child. Discard stimulable, early developing, relatively less marked targets. This will probably leave just late developing sounds and clusters. Given that intervention that targets clusters can be an efficient option, scrutinise all two-and-three-element clusters. Identify clusters with small sonority differences, excluding /sp, st, sk/. Consider prioritizing three-element clusters (e.g., /skw, spl/) only if the second and third consonants in the clusters (i.e., /k/ and /w/ in /skw/) are already serving as phonemes in the child's system (Morrisette et al., 2006). If that is not an option, consider targeting consonant clusters with small sonority difference scores such as /fl, sl, ʃɹ/, again based on your analysis of the child's phonological knowledge. See Gierut (2004), Morrisette et al. (2006) and Gierut and Hulse

(2010) for helpful cases and guidelines about the identification of complex targets for children with phonological impairment. Having identified your target, consider the characteristics of the words to be used in intervention, with respect to lexicality, frequency, age of acquisition and neighbourhood density. Finally and most crucially, although target selection guided by complexity and learnability theory offers predictive insight into possible system-wide changes, the predictions do not *guarantee* a child's response to intervention. As an evidence-based clinician, it is important that you collect phonological generalisation data regularly throughout intervention to monitor progress (Baker & McLeod, 2004). Watch for changes in children's systems, not just the target(s) you have selected for intervention. Pay particular attention to the singletons and clusters previously identified as absent from the child's inventory.

This has been a brief account of the complexity approach to theoretically principled target selection, a deeper understanding of which can be gained by reading the fascinating references suggested here. Readers should also appreciate that the complexity approach is not without its critics (Rvachew & Brosseau-Lapré, 2012, p. 656). It is also one of a range of approaches for identifying and prioritising intervention targets for children with phonological impairment. See Williams' (2005) systemic approach, Bernhardt & Stemberger's (2000) constraint-based nonlinear approach, Rvachew and Brosseau-Lapré's (2012) approach based on dynamic systems theory, Hodson's (2007, 2010) cycles approach and Stackhouse and Well's (1997) psycholinguistic approach for other perspectives.

Communicating with clients

In a much-thumbed chapter on terminology, Kenneth Scott Wood wrote:

All areas of scientific study are afflicted with a certain amount of ambiguity, duplication, inappropriateness, and disagreement in the use of terms. Like other sciences, speech pathology, audiology, and the entire cluster of studies associated with the production and perception of speech have been developing over the years a terminology and nomenclature that leave much to be desired in logic and stability. Many terms and their meanings are not well crystallized because the subject matter is always changing; concepts themselves are often tentative and fluid, and many writers have liberally coined new terms whenever they felt a need to do so. This growth of speech pathology and audiology, stimulated as it has been by so many workers, has generated hundreds of terms, some of which are interchangeable, some of which have different meanings to different people, some of which are now rare or obsolete, and some of which for various reasons have had only a short literary life (Wood, 1971, p. 3).

What might Wood have made of 'prioritising complex targets', 'linguistic universals', 'markedness theory', 'the sonority sequencing principle', 'implicational relationships', 'psycholinguistic structures', 'most' and 'least' productive phonological knowledge, 'phoneme collapse' and 'constraint-based nonlinear phonology'? Onerous and confusing though it may be, technical language is essential to professions like ours. It enables us to define precisely what we are talking about, so facilitating unambiguous communication within our profession, with other professions, and, when appropriate, with consumers of our services.

Meanwhile, a crucial role for SLPs/SLTs is that of clarifying jargon for consumers, if and when they want such explanations. Conveying such information can be difficult. The information itself may be distressing; it is not an easy thing, for instance, to explain the prognostic implications of CAS or dysarthria to a troubled parent. The recipient of the information may be upset, unprepared for answers, or have difficulty absorbing, understanding or accepting them. The situation in which the information is being transmitted may be unfavourable and the available time may be too short. And the manner in which the information is conveyed may be problematic: detailed written reports, for example, with no face-to-face verbal explanation, may be alienating and too confronting for many clients.

Many of us have had the unfortunate experience of trying unsuccessfully to explain complex concepts and issues, for clients or caregivers, without misinforming them by oversimplifying the message. At the same time, we know that, for some consumers, the use of correct terminology is a sign (to them) that professionals are prepared to share information openly and respectfully without making condescending value judgements about their capacity to understand, accommodate and 'use' such information appropriately. Indeed, numerous families (and clients, if they are old enough) prefer to be told the correct name of a disorder, symptom, anatomical feature, assessment procedure or therapy technique – especially if they want to look it up.

On the other hand, the last thing many families of children with communication difficulties want when they are attempting to understand and help their child's speech development is to be inundated with incomprehensible jargon. For a lot of families, this is particularly true in the early stages of diagnosis and at times when they are anxious and troubled. They want facts, but until they are confidently engaged in a constructive program for their child, most can do without the complications of having to understand the differences between, for example, the large number of 'speech pathology words' that start with 'phon' or 'dys'! We also have to bear in mind that people deal with the information we present in different ways and at different rates. In situations where just one parent brings a child to consultations, so that the other parent receives information by proxy, it is not uncommon for the accompanying parent to reach a degree of acceptance and insight into the child's difficulties ahead of their partner. In such a situation, the parent who meets with the clinician may be more prepared to 'trust' the information being conveyed. These and other issues around terminology, classification, description, assessment and 'breaking the news' are often highlighted in our engagement with the 'special populations' of children described in Chapter 3.

References

American Psychiatric Association. (2013). *Diagnostic and statistical manual of mental disorders (DSM-5)* (5th ed., pp. 44–45). Arlington, VA: American Psychiatric Publishing.

Andrews, N., & Fey, M. E. (1986). Analysis of the speech of phonologically impaired children in two sampling conditions. *Language, Speech, and Hearing Services in Schools, 17*, 187–198.

ASHA (2004a). *Auditory Integration Training* [Technical Report]. Retrieved 15 January 2014 from www.asha.org/policy.

ASHA (2004b). *Evidence-Based Practice in Communication Disorders* [Position Statement]. Retrieved 15 January 2014 from www.asha.org/policy/PS2005-00221/

ASHA. (2004c). Preferred Practice Patterns for the Profession of Speech-Language Pathology [Preferred Practice Patterns]. Retrieved 26 April 2014 from www.asha.org/policy.

ASHA (2007). *Childhood Apraxia of Speech* [Position Statement]. Retrieved 15 January 2014 from www.asha.org/policy.

ASHA. (2012). *2012 Schools Survey Report: SLP Caseload Characteristics*. Retrieved 26 April 2014 from www.asha.org/research/memberdata/schoolssurvey/

Austin, D., & Shriberg, L. D. (1996). *Lifespan reference data for ten measures of articulation competence using the Speech Disorders Classification System (SDCS)* (Technical Report 3). Phonology Project, University of Wisconsin-Madison.

Baker, E. (2004). Phonological analysis, summary and management plan. *ACQuiring Knowledge in Speech, Language and Hearing, 6*(1), 14–21.

Baker, E. (2007). *Using sonority to explore patterns of generalisation in children with phonological impairment*. Paper presented at the Speech Pathology Australia National Conference, Sydney, Australia.

Baker, E., & McLeod, S. (2004). Evidence-based management of phonological impairment in children. *Child Language Teaching and Therapy, 20*(3), 265–285.

Baker, E., & McLeod, S. (2011). Evidence-based practice for children with speech sound disorders: Part 1 Narrative review, *Language, Speech, and Hearing Services in Schools, 42*(2), 102–139.

Baker, E., & Munro, N. (2011). An overview of resources for assessing toddlers' productions of polysyllables. *Acquiring Knowledge in Speech, Language and Hearing, 13*(2), 58–62.

Bellon-Harn, M. L., Credeur-Pampolina, M. E., & LeBoeuf, L. (2013). Scaffolded-language intervention: Speech production outcomes. *Communication Disorders Quarterly, 34*(2), 120–132.

Bernhardt, B., & Stemberger, J.P. (2000). *Workbook in nonlinear phonology for clinical application*. Austin, TX: Pro-Ed.

Bernthal, J. E., & Bankson, N. W. (2004). *Articulation and phonological disorders* (5th ed.). Boston: Allyn & Bacon.

Bernthal, J. E., Bankson, N. W., & Flipsen, P., Jr. (2013). *Articulation and phonological disorders* (7th ed.). Boston, MA: Pearson Education.

Bird, J., Bishop, D. V. M., & Freeman, N. H. (1995). Phonological awareness and literacy development in children with expressive phonological impairments. *Journal of Speech and Hearing Research, 38*, 446–462.

Bishop, D. V. M., & Adams, C. (1990). A prospective study of the relationship between specific language impairment, phonological disorders and reading retardation. *The Journal of Child Psychology and Psychiatry, 31*(7), 1027–1050.

Bowen, C. (1998a). *Developmental phonological disorders: A practical guide for families and teachers*. Melbourne: The Australian Council for Educational Research.

Bowen, C. (1998b). *Speech-language-therapy dot com*. Retrieved 15 January 2014 from http://www.speech-language-therapy.com

Broomfield, J., & Dodd, B. (2004a). Children with speech and language disability: Caseload characteristics. *International Journal of Language and Communication Disability, 39*, 303–324.

Broomfield, J., & Dodd, B. (2004b). The nature of referred subtypes of primary speech disability. *Child Language Teaching and Therapy, 20*, 135–151.

Broomfield, J., & Dodd, B. (2005a). Epidemiology of speech disorders. In: B. Dodd (Ed.). *Differential diagnosis and treatment of speech disordered children* (2nd ed., pp. 83–99). London: Whurr Publishers.

Broomfield, J., & Dodd, B. (2005b). Clinical effectiveness. In: B. Dodd (Ed.). *Differential diagnosis and treatment of children with speech disorder* (2nd ed., pp. 211–229). London: Whurr Publishers.

Buschmann, A., Jooss, B., Rupp, A., Feldhusen, F., Pietz, J., & Philippi, H. (2009). Parent based language intervention for 2-year-old children with specific expressive language delay: A randomised controlled trial. *Archives of Disease in Childhood*, 94, 110–111.

Casby, M. W. (2001). Otitis media and language development: A meta-analysis. *American Journal of Speech-Language Pathology*, 10, 65–80.

Cattell, R. (2000). *Children's language. Consensus and controversy*. London: Cassell.

Crais, E. (2011). Testing and beyond: Strategies and tools for evaluating and assessing infants and toddlers. *Language Speech and Hearing Services in Schools*, 42, 341–364.

Cummings, A. E., & Barlow, J. A. (2011). A comparison of word lexicality in the treatment of speech sound disorders. *Clinical Linguistics & Phonetics*, 25(4), 265–286.

Davenport, M., & Hannahs, S. J. (2010). *Introducing phonetics and phonology* (3rd ed.). London: Hodder Education.

Dean, E. C., Howell, J., Waters, D., & Reid, J. (1995). *Metaphon*: A metalinguistic approach to the treatment of phonological disorder in children. *Clinical Linguistics and Phonetics*, 9, 1–19.

DeThorne, L. S., Deater-Deckard, K., Mahurin-Smith, J., Coletto, M., & Petrill, S. A. (2011). Volubility as a mediator in the associations between conversational language measures and child temperament. *International Journal of Language and Communication Disorders*, 46(6), 700–713.

DfE (2012). *Statutory framework for the early years foundation stage*. Runcorn: Crown Copyright.

Dhooge, I. J. (2003). Risk factors for the development of otitis media. *Current Allergy and Asthma Reports*, 3(4), 321–325.

Dodd, B. (1995). *Differential diagnosis and treatment of children with speech disorder*. London: Whurr Publishers.

Dodd, B. (2005). *Differential diagnosis and treatment of children with speech disorder* (2nd ed.). London: Whurr Publishers.

Dodd, B. (2011). Differentiating speech delay from disorder: Does it matter? *Topics in Language Disorders*, 31(2), 96–111.

Dodd, B., Crosbie, S., Zhu, H., Holm, A., & Ozanne, A. (2002). *Diagnostic evaluation of articulation and phonology (DEAP)*. London: Psychological Corporation.

Dodd, B., & McIntosh, B. (2010). Two-year old phonology: Impact of input, motor and cognitive abilities on development. *Journal of Child Language*, 37(5), 1027–1046.

DuBois, E., & Bernthal, J. E. (1978). A comparison of three methods of obtaining articulatory responses. *Journal of Speech and Hearing Disorders*, 43, 295–305.

Eisenson, J., & Ogilvie, M. (1963). *Speech correction in the schools*. New York: Macmillan.

Elbert, M. (1989). Generalisation in treatment of phonological disorders. In: L. McReynolds, & J. Spradlin (Eds.), *Generalisation strategies in the treatment of communication disorders* (pp. 31–43). Toronto: B. C. Decker, Inc.

Elbert, M., Dinnsen, D., & Powell, T. (1984). On the prediction of phonological generalisation learning pattern. *Journal of Speech and Hearing Disorders*, 49, 309–317.

Fey, M. E. (1985). Clinical forum: Phonological assessment and treatment. Articulation and phonology: Inextricable constructs in speech pathology. *Human Communication Canada*. Reprinted (1992) *Language, Speech, and Hearing Services in Schools*, 23, 225–232.

Fey, M.E. (1992). Phonological assessment and treatment. Articulation and phonology: An addendum. *Language Speech and Hearing Services in Schools*, 23, 277–282.

Flipsen, P., Jr. (2002, May). *Causes and speech sound disorders. Why worry?* Presentation at the Speech Pathology Australia National Conference, Alice Springs, Northern Territory, Australia.

Flipsen, P., Jr., Hammer, J. B., & Yost, K. M. (2005). Measuring severity of involvement in speech delay: Segmental and whole-word measures. *American Journal of Speech-Language Pathology*, 14, 298–312.

Fox, A.V., Dodd, B., & Howard, D. (2002). Risk factors for speech disorders in children. *International Journal of Language and Communication Disorders*, 37(2), 117–131.

Gascoigne, M. (2006). Supporting children with speech language and communication needs within integrated children's services. *RCSLT position paper*. London: RCSLT.

Gibbon, F. (2013). Therapy for abnormal vowels in children with speech disorders. In: M. J. Ball, & F. E. Gibbon (Eds.). *Handbook of vowels and vowel disorders* (pp. 429–446). Hove: Psychology Press.

Gierut, J. A. (1992). The conditions and course of clinically induced phonological change. *Journal of Speech and Hearing Research, 35,* 1049–1063.

Gierut, J.A. (1998). Treatment efficacy: Functional phonological disorders in children. *Journal of Speech, Language and Hearing Research, 41,* S85–S100.

Gierut, J. A. (1999). Syllable onsets: Clusters and adjuncts in acquisition. *Journal of Speech, Language and Hearing Research, 42,* 708–726.

Gierut, J. A. (2001). Complexity in phonological treatment: Clinical factors. *Language, Speech, and Hearing in Schools, 32,* 229–241.

Gierut, J. A. (2004, Summer). Clinical application of phonological complexity. *CSHA Magazine, 6–7,* 16.

Gierut, J. A. (2007). Phonological complexity and language learnability. *American Journal of Speech-Language Pathology, 16*(1), 6–17.

Gierut, J. A., & Champion, A. H. (2001). Syllable onsets II: Three-element clusters in phonological treatment. *Journal of Speech, Language, and Hearing Research, 44,* 886–904.

Gierut, J., Elbert, M., & Dinnsen, D. (1987). A functional analysis of phonological knowledge and generalisation learning in misarticulating children. *Journal of Speech and Hearing Research, 30,* 462–479.

Gierut, J. A., & Hulse, L. E. (2010). Evidence-based practice: A matrix for predicting phonological generalization. *Clinical Linguistics and Phonetics, 24*(4–5), 323–334.

Gierut, J. A., & Morrisette, M. L. (2010). Phonological learning and lexicality of treated stimuli. *Clinical Linguistics & Phonetics, 24*(2), 122–140.

Gierut, J. A., & Morrisette, M. L. (2012a). Age of word acquisition effects in treatment of children with phonological delays. *Applied Psycholinguistics, 33*(01), 121–144.

Gierut, J. A., & Morrisette, M. L. (2012b). Density, frequency and the expressive phonology of children with phonological delay. *Journal of Child Language, 39*(04), 804–834.

Gierut, J. A., Morrisette, M. L., & Champion, A. H. (1999). Lexical constraints in phonological acquisition. *Journal of Child Language, 26,* 261–294.

Gierut, J. A., Morrisette, M. L., Hughes, M. T., & Rowland, S. (1996). Phonological treatment efficacy and developmental norms. *Language, Speech and Hearing Services in Schools, 27,* 215–230.

Gierut, J. A., Morrisette, M. L., & Ziemer, S. M. (2010). Nonwords and generalization in children with phonological disorders. *American Journal of Speech-Language Pathology, 19*(2), 167–177.

Gierut, J. A., & O'Connor, K. M. (2002). Precursors to onset clusters in acquisition. *Journal of Child Language, 29,* 495–517.

Gillon, G. T. (1998). The speech-literacy link: Perspectives from children with phonological speech disorders. *New Zealand Speech-Language Therapists Association Biennial Conference Proceedings,* Dunedin, 14–17 April 1998. Supplementary (1) pp. 1–6.

Gillon, G. T. (2004). *Phonological awareness: From research to practice.* New York: Guilford Press.

Girolametto, L., Steig Pearce, P., & Weitzman, E. (1997). Effects of lexical intervention on the phonology of late talkers. *Journal of Speech, Language, and Hearing Research, 40,* 338–348.

Glaspey, A.M., & Stoel-Gammon, C. (2007). A dynamic approach to phonological assessment. *International Journal of Speech-Language Pathology, 9,* 286–296.

Glogowska, M., & Campbell, R. (2000). Investigating parental views of involvement in pre-school speech and language therapy. *International Journal of Language and Communication Disorders, 35*(3), 391–405.

Goldman, R., & Fristoe, M. (2000). *Goldman-Fristoe test of articulation* (2nd ed.). Circle Pines, MN: American Guidance Service.

Goldstein, B. (1996). Error groups in Spanish speaking children. In: Powell, T. W. (Ed.), *Pathologies of speech and language: Contributions of clinical phonetics and linguistics.* New Orleans, LA: International Clinical Phonetics and Linguistics Association.

Gruber, F. A. (1999). Probability estimates and paths to consonant normalization in children with speech delay. *Journal of Speech Language and Hearing Research, 42,* 448–459.

Grunwell, P. (1975). The phonological analysis of articulation disorders. *British Journal of Disorders of Communication, 10,* 31–42.

Grunwell, P. (1981). *The nature of phonological disability in children.* New York: Academic.

Grunwell, P. (1985). *Phonological assessment of child speech (PACS).* Windsor: NFER-Nelson.

Grunwell, P. (1987). *Clinical phonology* (2nd ed.). Baltimore, MD: Williams & Wilkins.

Grunwell, P. (1989). Developmental phonological disorders and normal speech development: A review and illustration. *Child Language Teaching and Therapy, 5,* 304–319.

Gussenhoven, C., & Jacobs, H. (2011). *Understanding phonology* (3rd ed.). London: Hodder Education.

Hall, D., & Elliman, D. (Eds.). (2003). *Health for all children* (4th ed.). Oxford University Press.

Hanson, M. L. (1983).*Articulation.* Philadelphia, PA: W.B. Saunders Co.

Harrison, L. J., & McLeod, S. (2010). Risk and protective factors associated with speech and language impairment in a nationally representative sample of 4- to 5-year-old children. *Journal of Speech, Language, and Hearing Research, 53*(2), 508–529.

Hase, M., Ingram, D., & Bunta, F. (2010). A comparison of two phonological assessment tools for monolingual Spanish-speaking children. *Clinical Linguistics and Phonetics, 24,* 346–356.

Hayden, D., Eigen, J., Walker, A., & Olsen, L. (2010). PROMPT: A tactually grounded model for the treatment of childhood speech production disorders. In: A. L. Williams, S. McLeod, & R. J. McCauley (Eds.), *Treatment for speech sound disorders in children* (pp. 453–474). Baltimore, MD: Paul H. Brookes Publishing Company.

Healy, T. J., & Madison, C. L. (1987). Articulation error migration: A comparison of single word and connected speech samples. *Journal of Communication Disorders, 20,* 129–136.

Hodge, M. (2010). Intervention for developmental dysarthria. In: A. L. Williams, S. McLeod, & R. J. McCauley (Eds.), *Interventions for speech sound disorders in children* (pp. 557–578). Baltimore, MD: Paul H. Brookes Publishing Company.

Hodson, B. (2004). *Hodson assessment of phonological patterns* (3rd ed.). Austin, TX: Pro-Ed.

Hodson, B. (2007, 2010). *Evaluating and enhancing children's phonological systems: Research and theory to practice.* Wichita, KS: PhonoComp Publishers.

Hodson, B. (2011). Enhancing phonological patterns of young children with highly unintelligible speech. *The ASHA Leader,* April 5, 16–19.

Hodson, B.W., & Paden, E. P. (1991). *Targeting intelligible speech: A phonological approach to remediation* (2nd ed.). Austin, TX: Pro-Ed.

Holm, A., & Dodd, B. (2011). *A novel intervention for non-developmental speech disorders: Preliminary evidence.* Child Language Seminar, July, City University, London.

Howell, J. & Dean. E. (1994). *Treating phonological disorders in children: Metaphon theory to practice.* London: Whurr Publishers.

Ingram, D. (1976). *Phonological disability in children.* London: Edward Arnold.

Ingram, D. (1981). *Procedures for the phonological analysis of children's language.* Baltimore, MD: University Park Press.

Ingram, D. (1989a). *Phonological disability in children* (2nd ed.). London: Whurr Publishers.

Ingram, D. (2002). The measurement of whole word productions. *Journal of Child Language, 29,* 1–21.

Ingram, D. (2012, November). *A comparison of two measures of correctness: PCC & PWP.* Paper presented at the annual meeting of the American Speech-Language-Hearing Association, San Diego.

Ingram, D., & Ingram, K. (2001). A whole word approach to phonological intervention. *Language, Speech and Hearing Services in Schools, 32,* 271–283.

International Expert Panel on Multilingual Children's Speech (2012). *Multilingual children with speech sound disorders: Position paper.* Bathurst, NSW: Research Institute for Professional Practice, Learning & Education (RIPPLE), Charles Sturt University. Retrieved 15 January 2014 from www.csu.edu.au/research/multilingual-speech/position-paper

Jakielski, K. J., Kostner, T. L., & Webb, C. E. (2006, June). *Results of integral stimulation intervention in three children.* Paper presented at the 5th International Conference on Speech Motor Control. Nijmegen: the Netherlands.

Johnson, C. A., Weston, A. D., & Bain, B. A. (2004). An objective and time-efficient method for determining severity of childhood speech delay. *American Journal of Speech-Language Pathology, 13,* 55–65.

Kamhi, A. G. (2006). Treatment decisions for children with speech-sound disorders. *Language, Speech, and Hearing Services in Schools, 37*(4), 271–279.

Katz, L. A., Maag, A., Fallon, K. A., Blenkarn, K., & Smith, M. K. (2010). What makes a caseload (un)manageable? School-based speech-language pathologists speak. *Language, Speech, and Hearing Services in Schools. 41*(2), 139–151.

Kaufman, N. (2005). *Kaufman speech praxis workout book.* Gaylord, MI: Northern Speech Services.

Khan, L. M. L., & Lewis, N. P. (2002). *Khan–Lewis. Phonological analysis* (2nd ed.). Circle Pines, MN: American Guidance Service.

Kiran, S. (2007). Complexity in the treatment of naming deficits. *American Journal of Speech-Language Pathology, 16*(1), 18–29.

Law, J., Boyle, J., Harris, F., Harkness, A., & Nye, C. (1998). Screening for speech and language delay: A systematic review of the literature. *Health Technology Assessment, 2*(9), 1–184.

Law, J., Reilly, S., & Snow, P. (2013). Speech, language and communication need in the context of public health: A new direction for the speech and language therapy profession. *International Journal of Language and Communication Disorders, 48*(5), 486–496.

Leahy, J., & Dodd, B. (1987). The development of disordered phonology: A case study. *Language and Cognitive Processes, 2*(2), 115–132.

Lowe, R. J. (2000). *ALPHA-R: Assessment link between phonology and articulation – Revised.* Mifflinville, PA: ALPHA Speech & Language Resources.

Masterson, J. A., Bernhardt, B. H., & Hofheinz, M. K. (2005). A comparison of single words and conversational speech in phonological evaluation. *American Journal of Speech-Language Pathology, 14*, 229–241.

McCormack, J., McLeod, S., Harrison, L. J., & McAllister, L. (2010). The impact of speech impairment in early childhood: Investigating parents' and speech-language pathologists' perspectives using the ICF-CY. *Journal of Communication Disorders, 43*(5),378–396.

McCurry, W. H., & Irwin, O. C. (1953). A study of word approximations in the spontaneous speech of infants. *Journal of Speech and Hearing Disorders, 18*(2), 133–139.

McIntosh, B., & Dodd, B. (2008). Two-year-olds' phonological acquisition: normative data. *International Journal of Speech-Language Pathology, 10*, 460–469.

McIntosh B., & Dodd, B. (2011). *Toddler phonology test*, London: Pearson Publishers.

McLeod, S., Baker, E. M., McCormack, J. M., Wren, Y. E., & Roulstone, S. E. (2013–2015). A sound start: Innovative technology to promote speech and pre-literacy skills in at-risk preschoolers (DP130102545). Australian Research Council (ARC) Discovery Grant.

McLeod, S. & Bleile, K. (2003). Neurological and developmental foundations of speech acquisition.

American Speech-Language-Hearing Association Convention, Chicago, November.

McLeod, S., Harrison, L. J., McAllister, L., & McCormack. J. (2013). Speech sound disorders in a community study of preschool children. *American Journal of Speech-Language Pathology, 22*, 503–522.

McLeod, S., Verdon, S., & Bowen, C. (2013). International aspirations for speech-language pathologists' practice with multilingual children with speech sound disorders: Development of a position paper. *Journal of Communication Disorders, 46*, 375–387.

Morrisette, M. L., Farris, A. W., & Gierut, J. A. (2006). Applications of learnability theory to clinical phonology. *International Journal of Speech-Language Pathology, 8*(3), 207–219.

Morrisette, M. L., & Gierut, J. (2002). Lexical organisation and phonological change in treatment. *Journal of Speech, Language, and Hearing Research, 45*, 143–159.

Morrison, C., Chappell, T., & Ellis, A. (1997). Age of acquisition norms for a large set of object names and their relation to adult estimates and other variables. *The Quarterly Journal of Experimental Psychology, 50A*(3), 528–559.

Morrison, J. A., & Shriberg, L. D. (1992). Articulation testing versus conversational speech sampling. *Journal of Speech and Hearing Research, 35*, 259–273.

Mullen, R., & Schooling, T. (2010). The national outcomes measurement system for pediatric speech-language pathology. *Language, Speech, and Hearing Services in Schools, 41*(1), 44–60.

Nathan, L., Stackhouse, J., Goulandris, N., & Snowling, M.J. (2004). The development of early literacy skills among children with speech difficulties: A test of the "Critical Age Hypothesis". *Journal of Speech, Language and Hearing Research, 47*(2), 377–391.

Nelson, H.D., Nygren, P., Walker, M., & Panoscha, R. (2006). Evidence review for the US preventive services task force for speech and language delay in preschool children. *Pediatrics, 117*, e298–e319.

O'Grady, W., Archibald, J., Aronoff, M., & Rees-Miller, J. (2005). *Contemporary linguistics: An introduction* (5th ed.). Boston: Bedford/St. Martin's.

Ohala, D. K. (1999). The influence of sonority on children's cluster reductions. *Journal of Communication Disorders, 32*, 397–422.

Overby, M. S., & Caspari, S. (2013). *Observed early characteristics of CAS via video research.* Paper presented to the CASANA Conference, Denver, CO.

Ozanne, A. (1995). The search for developmental verbal dyspraxia. In: B. Dodd (Ed.). *Differential diagnosis and treatment of children with speech disorder* (pp. 91–109). London: Whurr Publishers.

Ozanne, A. (2005). Childhood apraxia of speech. In: B. Dodd (Ed.), *Differential diagnosis and treatment of children with speech disorder* (2nd ed., pp. 71–82). London: Whurr Publishers.

Paul, D. (2013, August 01). A quick guide to DSM-5. *The ASHA Leader*.

Paul, R., & Roth, F. (2011). Characterising and predicting outcomes of communicative delays in infants and toddlers: Implications for clinical practice. *Speech and Hearing Services in Schools, 42*, 331–340.

Pickstone, C. (2007). Triage in speech and language therapy. In: S. Roulstone (Ed.). *Prioritising child health*. London: Routledge.

Pickstone, C., Hannon, P., & Fox, L. (2002). Surveying and screening preschool language development in community-focused intervention programmes: A review of instruments. *Child: Care Health & Development, 28*(3), 251–264.

Pollock, K. E. (2013). The Memphis vowel project: Vowel errors in children with and without phonological disorders. In: M. J. Ball, & F. E. Gibbon (Eds.), *Handbook of vowels and vowel disorders* (pp. 260–287). Hove: Psychology Press.

Pollock, K. E., & Berni, M. C. (2003). Incidence of non-rhotic vowel errors in children: Data from the Memphis vowel project. *Clinical Linguistics and Phonetics, 17*, 393–401.

Powell, T. W. (2003). Stimulability and treatment outcomes. *Perspectives on Language Learning and Education, 10*(1), 3–6.

Powell, T. W., Elbert, M., & Dinnsen, D. A. (1991). Stimulability as a factor in the phonological generalisation of misarticulating preschool children. *Journal of Speech and Hearing Research, 34*, 1318–1328.

Pring, T., Flood, E., Dodd, B., & Joffe, V. (2012). The working practices and clinical experiences of paediatric speech and language therapists: A national UK survey. *International Journal of Language and Communication Disorders, 47*(6), 696–708.

Reilly, S., Wake, M., Ukoumunne, O., Bavin, E., Prior, M., Cini, E., Conway, L., Eadie, P., & Bretherton L. (2010). Predicting language outcomes at 4 years of age: Findings from early language in Victoria study. *Pediatrics, 126*, e1530.

Rescher, N. (1998). *Complexity: A philosophical overview*. New Brunswick, NJ: Transaction.

Reynolds, A., Temple, J., Robertson, D., & Mann, E. (2001). Long-term effects of an early childhood intervention on educational achievement and juvenile arrest. A 15 year follow-up of low-income children in public schools. *Journal of the American Medical Association, 285*(18), 2339–2346.

Rice, M., Taylor, C., & Zubrick, S. (2008). Language outcomes of 7-year-old children with or without a history of late language emergence at 24 months. *Journal of Speech, Language, and Hearing Research, 51*, 394–407.

Robb, M. P., Bleile, K. M., & Yee, S. S. L. (1999). A phonetic analysis of vowel errors during the course of treatment. *Clinical Linguistics and Phonetics, 13*(4), 309–321.

Ruscello, D. R. (2008). *Treating articulation and phonological disorders in children*. St. Louis, MO: Elsevier.

Rvachew, S., & Bernhardt, M. (2010). Clinical implications of the dynamic systems approach to phonological development. *American Journal of Speech-Language Pathology, 19*, 34–50.

Rvachew, S., & Brosseau-Lapré, F. (2012). *Developmental phonological disorders: Foundations of clinical practice*. San Diego, CA: Plural Publishing.

Rvachew, S., & Nowak, M. (2001). The effect of target-selection strategy of phonological learning. *Journal of Speech, Language and Hearing Research, 44*, 610–623.

Scarborough, H. S., & Brady, S. A. (2002). Toward a common terminology for talking about speech and reading: A glossary of the 'phon' words and some related terms. *Journal of Literacy Research, 34*, 299–334.

Schmidt, A. M., & Meyers, K. A. (1995). Traditional and phonological treatment for teaching English fricatives and affricates to Koreans. *Journal of Speech and Hearing Research, 38*, 828–838.

Schonweiler, R., Ptok, M., & Radu, H. J. (1998). A cross-sectional study of speech- and language-abilities of children with normal hearing, mild fluctuating conductive hearing loss, or moderate to profound sensoneurinal hearing loss. *International Journal of Pediatric Otorhinolaryngology, 44*(3), 251–258.

Shelton, R. L. (1993). Grand rounds for sound system disorder. Conclusion: What was learned? *Seminars in Speech and Language, 14*, 166–177.

Shriberg, L. D. (1975). A response evocation program for /ɚ/. *Journal of Speech and Hearing Disorders, 40*, 92–105. Reprinted in *Contemporary readings in articulation disorders.* In: C. Bennett, N. Bountress, & G. Bull (Eds.). Dubuque, IA: Kendall-Hunt.

Shriberg, L. D. (1982). Diagnostic assessment of developmental phonological disorders. In: M. Crary (Ed.), *Phonological intervention, concepts and procedures.* San Diego, CA: College-Hill, Inc.

Shriberg, L. D. (1997). Developmental phonological disorders: One or many? In: B. W. Hodson, & M. L. Edwards (Eds.), *Perspectives in applied phonology* (pp. 105–132). Gaithersburg, MD: Aspen.

Shriberg, L. D. (2004). *Diagnostic classification of five sub-types of childhood speech sound disorders (SSD) of currently unknown origin.* Paper presented at the 2004 International Association of Logopedics and Phoniatrics Congress, Brisbane, Australia.

Shriberg, L. D. (2006, June). *Research in idiopathic and symptomatic childhood apraxia of speech.* Paper presented at the 5th International Conference on Speech Motor Control Nijmegen, The Netherlands.

Shriberg, L. D., Austin, D., Lewis, B. A., McSweeny, J. L. & Wilson, D. L. (1997). The percentage of consonants correct (PCC) metric: Extensions and reliability data. *Journal of Speech, Language, and Hearing Research, 40*(4), 708–722.

Shriberg, L.D., Campbell, T.F., Karlsson, H.B., McSweeney, J.L., Nadler, C.J. (2003). A diagnostic marker for childhood apraxia of speech: The lexical stress ratio. *Clinical Linguistics and Phonetics, 17*(7), 549–574.

Shriberg, L. D., Flipsen, P., Jr., Kwiatkowski, J., & McSweeny, J. L. (2003). A diagnostic marker for speech delay associated with otitis media with effusion: The intelligibility-speech gap. *Clinical Linguistics and Phonetics, 17*, 507–528.

Shriberg, L. D., Fourakis, M., Hall, S., Karlsson, H. K., Lohmeier, H. L, McSweeny, J., Potter, N. L., Scheer-Cohen, A. R., Strand, E. A., Tilkens, C. M., & Wilson, D. L. (2010). Extensions to the Speech Disorders Classification System (SDCS). *Clinical Linguistics & Phonetics, 24*, 795–824.

Shriberg, L. D., Kent, R. D., Karlsson, H. B., McSweeny, J. L., Nadler, C.J., & Brown, R. L. (2003). A diagnostic marker for speech delay associated with otitis media with effusion: backing of obstruents. *Clinical Linguistics and Phonetics, 17*(7), 529–547.

Shriberg, L.D., & Kwiatkowski, J. (1982). Phonological disorders III: A procedure for assessing severity of involvement. *Journal of Speech and Hearing Disorders, 47*, 256–270.

Shriberg, L. D., & Kwiatkowski, J. (1994). Developmental phonological disorders I: A clinical profile. *Journal of Speech and Hearing Research, 37*, 1100–1126.

Shriberg, L., & Widder, C. J. (1990). Speech and prosody characteristics of adults with mental retardation. *Journal of Speech and Hearing Research, 33*, 627–653.

Snowling, M., Bishop, D. V. M., & Stothard, S. E. (2000). Is pre-school language impairment a risk factor for dyslexia in adolescence? *Journal of Child Psychology & Psychiatry, 41*(5), 587–600.

So, L. K. H., & Dodd, B. (1994). Phonologically disordered Cantonese speaking children. *Clinical Linguistics and Phonetics, 8*, 235–255.

Speake, J., Stackhouse, J., & Pascoe, M. (2012). Vowel targeted intervention for children with persisting speech difficulties: Impact on intelligibility. *Child Language Teaching and Therapy, 28*(3), 277–295.

Stackhouse, J., & Wells, B. (1997). *Children's speech and literacy difficulties I: A psycholinguistic framework.* London: Whurr Publishers.

Stampe, D. (1969). *The acquisition of phonetic representation.* Papers from the 5th Regional Meeting of the Chicago Linguistic Society. 443–454.

Stein, C. M., Lu, Q., Elston, R. C., Freebairn, L. A., Hansen, A. J., Shriberg, L. D., Taylor, H. G., Lewis, B. A., & Iyengar, S. K. (2011). Heritability estimation for speech-sound traits with developmental trajectories. *Behavioral Genetics, 41*, 184–191.

Steriade, D. (1990). *Greek prosodies and the nature of syllabification (Doctoral dissertation, Massachusetts Institued of Technology, 1982).* New York: Garland Press.

Stoel-Gammon, C. (1988). *Evaluation of phonological skills in pre-school children.* New York: Thieme Medical Publishers.

Stoel-Gammon, C. (2007). Variability in speech acquisition. In: S. McLeod (Ed.) *International guide to speech acquisition* (pp. 55–60). Clifton Park, NY: Delmar Thomson Learning.

Stoel-Gammon, C., & Dunn, C. (1985). *Normal and disordered phonology in children.* Baltimore, MD: University Park Press.

Stoel-Gammon, C., & Pollock, K. E. (2008). Vowel development and disorders. In: M. Ball, M. Perkins, N. Müller, & S. Howard (Eds.), *Handbook of clinical linguistics.* Oxford: Blackwell Publishers.

Storkel, H. L., & Morrisette, M. L. (2002). The lexicon and phonology: Interactions in language acquisition. *Language, Speech and Hearing Services in Schools, 33*(1), 24–37.

Strand, E., Stoeckel, R., & Baas, B. (2006). Treatment of severe childhood apraxia of speech: A treatment efficacy study. *Journal of Medical Speech Pathology, 14*, 297–307.

Thompson, C. K. (2007). Complexity in language learning and treatment. *American Journal of Speech-Language Pathology, 16*(1), 3–5.

Thompson, C. K., & Shapiro, L. P. (2007). Complexity in treatment of syntactic deficits. *American Journal of Speech-Language Pathology, 16*(1), 30–42.

Ttofari Eecen, K. (2011). *Early identification, prediction, and classification of speech sound disorders in the preschool years* (PhD thesis). Department of Paediatrics, The University of Melbourne.

Van Riper, C. (1963). *Speech correction: Principles and methods*. New Jersey: Prentice Hall.

Van Riper, C., & Irwin, J. V. (1958). *Voice and articulation*. Englewood Cliffs, NJ: Prentice Hall.

Van Riper, R., & Emerick, L. (1984). *Speech correction: An introduction to speech pathology and audiology*. Englewood Cliffs, NJ: Prentice-Hall.

Vargha-Khadem, F., Watkins, K., Alcock, K., Fletcher, P., & Passingham, R. (1995). Praxic and nonverbal cognitive deficits in a large family with a genetically transmitted speech and language disorder. *Proceedures of the National Academy of Science USA, 92*, 930–933.

Velleman, S. L. (1998). *Making phonology functional: What do I do first?* Boston: Butterworth-Heinemann.

Waring, R., & Knight, R. (2013). How should children with speech sound disorders be classified? A review and critical evaluation of current classification systems. *International Journal of Language and Communication Disorders, 48*(1), 25–40.

Watt, N., Wetherby, A., & Shumaway, S. (2006). Prelinguistic predictors of language outcome at three years of age. *Journal of Autism and Developmental Disorders, 49*, 1224–1237.

Watts, N. (2004). Assessment of vowels summary. *ACQuiring Knowledge in Speech, Language and Hearing, Speech Pathology Australia, 6*(1), 22–25.

Weiner, F. (1981). Treatment of phonological disability using the method of meaningful contrast: Two case studies. *Journal of Speech and Hearing Disorders, 46*, 97–103.

Whitehouse, A., Robinson, M., & Zubrick, S. (2011). Late talking and the risk for psychosocial problems during childhood and adolescence. *Pediatrics, 128* (2), 324–332.

Williams, A. L. (2003). *Speech disorders: Resource guide for preschool children*. Clifton Park, NY: Thomson Delmar Learning.

Williams, A. L. (2005). From developmental norms to distance metrics: Past, present, and future directions for target selection practices. In: A. G. Kamhi, & K. E. Pollock (Eds.), *Phonological disorders in children: Clinical decision making in assessment and intervention* (pp. 101–108). Baltimore, MD: Paul. H. Brookes Publishing Company.

Williams, A. L. (2012). Intensity in phonological intervention: Is there a prescribed amount? *International Journal of Speech-Language Pathology, 14*(5), 456–461.

Winitz, H. (1969). *Articulatory acquisition and behavior*. New York: Appleton-Century-Crofts.

Winitz, H. (1975). *From syllable to conversation*. Baltimore, MD: University Park.

Wolk, L., & Meisler, A. W. (1998). Phonological assessment: A systematic comparison of conversation and picture naming. *Journal of Communication Disorders, 31*, 291–313.

Wood, K. S. (1971). Terminology and nomenclature. In: L. E. Travis (Ed.), *Handbook of speech pathology and audiology*. Englewood Cliffs, NJ: Prentice Hall.

Wren, Y., Hughes, T., & Roulstone, S. (2006). *Phoneme factory phonology screener*. London: NFER Nelson Publishing Company.

Wren, Y., & Roulstone, S. (2006). *Phoneme factory sound sorter*. Manchester: Granada Learning.

Wren, Y., Roulstone, S., & Miller, L. (2012). Distinguishing groups of children with persistent speech disorder: Findings from a prospective population study. *Logopedics, Phoniatrics & Vocology, 37*(1), 1–10.

Chapter 3

Special populations of children

All children with speech sound disorders (SSD) require 'special consideration', but there are certain individual clients and client-groups that seem to warrant *extra* special consideration. In this chapter, issues that manifest clinically for these individuals and groups and their families are examined. The topics are: children at the point of initial referral and their parents' perceptions of SSD and its impact; children with co-occurring speech *and* language disorders (McCauley, A14); families, children and counselling (Bitter, A15; Overby & Bernthal, A16); children with craniofacial anomalies, and velopharyngeal dysfunction (Golding-Kushner, A17); children who have been internationally adopted (Pollock, A18); and children with SSD who are multilingual (Goldstein, A19). Then, Zajdó (A20) writes about children acquiring speech in languages other than English; and Bleile (A21) reflects upon issues around children with speech impairments in culturally and linguistically diverse settings in the non-industrialised world. Finally in this chapter, Neilson (A22) discusses children who have speech *and* literacy difficulties.

Parents' initial perceptions of their child's SSD

In general SLP/SLT paediatric practice, some children whose parents bring them for initial screening and assessment have speech difficulties as their *only* voice, speech, language or fluency issue, and others have an SSD as their obvious and *primary* communication disorder perhaps in conjunction with minor language delays. For the majority of them, SLP/SLT management is straightforward from the therapist's perspective. In these cases, parents will have detected their child's speech issue and arranged for an assessment, whereupon the clinician assessed the child's speech and initiated an appropriate intervention regimen, suggested a 'watchful waiting' approach, or informed the parent that the child's speech was within normal limits (WNL) and discussed, reassuringly, normal expectations. Some parents contact the SLP/SLT indicating descriptively that their child has severe, moderate or mild speech issues. Within the 'mild' group, parents may report difficulties with one or two sounds: /k/ and /g/; /s/ and /z/;

Children's Speech Sound Disorders, Second Edition. Caroline Bowen.
© 2015 John Wiley & Sons, Ltd. Published 2015 by John Wiley & Sons, Ltd.
Companion website: www.wiley.com/go/bowen/speechlanguagetherapy

/ɹ/, /l/, or /θ/ and /ð/. When some of these children actually attend for assessment, it transpires that the parents' observations were accurate and sufficient, but often this turns out *not* to be the case. Most seasoned clinicians can probably produce examples of times when, given a parent's description during the intake process, they were expecting to evaluate a child with minimal speech difficulties, only to find a complex speech picture, on occasion with additional issues.

Similarly, parents may come to the SLP/SLT because, or partly because, they have been encouraged to do so by a nursery or daycare worker ('carer') or preschool teacher or school teacher ('teacher'), who all regularly assume an important role as screeners and referrers to SLP/SLT services (Roulstone, A8). Sometimes parents, suspecting a problem, will have approached the carer or teacher for referral advice ('I think Jason needs to see a speech therapist; do you agree?'; 'Is Erica's speech development on-track for a child of her age?'). On the other hand, sometimes the carer or teacher makes the first move, with the parents apparently unaware of any difficulty ('Jean-Paul's speech is difficult to understand; have you considered an assessment by a speech professional?'). Other parents notice a speech problem but actually *wait* for carers or teachers to spur them into action.

In these situations, carers and teachers can be understandably tentative and overly reassuring, not wanting to alarm parents or appear to be critical of their child-rearing prowess. So, when the parent contacts the SLP/SLT, they may quote the referring person as saying that the child's pronunciation errors are minor and that the referral is precautionary. They may even report to the SLP/SLT that the referrer mentioned that 'just a few sessions' of therapy or home management advice would quickly rectify the problem. Again, this sort of low-key initial presentation can herald the appearance on a caseload of children who prove to have complex intervention needs. The reverse happens, too, with parents reporting severe difficulties that turn out to be mild (though not necessarily 'mild' from the parents' perspective). Further, they may express concerns about *speech*

when issues with *language* or *fluency* appear, to the therapist, to be more in need of attention. Such circumstances may require a perceptual shift by parents and needed support while this occurs should be in place (Overby & Bernthal, A16). It may not be a big step for a parent to accept that he or she has been worrying unnecessarily, but it can be a painful adjustment for those who unexpectedly discover that a so-called mild problem is serious, especially when the advice of a trusted carer or teacher conflicts with the SLP's/SLT's expert advice. No matter how serious or mild the child's difficulty seems to be, it is the clinician's responsibility to determine the presence or absence of speech impairment, to diagnose the nature of it if there is one and to determine if any *other* types of communication disorder, or 'special considerations' are present.

Three special populations

Referral of children with co-occurring speech *and* language difficulties is a frequent occurrence and language-based approaches appear to be the best possible choice for them (Tyler, 2002; 2010). Even with timely, appropriate intervention, these children may be engaged in treatment for lengthy periods (Ruscello, St. Louis & Mason, 1991; Tyler & Watterson, 1991), so there is often a strong desire on everyone's part for therapy to start without delay. But there is a period for some children with speech *and* language impairment when, in the scheme of things, addressing their poor intelligibility warrants low priority. For example, first there are children with severe language issues, including pragmatic language limitations with accompanying, significant behaviour difficulties. For them, it can be exceptionally hard to know how to tame and engage with them, what to treat first and what combination of issues to address. Second, there are the sickest children with cleft palate and co-morbid craniofacial anomalies (Persson & Sjögreen, 2011), who run a physical and emotional marathon – with their families – of heroic medical management, surgical intervention, varying degrees of recovery and hard-won survival before they ever reach us (Kummer, 2008; Sell & Harding-Bell, 2010). Third, there are the internationally adopted infants, toddlers and children who may have travelled to foreign countries from places where SLP/SLT services are unavailable and for whom initial consultation may be late compared with usual industrialised-world standards (Glennen, 2007c; Price, Pollock & Oller, 2006).

All of these groups *may* contain *some* children who are behaviourally challenging: actively acting out, depressed or unduly passive, possibly as a consequence of their life experiences, in terms of health and wellbeing, surgery, trauma, malnutrition, dislocation and separation. Their communication challenges may have been exacerbated by insufficient stimulation in orphanages or hospitals, late identification, communicative frustration or shifting linguistic influences. There may be powerful co-morbidities, such as medical fragility and the complex of psychosocial disturbances, sensory issues and seizures, which appear to go hand in hand with some craniofacial anomalies and certain syndromes. The following five questions posed to our experts (Q14, Q15, Q16, Q17 and Q18) concern these special groups of children and their families.

Children with co-occurring speech and language disorders

In a thoughtful piece on spoken language, Kent (2006, p. 1) may have summed up the view of many parents about the elite status of speech, when he made this arresting statement:

> *Speech is but one modality for the expression of language; however, speech has special importance because it is the primary, first-learned modality for hearing language users. Speech is a system in the sense that it consistently and usefully relates the meanings of a language with the sounds by which a language is communicated.*

Many parents will wistfully tell SLPs/SLTs something along the lines of, 'If he could talk clearly, it would solve a lot of problems'. These same parents may be surprised or worried if a clinician appears not to be focused on speech, but more interested in evaluating a range of *other* aspects of the child's presentation, such as levels of comprehension in differing conditions. Then, when it comes to intervention, parents of children with speech *and* language impairment may feel that their genuine concerns about intelligibility are being sidelined, as they see it, while language objectives are given undue precedence.

In A14, Rebecca McCauley talks about the issues involved in assessment, treatment planning and intervention for severely involved children with co-occurring speech and language issues, including those with complex presentations and worrying behaviour, where families in particular, but also at times, trans-disciplinary team members, find it hard to come to grips with customary, evidence-based SLP/SLT intervention priorities and hierarchies.

Dr. Rebecca McCauley is a Professor in the Department of Speech and Hearing Science at the Ohio State University. She is a Board-Recognized Specialist in Child Language and a Fellow of the American Speech–Language–Hearing Association. Her primary interests are in SSD in children, especially severe speech disorders such as childhood apraxia of speech (CAS), and in the nature of interventions, especially those used for children with a variety of communication disorders. Publications related to these topics include six books, five of which are edited volumes, including, in 2010, *Interventions for speech sound disorders in children*, which she co-edited with A. Lynn Williams and Sharynne McLeod.

Q14. Rebecca McCauley: Children with co-occurring speech and language issues

How would you set about prioritising and implementing speech *and* language treatment; in what ways would you involve parents and the wider family in the intervention team? Sometimes parents' or other team members' perception of the SLP/SLT needs of the child, and their expectations of the focus that therapy will have, are at odds with the speech–language clinician's findings and recommendations. In such instances, how would you approach the task of information sharing and reaching consensus treatment priorities and goals?

A14.   Rebecca McCauley: Prioritising goals for children with speech and language disorders

Children with severe language delays and disorders who also show evidence of SSD represent a large heterogeneous group with diagnoses such as specific language impairment (SLI), autism spectrum disorder or developmental delay. Almost invariably, these children find it difficult to make what they say understood in everyday communication – in fact, usually that is the reason they have been found eligible for intervention. In addition, such children may exhibit co-occurring or core challenges in attention or behaviour (e.g., tantrums or withdrawal) that negatively affect their lives at home and at school. Prioritising intervention goals for children whose needs span speech, language, communication – and sometimes management of problem behaviours – represents a delicate balancing act.

That balancing act is both facilitated, in the long run, and complicated, in the short run, by the involvement of teams of educators, health professionals, SLPs/SLTs and families. Parents or other primary caregivers play a central role in the teams constituted to address the child's communication needs. Within a philosophy of family-centred practice (Pappas, McLeod, McAllister & McKinnon, 2007), parents' expertise about, investment in and access to the child are recognised as invaluable resources. In order

to help establish a strong alliance among the team members, I find it helpful to introduce at least three concepts: *speech production* (what sounds were used and whether they were used for communicative purposes), *language* (words and larger units of meaning that were understood or attempted in production) and *communication* (verbal and nonverbal means of sharing and receiving information). Ideally, I incorporate examples from our shared observations of the child to illustrate these concepts and their interrelationships. For children exhibiting problem behaviours, I would also point out that such behaviours probably represent efforts to communicate that can be replaced when more conventional communications are identified, learned and rewarded (Halle, Ostrosky & Hemmeter, 2006)

To the extent that all members of the child's team share a common understanding of *speech, language* and *communication*, they are in a better position to react to any plan that I might propose based on evaluation results and my knowledge of what research exists to support a given set of intervention goals and strategies. Team collaboration on such a plan facilitates changes ranging from subtle refinements to everyday interactions with the child, to major modifications that more effectively incorporate knowledge of the child, his or her surroundings (including his or her family's needs and values) and team members' abilities to contribute.

Plans for children with significant speech and language needs often incorporate two kinds of strategies: (a) augmentative alternative communication (AAC) strategies for optimising the child's current communicative effectiveness and (b) specific intervention strategies for improving the child's more specific speech and language skills. Initially, parents are sometimes reticent about using AAC strategies (e.g., a communication board or signing) because of fears that it represents a lowering of expectations and may hamper speech and language development.

However, reassurance on two fronts usually allays those fears. First, available evidence suggests that the use of AAC is more likely to facilitate than retard advances in other forms of communication. Second, the child's becoming a more effective communicator can produce immediate improvements in the quality of his life and the lives of those around him—a valuable outcome independent of future effects.

Intervention methods used for speech and language facilitation vary depending on the child's level of development in each area, but often include those described by Hodson (A5), and Strand (A45) in their contributions to this volume as well as a variety of methods described in McCauley and Fey (2006). How I involve parents in implementing an intervention plan depends on their interest and resources. Often, at the outset of therapy, I will suggest that we start small and consider greater involvement as we go. At the most basic level, I ask that parents keep me abreast of times when they see advancement or suspect special unanticipated challenges that might affect the course of our work. Most parents are also happy to reward the spontaneous use in the home setting of target behaviours that I can let them know are emerging in treatment sessions.

For children whose communication and language are in relatively early stages of development, parent-implemented programs are especially appropriate and well supported by evidence if parents are interested and able to take the time. In such programs, parents are taught several facilitating strategies to use in play and/or book reading with their child (Girolametto & Weitzman, 2006). For other parents with similar children but less time or interest, I might teach them a specific strategy (e.g., focused stimulation; Ellis Weismer & Robertson, 2006). Yet another area in which parents and I have had success is in approximating stimulability activities such as those described by Williams and Miccio (2010) or phonological awareness (PA) activities such as those described by Neilson (A22) and Hesketh (A28).

Working with parents and other professionals in a team context can be an immensely satisfying process, even as it is a challenging. The team's diverse perspectives not only produce a better plan for the child, but also help me do my job better. When children have many missing speech and language skills, it is very easy to get lost in the 'trees' of their many potential goals. Other team members, especially parents, can help us all keep track of the 'forest', that is, the child's overall communicative effectiveness.

Children with difficult behaviour

There are promising indications in the literature that it is possible to reduce behaviour difficulties by targeting communication skills (Law, Plunkett & the Nuffield Speech and Language Review Group, 2009; Law, Plunkett & Skinner, 2012), but to date studies have focused on children with autism and/or severe speech, language and communication needs (commonly abbreviated SLCN in the United Kingdom) and not discrete populations of children with SSD plus behavioural issues. Clinicians and parents, however, have reported improvements in behaviour as children's intelligibility increases and this is often attributed to a corresponding reduction in communicative frustration. Conversely, some parents say that behaviour becomes more overtly difficult when a taciturn child comes out of his or her shell and becomes more assertive and 'verbal'.

For example, my client Harriet who presented at 4;0 with a percentage of consonants correct (PCC) of 35% was a passive, 'good' little girl whose mother said compensated for her intelligibility difficulties by being 'everybody's helper' to the point where she earned the family nickname 'Helpful Harry'. By 5;6 her speech approached normal expectations and she began 'answering back' with, 'No! Why should I?' and the like when asked to do something. She had also become accustomed to holding the floor at home and when visiting friends and relatives because people close to her dreaded 'inhibiting' her further speech progress. If anyone suggested that it might be someone else's turn to talk, she would react angrily ('you don't care what I think!', 'You never let me talk', and so on). Around this time her mother called me, sounding shocked with herself, to say guiltily, 'I never thought I would tell Harry to "shut up" – but I just did!' We talked about the factors involved, and over a period of two or three months, Harry's speech normalised, and her behaviour improved, along with her pragmatics. But it is not always that easy to deal with children's difficult behaviour.

McCauley (A15) talked about the satisfying, challenging experience of working in a team context. Multidisciplinary, cross-disciplinary and transdisciplinary team members may include social workers, psychologists, family therapists and people from a range of different backgrounds, who have special expertise in counselling. SLPs/SLTs regularly engage in information sharing and counselling, but in their work with the following three groups children with SSD they sometimes encounter troubling behavioural, practical issues and ethical concerns that are beyond their remit as counsellors. The three are:

1. Children who *are able* to demonstrate co-operation and good rapport with adults in other situations who exhibit 'difficult' non-compliant behaviour, including refusal to cooperate in assessment and intervention sessions; or those who show good cooperation in the treatment room coupled with refusal to do homework.
2. Children who are *unable* to demonstrate co-operation and good rapport with adults in speech assessment and intervention settings, and in other situations. These children may present for SLP/SLT assessment and intervention with parents 'expecting' the SLP/SLT to manage both the difficult behaviour and the speech disorder. Some conscientious SLPs/SLTs make themselves miserable by trying unsuccessfully to manage behavioural issues with no relevant background in social work, psychology, family therapy, counselling and so on.
3. Children who do not have the potential for speech who are referred by their families. Young, inexperienced or newly qualified SLPs/SLTs, especially those in private practice, often have great difficulty talking to parents openly about children who are more suited to AAC – or indeed, may not have the capacity even to benefit from simple, low-tech augmentative devices – and the parents themselves often take the position that if they are prepared to bring the child to therapy and pay for it, then the SLP/SLT is obliged to work with the child.

Who better to ask about working with these 'difficult' children and their families than Dr. James Robert Bitter, Professor of Family Counselling at East Tennessee State University in Johnson City, Tennessee, USA. Dr. Bitter is the author of *Theory and Practice of Family Therapy and Counseling* (Bitter, 2013). Over the course of his career, he has worked with the late pioneer of family therapy, Virginia Satir, as well as the master Adlerian family therapists, Manford Sonstegard and Oscar Christensen. He has written more than 70 articles and 4 books, and he is a founding faculty member of the Adlerian Training Institute in Port St. Lucie, Florida.

Q15.   James Bitter: Children with problematic behaviour and their families

Thinking about the above three groups of children and their families, can you explore for the reader the reasons why these behaviours might manifest, the first steps in setting counselling goals that an SLP/SLT might take, basic management strategies, and indicators as to when to refer to a specialist in counselling, and ways that SLPs/SLTs who are not normally engaged in multi-, cross- or trans-disciplinary teams can liaise productively with such specialists?

A15.   James Bitter: Counselling children and their families experiencing SSD: systemic interventions for speech–language professionals

Despite Western culture's emphasis on individuality, all humans are relational beings (Gergen, 2009). Human life is social, purposeful, subjective and interpretive in nature (Sweeney, 2009). Without this orientation to life, and the social, physical and emotional nurturing provided by adults, no infant would survive. Moreover, the quality of attachment experienced by a child plays a significant role in the child's development across the lifespan (Bowlby, 1988).

When individuals choose to couple, they do so hoping that they can build a better life together than either of them might have had separately. Individuals or couples who choose parenthood usually want a happy, *healthy* child with whom they can bond and travel through life. What happens when the dream of a happy, healthy child does not occur at birth or is de-railed by the revelation of protracted or atypical speech development? Initially, the family experiences shock (Holland, 2007).

The reality of diagnosis

Diagnosis of a significant SSD shocks the family system, forcing its members to deal with a new reality, with the SSD becoming the focus of everyone's attention. Many families are in chaos at this point and unable to mobilise the internal and external resources needed to deal constructively with the problems they face. This is not a good time for the SLP/SLT to give family members information about the SSD and its implications, because their shock and chaos will prevent them from absorbing it. Indeed, when information is provided prematurely, many family members will later say that they never received any information about the disorder.

Acknowledgment and acceptance take time. A significant SSD constitutes the *loss* of the dream of a healthy child, and that process of loss is well documented (Goldberg, 2006; Kabat-Zinn, 2005; Kleinman, 1988; Kubler-Ross, 1969). Commonly, the initial shock of diagnosis slowly evolves into a realisation that the problem will not be *wished* away, easily remediated or evaporate with time. This realisation often results in a *retreat*, into some combination of denial, prayer, bargaining, depression or anger. Family members will react differently from each other, too often leaving individuals feeling alone or disconnected. All of this can be happening while the SLP/SLT endeavours to help the child and the family address the reality of a significant SSD.

Listening

The first step, therefore, in counselling an individual client or a client family is to stay present and *listen*. Staying present means staying in the moment, asking what it is like to hear difficult news and remaining alert to how people are feeling; it means employing *reflection* or *active listening*. Active listening is paraphrasing to clients what you hear them say and what you empathically believe they might be feeling. 'Hearing that Beatrice is developing speech that is quite different from others her age, and from what she will need as an adult, is hard. You must be worried about all that lies ahead of you'. Notice that these two sentences avoid the use of technical language and focus on what the family feels. Active listening will likely promote further sharing, and the SLP/SLT continues paraphrasing – perhaps for quite some time.

Acknowledgment changes the family system at multiple levels. It focuses the *family atmosphere* and it influences the manner in which *mistaken goals and mistaken interactions* develop. Let us look at each of these separately – even though they develop concurrently and have recursive effects on each other.

Family atmosphere

In each family, an atmosphere or climate develops that can be said to characterise how the family members relate to each other. Let us say that a child is born with an unexpected cleft palate, requiring surgery with the anticipation of years of speech therapy. The initial experience of cleft palate throws the family into shock. Initially, the parents are incapable of hearing any important information. The key professional attributes that an SLP/SLT can bring to a first meeting with the family are patience, presence, empathy and active listening skills. It is by staying present and listening empathically that *shock* and *retreat* eventually give way to *realization* and *acknowledgment* (Holland, 2007). When these latter stages occur, professional information is more easily received. This informational delivery will affect the development of the family atmosphere over many years. Over time, the family will evolve into some version of a 'cleft palate' family as the craniofacial anomaly significantly influences who they are. It may pull the parents together or push them apart. The family may feel supported or abandoned in the frustration of dealing with doctors, insurers, parents and children of other families, social support systems and other agencies including school and advocacy groups. The family atmosphere emerges within the domain of the disorder, impacting who takes charge and who retreats; the emotions expressed with whom and towards whom; the expectations developed for the child with the cleft compared to typically developing children. All of these aspects contribute to the model the child receives for handling life.

A debilitating family atmosphere results when parents lapse into feeling sorry for both themselves and their child. Such an atmosphere robs family members of courage, removes confidence, blocks resilience and may lead to pampering or over-protection. In intervention sessions, these parents will want to hover, intervene and/or block sadness, challenge or discomfort in the child. This counterproductive stance, relative to their child and the disorder, emanates from the belief that the child has already suffered enough and should experience no additional difficulties. The family has not yet come to terms with what Holland (2007), quoting Kabat-Zinn (2005), calls *the full catastrophe*: . . . it is not a disaster to be alive just because we feel fear and we suffer . . . [to understand] that there is joy as well as suffering, hope as well as despair, calm as well as agitation, love as well as hatred, health as well as illness . . . (p. 5).

Mistaken goals of children's misbehaviour

Some children with SSD also exhibit challenging and disrupting behaviours. When such conduct interrupts or overwhelms therapeutic practices, addressing the behaviours *per se* must become an explicit therapy goal. Dreikurs (1940a,b) first delineated four goals of children's misbehaviour as a motivational typology for the everyday behaviours of children. These goals are *attention getting*, *power struggle*, *revenge* and a *demonstration of inadequacy* (also called an *assumed disability and signifying the goal of withdrawal*). Dreikurs (1948, 1950) and Dreikurs and Soltz (1964) described the behaviours associated with these four goals and these are displayed in Figure A15.1.

There are two ways in which an SLP/SLT can determine the goal of a child's misbehaviour. First, by observing what happens when a child is corrected; and second by asking what the adult feels in the midst of the misbehaviour. These indicators are noted by goal in Table A15.1.

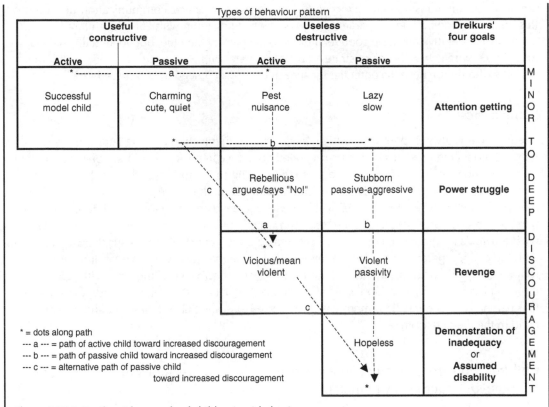

Figure A15.1 Dreikurs' four goals of children's misbehaviour

Applications to specific situations

As a profession, SLP/SLT has its own set of best practices, ethical codes and goals and objectives. Training in counselling does not seek to turn SLPs/SLTs into professional counsellors. Rather, the goal is to learn enough about the counselling process and systemic development to aid clients and

Table A15.1 Identifying the mistaken goals of children's misbehaviour

Mistaken goals	Observed behavior	Adult response	What the child does when corrected
Attention getting	Model child cute and charming pest and nuisance lazy	Irritated annoyed frustrated	Stops for a short while when corrected–even just a few moments or minutes
Power struggle	Rebellious argues and fights stubborn passive-aggressive	Angry challenged defeated	Keeps going even when told to stop and may even intensify the misbehavior
Revenge	Vicious or violent vandalism meanness violent passivity	Hurt	Intensifies the misbehavior and the misbehavior becomes mean
Assumed disability	Acts hopeless gives up is discouraged acts incompetent	Despair helplessness	Limited or no interaction Adults start to give up too Won't try

families with the transition into effective therapy for the presenting communication disorder. To this end, let us look at three separate situations involving children with SSD: (a) children who are generally cooperative and have good relations in other parts of their life, but not initially in therapy; (b) children who generally demonstrate a lack of cooperation in most settings; and (c) children or families who do not have the potential for speech therapy and need to be referred.

Some basics

The first goal is always to form a positive relationship with the child and the family. If the service delivery model requires the child to be separated from the parents for all, or part, of an assessment or intervention session, SLPs/SLTs who go to the waiting room and greet the family in a friendly manner are off to a good start. Providing information about the process facilitates a transition to therapy, including where the SLP/SLT will be taking the child and how long it will take; where the parents can wait, or if possible, where they can watch the assessment or therapy in process; and what the goals for the session might be. In general, we want the SLP/SLT to leave the waiting room with the child, separating from the parents even if the parents, too, will leave for another viewing room. During this process, parents may raise worries or concerns regarding what will happen with their child. An effective transition is usually facilitated via active listening followed by reassurance that parental concerns will be more easily addressed after the SLP/SLT has met and assessed the child in the therapy room.

Children who are generally cooperative and have good relations in other parts of their life, but not initially in therapy

Some children can initially be frightened in new situations or when meeting new people. This is especially true for children in a family atmosphere where parents feel sorry for their child or are trying to protect them from further hardships. The child's non-cooperative behaviour may reflect the parents' apprehension as much as that of the child. Some children are fine for several sessions, a honeymoon period, and then suddenly become upset. When children start to cry, the SLP/SLT may hear the parents coax the child or make excuses for the behaviour or express surprise or embarrassment ('She doesn't generally act this way at home'). A statement of understanding goes a long way: 'You know, new situations can be hard at first, but I am sure we will be fine when we get to know each other [engaging with the child at eye level, and smiling]. Would you like to take my hand and walk with me to the room or would you like to walk like a big girl on your own?'

In the therapy room, take time to build a relationship with the child. Even in a 30-minute session, 5–10 minutes can be devoted to exploring the room with the child, asking about what the child likes or dislikes, talking calmly with each other, and perhaps even playing a short game. When it is time to engage in a task, say clearly what the task is, have only that task in front of the child, and then notice what the child does in response and what feelings emerge in you (the SLP/SLT). Is the child seeking attention, power or revenge (the three most common)? If the child is seeking attention, the SLP/SLT will only want to provide it for on-task behaviour: ignore the rest. If the child is seeking power or revenge, the SLP/SLT, having explained what is required in the task, can say, 'Let me know when you are ready to begin' and then stay quiet. If the child moves towards the door, the SLP/SLT might move to sit quietly in front of the door. If the child lets the SLP/SLT know that she/he is ready to cooperate, the SLP/SLT begins the process again provided the child stays on task. End the session with a game or joint play. It may take a whole session to build rapport, and this is time well invested. Whether parents participate in assessment and intervention sessions or stay in a waiting room, it is important to update them on the process of therapy and to be open to answering their questions. This builds cooperation between the family and the therapist. As the parents relax about the process, the child will also tend to do so.

Children who generally demonstrate a lack of cooperation in most settings

An SLP/SLT working with a child who is uncooperative in most settings is forced into pitting control against power. But let us be clear about what the therapist can control. Therapists can control themselves and the situation, but not the child. Indeed, the child is probably out of control because the family has used ineffective responses in attempting to control him or her. The SLP/SLT must first control the room. Remove or secure any items or objects that will not be a direct part of either the therapy task or a single play event. A general rule is: if you do not want it damaged, do not have it in the room. In the therapy room, prepare for a child to throw a temper tantrum that might include yelling, crying, falling on the floor, pounding on doors or windows and attempts at hitting or kicking. Bring a book or something else to occupy you during periods of temper. If a temper tantrum starts (whining counts), say, 'Let me know when you are ready to work'. Say this once, and sit in a chair in front of the therapy room door. Read, do your crossword, or pursue some other peaceful activity, stay calm and stay quiet.

Some SLPs/SLTs have had to invest two to three therapy sessions in winning a child over. It is useful to assure the parents that this has happened before and that the SLP/SLT expects to catch up rather quickly once the child loses steam and becomes cooperative. Taking an indirect approach, the SLP/SLT models for the parents the setting of limits with the child. Children do what works, and they will eventually stop what does not work. When SLPs/SLTs work with a very uncooperative child they can expect the child to try everything that has worked at home. Behaviour will get worse before it gets better. Riding it out can seem difficult, but it seldom takes more than three half-hour sessions, after which the child and the parents tend to be much more cooperative. Children will test SLPs/SLTs subsequently. The child may cooperate for several sessions and then come into a session with anger and rage flying. It is important that the therapist set their practice goals aside and return to waiting the child out, calmly requesting that the child let the SLP/SLT know when he or she is ready to work.

Children or families who do not have the potential for speech therapy and need to be referred

There are two general types of families who may need referral. First, there are the families whose psycho-social-behavioural problems overwhelm any treatment possibilities. Second, those families with a child who has an SSD that requires outside services, or who has no speech and no apparent capacity for speech, again requiring appropriate referral. Parents sometimes bring their children who have severe cognitive challenges to the SLP/SLT thinking the child can be 'taught to speak'. It is surprising how often these families can slip through the screening process and arrive at the office of the SLP/SLT as inappropriate referrals.

In the first category are children whose misbehaviour is consistently aimed at a goal of revenge or a demonstration of inadequacy (extreme withdrawal). The former includes consistent attempts to hit, bite, kick or hurt as well as acts of vandalism or vicious attacks on pets or other humans. The latter will most likely be expressed in extreme feelings of anxiety, depression, encopresis or enuresis or phobic reactions. Under such circumstances, referral to a child psychologist or family therapist should become a pre- or co-requisite for speech services.

In the second category are children with SSD that may need additional referrals for assessment and treatment planning, perhaps to an ENT specialist. Further, there may also be a need for referral when speech therapy will be coupled with either medical (as in cleft palate) or audiology (say, for hearing aids) services – or when the child and family are more appropriately seen by a clinician from a totally different profession. Referral is nothing more than the involvement of other professionals in service to the child and the family. Having a fully developed, local referral list is essential to good practice.

In general, the more severe and chronic the disorder, the greater the impact will be on family dynamics. As in any serious medical illness (e.g., cancer or heart problems), families tend to coalesce around family members who have special needs. When these special needs are severe and ongoing, it is not a child with an SSD; it is a family with an SSD. In larger communities, there are usually support groups for all sorts of difficulties. Even in smaller communities, there are professional counsellors and social workers that can help families set new goals and priorities and still live a life characterised by acceptance, happiness, success and fulfilment.

Referral

When meeting with a family in need of a referral, it is important to take the process in steps. Ideally, preparation would see the SLP/SLT with a choice of options for any referral or set of referrals that might be made. This includes a written list of the specialists and agencies, as the case may be, including addresses and phone numbers. Meeting the family starts with a simple inquiry about how people are doing and how they are feeling. The SLP/SLT should respond with active listening. When the family is ready, the SLP/SLT calmly reviews what has been learned and where the child and family 'are' in the process of facing the tasks ahead. The SLP/SLT thereby lays the foundation for why a referral is necessary and potentially useful – and ultimately, the likely next steps following the referral. It is important to check that the information is understandable to the family and to ask how they feel about it. Provision of additional information or further planning may be needed at this point, usually requiring more active listening. Towards the end of the referral session, the SLP/SLT ascertains whether the child and the family need support in enacting the referral. Do they need letters or paperwork from the SLP/SLT? Do they know where they need to go and how they will get there? Do they need phone calls or other support services? An effective referral is one in which all parties see the need, have a plan and have the possibility of enacting the plan. Finally, SLPs/SLTs who sets a time to follow up with the family after the referral date are more likely to ensure treatment adherence and prevent treatment interruption and derailment.

Not all children and their families will be difficult clients. Many will fall right into speech therapy and benefit greatly from it. My aim here has been to identify ways of understanding and working with children and families who may not accept therapy interventions quite so smoothly. Because individuals, children and adults are always in relationship, always part of systems, learning to interact with and treat the whole family is the surest way to support positive outcomes in therapeutic practice with less than cooperative clients.

An SLP/SLT view of counselling

Responding to a different question, Megan Overby and John Bernthal offer another perspective on SLPs/SLTs as counsellors that complements the information and reflections provided by James Bitter, who wrote from an Adlerian Family Therapy perspective in A15.

Dr. Megan Overby is an Associate Professor at Duquesne University in Pittsburgh, Pennsylvania, USA. Dr. Overby has authored three publications and frequently presents on children's SSD. Her current research focuses on aspects of CAS, as well as issues of literacy and counselling in SSD.

Dr. John Bernthal is an ASHA past president and recipient of ASHA Honors. He is also Professor Emeritus, past chair of the Department of Special Education and Communication Disorders and past director of the Barkley Memorial Center at The University of Nebraska-Lincoln in Lincoln, Nebraska, USA. He is co-author with Dr. Nicholas Bankson of five editions of *Articulation and Phonological Disorders*, and with Bankson and Peter Flipsen, Jr. of the sixth and seventh editions (Bernthal, Bankson & Flipsen, Jr., 2013).

Q16.   Megan Overby and John Bernthal: Counselling and children with SSD

What is your take on the role of, and related literature associated with, counselling in communication sciences generally, and in SSD in particular? What are the signs the SLP/SLT should be alert to in deciding whether to refer a child with an SSD (or his/her parents) to a professional counsellor? Do you see a place for counselling adolescents and adults with persisting, or residual speech difficulties and/or related literacy issues?

A16.   Megan Overby and John Bernthal: The role of counselling in the treatment of children with SSD

In the literature, counselling is defined in a variety of ways, reflecting different authors' perspectives (Wolter, DiLool & Apel, 2006). It has been described as a clinician's facilitation of a client's adjustment to the consequences of a significant problem (Webster, 1977), empowering clients to make informed decisions (Luterman, 2008) or helping others to understand their thoughts and motivations so they are more able to cope with their problems (Kuo & Hu, 2002). In the context of SLP/SLT practice, the role of counselling includes helping a client's family members better understand the communication disorder as well as 'preventing, managing, adjusting to, or coping with these disorders' (Flasher & Fogle, 2012, p. 5). Although the American Speech–Language–Hearing Association 2007 Scope of Practice (ASHA, 2007) identifies counselling as an appropriate and important role for speech–language pathologists, obviously SLP/SLT practitioners are not professional 'counsellors', and thus do not usually have the specific education and training requirements for counselling certification or licensing. Rather, the role for the SLP/SLT is to communicate with the client and/or the family about the communication delay or disorder, provide appropriate referrals and engage the clients in 'problem-solving strategies to enhance the (re)habilitation process' (ASHA, 2004, Counselling section, paragraph 1).

Counselling has been reported to be both important and effective for several types of communication disorders. For a child with fluency problems, counselling is an integral part of treatment. Guitar (2014) notes that the clinician must listen to the child and his/her family, acknowledge any feelings of discouragement, frustration and guilt about stuttering but resist giving 'simple reassurance'. For those with language-literacy delays, counselling can address feelings of decreased self-esteem, blame, disillusionment and fear of failure (Wolter, DiLollo & Apel, 2006). When counselling older adults and caregivers or those who have experienced strokes, addressing the client and family's social and economic concerns, life experiences, fears, psychological disorientation and the physical and cognitive effects of ageing can have important therapeutic value for clients and their family members (Holland & Fridricksson, 2001; Toner & Shadden, 2002). The need for effective counselling in clients with hearing loss is well documented (Luterman & Kurtzer-White, 1999; von Almen & Blair, 1989; English, Mendel, Rojeski & Hornak, 1999), and several effective counselling strategies (e.g., the Readiness Scale and self-assessments) for clients with impaired hearing have been described (Flasher & Fogle, 2012; English, 2008).

There is little research, however, that has explored the need for or the effectiveness of counselling for clients and families facing a significant SSD. Yet, as with other communication disorders, young children (and their families) facing an SSD experience a variety of emotional responses for which counselling may be required, including grief, denial, anger, bargaining, depression, accepting the SSD, anxiety, guilt (Luterman, 2008; Miron, 2012). In the following narrative relayed to the first author, consider the range of emotions expressed by a parent after her daughter was diagnosed with CAS:

You don't want to think that this is true, that there's something really wrong. And even though I was denying it until I sat in your office down here, I knew that this was what she had. You have a baby and you want the best for them. You want them to have every opportunity possible… Can I not help her reach her goals because of

this (disorder)? That terrifies me because I think she's so special. The worst is some adults don't give her a chance because she can't communicate with them and that hurts my feelings for her and it worries me. I worry because kids can be so cruel that it's going to start affecting her internally. I have hope because every day she's smiling and she does something new almost every day. It's just sometimes when I'm trying to be her mother and give her lunch, she's screaming because she can't tell me what she wants. You lose it a little bit. But I'm thankful that all of her caregivers don't lose hope. But you know, I won't relax ever. Until she's in a typical kindergarten and there's no aide sitting next to her and she's talking to her peers and no one knows except for her what's going on – I might relax then… I'm getting there. I feel myself much more Zen, I guess, much more at peace because I'm accepting that if I give to myself a little bit, everything is easier. So I'm trying to make myself happy and peaceful and I think it will help her reach her potential.

Clearly, this parent is experiencing a profound sense of loss, as well as feelings of anxiety and fear, sadness and worry. In a study of 60 self-identified parents of children with CAS, the most common (18.3%) emotion at the time of diagnosis was fear, followed by grief (16.1%), anxiety (18.5%), loss (15.7%) and guilt (16.3%) (Carroll & Overby, 2010). Out of 14 possible concerns about parenting a child with CAS, the greatest concern appeared to be worry about the child's future. Despite this need for information and support, only 19.5% of parents indicated that SLPs provided them adequate emotional support. In another study of parents of children with CAS, the most common initial reactions to the diagnosis of CAS were feeling proactive (86.2%), sadness (81.9%) and anxiety (80.4%) (Boh, Csiacsek, Duginske, Meath & Carpenter, 2006).

Miron (2012) interviewed 11 parents of children with a CAS diagnosis and found that the parents experienced an initial reaction phase (lasting 3–6 months) during which time they experienced fear, uncertainty and helplessness. However, these feelings were diminished by a positive relationship with an important service provider (such as a teacher, paediatrician or SLP/SLT) who provided encouragement and information about working with complex educational and medical systems. Interestingly, even though a clear majority (98%) of SLPs/SLTs providing therapy to children agreed that parent involvement is critical for speech therapy to be effective, only 42% of those practitioners agreed that parents should have 'the final say' on the content of their child's intervention goals and activities (Watts Pappas, McLeod, McAllister & McKinnon, 2008).

For many clients with a communication disorder, initial denial of the problem is not unusual; they believe either that theirs is a special case, the problem is not that serious or that there is an ultimate cure (Spillers, 2007). In such situations, an individual with a disorder and/or their families may seek medications or devices that can bring about a cure. For clients with an SSD, proposed cures for the disorder have included a gluten-free diet and/or dietary supplements such as fish oil, but there is currently no empirical evidence to support their use. A particular SLP/SLT may also be viewed as 'the solution'. The senior author of this essay has had several clients whose parents, upon initial diagnosis of a significant SSD for their child, considered relocating to receive services from a particular SLP. Both authors of this essay have had clients and families who seek out multiple opinions in hope that the diagnosis was wrong and/or there really was not a problem. Others seek information on the Internet and then come to the SLP/SLT with their own assessments and opinions.

Several types of counselling can be used with clients with communication disorders: informational counselling, humanistic therapy, interpersonal therapy, behavioural therapy, cognitive therapy, family systems therapy, existential therapy and multicultural therapy among others (Flasher & Fogle, 2012). Although the extent to which SLPs/SLTs should engage in these types of counselling is unclear (Crowe, 1997), didactic, informational counselling (or 'teaching') is arguably one of the most common types of counselling used by SLPs/SLTs (English, 2008; Masterson & Apel, 1997). In this type of counselling, facts and opinions about the disorder are first typically elicited from the client and or family through an intake form and/or during an interview, after which the SLP/SLT provides needed diagnostic and/or treatment information. For example, clients and their families may know little about the disorder, its causes, the prognosis or treatment options. Even though little has been reported in the literature about what type of specific information clients with SSDs and their families need or desire, SLPs/SLTs should be aware that clients recall only 50% of the information they hear from health care professionals and can convey only half of that to loved ones (Margolis, 2004).

Masterson and Apel (1997) allude to some issues the SLP/SLT should be alert to when deciding whether to provide counselling to a client and/or family member or to make a referral to a professional counsellor (Bitter, A15). If either the child or the family has a significant or unexpected reaction to the speech sound production disorder, to the child's unintelligibility, or has unrealistic expectations of therapy, counselling by the SLP/SLT may not provide adequate emotional support. If the focus of the counselling is no longer the communication issue (SSD), referral to a counsellor is appropriate and we recommended it in most cases. Examples of this loss of focus might include when one parent blames the other for 'not doing enough', when a parent 'babies' the child or if the emotional and physical demands of the child's

SSD interferes with the relationship between the child's parents.

To date, there is no research available exploring the need for and effectiveness of counselling in adolescents and adults who have persisting or residual speech sound difficulties. In the case of an adolescent with residual speech sounds errors, the SLP/SLT may need to engage in client-centred discussions to explore potential issues of frustration, ambivalence and motivation. This process, known as motivational interviewing (McFarlane, 2012; Miller & Rollnick, 2002), can help the SLP/SLT identify whether the adolescent's limited progress is a matter of fatigue with therapy or lack of intrinsic motivation. In such situations, the SLP/SLT should counsel the client about these feelings, or perhaps terminate therapy, because without internal motivation, speech change is unlikely. If an adult with residual speech production errors seeks therapy, counselling (at least to some degree) is probably important because the client has embraced a need for change and this internal motivation should be explored so that therapy is as productive as possible.

As SLPs/SLTs reflect on their roles and responsibilities to counsel clients and families coping with an SSD, we see three challenges. First, there is the obvious gap in the literature for evidence-based guidelines when providing effective counselling to clients with this disorder and their families. Second, as the role of genetics in SSDs becomes increasingly important in our understanding of at least some SSDs, practitioners need to be prepared for the realities that genetic testing may have on health care (McDaniel, 2005) and the responsibilities SLPs/SLTs will have in counselling clients and families in this area. Finally, the emergence of telepractice as a service delivery model will require SLPs/SLTs to identify whether online counselling is efficacious and, and if so, which counselling techniques are most effective in this type of delivery. For some clients, technical difficulties and the loss of face-to-

face interaction during online client sessions may make it difficult to develop a productive and supportive relationship (Haberstroh, Duffey, Evans, Gee & Trepal, 2007).

Children with cleft palate, craniofacial anomalies and velopharyngeal dysfunction

Whereas children with co-occurring speech and language difficulties form a typical component of the generalist child SLP/SLT caseload, children with cleft lip and palate, craniofacial anomalies and velopharyngeal dysfunction (or velopharyngeal insufficiency, VPI) may or may not be frequent referrals. In Australia, Canada, New Zealand, the United Kingdom and the United States, and in most other parts of the industrialised world, the majority of children with cleft palate and craniofacial disorders receive speech and/or language therapy at school or in the community, and not from cleft palate 'specialists'. The flow of referrals to generalist settings is likely to increase as the most fragile babies increasingly survive infancy. In the United States, there are public laws (e.g., Public Law 107-110, *No child left behind*, of 2001) *requiring* school personnel to meet the needs of children with all types of impairments and legislation (Individuals with Disabilities Education Improvement Act [IDEA], 2004) that ensures that, if they desire it, parents are full participants in the process (Gretz, A7).

Fortunately located generalist SLPs/SLTs have opportunities to refer to, or consult with by phone, teleconference, e-mail or in person, more experienced colleagues; collaborate with a craniofacial team; or seek the opinion of a specialist in velopharyngeal dysfunction. But many do not have such resources to call upon and are left to handle the task of reading up on and then managing a wide range of difficulties related to cleft lip, cleft palate, submucous cleft, maxillary retrusion, malocclusion and nasal and nasal cavity abnormalities (Persson & Sjögreen, 2011).

It is generally advised that a child who has had early palate surgery should be reviewed at least annually by an SLP/SLT to monitor speech development. The majority of these children will require 'some' through to 'intense' SLP/SLT intervention, and about one in five requires additional (secondary) palate surgery to optimise their potential for typical voice quality, resonance (eliminating hypernasality) and speech. In terms of speech output, the therapy itself may target articulation, phonology and voice quality and aim to expand restricted sound repertoires and eliminate or reduce abnormal compensatory articulation patterns. Children with craniofacial anomalies often have concomitant difficulties with hearing, including chronic otitis media and all that it implies (Purdy, Fairgray & Asad, A52) and additional health and medical issues (Persson & Sjögreen, 2011).

Dr. Karen Golding-Kushner tackles Q17, lending her extraordinary expertise to the important questions that immediately arise for practitioners who see youngsters with craniofacial anomalies infrequently. Known for her role as the past Executive Director of the Velo-Cardio-Facial Syndrome Educational Foundation, Inc., Dr. Golding-Kushner is the former Clinical Director of the Center for Craniofacial Disorders at the Montefiore Medical Center, Bronx, NY, and is currently owner of the Golding-Kushner Speech Center, LLC, a private practice in central New Jersey, USA. An ASHA Fellow, she has specialised in craniofacial disorders, cleft palate and velopharyngeal function for the best part of 30 years.

Q17. Karen Golding-Kushner: Children with craniofacial anomalies

For the generalist SLP/SLT and others who are inexperienced with craniofacial disorders, cleft palate and velopharyngeal function, what are the important issues in speech development, assessment and intervention? Are there circumstances in which the generalist is best advised to step back and rec-

ommend to families that they seek experienced, expert guidance? Some children with craniofacial anomalies have been adopted nationally or internationally, often by parents who have already raised a family and feel they have something to offer a child with special challenges, and in so doing they can face unexpected complications. How would you guide these parents?

A17. Karen Golding-Kushner: Issues in speech development and management of children with craniofacial disorders, cleft palate and velopharyngeal dysfunction

Soon after a new baby with a cleft is born, and prior to any surgery, the SLP/SLT should meet baby and parents, providing information on normal communication development and guidelines for stimulating oral sound development and feeding. Every child with a cleft palate or craniofacial disorder should have a complete speech and language evaluation by the age of 1 year. In the industrialised world, cleft palate is usually repaired at around 12 months, and because of the high risk in this population for *otitis media*, pressure-equalising tubes (ventilation tubes or 'grommets') are frequently surgically inserted at the same time. It is important that both middle-ear health and hearing be closely monitored. Provided these things happen in a timely manner, for the majority of children with cleft lip only, or non-syndromic cleft palate, speech and language development proceeds along typical lines. For about 20% of children with cleft palate, however, and for children with craniofacial disorders associated with certain syndromes, development of language and speech and the quality of voice and resonance may be compromised by risks related to associated anomalies potentially affecting hearing, cognition, morphological (anatomic) structure, physiology (function or movement of structures) and dentition (Hall & Golding-Kushner, 1989; Golding-Kushner, 2001). Some studies have suggested the number of children with speech disorders related to cleft palate, velopharyngeal insufficiency (VPI), or both, is as high as 75%, and that those disorders may even persist into adolescence (Peterson-Falzone, Hardin-Jones & Karnell, 2001; Peterson-Falzone, Trost-Cardamone, Hardin-Jones & Karnell, 2006). Further, some syndromes are associated with *specific* patterns of articulation, voice, resonance and language disorders.

Hearing

The association between palatal clefts, even submucous clefts, and middle ear disease is strong, because the *levator veli palatine, tensor palatine* and other palatal and pharyngeal muscles are abnormally positioned and oriented. The eustachian tube, designed to ventilate the middle ear, leads from each middle ear to the back of the throat. The *tensor palatini* is responsible for opening the eustachian tube orifice, and its abnormal placement and function limits or prevents ventilation. In some cases, the eustachian tube itself may be angled or positioned abnormally. To make matters worse, the belly of the *levator veli palatini* often elevates to fill the opening to the eustachian tube, occluding it during speech and swallowing, preventing it from fulfilling its proper function of ventilating and equalising pressure on either side of the middle ear cavity (Shprintzen & Croft, 1981; Gereau et al. 1988; Shprintzen & Golding-Kushner, 2008). Some syndromes, such as Treacher Collins syndrome, are associated with severe conductive hearing loss. Others, such as Stickler syndrome, are associated with sensorineural hearing impairment. For affected infants and toddlers, early detection, medical or surgical treatment, and, if appropriate, amplification are essential (Purdy, Fairgray & Asad, A52).

Associated syndromes

Over 400 syndromes are associated with cleft palate, and some, including velo-cardio-facial syndrome (VCFS) and foetal alcohol syndrome, are known to be associated with cognitive impairment, language delays or disorders and/or significant hearing loss. These risks, caused by the same genetic defect responsible for the cleft, are inherent to the particular syndrome under consideration. Further, some syndromes, such as VCFS which is caused by a microdeletion on chromosome 22 in the 22q11.2 region, are associated with syndrome-specific patterns of speech and language disorders (Golding-Kushner, 2005, 2012; Shprintzen & Golding-Kushner, 2008; Golding-Kushner & Shprintzen, 2011).

Voice

Vocal quality, pitch and volume each reflect activity at the level of the larynx. Although cleft palate is not a direct risk factor for any of these features, it appears that individuals with borderline velopharyngeal competence may exhibit degrees of hyperfunctional voice use, vocal fold changes and dysphonia (hoarseness), due to attempts to compensate for loss of intraoral air pressure (D'Antonio, Muntz, Marsh, Marty-Grames & Backensto-Marsh, 1988; Lewis, Andreassen, Leeper, Macrae & Thomas, 1993). Some syndromes are associated with laryngeal anomalies that result in voice disorders. For example, among the characteristics of VCFS are unilateral vocal fold paralysis and laryngeal asymmetry, both of which may cause hoarseness; and, laryngeal web, which may cause elevated vocal pitch and loss of volume (loudness) (Chegar, Tatum, Marrinan & Shprintzen,

2006; Miyamoto et al. 2004; Shprintzen, 1999; Shprintzen & Golding-Kushner, 2008; Golding-Kushner & Shprintzen, 2011). Vocal loudness also may be reduced in speakers with conductive hearing loss and increased in speakers with sensorineural hearing loss, both of which might be associated with specific syndromes.

Oral resonance

Very severe oral crowding or hypertrophy (enlargement) of the gingival tissue, or more commonly tonsillar hypertrophy, can cause oral damping of the acoustic signal and muffled resonance. Enlarged tonsils may or may not appear to be infected, but in most cases, removal and pathology analysis reveals they are bacteria-laden. Infection aside, their presence can cause a 'potato-in-the-mouth' tone or *cul-de-sac* resonance. Extremely hypertrophied tonsils in toddlers acquiring speech are also associated with habitual forward tongue carriage as the child works to open the airway by maintaining the tongue in an anterior position. Tonsil size appears different when comparing the view looking in the mouth with the view looking into the airway 60% of the time (Traquina, Golding-Kushner & Shprintzen, 1990). Therefore, in many cases, diagnosis is based on imaging of the vocal tract by nasoendoscopy or, if that is not possible, lateral fluoroscopy with a good barium coat and cannot be based on oral view of the tonsils alone. Oral resonance abnormalities typically require physical management (e.g., tonsillectomy) and are not amenable to speech therapy.

Hyponasality

Too little nasal resonance may result from adenoid hypertrophy, deviated septum, other nasal anomalies or obstruction of the nasopharynx following pharyngoplasty (secondary surgery to eliminate VPI). Because hyponasality can co-occur with hypernasality, both should be rated separately during evaluation (see Table A43.1 in Chapter 6). While the treatment of hyponasality is usually medical or surgical, increasing the duration of nasal consonants during connected speech may effectively reduce the perception of hyponasality (Golding-Kushner, 2001).

Hypernasality

Excessive nasal resonance during vowel production, due to communication between the oral and nasal cavities, is one of the greatest risks associated with cleft palate. Hypernasality, the consequence of VPI, discussed below, is best diagnosed by a trained listener and not instrumentally, because it is *only* of significance if it can be perceived. On the other hand, velopharyngeal dysfunction can *only* be diagnosed using instrumentation to visualise the region, as discussed below. Hypernasality permeates connected speech and occurs when the speaker is unable to fully separate the oral and nasal cavities at the right time during connected speech due to a physical inability to effect velopharyngeal closure, timing errors or both. Hypernasality is a vowel phenomenon but commonly co-occurs with a consonant event also caused by VPI: nasal emission, which is nasal air escape through the nose during speech, especially during production of pressure consonants. Nasal air escape is an obligatory articulation error that occurs in the presence of VPI.

VPI: Velopharyngeal insufficiency, velopharyngeal incompetence, velopharyngeal dysfunction

VPI (or VPD) primarily requires physical management and has several causes including deficient velar tissue, abnormal or asymmetric movement of the velum, lateral pharyngeal walls, or posterior pharyngeal wall, tonsillar hypertrophy (Shprintzen, Sher & Croft, 1987) and errors in learning. If present, an oronasal fistula may exacerbate the effects of VPI (Isberg & Henningsson, 1987). The presence of compensatory articulation errors may also exacerbate VPI (Hoch, Golding-Kushner, Sadewitz & Shprintzen, 1986; Henningsson & Isberg, 1986; Golding-Kushner, 2001). Neuromotor problems may also cause VPI, but cleft palate is not a risk factor for neuromotor problems, and neuromotor problems, such as dysarthria and dyspraxia, occur rarely in children with cleft palate.

Treatment efficacy always rests on accurate diagnosis, and diagnosis of VPI requires direct visualisation of velopharyngeal function during unimpeded connected speech. The gold standard for assessing velopharyngeal closure is direct visualisation using both flexible fibreoptic nasopharyngoscopy to analyse anatomy and airway patency (openness) and multiview videofluoroscopy to view pharyngeal wall motion and tongue activity during speech. Unfortunately, my experience has been that many clinicians continue to rely upon indirect measures like pressure-flow techniques or nasometry to diagnose disorders of resonance and velopharyngeal function. They confuse data that appear 'objective' with an assessment that is valid (relevant). Indirect assessment techniques such as these provide no information about the location, configuration, consistency or cause of VPI and so their value in treatment planning is controversial (Peterson-Falzone et al. 2001).

People often ask, 'Why not do trial therapy to see if hypernasality can be reduced without surgery?' There is no therapy technique to eliminate velopharyngeal closure when VPI is consistently present. Other than for errors of learning (see below), speech therapy is ineffective in eliminating VPI. Never-

theless, despite an absence of evidence in their favour (Lof, A35; Powell, A39), clinicians persist with NS-OME (horn-tooting, whistle-blowing, bubble blowing, pushing manoeuvres), electrical stimulation, palatal massage and other nonsense, wasteful of time and resources. Regrettably, I have seen more than a few patients in whom these procedures caused additional, *avoidable* problems including habituated abnormal tongue position; substitution of /m/ for /n/ because of the focus on lip closure around chewy tubes and wind instruments; and, vocal fold nodules due to excessive laryngeal tension during blowing exercises. A few reports (Kuehn, 1991, 1997) indicate that, under very specific conditions involving inconsistent closure, *improvement* has occurred with continuous positive airway pressure (CPAP) or nasopharyngoscopic biofeedback. However, results were inconsistent across subjects, and it was not clear that VP closure could be completely established or maintained long term. If closure is short term, or 'improved' but not eliminated, hypernasality will persist, so the use of CPAP at this time must be considered experimental (Kummer, 2001).

Errors in learning

Some speech learners, with or without clefts, exhibit adequate velopharyngeal closure on all but one phoneme or sound class, typically involving a nasal snort or nasal fricative substitution for /s, z, f, v, ʃ, ʒ, tʃ, dʒ/. Occluding the nares during stimulability testing results in production of /k/ or nothing at all, and the speaker may exhibit discomfort at not being able to emit air. Such errors in learning are easily treatable with speech therapy, and physical management is inappropriate and unwarranted. In contrast, a speaker with nasal emission, that is, passive loss of air through the nose, sounds better with the nares occluded because he or she was directing air orally and closing the nose eliminated the passive 'leak'. This sometimes occurs in people without history of structural anomalies, in which case it is known as 'phone-specific' or 'sound-specific' VPI. Clinicians are sometimes baffled by this phenomenon and rush to refer to ENT for assessment. However, when nasal symptoms are isolated to a single sound or single group of sounds, it is clear that this is a therapy situation. If, for some reason, further medical assessment were desired, the appropriate referral would be to a craniofacial team who, at intake, would likely identify this as a non-surgical situation and recommend speech therapy.

Articulation

Articulation errors in children with cleft palate, VPI and craniofacial syndromes may be obligatory, maladaptive, developmental or compensatory (Golding-Kushner, 1995, 2004). Of these, all but developmental errors may be related to malocclusion, palatal fistulae, VPI, severe oral crowding or hearing loss. It is important to note that children with cleft palate do *not* typically have CAS, oral-motor weakness, dysarthria or other speech problems of neuromuscular origin. Extensive clinical experience shows that, unfortunately, they are very frequently misdiagnosed with these disorders, leading to the application of inappropriate therapy procedures (Golding-Kushner, 2001). Even when correctly diagnosed, many SLPs/SLTs persist in the inappropriate use of non-speech oral motor exercise. This, in spite of a complete lack of evidence of any benefit (Powers & Starr, 1974; Ruscello, 1982; Starr, 1990; Van Demark & Hardin, 1990; Lof, 2011), and see Ruscello (A48).

Expert guidance

Before starting treatment, it is incumbent on the speech pathologist to sort out which part of the speech disorder can be treated ther-apeutically and which part cannot. Unfortunately, most SLPs/SLTs lack specific training in cleft palate and VPI. When a cleft palate team follows the child in question, the therapist can consult with the SLP/SLT who is part of the team for guidance. I have had excellent results working with children (and their parents) who live long distances from my office using videoconferencing (Golding-Kushner, 2007). Teletherapy, which is gaining in application and popularity in many aspects of medicine, habilitation and rehabilitation, is beyond the scope of this contribution, but is an exciting new frontier. In addition to providing direct therapy services at a distance, telepractice enables SLPs/SLTs with less experience in treating specific disorders and families to access services of a specialist to consult about treatment (Shprintzen & Golding-Kushner, 2012; Tindall, Cohn, Campbell, Golding-Kushner & Christiana, 2012). More information on telepractice as a delivery model for speech and language therapy is available on the American Speech–Language–Hearing Association website (www.asha.org) and on the discussion boards for ASHA's Special Interest Group on Telepractice, SIG 18, accessible to ASHA members and International Affiliates.

What about children who are not known to have a cleft or VPI? The mouth may appear normal on oral examination but that does not mean occult submucous cleft or VPI can be ruled out. A decision tree can be helpful. If you hear hypernasality and all speech errors are obligatory, refer for velopharyngeal imaging. If you hear nasal airflow on only one sound, one cognate pair or one sound class, but nasal airflow is appropriate on other sounds, the problem is likely nasal snorting (also called nasal fricative or phone-specific VPI), treatable with speech therapy. In that situation, referral to a craniofacial team is not necessary, because phone-specific VPI is only treated with speech therapy. Physical management would be inappropriate and would not solve the speech problem.

Nasal airflow can be detected easily by holding a sensitive mirror beneath the nares while the child produces words that exclude nasal phonemes or by holding one end of a drinking straw at the edge of a nostril and holding the other end of the straw to your ear (Skinder-Meredith, A43). If you are not sure, pinch the nose and see if speech (excluding nasal sounds /m, n, ŋ/) seems better. If it is better, the airflow was likely obligatory. If it sounds the same or even worse, the error was likely phone specific, requiring speech therapy. If one is unsure, a referral to an SLP/SLT with expertise in this area, to a craniofacial team or both should be made. Similarly, an SLP/SLT treating a child with a compensatory articulation disorder may lack training in this area. While the basic procedures are those used in 'traditional' articulation therapy, an SLP/SLT with expertise in this area will be able to offer special techniques and 'tricks' to the treating clinician (Golding-Kushner, 2001; Ruscello, A48).

International adoption

I have worked with many families who adopted a child they were told had a repaired cleft palate, only to discover at the time of, or even after, the adoption that the palate had not been repaired, that it was poorly repaired or that the repair had dehisced (ruptured or broken open). This might have been due to poor surgical technique or inadequate post-operative care. These adoptive families are faced with making a decision about surgery while, at the same time, helping their child adjust to their new family, culture and life (Pollock, A18). In many instances, these children were 3 years old or even older when the palate repair was finally done, invariably leading to the development of a severe compensatory articulation disorder. With the support of their family, the ultimate speech outcome for these children has a good prognosis.

Most of the time, children waiting for adoption have not had the benefit of examination by a clinical geneticist, and biological family history may be unknown. This means that, at times, a cleft palate is 'just' a cleft palate, but at others, the cleft may be only one feature of a syndrome. This may or may not be apparent until after the child has been placed, and those considering adoption should be prepared for that possibility.

Summary

The prognosis for normal speech in children with cleft palate is excellent, but is often dependent on a combination of surgery and speech therapy. There are many different surgical procedures and the one that will work best for an individual patient should be determined by the configuration of the velopharyngeal gap as visualised according to the procedures described above.

Children who have been internationally adopted

International, 'inter-country', or 'overseas' adoption is a prevalent practice throughout the industrialised world (Pollock, 2007). Anecdotally, most of these children acquire their new home language with relative ease, even though they may have been quickly transported from orphanage to family home, and from one language to another. A contrary view, well supported by evidence, comes from research effort by Karen Pollock and others into language acquisition of adopted children from non-English-speaking environments, showing that they can have significant difficulties, necessitating SLP/SLT assistance. Dr. Pollock emphasises the need for more research into why, when and how to intervene with these children, stressing the urgent need for both early normative data on language development in internationally adopted children as well as studies identifying predictors of later (school-age) outcomes.

Head of the Child Phonology Laboratory at the University of Alberta in Edmonton, Canada, Dr. Karen Pollock is a professor and chair of the Department of Speech Pathology and Audiology. With a background in both linguistics and SLP, she is co-editor of one of *my* favourite child speech references (Kamhi & Pollock, 2005). Karen received the Honours of the College from the Alberta College of Speech-Language Pathologists and Audiologists in 2009. Her recent research has been concerned with vowel errors in children with phonological disorders and speech–language acquisition in internationally adopted children. Suppressing, with some difficulty, the urge to ask about her important vowel research as well, I asked her to cover some of the international adoption issues that are important for SLPs/SLTs to understand.

Q18.   Karen E. Pollock: Speech–language acquisition of international adoptees

What do we now know about the nature and course of speech–language acquisition in typically developing internationally adopted children? When should we encourage parents to seek professional services, such as speech–language therapy or early intervention, and how can they be supported in the process? And what preparation, in terms of professional consultation, might parents undertake if they are planning to adopt a child from overseas with a known cognitive or communication disability?

A18.   Karen E. Pollock: Internationally adopted children learning English as a second first language

Children adopted internationally experience a unique pattern of linguistic exposure. They typically hear only the language of their birth country prior to adoption, and then, because most English-speaking adoptive parents do not speak the child's birth language, they hear only English after adoption. Consequently, children lose their birth language abilities rapidly; within weeks according to some estimates. In essence, they become monolingual English speakers shortly after adoption, but have not yet had sufficient time to acquire age-appropriate English skills. Obviously, the older the child at adoption, the more linguistic catching up is required to match monolingual non-adopted peers, and the more likely their overall language proficiency and academic success will be affected. Because language acquisition in children adopted internationally differs from that of other bilingual or second language learners, the term 'second first language learners' has been proposed (e.g., Glennen, 2002; Roberts et al. 2005). Lacking ongoing first language capabilities as a scaffold, the reality for these children is that they have to 'start over' with learning the new language (Geren, Snedeker & Ax, 2005).

Early empirical investigators of second first language acquisition anticipated various delays based on two assumptions. First, they believed the second first language-learning situation was bound to impact development detrimentally. Second, they expected early environmental deprivation related to orphanage care to evoke significant delays in cognition and language. Indeed, studies of children adopted from Romania during the early 1990s supported these hypotheses, with the prevalence of language delays extending from 60 to 94% (e.g., Johnson, 2000; Rutter & The English and Romanian Adoptees Study Team, 1998).

Optimistic findings from subsequent studies of children adopted from Russia, China and elsewhere suggest that the Romanian situation was extraordinary. The extreme neglect/deprivation suffered by Romanian orphans and their struggles post-adoption appear to be atypical of internationally adopted children generally. In fact many internationally adopted children have been found to demonstrate average or better English language skills within a year or two post-adoption (see summary of studies reviewed below), demonstrating that for many children second first language learning proceeds relatively smoothly and the effects of early institutionalization may be counteracted by placement in an enriched environment (Glennen, 2007b; Windsor, Glaze, Koga & the Bucharest Early Intervention Project Core Group, 2007).

Language acquisition in internationally adopted children

Most communication research with this population deals with lexical and syntactic development. Results show that for children adopted under 2;0, vocabulary and morphosyntax increase rapidly during the first year home, continuing to improve during the preschool years. For example, Glennen (2007a) found that 78% of a group of children adopted from Eastern Europe had language abilities that were comfortably WNL, using standard monolingual English norms, by 1 year post-adoption. Similarly, Pollock, Chattaway, Fast, Reay and Zmijewski (2006) reported that 82% of a group of children adopted from Haiti showed abilities WNL one or more years post-adoption. In addition, 29% of their children showed exceptional language abilities (more than 1.25 SD above the test mean). Roberts et al. (2005) found that 95% of the adopted Chinese preschoolers they studied, all of whom had been in their permanent homes for two or more years, scored within or above the normal range on standardised speech and language measures, and 27% demonstrated exceptional language skills. Thus, it appears that although there is a wide range of abilities, most children adopted as infants or toddlers 'catch up' to norms for non-adopted monolingual peers following a year or two of expo-

sure to English. Less research has been completed on children adopted at older ages (2–5 years), but preliminary studies (e.g., Glennen, 2007c) indicate equally impressive progress, with most children scoring WNL on standardised test measures from 1 to 2 years post-adoption. However, despite the promising group trends, most studies have reported a number of children (from 5 to 22%) who continue to struggle with the acquisition of English beyond 2 years post-adoption.

Results of recent investigations of longer-term outcomes (early elementary school) for language and literacy skills in children adopted under 2;0 are mixed. For example, Scott, Roberts and Krakow (2008) found that 92% of a group children adopted from China who had completed Grade 1 or 2 performed at or above average on direct measures of oral and written language, compared to 77% of the Grade 1–7 children adopted from Haiti reported by Pollock, Bylsma, Perry, and Yam (2010). Pollock and Yan (2011) reported that 86% of children adopted from China and currently in Kindergarten to Grade 4 (in the United States) had acceptable general language scores on a parent report measure. By contrast, Glennen and Bright (2005) found a higher incidence of pragmatic and higher-level language skills difficulties in school-age children adopted from Eastern Europe. Approximately 11% of them received diagnoses of either a speech—language impairment or learning disability, and 25% had attention deficits and/or were considered hyperactive. These discrepant results may relate to the different birth countries, gender (all girls in the group adopted from China), age at testing or methodology (hands-on assessments vs. parent/teacher surveys).

Speech acquisition in internationally adopted children

There is little research on speech (i.e., phonetic or phonological) development in these children, with Pollock (2007) and Pollock and Price (2005) providing detailed summaries of the available studies. Two longitudinal small-N group studies (Pollock, Price & Fulmer, 2003; Price, Pollock & Oller, 2006) of children adopted from China as infants/toddlers found considerable individual variation in early phonological measures, such as canonical babbling ratio, phonetic inventory size and diversity and proportion of monosyllables. However, the majority (seven out of eight) of participants performed WNL on the *Goldman Fristoe Test of Articulation – 2nd Edition* (GFTA-2) (Goldman & Fristoe, 2000) at 3;0 and/or had normal range PCCs. Errors were primarily familiar developmental ones seen in monolingual English-speaking children, like cluster reduction, gliding, stopping and derhotacisation. The one child whose GFTA-2 score was below average also had a low PCC, explained by prevalent cluster reduction and stopping, and an idiosyncratic pattern of consonant addition. Interestingly, none of the early speech measures taken at 6 months post-adoption appeared to predict performance at 3;0.

Several larger group studies of toddlers/pre-schoolers one or more years post-adoption included a standardized measure of articulation proficiency, the GFTA-2, in their assessment battery. Glennen (2007c) found that 3 (or 11%) of 27 2 year olds adopted from Eastern Europe scored below average and Pollock et al. (2006) reported low scores for 2 of 17 (12%) 2- to 7-year-old children adopted from Haiti. Similarly, in their study of 55 3- to 6 year olds adopted from China under 2;0, Roberts et al. (2005) found that only 4 of the 55 (or 7%) had below average standard scores. Although studies of school age internationally adopted children have not included expressive phonology measures, Scott et al. (2008) reported that 3 of the 24 first- and second-grade children studied were receiving services for mild articulation disorders.

Aiming to explore phonological abilities in more detail, Pollock, Chow, and Tamura (2004) phonetically transcribed spontaneous language samples from a subset (25) of the pre-schoolers in the Roberts et al. (2005) study. Analyses included PCC-Revised (PCC-R), phonological mean length of utterance (PMLU) and phonological process incidence. Three children (12%) had low scores on one or more measures, but no common trends emerged. Mostly, they produced developmental errors commonly seen in non-adopted monolingual English-speaking peers, and evidence of cross-linguistic interference from Chinese was absent. Similar findings were reported by Balding and Smith (2008) for children adopted from Haiti. In summary, the bulk of children studied demonstrated age-appropriate phonology following 1 or 2 years of English exposure. The error types of those with delays were comparable to those often seen in their monolingual English-speaking peers with phonological delay.

Implications for assessment

Parents considering adoption or waiting for a child's arrival need to gather all available information about the child's communication status in their birth language. Such information is not routinely provided, but can be critical in diagnosing true disorders and determining eligibility for services. Glennen (2002) provided a comprehensive list of suggested questions about language development and abilities to ask caregivers during pre-adoption interchanges or at the time of adoption, and communication skills to observe during initial meetings.

Communication assessment of internationally adopted children presents challenges for SLPs/SLTs, particularly during the first-year post-adoption. While the birth language is undergoing rapid attrition and the transition to the emerging adopted language is proceeding, it is difficult (if not impossible) to determine whether apparent delays relate to this natural transition or are evidence of developmental communication delays that predated adoption.

Glennen (2005, 2007a) proposed guidelines for the assessment of speech–language skills in newly adopted children, combining prelinguistic (foundational) measures like joint attention, gestures and symbolic play (using the Communication and Symbolic Behaviour Skills-Developmental Profile) (Weatherby & Prizant, 2002) and linguistic measures like vocabulary comprehension (using the MacArthur Communicative Development Inventories) (Fenson et al. 1993). Applied to a group of 27 toddlers (aged 11–23 months) adopted from Eastern Europe, these guidelines accurately predicted those with persistent language delays at 2;0. Glennen stressed the benefit of including prelinguistic measures in early assessments, noting that they are not language specific and remain unchanged post-adoption. When using language-specific measures with newly adopted children, comprehension measures are more likely to accurately reflect abilities, as comprehension typically precedes production. Pollock and Price (2005) offered similar suggestions for phonetic/phonological assessment, emphasizing that during the first weeks or months post-adoption, observations of the quality and quantity of vocalisations (whether actual words or not) and size and diversity of the phonetic inventory could yield important diagnostic information. For example, typically developing children, regardless of adoption status or language environment, are expected to produce canonical syllables by 10 months of age.

Over the first year or two post-adoption, preliminary normative data are available for vocabulary size and utterance length from two longitudinal studies. Glennen and Masters (2002) followed 130 children adopted from Eastern Europe, and Pol-

lock (2005) provided similar data for 141 children adopted from China. These data, organized by chronological age or months post-adoption, can be used to compare a child's scores to those of other children adopted at similar ages. In terms of phonetic/phonological development, Pollock and Price (2005) suggest periodic reassessments to monitor the size, diversity and distribution of sounds in the phonetic repertoire to monitor the rate and amount of change over time. These measures may also be compared to normative data for monolingual children, but interpreted according to length of exposure to English rather than chronological age.

Finally, based on the results of numerous studies of preschool and school-aged children adopted from China and Eastern Europe as infants/toddlers (e.g., Glennen & Bright, 2005; Pollock et al., 2004; Roberts et al., 2005; Scott et al., 2008), it appears that standard English tests can be used (although cautiously) 1 or more years post-adoption. Children adopted as pre-schoolers may be assessed with such instruments 2 or more years post-adoption (Glennen, 2007c).

Any child adopted internationally is potentially 'at risk' for speech–language delays, by virtue of the abrupt language switch and inadequate stimulation in orphanages. This necessitates parents being watchful regarding development during the first-year home, and, if concerns emerge, seeking an SLP/SLT opinion. As a rule of thumb for families, if vocabulary, utterance length and intelligibility gains are sluggish, a comprehensive speech–language evaluation is indicated, and intervention may be necessary.

Well-established guidelines for determining eligibility for speech–language intervention services for children adopted internationally are currently unavailable, with intervention decisions often made randomly (Glennen, 2007b). Glennen found that about half of the newly adopted toddlers she followed were assessed by early intervention teams and provided speech–language intervention, even though many were *already* functioning at the top of their peer group. At the other extreme, stories of older internationally adopted children being denied services are even more concerning. For example, Glennen (2007b) shared an example of a girl aged 8;0, floundering academically 4 years post-adoption, who was denied assessment and treatment services in English because she was classified as an English as a Second Language (ESL) student. Incredibly, even though she had not been exposed to her birth language for 4 years, the school insisted on testing her in that language. I also have personal knowledge of a child for whom a school postponed speech–language assessment until the child had 'graduated' from their ESL program: a glaring catch-22! The ESL program was not designed to meet the needs of second first language learners or children with language delays/impairments.

It is unclear whether such stories are common, but there is a clear need for the development and implementation of evidence-based guidelines for assessment and intervention. Meanwhile, when such situations arise, parents and SLPs/SLTs should advocate for appropriate services and educate other professionals about the unique circumstances of children adopted internationally and the nature of second first language acquisition. Just as it is inappropriate to hold newly adopted children to unreasonable expectations based on non-adopted monolingual speech–language norms, service eligibility guidelines developed for bilingual and ESL children cannot simply be generalised to children adopted internationally.

To date, there have been no investigations of treatment efficacy for internationally adopted children with speech–language delays/disorders, but we do have descriptions of such children with true speech–language disorders (Pollock, 2007). They include little evidence of either cross-linguistic (birth language) interference or communication patterns unique to this population. Apparently the children mimic the same process of development as monolingual English-speaking children, but at later ages. Thus, when intervention is warranted, it is appropriate to employ the procedures and materials commonly used with monolingual clients. As Glennen (2007b) notes, intervention should 'target each child's diagnosis and symptoms, not the adoption status' (p. 6).

Children learning more than one language

The publication of a position paper on *Multilingual children with speech sound disorders* (International Expert Panel on Multilingual Children's Speech, 2012) marked the culmination of a huge collaborative effort, described by McLeod, Verdon & Bowen (2013), and the launch of further work in this fascinating area. The panel's position statement (p. 1) reads: 'The International Expert Panel on Multilingual Children's Speech recommends that:

1. Children are supported to communicate effectively and intelligibly in the languages spoken within their families and communities, in the context of developing their cultural identities.
2. Children are entitled to professional speech and language assessment and intervention services that acknowledge and respect their existing competencies, cultural heritage, and histories. Such assessment and intervention should be based on the best available evidence.
3. SLPs aspire to be culturally competent and to work in culturally safe ways.
4. SLPs aspire to develop partnerships with families, communities, interpreters, and other health and education professionals to promote strong and supportive communicative environments.
5. SLPs generate and share knowledge, resources, and evidence nationally and internationally to facilitate the understanding of cultural and

linguistic diversity that will support multilingual children's speech acquisition and communicative competency.

6. Governments, policy makers, and employers acknowledge and support the need for culturally competent and safe practices and equip SLPs with additional time, funding, and resources in order to provide equitable services for multilingual children.'

The 57 members of the International Expert Panel on Multilingual Children's Speech had worked in the following 31 countries: Australia, Austria, Brazil, Canada, China, Ecuador, Finland, France, Germany, Greece, Hong Kong, Hungary, Ireland, Israel, Jamaica, Japan, Korea, Malta, New Zealand, Paraguay, Peru, Russia, Slovakia, Singapore, South Africa, Sweden, Switzerland, Turkey, United Kingdom, United States of America and Viet Nam. The members used the following 26 languages in a professional capacity: Afrikaans, Arabic, Australian Sign Language (Auslan), Bulgarian, Cantonese, Danish, Dutch, English, Finnish, French, German, Greek, Hebrew, Hungarian, Icelandic, Italian, Jamaican, Korean, Mandarin, Portuguese, Russian, Spanish, Swedish, Turkish, Yiddish and Welsh plus many other languages in non-professional capacities.

The panel included several of the contributors to *Children's Speech Sound Disorders*, Second Edition: Elise Baker (A13), Martin Ball (A3), B. May Bernhardt (A37), Caroline Bowen, Brian Goldstein (A19), Anne Hesketh (A28), David Ingram (A6, A12), Sharynne McLeod (A1), Benjamin Munson (A51), Michelle Pascoe (A2), Carol Stoel-Gammon (A9), A. Lynn Williams (A26) and Krisztina Zajdó (A20). The reader will see that the authors of the next two essays, Brian Goldstein and Krisztina Zajdó, appear on this list.

Dr. Brian Goldstein is Dean and Professor, School of Nursing and Health Sciences, La Salle University, Philadelphia, USA. Dr. Goldstein is well published in the area of communication development and disorders in Latino children focusing on speech sound development and disorders in monolingual Spanish and Spanish-English bilingual children. He is the former editor of *Language, Speech and Hearing Services in Schools*, is a Fellow of the American Speech-Language-Hearing Association (ASHA), and received the Certificate of Recognition for Special Contribution in Multicultural Affairs from ASHA.

Q19.   Brian Goldstein: Children with SSD who are multilingual

SLPs/SLTs who work with culturally and linguistically diverse families field an unending array of frequently asked questions about normative expectations, and when and why to refer a child growing up bilingual for speech assessment. For example, should all bilingual preschoolers be assessed 'just in case'; should a child hear one language or two if he or she has speech and language difficulties; do multilingual children acquire speech differently from monolingual peers; are they typically 'behind' in both languages for a period; do some combinations of languages pose more difficulties in acquisition than others; what significant speech characteristics should parents and teachers be alert to as a child who is to grow up multilingual acquires speech; and should the family seek out a multilingual clinician? Can you guide the reader as to expected developmental pathways for speech acquisition; suggest appropriate screening and assessment procedures, and describe suitable intervention methodologies for multilingual children with SSD and ways of managing homework. Certain concerns can arise in cases of bilingualism in families where the language(s) other than English are indigenous, perceived as low-status, unusual or endangered. Can you comment on this and also reflect on the potential impact upon service delivery of attitudes, preconceptions and beliefs, held by the clinician, and how a clinician might enhance his or her cultural competence in clinic and education settings.

A19. Brian Goldstein: Providing clinical services to multilingual children with SSD

Many parents who are raising multilingual children question the rate and quality of their children's speech and language development. They do so, in part, because they are concerned that the acquisition of more than one language will 'confuse' their children and result in delayed, or at least slowed, language development in both languages. SLPs/SLTs also might hold this view, especially if they do not believe they have the requisite knowledge and skills to provide services to those who are culturally and linguistically diverse (Guiberson & Atkins, 2012), particularly if they are multilingual (Williams & McLeod, 2012). *Intuitively*, acquiring two of anything should be more complex than acquiring only one of something, but given that a majority of the world's speakers are multilingual (Grosjean, 2010), such unease is fortunately unfounded.

The literature on speech and language development unambiguously reports that multilingual children are not at-risk for SSD simply because they are multilingual or because of the constellation of languages they are acquiring (see Kohnert, 2008 for a comprehensive review). That is, from an acquisition perspective, no one language is more difficult to acquire than another, assuming that children have significant opportunity to hear and speak each language.

That said, it is critical to know that language development, in general, and speech development, in particular, is not the same as it is for monolingual children. Multilinguals will exhibit dissimilar speech sound skills/phonological patterns across languages (Goldstein & McLeod, 2012), exhibiting differing skills, patterns and/or errors in each of their languages. For example, a child acquiring English and Italian will demonstrate a higher frequency of final consonant deletion in English than in Italian because of the phonotactic (structural) properties of English compared to Italian. Thus, clinicians should not expect to see errors/patterns in one language duplicated in the other(s) in either multilinguals with SSD or those who are typically developing.

Speech sound development in typically developing multilinguals

Speech sound development in multilinguals results in positive transfer and negative transfer (McLeod & Goldstein, 2012).

Positive transfer occurs when speech sound development occurs at a faster rate in multilinguals than in monolinguals. For example, Grech and Dodd (2008) examined speech sound skills in 2- to 6-year-old Maltese and English speakers, finding that their bilingual participants exhibited more advanced skills compared to monolingual speakers as exemplified by consonant accuracy, consistency and a fewer error patterns. The same has been noted in 3 year olds (Fabiano-Smith & Goldstein, 2010). Several other studies have shown that speech sound skills were not significantly different in multilinguals compared with monolinguals (e.g., Arnold, Currio, Miccio & Hammer, 2004; Goldstein & Bunta, 2012). So, children acquiring multiple languages are able to maintain speech sound skills that are WNL relative to monolinguals, indicating a type of positive transfer (see Fabiano-Smith & Goldstein, 2010 for more details).

Negative transfer occurs when speech sound skills develop at a slower rate in multilinguals than in monolinguals. Studies have indicated that the phonetic inventories in bilingual children were not age-appropriate compared to monolinguals (Holm & Dodd, 2006), that multilinguals exhibited lower accuracy and a higher number of errors than did monolinguals (Gildersleeve-Neumann,

Kester, Davis & Peña, 2008) and that multilingual children made more errors and produced more uncommon error patterns than monolinguals (Gildersleeve, Davis & Stubbe, 1996).

Importantly, over time, typically developing multilingual children achieve speech skills commensurate with those of monolinguals (Holm & Dodd, 2006).

Speech development in multilinguals with SSD

Not all multilinguals develop speech sound skills typically. Multilingual children will exhibit SSD, but SSD in this population do *not* result from *being multilingual*. That is, multilingualism is *not* a risk factor for SSD. Studies of SSD in multilingual children indicate the following characteristics (Dodd, Holm & Li, 1997; Holm & Dodd, 1999a; Goldstein, 2000; Holm, Dodd, Stow & Pert, 1998):

- Low intelligibility to family and non-family members.
- Low consonant accuracy in *both* languages.
- Similar, although not identical, phonological skills to monolinguals with SSD.
- Similar phonological patterns in both languages.
- Dissimilar phonological patterns in both languages.
- Phonetic inventories consisting of mainly early developing sounds, although some later developing phonemes will occur as well.
- Numerous substitution errors in both languages when cross-linguistic effects and dialect features are taken into account during scoring.
- Substitutions for both early developing and later developing phonemes in all languages.

Assessing speech sound skills in multilinguals

In assessing and subsequently treating (if necessary) multilingual children with SSD, some clinicians mistakenly believe that best practices they have learned and utilized with monolinguals should be abandoned simply because a child is acquiring more than one language. Best practices in providing clinical services are invariable regardless of the number of languages a child is acquiring. Moreover, clinical services should conform to the International Classification of Functioning, Disability and Health: Children and Youth Version (ICF-CY) (World Health Organization, WHO, 2007; International Expert Panel on Multilingual Children's Speech, 2012).

Regardless of the constellation of languages the child speaks, or the perceived status of the languages by the larger community, intervention emanates from comprehensive assessment (Goldstein & Fabiano, 2006) that takes all of them into account. Similarly, all languages spoken by the child need to be accounted for in the intervention processes. A monolingual approach to either assessment or intervention is untenable. As Kohnert (2008) has noted, a disorder in bilinguals is not caused by bilingualism or cured by monolingualism.

Ideally, a clinician who speaks all the child's languages performs assessment, but typically, this is not feasible. Most clinicians will need the help of support personnel such as interpreters and translators (see Langdon & Cheng, 2002) in an assessment that covers language status, hearing status, the oral-peripheral mechanism and speech sound skills. The latter is emphasised here.

Assessment begins with a case history that encompasses questions added about language history, language use and language proficiency: dimensions that change over time and affect speech sound skills in multilinguals (Goldstein, Bunta, Lange, Rodriguez & Burrows, 2010). The clinician then obtains single word and connected speech samples in all languages using tools designed for that population (International Expert Panel on Multilingual Children's Speech, 2012). Assessments for languages other than English are listed in McLeod and Goldstein (2012) and McLeod (2007). Sampling all languages is paramount because multilingual children exhibit discrepant skills, errors and error patterns that are distributed across their languages (Goldstein, Fabiano & Washington, 2005). Thus, measuring skills in only one language provides an incomplete picture of the child's phonological *system*. The samples are subjected to independent and relational analyses (Stoel-Gammon, A9). Independent analyses examine the child's speech sound system without reference to the adult targets. Clinicians should create a phonetic inventory in each language consisting of, for example, singleton consonants, clusters, syllable types, syllable shapes and word length. Then, relational analyses (referencing the child's productions against the adult target) should be completed. Common relational analyses include consonant accuracy, vowel accuracy, whole word accuracy (Ingram, 2012; A12) and phonological patterns (e.g., final consonant deletion, velar fronting, unstressed syllable deletion). For multilingual children, also examine accuracy of shared elements (i.e., those common to all languages, such as /m/ between Italian and English) and unshared elements (i.e., unique to each language, such as the trill, which occurs in Spanish but not in English) (Fabiano-Smith & Goldstein, 2010). Finally, complete an error analysis, examining for substitution and syllable structure errors.

In each analysis, it is vital to account for both cross-linguistic effects (using an element specific to one language in the production of the other language; e.g., a child producing the Spanish trill /r/ in the production of an English word) and dialect features (Goldstein & Iglesias, 2001). Neither cross-linguistic effects nor dialect features should be scored as errors or considered to be appropriate intervention targets.

Providing intervention to multilinguals with SSD

In this age of evidence-based practice in communication sciences and disorders (Dollaghan, 2007), clinicians base their intervention decisions on literature-supporting approaches and techniques that are reliable and valid. Doing so for multilingual children with SSD is difficult, if not impossible, given the paucity of relevant intervention studies. The available few include Holm and Dodd (1999b); Holm, Dodd and Ozanne (1997), Holm, Dodd, Stow and Pert (1998) and Ray (2002) in which only English was utilised as the language of intervention. Their results indicate that intervention in English generally positively influences speech sound skills in the other language. Thus, speech sound skills in all languages should be monitored throughout intervention in order to track cross-linguistic generalisation flowing from interdependence between the two languages (Paradis, 2001).

Clinicians, with little evidence to guide them, often mistakenly believe that the first treatment decision for multilingual should be focused on the language of intervention. They should really be asking themselves, 'When do I treat in each of the two languages?' (Goldstein, 2006). Answering this clinical question begins with a broad and deep understanding of the child's phonological system in each language. As with a monolingual child with an SSD, initial speech sound goals for the multilingual child are determined. Determining those goals can be completed through a bilingual approach and a cross-linguistic approach (Kohnert & Derr, 2012; Kohnert et al. 2005). In a *bilingual approach* speech sound skills, errors or error patterns common to all the languages spoken by the child (e.g., stopping of fricatives) should be targeted initially because, theoretically, this may promote cross-linguistic generalisation from one language to the other language(s) (Yavaş & Goldstein, 1998). Once speech sound skills, errors or error patterns common to all languages have been targeted, the clinician would introduce a *cross-linguistic approach* to focus on speech sound skills, errors or error patterns that occur in only one of the child's languages. This approach is adopted because, for example, Language A will contain a phoneme such as the palatal nasal in Amharic that does not exist in the other language (English). Additionally, clinicians might target errors or error patterns that are exhibited with unequal frequency in each language. For example, unlike English, Korean does not contain word-initial clusters (Kim & Pae, 2007). Thus, remediation of cluster errors could occur only for English and in English.

Once the approach is chosen, the goal attack strategy can be determined. Fey (1986) outlined three goal attack strategies: vertical, horizontal and cyclical. A vertical strategy focuses on one goal until a specified criterion is reached. The multilingual correlate would be focusing on a goal that is specific to one language but also measuring how it generalizes to the other language(s). For example, /s/ would be remediated in English and monitored in Cantonese. A horizontal strategy is one in which more than one goal is addressed in each session. The bilingual correlate is to target one goal in Language A and one goal in Language B within the same session, although the targets would be divergent. For example, the clinician might target final consonants in English and aspirated affricates in Hmong. In a cyclical strategy several goals are addressed in rotation, but only one goal is incorporated at a time within a session. The bilingual correlate would be to alternate both targets *and* languages. For example, in cycle 1, the clinician might target /s/ in Language A and clusters in Language B; in cycle 2, the

clinician might focus on clusters in Language A and /s/ in Language B.

The language of intervention will probably be determined during the process of choosing the intervention approach goals and goal attack strategy. There might be, however, additional factors to consider in deciding the language of intervention. Such factors might include language history, language use, language proficiency and the family's goals (Goldstein, 2006).

Summary and conclusions

The world is becoming more 'flat' (Friedman, 2005). Because of global interconnection, and a host of other factors, the number of multilingual children appears to be increasing making it more likely that clinicians will have to provide services to this population. Doing so might necessitate changed perspectives, enhanced cultural competence and a need for updated information and knowledge.

SLPs/SLT clinicians are trained in the foundation of language and linguistics for a reason. That is, they are grounded in phonetics and phonology so that they can bring that knowledge to bear in the assessment and intervention of children with SSD, regardless of the type and number of languages they are acquiring. That knowledge can be reviewed and upgraded, or acquired, in order to assess and treat multilingual children with SSD.

Providing clinical services to multilingual children with SSD can be daunting because of a general lack of research with this population, little to no pre-service training and scant resources. Despite these limitations, it is possible to provide reliable, valid clinical services to multilingual children with SSD by keeping an open mind, knowing what you do not know, doing your homework at the pre-referral and pre-assessment stages, reaching out to others (interpreters, translators, cultural brokers), completing a comprehensive assessment in all languages, providing intervention based on bilingual and cross-linguistic approaches and monitoring cross-linguistic generalisation. Finally, remember to do the 'right' thing as 'this will gratify some and astonish the rest' (Mark Twain).

Non-English-speaking children

In A19, Brian Goldstein discusses assessment and intervention with children with SSD who are multilingual in English and one or more other languages. Extending the information he provides, Dr. Krisztina Zajdó reviews, in A20, research into speech acquisition in non-English-speaking children, reflecting on what it reveals about speech development in general, and how it can help to inform SLP's/SLT's assessment and intervention decisions.

Krisztina Zajdó, PhD, is a linguist and speech scientist in Hungary, where she currently works as an associate professor in Special Education/Speech-Language Pathology at the University of West Hungary in Győr. She studied speech and hearing sciences at the University of Washington in Seattle under the direction of Dr. Carol Stoel-Gammon. Her primary research interests are the acquisition of vowels in children and developmental changes in children's speech timing patterns cross-linguistically. She also studies phonetic differences in adult directed vs. child-directed speech. After returning from the United States to her native Hungary in 2008, she directed the development of a new speech–language pathology program at UWH. Recently, she developed an interest in studying speech, language and cognitive development in children with mild intellectual disability being reared in both segregated and integrated learning environments.

Q20.   Krisztina Zajdó: Speech acquisition in non-English-speaking children

There are differences in the speech acquisition process between children who are monolingual and children who are multilingual (Goldstein, A19). Are there implications from contemporary research relating to non-English-speaking children that SLPs/SLTs might usefully take into account when planning and delivering intervention for multilingual children with SSD?

A20.   Krisztina Zajdó: What cross-linguistic studies can teach us about vowel and consonant acquisition

A fundamental goal in speech–language pathology is to help children with SSD learn to generate and use language-specific speech patterns spontaneously. An important requirement is that children's speech should be intelligible to native speakers of the environmental language or languages. By definition, multilingual children who are in the process of becoming equipped with the capability to communicate successfully must acquire speech sounds, sequences and patterns in the languages they speak.

The majority of speech acquisition studies published in the twentieth century focus on elucidating the acquisition process in children acquiring English. Major textbooks and professional publications contain information on children's speech production skills based on studies carried out by monolingual English SLPs/SLTs as experimenters studying monolingual English-speaking participants. It is only recently that more emphasis has been given to understanding speech acquisition in non-English-speaking language communities and bilinguals speaking a non-English language. Overall, there is a scarcity of data on speech acquisition in children acquiring non-English languages, including major non-standard dialects of those languages. An additional difficulty is that studies on speech sound acquisition in languages other than English apply considerably different research methodologies. Thus, results need to be reviewed and interpreted with caution.

Recent research has uncovered new information about speech acquisition in various language environments, enriching our understanding of speech acquisition. Cross-linguistic studies shed light both on universal and more restricted tendencies in speech sound acquisition. Many well-established 'truths', based solely on inter-pretations of data from monolingual English-speaking children, are proving to be valid for specific language environments, rather than simply being constituent representatives of universal trends.

Ages of vowel acquisition

An example is the once widely held the-ory pertaining to the so-called 'early' acquisi-tion of vowels. For Cantonese-speaking chil-dren, percentage of vowels correct (PVC) is reported to be 98.8% for the age range 2;0–2;5 (So & Dodd, 1995). At these ages, chil-dren acquiring Putonghua produce 82.4% of vowels correctly (Zhu & Dodd, 2000). By contrast, Hungarian-speaking children's vowel accuracy is 85.2% at 2;0 (Zajdó, 2002). In American English-speaking young children's single word productions, vowel errors are relatively rare, with the exception of r-coloured vowels (Pollock & Berni, 2003). However, the authors report occasional non-rhotic vowel errors for the age range 6;6–6;11. Cross-linguistic research indicates that the acquisition of non-rhotic vowels in some languages takes considerably longer than once supposed. For example, in Hungar-ian, vowel errors are still expected in typi-cally developing children of 7;0–8;0 in single word productions, especially during the pro-duction of mid front rounded vowels (Nagy, 1980). Thus, cross-linguistic data demon-strate that accurate vowel production poses more challenge, and therefore takes longer

to perfect, for children than once thought (Zajdó, 2013).

Order of vowel acquisition

Another theory called into question in light of cross-linguistic research pertains to the order of acquisition in vowel categories proposed by Jakobson (1941/1968). He speculated that children first acquire unrounded vowels, fol-lowed by back rounded ones and then front rounded ones. The findings of a detailed study on Putonghua (Modern Standard Chi-nese; Zhu, 2002), however, indicate that chil-dren in this language community acquire the front rounded vowel /y/ prior to the back rounded vowel /o/. Thus, cross-linguistic data in this case challenge old beliefs that were once considered 'language (speech) univer-sals'. Obviously, further research is needed with regard to vowel development in mono-lingual and multilingual children.

Singleton consonant acquisition

Widely held beliefs around the acquisition of consonants have also been called into ques-tion. First, in terms of accuracy of conso-nant production, it was thought that children produce perceptually accurate consonants accurately, with very few exceptions, by the time they are 6;0. While this observation seems to be valid for many languages includ-ing Cantonese, Turkish, Putonghua, German and Sesotho, where PCC measures for chil-dren at this age exceed 98% (Zajdó, 2013), Jordanian Arabic appears to be an excep-tion. Results from children acquiring this lan-guage show PCC results that are at 90% in the 6;0–6;10 age range (Amayreh & Dyson, 1998). Thus, a clinician might expect some-what lower speech sound accuracy results from multilinguals that speak Jordanian Ara-bic. We can draw from this information that the acquisition of accurate consonant production appears to be language specific rather than universal.

The second belief that has recently been shown to be unfounded is that consonants across languages are acquired roughly by the same age by children from diverse language backgrounds. For example, it has long been known that the voiced palatal approximant /j/ is present in many of the world's languages, including child speech. Recent results suggest that age of acquisition for this consonant in monolingual children is reported to be different from language to language. In Cantonese, several studies established a very early age of acquisition, between 1;3 and 2;1 (Cheung, 1990; So & Dodd, 1995; Tse, 1991; Tse, 1982). Similarly, the approximant is acquired early, by the age of 2;0 in Maltese by 75% of children (Grech, 1998). The same sound is reported to be produced correctly somewhat later in Thai, where its age of acquisition at the 80% level is between 2;1–2;6 and 3;1–3;6 by Boonyathitisuk (1982). German children learn this sound by 3;0–3;5 (Fox & Dodd, 1999). Children learning Hungarian acquire /j/ between 3;0 and 4;0 (Nagy, 1980). Diverse ages of acquisition are reported for Japanese, ranging from 2;10–3;0 (Takagi & Yasuda, 1967) to 4;0–4;5 (Nakanishi, Owada & Fujita, 1972). By contrast, the voiced palatal approximant is acquired late, between 6;0 and 6;6, in Jordanian Arabic (Amayreh & Dyson, 1998; Amayreh, 2003). Taken together, these data suggest that the age of acquisition is language specific for this consonant in monolingual children. In Cantonese, it is acquired early while in Jordanian Arabic it is acquired quite late. Cross-linguistically, 4 years of difference can be detected in the age of acquisition of the voiced palatal approximant.

A similar example is the acquisition of the alveolar lateral approximate /l/ across languages. In both German (Fox & Dodd, 1999) and Cantonese (Tse, 1982; Cheung, 1990), it is acquired during the third year of life. In Jordanian Arabic (Amayreh & Dyson, 1998),

Greek (Papadopoulou, 2000) and Hungarian (Nagy, 1980), it is acquired during the fourth year of life. Korean-speaking children, however, learn to produce /l/ correctly during their fifth year (Kim & Pae, 2005). Depending on the language environment, children learn to produce this sound correctly at various ages. Thus, SLPs/SLTs need to take into account language-specific patterns in acquisition in their evaluations of multilingual children's speech.

Consonant cluster acquisition

Considering the language background of multilingual children is important for clinicians' expectations of the acquisition of clusters too. For example, results of a study by Yavaş (2013) suggest that children acquiring different languages vary in correctly producing word-initial /#sC/ clusters. Children learning Germanic languages (such as English, Dutch and Norwegian) are more successful in producing accurate consonant clusters where the second element is a continuant rather than a non-continuant. In contrast, children acquiring non-Germanic languages (such as Hebrew, Croatian and Polish) show no such dichotomy in consonant cluster accuracy. Here, we see an example of a *language-group pattern in acquisition* (a specific pattern for children learning Germanic languages) that needs to be taken into consideration by SLPs/SLTs when assessing and evaluating cluster accuracy in multilingual children with one or more Germanic languages.

Syllable-shape/phonotactic acquisition

SLPs/SLTs may also benefit from studying age-of-acquisition differences between monolingual and multilingual children learning to produce speech sounds in specific syllable and word positions. Studies on the speech of Spanish–German bilinguals demonstrated a higher rate of coda productions in Spanish bilinguals than Spanish monolinguals. A possible explanation for this phenomenon (Kehoe, Trujillo & Lleó, 2001; Lleó, Kuchenbrandt, Kehoe & Trujillo, 2003) is that, German, unlike Spanish, has fewer restrictions against coda consonants. Therefore, coda consonants in Spanish are acquired earlier in bilingual than in monolingual children. This is an example of an acceleration process, meaning that interlanguage effects in this case make the acquisition of coda consonants in bilinguals achieved earlier than in monolinguals (see Goldstein, A19 regarding positive transfer).

Research need

Research from additional language communities is needed to map out important differences in speech acquisition. It is hoped that future studies will uncover trends in speech sound acquisition in multilingual children. Such studies should include research into 'interlanguage' effects (Dickerson, 1975) such as segmental transfer phenomena (Fabiano-Smith & Goldstein, 2010), the occurrence of segments specific to one of the languages in another language in multilinguals. In some cases, segmental transfer has been shown to decrease accuracy in bilinguals.

In addition to applying perceptual measures, the importance of narrow transcription and fine-grained phonetic analysis in assessment and treatment of multilinguals cannot be emphasised enough, particularly in light of recent research on the development of voice onset time in bilingual Korean–English as opposed to monolingual Korean and English-speaking children. Research indicated that bilingual children's stop systems are not fully separate at the age of 5;0 years but rather show interlanguage effects

in their categorical organisation (Lee & Iverson, 2012). There is a pressing need to gather and analyse more data from diverse language communities, from both monolingual and multilingual children, to inform clinicians aspiring to implement theoretically sound and evidence-based procedures in the management of SSD in children speaking one or more non-English languages.

Children with speech impairments in culturally and linguistically diverse settings

Our next 'special' population comprises children with speech impairments in culturally and linguistically diverse settings, in the majority world, where many SLPs/SLTs, including student clinicians, have had the privilege of volunteering. There is a reciprocal relationship between culture and communication, each influencing the other. One of the effects of population migration, relocation and dislocation throughout the world has been to add a new dimension to SLPs'/SLTs' attention to the individual differences of our clients, and most clinicians need to take diversity and multiculturalism into account to ensure that clinical management leads to functional and meaningful outcomes for *all* the clients we see.

Dr. Ken Bleile is an internationalist, a professor in the Department of Communicative Disorders at the University of Northern Iowa, and the author of several practical child speech publications, including the second edition of *The Late Eight* (Bleile, 2013) and the *Manual of Articulation and Phonological Disorders* (Bleile, 2004), among many scholarly publications. Passionately interested in the impact of communication impairment on people living in the non-industrialised world, he has taken students on field trips to places as diverse as New Zealand (which is industrialised) and Nicaragua – and that is just the Ns! As well, he is vitally interested in the SLP issues that affect culturally and linguistically diverse populations in the United States.

Q21.   Ken M. Bleile: Humanitarian SLP/SLT outreach and the ICF-CY

The International Classification of Functioning, Disability and Health – Children and Youth (ICF-CY; WHO, 2007) is a classification system to be used throughout the world to support the health and wellness of all people (McLeod & Bleile, 2004, 2007). In Bleile (2002), you outlined an assessment procedure for speech you would use if time were short. How would you tackle the same exercise with culturally and linguistically diverse test subjects, taking into account the ICF-CY criteria?

A21.   Ken M. Bleile: A Nicaraguan experience

How would I tackle an assessment for speech with culturally and linguistically diverse test subjects if the time were short, taking into account the ICF-CY criteria? For reasons given shortly, the quick answer is: with humility.

I have provided speech–language services in six different countries. Most recently, students and I spent a good portion of summer preparing for and then providing services (including many short speech and language assessments) to children with communication disorders in Nicaragua. Nicaragua is a beautiful country of volcanoes, lakes and widespread poverty surrounding small islands of great wealth. It is the second poorest country in Latin America, second only to Haiti, and 4-hour electrical blackouts, armed guards and emaciated animals are part of daily life. We worked in the outskirts of Managua in a school and an orphanage for children with developmental disabilities, the country's only orphanages and schools for such children. Many children we assessed were

from families that were impoverished even by Nicaraguan standards.

On assessment days, we saw children as long as there were children to see, which usually meant from early morning to late afternoon. Assessments typically lasted approximately 30 minutes and were undertaken by a team that included a Nicaraguan special educator (the professions of communication disorders are only beginning to be developed in Nicaragua), the child, a caregiver, a translator, several American students and myself. The assessment location typically was an area set off from a noisy play area, and, because it was the rainy season, the room was hot, steamy and buggy, even during those rare occasions when the electricity and fans were on and working simultaneously. The children typically had severe developmental disabilities. Injuries from head trauma and malnutrition were present, though less prevalent.

Although chronologically many children were between 5 and 10 years old, this was the first communication assessment most had received. Much of what the team did would seem familiar to individuals trained in our profession. First, a case history was obtained to determine what factors in the child's past might influence present functioning and prognosis for future development. Current functioning in speech and language was obtained through a combination of observation and parent report. Because no standardised assessment instruments exist for Nicaraguan children, 90% of whom speak Central American Spanish, only non-standardised testing was performed. However, this was not much different from procedures in countries in which normative speech and language information is available, because children with such severe levels of disability typically are unable to perform on standardised tests. In addition to assessing speech and language development, we listened for voice and fluency problems and screened for feeding and oral motor difficulties. A hearing screening was performed separately.

The most challenging assessment task was determining long-term prognosis and developing therapeutic recommendations. Among other factors, prognosis depends on the nature of the developmental disability and availability of services. Many times the nature of the developmental disability was unknown, stated in vague terms ('brain problems'), or involved a disease for which little or no information on developmental disorder exists (e.g., what is the developmental outcome in speech and language for Dengue Fever?). Limited medical care and poor health conditions also impacted prognosis. To illustrate, most children were observed to cough and show other signs of aspiration after feeding, and caregivers reported frequent episodes of pneumonia. Even for children with well-studied disabilities, prognosis could be difficult to determine. What, for instance, is the prognosis in speech and language for a 10-year-old orphan with Down syndrome in a country in which the professions that treat communication disorders are scarcely older than the youngest children they serve, where developmental services for adults are virtually nonexistent, and where most children leave an orphanage at 18 years to enter the community, where life for the homeless often is brutal and short?

Most caregivers wanted their child to receive a speech and language assessment for the therapeutic recommendations they hoped to receive. This critical aspect of the assessment would have been impossible to provide were it not for our Nicaraguan special educators and for the caregivers themselves. Our Nicaraguan team members knew the children, their families, and the types of available services. They were our leaders in turning general recommendations into plans of action. The special educators helped caregivers to identify aspects of communication about which they wanted additional information. One highlight of our experience in Nicaragua was a meeting with approximately 30 parents and their children in a school for children with disabilities. Prior to the meeting, family members selected topics about which they wanted information, and, during the meeting, guided us further with questions and ideas. We provided the information orally and demonstrated techniques and approaches.

Why 'with humility'?

'With humility' because performing a speech evaluation in another language and culture is challenging work. 'With humility' because we were conscious of the differences between providing the 'best service' versus providing the 'best service possible under the circumstances'. 'With humility' because we often worked hand-in-hand with professionals, both Nicaraguan and from other countries, providing excellent services, year in and year out, with a positive spirit under challenging conditions. 'With humility' because many families, though living sometimes in dire poverty, give their children lives that are rich, nurturing and filled with love. 'With humility' because the world is an uneven playing field for a person with a communication disorder, and the extent to which disability isolates socially and educationally and limits access to medical care in large measure is determined by the accident of where one is born.

ICF-CY

ICF-CY is the abbreviation for the *International Classification of Functioning, Disability and Health–Children and Youth* (McLeod, A1), a classification and diagnostic system developed by the World Health Organization for use with persons who experience developmental disabilities (WHO, 2001). The

ICF-CY is intended to serve the needs for professionals from many different disciplines, including those who assess and treat children with speech, language, swallowing and hearing disorders. Within the field of communication disorders it has found some use both as a general orientation and as a specific diagnostic system and the ICF (the adult version) has been especially relevant for adults who have experienced strokes and voice disorders.

The ICF-CY provided a general mindset for our work in Nicaragua. Because the ICFCY was developed by an international organisation (the World Health Organization) for professionals from many different countries and cultures, it did not impose an American system on our Nicaraguan colleagues. Use of the ICF-CY was in accordance with the view that international work is collaboration between colleagues from different cultures and countries on topics of mutual concern, rather than an imposition of the perspective of one country on the care provided in a different country.

The ICF-CY system distinguishes between biological, psychological and social aspects of health. This distinction is critically important in international work in communication disorders, because culture plays an enormous role in determining consequences of a deficit. For example, two children may be born with similar hearing deficits, one in a country with well-developed hearing services and another in a country without such services. In the country with well-developed hearing services, a child may elect to enter the deaf community or receive a cochlear implant, whereas in a country without such services, a child may effectively be denied access to education, health services and community (Jewett, 2003). When performing international work, the ICF-CY also provides a useful mind-set for considering degree of impairment. This is because whether a communication disorder is 'milder' and 'more serious' depends in large measure on

cultural and economic factors. To illustrate, in many developed countries, a 7 year old who mispronounces /s/ is considered to have a mild communication disorder. In a country with limited economic and educational resources, the same communication disorder may result in serious consequences, including early death. This is because in countries with intense poverty, a family may need to select among its children who is allowed to attend school. A child with a communication difficulty, even one as seemingly minor as difficulty pronouncing /s/, may not be deemed by the family to be the best educational candidate. A disability that limits a person's educational and vocational opportunities, including those in communication, contributes to poverty and, consequently, to higher childhood mortality (UN Millennium Project, 2005). In recognition of the importance of education and disability on childhood mortality, the Millennium Project's five-point agenda includes improving human development services by rapidly increasing the supply of skilled workers in health and education (UN Millennium Project, 2005).

A case study

The child described in this brief case study will be called 'Olaf', after a poem by E. E. Cummings (Cummings & Firmage, 1994), which begins, 'I sing of Olaf glad and big'. In the poem, Olaf is undone in part because he is glad and big, and the same may prove true for the child described here. The case study is offered to illustrate some of the challenges that may face a child with communication disorder in a country with limited financial resources.

When we met Olaf, he was 14 years old and living in an orphanage, in a room apart from the main group of children. His room was attached to the outside of an outlying building and was a cage-like structure with a dirt floor, a barred glassless window and a concrete ceiling over one-half of the room and open sky over the other half. At that first meeting, Olaf was naked from the waist up, a large thickset boy with short-cropped hair. An attendant stood nearby, encouraging him to dress. When Olaf saw us, he half stumbled, half ran over to give us welcoming hugs, nearly knocking us over.

Olaf was evaluated and was found to communicate largely through grunts, eye gaze and reaching. He spoke no words. Olaf appeared to have a severe cognitive impairment, though no standardised testing was available to confirm this impression. Olaf's nearly constant movement was consistent with hyperactivity. Hearing could not be assessed. The staff reported that Olaf received medications to reduce his restlessness, though they believed none of them were effective. Trials of sign language and picture communication systems were undertaken, without effect.

In a country with greater financial resources, a child with similar apparent intellectual disabilities and attention difficulties might have received extensive therapy and effective medications to maximise his learning potential. These were not available to Olaf. Instead, what Olaf had was a home away from the dangers of the streets and freedom from abuse and malnutrition. He lived through the care and sometimes-heroic efforts of the orphanage staff. Discussions with orphanage caregivers revealed that Olaf was housed in his cage-like room because he frequently wandered, and the orphanage had no other structure that might hold him. Because Olaf was big and affectionate, he posed a significant threat to the many much smaller children in the orphanage, and so was largely kept apart under the care of an aide, who provided for his daily needs and watched carefully when Olaf interacted with other children.

Olaf's future is unknown. The orphanage keeps children until age 18, and no settings exist for adults with Olaf's level of disability.

The orphanage, recognising the need to work quickly, is attempting to develop and build a setting for adults with disabilities. The hope is that the setting will exist when Olaf turns 18. If it does not, Olaf will likely live on the street or in the Managua city dump among the approximately 5000 people who make their home there.

Children with speech and literacy difficulties

Phonological Awareness (PA) is the ability to reflect on and manipulate the structure of an utterance as distinct from its meaning (Stackhouse 1997, p. 157), and children with impaired phonological output are at greater risk for impaired PA skills (Snowling, Goulandris & Stackhouse, 1994). Having said that, it is important to mention Larrivee and Catts (1999), who cautioned that phonological disorder *alone* is not closely related to problems with early reading skills, but that when phonological disorder is accompanied by another speech or language impairment, such as CAS or SLI, reading and writing disabilities may emerge. This takes us to school and to the interface between teachers, mentioned previously in this chapter for their frequent role in making referrals, and clinicians.

Dr. Roslyn Neilson is a Private Speech Pathologist who has, over many years, completed a PhD in Psychology in the area of PA and reading difficulties, taught in the Faculty of Education at the University of Wollongong in Australia, lectured in the Speech Pathology Departments at Sydney and Macquarie Universities, published two innovative tests of PA, and presented numerous in-services to working teachers, educational psychologists and SLPs/SLTs. Her clinical specialty is children with reading difficulties, and, with characteristic modesty, she says she 'continues to do her best' to learn from them in the assessment and intervention process. In A22, she explores issues around teacher–clinician communication, and the final special population to be discussed in Chapter 3, children with speech *and* literacy difficulties.

Q22.   Roslyn Neilson: School children: clinician–schoolteacher collaborations

Although it is firmly established that the most important factors associated with literacy difficulties in children include histories of speech–language delay and current weaknesses in phonological skills, literacy teaching (including 'remedial reading') is a traditional province of schoolteachers, and not SLPs/SLTs, especially in the eyes of teachers. Meanwhile, it can be argued that speech is our business, especially in the eyes of SLPs/SLTs. In your clinical research (Neilson, 2009), publishing (Neilson, 2003a,b), and academic teaching roles, you have spent more time than most engaging with teachers around the topic of children's SSD, phonology, PA and early literacy. Some of these teachers have been your clients' parents or your clients' teachers. Others have been graduate students in your university classes or participants in continuing education and in-service events. You also talk at SLP/SLT student and CPD/CEU gatherings about the key points to consider in engaging collaboratively and co-operatively with teachers. What role can teachers play in the screening and management of speech disorder? What are the interrelated speech and language weaknesses that place children in an at-risk category for literacy difficulties? What can be done to help, and what are the implications for the collaborative classroom? Are there regularly recurring issues of epistemology, terminology, ethos and culture that need to be addressed before SLPs/SLTs can best support the knowledge base that teachers bring to literacy teaching and place themselves in a good position to receive support from them?

A22.   Roslyn Neilson: Teachers and speech–language professionals: communicating at the chalkface

Like many practising SLPs/SLTs, I have had my share of ups and downs when communicating with the teachers of school-age clients. Although collaborating at the chalkface is not always easy, I do feel that, at least with one group of clients, working constructively with teachers is one of the most important clinical goals we can set ourselves.

I specialise in therapy with school-age children who are experiencing serious literacy difficulties. The core of their problem typically involves word recognition and spelling – laborious, inefficient handling of the alphabetic code. This decoding weakness invariably flows on to affect their reading fluency and comprehension, although their comprehension may be compromised in its own right as well (Nation & Norbury, 2005).

Many of these children experienced speech and/or language difficulties as pre-schoolers. The presence of early oral language weaknesses represents a major risk for literacy difficulties, as does a familial history of dyslexia (Pennington & Bishop, 2009). Nathan, Stackhouse, Goulandris and Snowling (2004) report that children who have even mild or isolated speech sound difficulties past the age of 6;9 are at risk for complications in their literacy development. But by school age, the children who make up my caseload often present with their speech and language weaknesses having 'gone underground', so that their conversation sounds 'normal to the naked ear' (Paul & Norbury 2012, p. 394). In terms of their literacy development, however, there are usually subtle but very important difficulties with the interface between their phonological systems and their efforts at learning to read. Terms like 'weak phonological coding' (Stackhouse, 1996; Vellutino, Fletcher,

Snowling & Scanlon, 2004) are often used to explain how apparently subtle speech and language difficulties can underlie serious literacy problems.

What are the overt 'phonological' symptoms for children with literacy difficulties? If they do have a speech problem in conversation it often involves difficulty pronouncing and remembering complex words (e.g., 'ask' and 'twelfth') or words of three or more syllables (e.g., 'congratulations' and 'extinguisher'). Weak syllable deletion is common, and consonant sequences are often confused in complex phrases, such as 'fly free in the air force' (Catts, 1986). More formal assessment of their expressive language typically reveals slow, inaccurate word retrieval, with sentences getting lost in 'mazes' (Dollaghan & Campbell, 1992) that involve false starts, repetitions and revisions (e.g., 'My brother, I mean my sister is here'). Phonological working memory is a consistent problem for these children (Gathercole, Alloway, Willis & Adams, 2006); they struggle to hold sequences of sounds in their minds as they process information. Many of them have difficulty with the rapid automatic naming of known words (Wolf, Bowers & Biddle, 2000), and when under pressure they show characteristics of word retrieval difficulty (Messer & Dockrell, 2006). Stackhouse (1966) and many others (e.g., Claessen & Leitaõ, 2012) have posited that the core of all these symptoms involves the quality of lexical representations, where the phonological specifications for the representations of words may be unstable, coarse-grained or imprecise. Importantly, these phonological difficulties seem to permeate many aspects of higher-level language functioning, including those functions upon which literacy development depends.

The flow-on effect of underlying phonological difficulty typically includes weak phonemic awareness, with children being slow or inefficient at segmenting, blending or manipulating sounds in words. Mastering the English alphabetic code, with its complex and often opaque system of mapping letters onto sounds, places extraordinary demands on the phonological system.

SLPs/SLTs can play a useful role in alerting teachers and parents to both the presence and relevance of subtle phonological difficulties. It may be necessary to assume a degree of naivety on teachers' part in that Overby, Carrell and Bernthal (2007) report that half of a group of teachers listening to recordings of moderately intelligible second graders (in their third year of school) judged that the children were not at risk for literacy difficulties. This finding suggests that large numbers of teachers may be oblivious to the associated learning implications of expressive phonological difficulties, whereas they may recognise the social repercussions (Nathan, 2002).

What are the implications for therapy? There has been a general move in most English-speaking countries towards explicit code-based instruction in the early years of literacy teaching (NICHD, 2000; Rowe, and the National Inquiry into the Teaching of Literacy (Australia), 2005; Rose, 2006), and many schools now include at least some systematic phonics teaching in their early literacy programs. This is a welcome break-through for those children with weak phonological skills, who demonstrably need explicit support (Chapman, Tunmer & Prochnow, 2001). But questions about the role of SLPs/SLTs remain. Should we be responsible for suggesting extra adaptations to teaching practices that include systematic phonics to help children to compensate for phonological weaknesses, and should we be offering to work with the children ourselves? Are we really needed in the management of these children's learning, or is the business of remedial reading best left to classroom teachers and reading specialist teachers?

I contend that SLPs/SLTs currently do have a key role to play. The problem is that most school literacy programs – even the most explicit systematic phonics programs – are based on the assumption that learners have normal underlying phonological skills. Teachers assume that children know what is meant when they are asked to 'sound out' words, and that children are able to retrieve the sounds and hold them in working memory as they do the 'sounding out'. When things go wrong, however – as they do for our clients with subtle phonological difficulties – it is difficult for teachers to pinpoint the exact problem, let alone work out ways to scaffold the children's attempts.

I believe this gap in teaching practice may be a result of current teacher training practices. It can be difficult to teach phonics, or phoneme–grapheme relationships, to children who have not grasped phonemic awareness, partly because the phonemic level of language is surprisingly inaccessible to many of the teachers themselves. Once one has learned to read and write in an alphabetic script such as English, phonemic awareness easily gets subsumed into thinking about spelling patterns in words (Ehri, 1989). It is common, for example, for teachers to think that when children are asked to blend /æ/ and /s/, the word 'as', rather than 'ass', will emerge. SLPs/SLTs may shake their heads at teachers' apparently poor phonemic awareness, but it must be remembered that teachers are quite 'normal' in their tendency to think of letters rather than phonemes. Teachers do, fortunately, generally have all the implicit phonemic awareness they need to be able to read and spell unfamiliar words themselves, but they can become confused about distinctions we draw between spelling and sounds and are often unaware of issues relating to allophones and coarticulation. Given that phonemic analysis is such a useful tool in working with SSD *and* with early reading and spelling (Fielding-Barnsley & Purdie, 2005), I predict that teacher training undergraduate curricula will eventually include basic phonetics and phonology. Until then, however, SLPs/SLTs can usefully provide in-services about the phonemic structure of lan-

guage to bridge the gap in teachers' knowledge base (Moats, 1994), in order to help them to make their own phonemic awareness explicit. SLP/SLT in-services can also highlight for teachers the phonological processing demands involved in segmenting and blending phonemes. It can be useful, that is, to remind teachers that some children find it extraordinarily difficult to retrieve sounds automatically and hold them in working memory while mapping the sounds onto letters.

There is also, I think, a role for SLPs/SLTs to work directly with school-age clients who have literacy-related problems, complementing what they receive at school. It goes beyond working on phonemic awareness; individual or small-group therapy can usefully target the remnants of the phonological difficulty in children's oral language and develop strategies for sharpening their phonological representations, while respecting their phonological working memory problems. This kind of targeted support for reading and spelling is very difficult for a teacher to offer in the whole-class setting.

It can be rewarding to join forces and plan remedial strategies with teachers, parents and the children themselves as part of the therapy process. Collaboration must be an ongoing process, however, because the child is part of a classroom context where the curriculum, not the child's rate of learning, drives the pace and the content of what is being taught. When collaboration succeeds, it involves regular meetings at which current concerns and achievements are discussed, goals are set or revised and strategies are reinforced. Perhaps most importantly, meetings can serve to negotiate ways for the teacher to adapt regular classroom activities to suit the child and to make sure that parents are involved constructively in reasonable homework activities.

And the ups and downs mentioned in the opening paragraph? One source of discomfort that I have encountered involves a focus on 'sounding out' words during the process of reading, especially where the teacher has a preference for drawing children's attention to meaning-related strategies for decoding. In such circumstances I usually choose to work on the spelling side of literacy, rather than on reading; this avoids the confrontation and is also, I find, at least as effective.

Another interesting professional difference often involves terminology: the 'D' word, 'dyslexia'. The term 'dyslexia' is regarded by most community support groups as a politically useful and socially acceptable characterisation of the difficulty that intelligent individuals may have with handling the alphabetic code. The label, however, draws a mixed reception (at best) in many teaching circles. This reluctance may be based on the grounds that the term connotes unwanted and confusing *medical* baggage; teachers would rather view reading difficulty as a *teaching* problem. By contrast, SLPs/SLTs accept that children may bring intrinsic processing difficulties to the language-learning task, and we are therefore more comfortable with medical-sounding labels like 'dyslexia'.

I often feel that this labelling tendency of ours brings some vulnerability with it – vulnerability that we share with parents, who are not willing to leave any stone unturned in their efforts to find help for their children. We are often attracted to the idea of treating the underlying processing difficulties in their own right, and we can be distracted by the 'cures' that frequently crop up in the popular media (Rosen & Davidson, 2003), including physiologically plausible treatments claiming to rewire the child's brain. These programs have been appearing even more frequently since the term 'neural plasticity' came into vogue (Castles & Macarthur, 2012). SLPs/SLTs and parents do well, I feel, to take a leaf from the teachers' book and remind ourselves that there is so far little evidence for the effectiveness of anything other than careful, analytical, systematic and motivating experience

with reading and writing for helping children with phonological difficulties to master the alphabetic code (Snowling & Hulme, 2012).

Special issues and concerns

Matters associated with several special groups of children have been surveyed in this chapter. Included have been children with concomitant speech *and* language issues; co-occurring speech *and* literacy difficulties; and children with cleft palate, craniofacial anomalies and velopharyngeal dysfunction. As well we have considered counselling and how it relates to children with difficult-to-manage behaviour; its role in supporting and informing families' understanding of communication disorder; and the part that SLPs/SLTs can play in prevention, referral to specialist counsellors and in applying counselling skills to assist clients and families to manage, adapt to, or cope with SSD. Issues for children who have been internationally adopted were also included, with two essays about the needs and characteristics of multilingual children, with and without SSD, and one essay exploring the factors involved in humanitarian outreach in serving speech-impaired infants, children and youth in the majority world. To varying degrees, the interventions described in Chapter 4 will have a place in the management of the special populations of children considered here.

References

Amayreh, M. M. (2003). Completion of the consonant inventory of Arabic. *Journal of Speech, Language and Hearing Research*, *46*, 517–529.

Amayreh, M. M., & Dyson, A. T. (1998). The acquisition of Arabic consonants. *Journal of Speech, Language and Hearing Research*, *41*, 642–653.

Arnold, E., Curran, C., Miccio, A., & Hammer, C. (2004, November). *Sequential and simultaneous acquisition of Spanish and English consonants*. Poster presented at the convention of the American Speech-Language-Hearing Association, Philadelphia, PA.

ASHA. (2004). *Preferred Practice Patterns for the Profession of Speech-Language Pathology* [Preferred Practice Patterns]. Retrieved 26 April 2014 from http://www.asha.org/policy.

ASHA. (2007). *Scope of Practice in Speech-Language Pathology* [Scope of Practice]. Retrieved 26 April 2014 from http://www.asha.org/policy

Balding, M. A., & Smith, J. T. (2008). *Prosodic and phonological skills of children adopted from Haiti* (Unpublished master's research project). University of Alberta.

Bernthal, J. E., Bankson, N. W., & Flipsen, P., Jr. (2013). *Articulation and phonological disorders* (7th ed.). Boston, MA: Pearson Education.

Bitter, J. R. (2013). *Theory and practice of family therapy and counseling* (2nd ed.). Belmont, CA: Brooks Cole–Cengage Learning.

Bleile, K. M. (2002). Evaluating articulation and phonological disorders when the clock is running. *American Journal of Speech-Language Pathology, 11*, 243–249.

Bleile, K. M. (2004). *Manual of articulation and phonological disorders: Infancy through adulthood* (2nd ed.). Clifton Park, NY: Thomson Delmar Learning.

Bleile, K. M. (2013). *The late eight* (2nd ed.). San Diego, CA: Plural Publishing.

Boh, A., Csiacsek, E., Duginske, R., Meath, T., & Carpenter, L. (2006). *Counseling parents of children with CAS.* American Speech-Language-Hearing Association, Boston, MA.

Boonyathitisuk, P. (1982). *Articulatory characteristics of kindergarten children aged three to four years eleven months in Bangkok* (Unpublished Master's thesis). Mahidol University, Bangkok, Thailand.

Bowlby, J. (1988). *A secure base: Parent-child attachment and healthy human development.* New York, NY: Basic Books.

Carroll, K., & Overby, M. (2010). *Social and emotional needs of parents of children with childhood apraxia of speech.* Philadelphia, PA: American Speech-Language-Hearing Association.

Castles, A., & Macarthur, G. (2012). *Brain Training – or Learning as We Like to Call It.* Retrieved 1 April 2013 from http://theconversation.com/brain-training-or-learning-as-we-like-to-call-it-9951

Catts, H. W. (1986). Speech production/phonological deficits in reading-disordered children. *Journal of Learning Disabilities, 19*, 504–508.

Chapman, J. W., Tunmer, W. E., & Prochnow, J. E. (2001). Does success in the Reading Recovery program depend on developing proficiency in phonological processing skills? A longitudinal study in a whole language instructional context. *Scientific Studies in Reading, 5*, 141–176.

Chegar, B. E., Tatum, S. A., Marrinan, E., & Shprintzen, R. J. (2006). Upper airway asymmetry in velo-cardio-facial syndrome. *International Journal of Pediatric Otorhinolaryngology, 70*, 1375–1381.

Cheung, P. (1990). *The acquisition of Cantonese phonology in Hong Kong: A cross-sectional study* (Unpublished final year B.Sc. project). University College, London.

Claessen, M., & Leitão, S. (2012). Phonological representations in children with SLI. *Child Language Teaching and Therapy, 28*(2), 211–223.

Crowe, T. (1997). Counseling: Definition, history, rationale. In: T. Crowe, *Applications of counseling in speech-language pathology and audiology* (pp. 3–29). Baltimore, MD: Williams & Wilkins.

Cummings, E. E., & Firmage, J. G. (1994). *E. E. Cummings: Complete poems 1904–1962.* New York: Vintage.

D'Antonio, L. L., Muntz, H. R., Marsh, J. L., Marty-Grames, L., & Backensto-Marsh, R. (1988). Practical application of flexible fiberoptic nasopharyngoscopy for evaluating velopharyngeal function. *Plastic and Reconstructive Surgery, 82*, 611–618.

Dickerson, L. J. (1975). The learner's interlanguage as a system of variable rules. *TESOL Quarterly, 9*(4), 401–407.

Dodd, B., Holm, D., & Li, W. (1997). Speech disorder in preschool children exposed to Cantonese and English. *Clinical Linguistics and Phonetics, 11*, 229–243.

Dollaghan, C. A. (2007). *The handbook for evidence-based practice in communication disorders.* Baltimore, MD: Paul H. Brookes Publishing Co.

Dollaghan, C. A., & Campbell, T. (1992). A procedure for classifying disruptions in spontaneous language samples. *Topics in Language Disorders, 12*, 56–68.

Dreikurs, R. (1940a, November). The importance of group life. *Camping Magazine,* 3–4, 27.

Dreikurs, R. (1940b, December). The child in the group. *Camping Magazine,* 7–9.

Dreikurs, R. (1948). *The challenge of parenthood.* New York: Duell, Sloan, & Pearce.

Dreikurs, R. (1950). The immediate purpose of children's misbehavior, its recognition and correction. *Internationale Zeitschrift fur Individualpsychologie, 19*, 70–87.

Dreikurs, R., & Soltz, V. (1964). *Children: The challenge*. New York: Hawthorn.

Ehri, L.C. (1989). The development of spelling knowledge and its role in reading acquisition and reading disability. *Journal of Learning Disabilities, 22*, 356–365.

Ellis Weismer, S., & Robertson, S. (2006). Focused stimulation. In: R. J. McCauley, & M. E. Fey (Eds.), *Treatment of language disorders in children* (pp. 175–202). Baltimore, MD: Paul H. Brookes Publishing Co.

English, K. (2008). Counseling issues in audiologic rehabilitation. *Contemporary Issues in Communication Science and Disorders, 35*, 93–101.

English, K., Mendel, L., Rojeski, T., & Hornak, J. (1999). Counseling in audiology, or learning to listen: Pre-and post-measures from an audiology counseling course. *American Journal of Audiology, 8*, 34–39.

Fabiano-Smith, L., & Goldstein, B. (2010). Phonological acquisition in bilingual Spanish-English speaking children. *Journal of Speech, Language, and Hearing Research, 53*, 160–178.

Fenson, L., Dale, P. S., Reznik, J. S., Thal, D., Bates, E. Hartung, J., Pethick, S., & Reilly, J. (1993). *MacArthur communicative development inventories*. San Diego, CA: Singular.

Fey, M. E. (1986). *Language intervention in young children*. San Diego, CA: College Hill Press.

Fielding-Barnsley, R., & Purdie, N. (2005). Teachers' attitude to and knowledge of metalinguistics in the process of learning to read. *Asia-Pacific Journal of Teacher Education, 33*(1), 65–76.

Flasher, L. V., & Fogle, P. T. (2012). *Counseling skills for speech-language pathologists and audiologists*. Clifton Park, NY: Delmar-Cengage.

Fox, A. V., & Dodd, B. (1999). Der Erwerb des phonolo- gischen Systems in der deutschen Sprache. *Sprache-Stimme-Gehör, 23*, 183–191.

Friedman, T. (2005). *The world is flat: A brief history of the twenty-first century*. New York: Farrar, Straus & Giroux.

Gathercole, S. E., Alloway, T. P., Willis, C., & Adams, A. (2006). Working memory in children with reading disabilities. *Journal of Experimental Child Psychology, 93*, 265–281.

Gereau, S. A., Steven, D., Bassila, M., Sher, A. E., Sidoti, E. J., Jr., & Morgan, M. (1988). Endoscopic observations of Eustachian tube abnormalities in children with palatal clefts. In: D. J. Lim, C.

D. Bluestone, J. O. Klein, & J. D. Nelson (Eds.), *Symposium on otitis media* (pp. 60–63). Toronto: B. C. Decker.

Geren, J., Snedeker, J., & Ax, L. (2005). Starting over: A preliminary study of early lexical and syntactic development in internationally adopted preschoolers. *Seminars in Speech and Language, 26*, 44–53.

Gergen, K. J. (2009). *Relational being: Beyond self and community*. New York: Oxford University Press.

Gildersleeve, C., Davis, B., & Stubbe, E. (1996, November). *When monolingual rules don't apply: Speech development in a bilingual environment.* Paper presented at the annual convention of the American Speech-Language-Hearing Association, Seattle, WA.

Gildersleeve-Neumann, C., Kester, E., Davis, B., & Peña, E. (2008). English speech sound development in preschool-aged children from bilingual English-Spanish backgrounds. *Language, Speech, and Hearing Services in Schools, 39*, 314–328.

Girolametto, L., & Weitzman, E. (2006). It takes two to talk – The Hanen program for parents – Early language intervention through caregiver training. In: R. McCauley, & M. Fey (Eds.), *Treatment of language disorders in children* (pp. 77–104). Baltimore, MD: Paul H. Brookes Publishing Co.

Glennen, S. (2002). *Pre-adoption Questions for Parents*. Retrieved 19 February 2008 from http://pages .towson.edu/sglennen/PreAdoptionQuestions.htm

Glennen, S. (2005). New arrivals: Speech and language assessment for internationally adopted infants and toddlers within the first months home. *Seminars in Speech and Language, 26*, 10–21.

Glennen, S. (2007a). Predicting language outcomes for internationally adopted children. *Journal of Speech-Language-Hearing Research, 50*, 529–548.

Glennen, S. (2007b). International adoption speech and language mythbusters. *Perspectives on Communication Disorders and Sciences in Culturally and Linguistically Diverse Populations, 14*(3), 3–8.

Glennen, S. (2007c). Speech and language in children adopted internationally at older ages. *Perspectives on Communication Disorders and Sciences in Culturally and Linguistically Diverse Populations, 14*(3), 17–20.

Glennen, S., & Bright, B. (2005). Five years later: Language in school-age internationally adopted children. *Seminars in Speech and Language, 26*, 86–101.

Glennen, S., & Masters, G. (2002). Typical and atypical language development in infants and toddlers adopted from Eastern Europe. *American Journal of Speech-Language Pathology, 11*, 417–433.

Goldberg, S. (2006). Shedding your fears: Bedside etiquette for dying patients. *Topics in Stroke Rehabilitation, 13*, 63–67.

Golding-Kushner, K. J. (1995). Treatment of articulation and resonance disorders associated with cleft palate and VPI. In: R. J. Shprintzen, & J. Bardach (Eds.), *Cleft palate speech management: A multidisciplinary approach* (pp. 327–351). St. Louis, MO: Mosby.

Golding-Kushner, K. J. (2001). *Therapy techniques for cleft palate speech and related disorders.* San Diego, CA: Singular.

Golding-Kushner, K. J. (2004). Treatment of sound system disorders associated with cleft palate speech. *SID 5 Newsletter, 14*, 16–19.

Golding-Kushner, K. J. (2005). Speech and language disorders in velo-cardiofacial syndrome. In: K. Murphy, & P. Scambler (Eds.), *Velo-cardio-facial syndrome: A model for understanding microdeletion disorders* (pp. 181–199). Cambridge: Cambridge University Press.

Golding-Kushner, K. J. (2007, July). *Teletherapy: Using technology to solve the problem.* Paper presented at fourteenth international scientific meeting of the Velo-Cardio-Facial Syndrome Educational Foundation, Inc., Plano, Texas.

Golding-Kushner, K. J. (2012). Communication in velo-cardio-facial syndrome. In: D. Landsman (Ed.), *Educating children with velo-cardio-facial syndrome (also known as 22q11.2 deletion syndrome and DiGeorge syndrome)* (2nd ed.). San Diego, CA: Plural Publishing.

Golding-Kushner, K. J. & Shprintzen, R. (2011). *Velo-cardio-facial syndrome Volume 2: Treatment of communication disorders.* San Diego, CA: Plural Publishing, Inc.

Goldman, R., & Fristoe, M. (2000). *Goldman-Fristoe test of articulation* (2nd ed.). Circle Pines, MN: American Guidance Service.

Goldstein, B. (2000, November). *Bilingual (Spanish-English) children with phonological disorders.* Seminar presented at the Convention of the American Speech-Language-Hearing Association, Washington, DC.

Goldstein, B. (2006). Clinical implications of research on language development and disorders in bilingual children. *Topics in Language Disorders, 26*, 318–334.

Goldstein, B., & Bunta, F. (2012). Positive and negative transfer in the phonological systems of bilingual speakers. *International Journal of Bilingualism, 16*, 388–401.

Goldstein, B., Bunta, F., Lange, J., Rodriguez, J., & Burrows, L. (2010). The effects of measures of language experience and language ability on segmental accuracy in bilingual children. *American Journal of Speech-Language Pathology, 19*, 238–247.

Goldstein, B. A., & Fabiano, L. (2006, February 13). Assessment and intervention for bilingual children with phonological disorders. *The ASHA Leader, 12*(2), 6–7, 26–27, 31.

Goldstein, B., Fabiano, L., & Washington, P. (2005). Phonological skills in predominantly English, predominantly Spanish, and Spanish-English bilingual children. *Language, Speech, and Hearing Services in Schools, 36*, 201–218.

Goldstein, B., & Iglesias, A. (2001). The effect of dialect on phonological analysis: Evidence from Spanish-speaking children. *American Journal of Speech-Language Pathology, 10*, 394–406.

Goldstein, B., & McLeod, S. (2012). Typical and atypical multilingual speech acquisition. In: S. McLeod, & B. Goldstein (Eds.), *Multilingual aspects of speech sound disorders in children* (pp. 84–100). Clevedon, UK: Multilingual Matters.

Grech, H. (1998). *Phonological development of normal Maltese speaking children* (Unpublished doctoral dissertation). University of Manchester, UK.

Grech, H., & Dodd, B. (2008). Phonological acquisition in Malta: A bilingual learning context. *International Journal of Bilingualism, 12*, 155–171.

Grosjean, F. (2010). *Bilingual: Life and reality.* Cambridge, MA: Harvard University Press.

Guiberson, M., & Atkins, J. (2012). Speech-language pathologists' preparation, practices, and perspectives on serving culturally and linguistically diverse children. *Communication Disorders Quarterly, 33*(3), 169–180.

Guitar, B. (2014). *Stuttering: An integrated approach to its nature and treatment* (4th ed.). Philadelphia, PA: Lippincott Williams & Wilkins.

Haberstroh, S., Duffey, T., Evans, M., Gee, R., & Trepal, H. (2007). The experience of online counseling. *Journal of Mental Health Counseling, 29*, 269–282.

Hall, C., & Golding-Kushner, K. J. (1989, June). *Long-term follow-up of 500 patients after palate repair performed prior to 18 months of age.*

Paper presented at Sixth International Congress on Cleft Palate and Related Craniofacial Anomalies, Jerusalem, Israel. D. M. B.

Halle, J. W., Ostrosky, M. M., & Hemmeter, M. L. (2006). Functional communication training: A strategy for ameliorating challenging behavior. In: R. J. McCauley, & M. E. Fey (Eds.), *Treatment of language disorders in children* (pp. 509–546). Baltimore, MD: Paul H. Brookes Publishing Co.

Henningsson, G., & Isberg, A. (1986). Velopharyngeal movements in patients alternating between oral and glottal articulation: A clinical and cineradiographical study. *Cleft Palate Journal, 23,* 1–9.

Hoch, L., Golding-Kushner, K. J., Sadewitz, V., & Shprintzen, R. J. (1986). Speech therapy. In: B. J. McWilliams (Eds.), *Seminars in speech and language: Current methods of assessing and treating children with cleft palates* (7(3), pp. 313–326). New York: Thieme Inc.

Holland, A. L. (2007). *Counseling in communicative disorders: A wellness perspective.* San Diego, CA: Plural Publishing.

Holland, A., & Fridriksson, J. (2001). Aphasia management during the early phases of recovery following stroke. *American Journal of Speech-Language Pathology, 10,* 19–28.

Holm, A., & Dodd, B. (1999a). A longitudinal study of the phonological development of two Cantonese-English bilingual children. *Applied Psycholinguistics, 20,* 349–376.

Holm, A., & Dodd, B. (1999b). An intervention case study of a bilingual child with a phonological disorder. *Child Language Teaching & Therapy, 15,* 139–158.

Holm, A., & Dodd, B. (2006). Phonological development and disorder of bilingual children acquiring Cantonese and English. In: H. Zhu, & B. Dodd (Eds.), *Phonological development and disorders in children: A multilingual perspective* (pp. 286–325). Clevedon, UK: Multilingual Matters.

Holm, A., Dodd, B., & Ozanne, A. (1997). Efficacy of intervention for a bilingual child making articulation and phonological errors. *International Journal of Bilingualism, 1,* 55–69.

Holm, A., Dodd, B., Stow, C., & Pert, S. (1998). Speech disorder in bilingual children: Four case studies. *Osmania Papers in Linguistics, 22–23,* 46–64.

Ingram, D. (2012, November). *A comparison of two measures of correctness: PCC & PWP.* Paper presented at the annual meeting of the American Speech-Language-Hearing Association, San Diego.

International Expert Panel on Multilingual Children's Speech (2012). *Multilingual children with speech sound disorders: Position paper.* Bathurst, NSW: Research Institute for Professional Practice, Learning & Education (RIPPLE), Charles Sturt University. Retrieved 15 January 2014 from http://www.csu.edu.au/research/multilingual-speech/position-paper.

Isberg, A., & Henningsson, G. (1987). Influence of palatal fistulas on velopharyngeal movements: A cineradiographic study. *Plastic and Reconstructive Surgery, 79,* 525–530.

Jakobson, R. (1941/1968). *Child language, aphasia and phonological universals.* The Hague: Mouton.

Jewett, J. (2003, May 23). A labor of love in Bosnia, *The ASHA Leader, 11*(7), 20–21, 27.

Johnson, D. E. (2000). Medical and developmental sequelae of early childhood institutionalization in Eastern European adoptees. In: C. A. Nelson (Ed.), *The Minnesota symposia on child psychology: The effects of early adversity on neurobehavioral development* (Vol. 31, pp. 113–162). Mahwah, NJ: Lawrence Erlbaum.

Kabat-Zinn, J. (2005). *Full catastrophe living: Using the wisdom of your body and mind to face stress, pain, and illness* (15th anniv. ed.). New York: Delta.

Kamhi, A. G., & Pollock, K. E. (Eds.). (2005). *Phonological disorders in children: Clinical decision making in assessment and intervention.* Baltimore, MD: Paul H. Brookes Publishing Co.

Kehoe, M., Trujillo, C., & Lleó, C. (2001). Bilingual phonological acquisition: An analysis of syllable structure and VOT. In: K. F. Cantone, & M. O. Hinzelin (Eds.), *Proceedings of the colloquium on structure, acquisition and change of grammars: Phonological and syntactic aspects* (pp. 38–54). Hamburg: Arbeiten zur Mehrsprachigkeit-Universität Hamburg.

Kent. R. (2006). Normal aspects of articulation. In: J. E. Bernthal, & N. W. Bankson (Eds.), *Articulation and phonological disorders* (4th ed., pp. 1–62). Boston, MA: Allyn & Bacon.

Kim, M., & Pae, S. (2005). The percentage of consonant correct and the ages of consonantal acquisition for [the] "Korean Test of Articulation for Children" [in Korean]. *Korean Journal of Speech Sciences, 12*(2), 139–152.

Kim, M., & Pae, S. (2007). Korean speech acquisition. In: S. McLeod (Ed.), *The international guide to speech acquisition* (pp. 472–482). Clifton Park, NY: Thomson Delmar Learning.

Kleinman, A. (1988). *The illness narratives: Suffering, healing, and the human condition.* New York: Basic Books.

Kohnert, K. (2008). *Language disorders in bilingual children and adults.* San Diego, CA: Plural Publishing.

Kohnert, K., & Derr, A. (2012). Language intervention with bilingual children. In: B. Goldstein (Ed.), *Bilingual language development and disorders in Spanish-English speakers* (2nd ed., pp. 337–356). Baltimore, MD: Paul H. Brookes Publishing Co.

Kohnert, K., Yim, D., Nett, K., Kan, P. F., & Duran, L. (2005). Intervention with linguistically diverse preschool children: A focus on developing home language(s). *Language, Speech, and Hearing Services in Schools, 36,* 251–263.

Kubler-Ross, E. (1969). *On death and dying.* New York: Macmillan.

Kuehn, D. (1991). New therapy for treating hypernasal speech using continuous positive airway pressure (CPAP). *Plastic and Reconstructive Surgery, 88*(6), 959–966.

Kuehn, D. (1997). The development of a new technique for treating hypernasality: CPAP. *American Journal of Speech-Language Pathology, 6*(4), 5–8.

Kummer, A. W. (2001). Speech therapy for effects of velopharyngeal dysfunction. In: A. W. Kummer (Ed.), *Cleft palate and craniofacial anomalies: The effects of speech and resonance* (pp. 459–482). San Diego, CA: Singular.

Kummer, A. W. (2008). *Cleft palate and craniofacial anomalies: Effects on speech and resonance* (2nd ed.). Clifton Park, NY: Thomson Delmar Learning.

Kuo, J., & Hu, X. (2002). Counseling Asian American adults with speech, language, and swallowing disorders. *Contemporary Issues in Communication Science and Disorders, 29,* 35–42.

Langdon, H. W. & Cheng, L. L (2002). *Collaborating with interpreters and translators in the communication disorders field.* Eau Claire, WI: Thinking Publications.

Larrivee, L. S., & Catts, H. W. (1999). Early reading achievement in children with expressive phonological disorders, *American Journal of Speech-Language Pathology, 8,* 118–128.

Law, J., Plunkett, C., & The Nuffield Speech and Language Review Group (2009). *The interaction between behaviour and speech and language difficulties: Does intervention for one affect outcomes in the other?* London: Evidence for Policy and Practice Information and Co-ordinating Centre (EPPI Centre).

Law, J., Plunkett, C. C., & Stringer, H. (2012). Communication interventions and their impact on behaviour in the young child: A systematic review. *Child Language Teaching and Therapy, 28*(1), 7–23.

Lee, S. A. S., & Iverson, G. K. (2012). Stop consonant productions of Korean-English bilingual children. *Bilingualism: Language and Cognition, 15*(2), 275–287.

Lewis, J. R., Andeassen, M. L., Leeper, H. A., Macrae, D. L., & Thomas, J. (1993). Vocal characteristics of children with cleft lip/palate and associated velopharyngeal incompetence. *Journal of Otolaryngology, 22:* 113–117.

Lleó, C., Kuchenbrandt, I., Kehoe, M., & Trujillo, C. (2003). Syllable final consonants in Spanish and German monolingual and bilingual acquisition. In: N. Müller (Ed.), *Vulnerable domains in multilingualism* (pp. 191–220). Amsterdam, Philadelphia: John Benjamins.

Lof, G. L. (2011). Science-based practice and the speech-language pathologist. *International Journal of Speech-Language Pathology, 13*(3), 189–196.

Luterman, D. M. (2008). *Counseling persons with communication disorders and their families* (5th ed.). Austin, TX: Pro-Ed.

Luterman, D., & Kurtzer-White, E. (1999). Identifying hearing loss: Parents' needs. *American Journal of Audiology, 8,* 13–18.

Margolis, R. (2004). What do your patients remember? *Hearing Journal, 57*(6), 10–17.

Masterson, J., & Apel, K. (1997). Counseling with parents of children with phonological disorders. In: T. Crowe. *Applications of counseling in speech-language pathology and audiology* (pp. 3–29). Baltimore, MD: Williams & Wilkins.

McCauley, R. J., & Fey, M. (Eds.). (2006). *Treatment of language disorders in children.* Baltimore, MD: Paul H. Brookes Publishing Co.

McDaniel, S. (2005). The psychotherapy of genetics. *Family Process, 44,* 25–44.

McFarlane, L. (2012). Motivational interviewing: Practical strategies for speech-language pathologists and audiologists. *Canadian Journal of Speech-Language Pathology and Audiology, 36,* 8–16.

McLeod, S. (Ed.). (2007). *The international guide to speech acquisition.* Clifton Park, NY: Thomson Delmar Learning.

McLeod, S., & Bleile, K. M. (2004). The ICF: A framework for setting goals for children with speech impairment. *Child Language, Teaching and Therapy, 20*(3), 199–219.

McLeod, S., & Bleile, K. M. (2007). The ICF and ICF–CY as a framework for children's speech acquisition. In: S. McLeod (Ed.), *The international guide to speech acquisition.* Clifton Park, NY: Thomson Delmar Learning.

McLeod, S., & Goldstein, B. (Eds.) (2012). *Multilingual aspects of speech sound disorders in children.* Clevedon, UK: Multilingual Matters.

McLeod, S., Verdon, S., & Bowen, C. (2013). International aspirations for speech-language pathologists' practice with multilingual children with speech sound disorders: Development of a position paper. *Journal of Communication Disorders, 46,* 375–387.

Messer, D., & Dockrell, J. E. (2006). Children's naming and word-finding difficulties: Descriptions and explanations. *Journal of Speech, Language and Hearing Research, 49,* 309–324.

Miller, W. R., & Rollnick, S. (Eds.) (2002). *Motivational interviewing: Preparing people for change* (2nd ed.). New York: Guilford Press.

Miron, C. (2012). The parent experience: When a child is diagnosed with childhood apraxia of speech. *Communication Disorders Quarterly, 33*(2), 96–110.

Miyamoto, R. C., Cotton, R. T., Rope, A. F., Hopkin, R. J., Cohen, A. P., Shott, S. R., & Rutter, M. J. (2004). Association of anterior glottic webs with velocardiofacial syndrome (chromosome 22q11.2 deletion). *Otolaryngology–Head & Neck Surgery, 130,* 415–417.

Moats, L. C. (1994). The missing foundation in teacher education: Knowledge of the structure of spoken and written language. *Annals of Dyslexia, 44,* 81–102.

Nagy, J. (1980). *Öt-hat éves gyermekeink iskolakészültsége* [*Preparedness for school of our five-six years old children*]. Budapest: Akadémiai Kiadó.

Nakanishi, Y., Owada, K., & Fujita, N. (1972). K_onkensa to sono kekka ni kansuru k_satsu. *Tokyo Gakugei Daigaku Tokushu Kyoiku Shisetsu Hokoku, 1,* 1–19.

Nathan, L. (2002). Functional communication skills of children with speech difficulties: Performance on Bishop's children's communication checklist. *Child Language Teaching and Therapy, 18,* 213–231.

Nathan, L., Stackhouse, J., Goulandris, N., & Snowling, M. J. (2004). The development of early literacy skills among children with speech difficulties: A test of the "Critical Age Hypothesis". *Journal of Speech, Language and Hearing Research, 47*(2), 377–391.

Nation, K., & Norbury, C. F. (2005). Why reading comprehension fails. *Topics in Language Disorders, 25,* 21–32.

Neilson, R. (2003a). *Astronaut invented spelling test (AIST).* Wollongong: Author.

Neilson, R. (2003b). *Sutherland phonological awareness test – Revised.* Wollongong: Author.

Neilson, R. (2009). Assessment of phonological awareness in low-progress readers, *Australian Journal of Learning Difficulties, 14*(1), 53–66.

NICHD (2000). *Teaching children to read: an evidence-based assessment of the scientific research literature on reading and its implications for reading instruction* (National Institute of Child Health and Human Development Report of the National Reading Panel). Retrieved 26 September 2013 from http://www.nichd.nih.gov/publications/nrp/smallbook.htm.

Overby, M., Carrell, T., & Bernthal, J. (2007). Teachers' perceptions of students With speech sound disorders: A quantitative and qualitative analysis. *Language, Speech, and Hearing Services in Schools, 38*(4), 327–341.

Papadopoulou, K. (2000). *Phonological acquisition of modern Greek* (Unpublished BSc Honours dissertation). University of Newcastle upon Tyne, UK.

Pappas, N. W., McLeod, S., McAllister, L., & McKinnon, D. H. (2007). Parental involvement in speech intervention: A national survey. *Clinical Linguistics and Phonetics, 22*(4–5), 335–344.

Paradis, J. (2001). Do bilingual two-year-olds have separate phonological systems? *The International Journal of Bilingualism, 5*(1), 19–38.

Paul, R., & Norbury, C. F. (2012). *Language disorders from infancy through adolescence: Listening, speaking, reading, writing and communicating* (4th ed.). Missouri: Elsevier.

Pennington, B. F., & Bishop, D. V. B. (2009). Relations among speech, language and reading disorders. *Annual Review of Psychology, 60,* 283–306.

Persson, C., & Sjögreen, L. (2011). The influence of related conditions on speech and communication. In: A. Lohmander, & S. Howard (Eds.), *Cleft lip and palate: Speech assessment, analysis and intervention* (pp. 41–53). Oxford, UK: Wiley-Blackwell.

Peterson-Falzone, S., Hardin-Jones, M., & Karnell, M. (2001). *Cleft palate speech* (3rd ed.). St. Louis, MO: Mosby.

Peterson-Falzone, S., Trost-Cardamone, J., Hardin-Jones, M., & Karnell, M. (2006). *The clinician's guide to treating cleft palate speech*, St. Louis, MO: Mosby.

Pollock, K. E. (2005). Early language growth in children adopted from China: Preliminary normative data. *Seminars in Speech and Language, 26*, 22–32.

Pollock, K. E. (2007). Speech acquisition in second first language learners (children who were adopted internationally). In: S. McLeod (Ed.), *International guide to speech acquisition* (pp. 137–145). Clifton Park, NJ: Thomson Delmar Learning.

Pollock, K. E., & Berni, M. C. (2003). Incidence of non-rhotic vowel errors in children: Data from the Memphis Vowel Project. *Clinical Linguistics and Phonetics, 17*, 393–401.

Pollock, K. E., Bylsma, K., Perry, A., & Yam, C. (2010). *Speech-language skills of children adopted from Haiti: School-age follow-up.* Poster presented at the annual convention of the American Speech-Language-Hearing Association, November.

Pollock, K. E., Chattaway, K., Fast, R., Reay, M., & Zmijewski, C. (2006). English speech and language skills of children adopted from Haiti. Poster presented at the annual convention of the American Speech-Language-Hearing Association, November.

Pollock, K. E., Chow, E., & Tamura, M. (2004). *Phonology and prosody in preschoolers adopted from China as infants/toddlers.* Poster presented at the annual convention of the American Speech-Language-Hearing Association, Philadelphia, PA, November.

Pollock, K. E., & Price, J. R. (2005). Phonological skills of children adopted from China: Implications for assessment. *Seminars in Speech and Language, 26*, 54–63.

Pollock, K. E., Price, J. R., & Fulmer, K. (2003). Speech-language acquisition in children adopted from China: A longitudinal investigation of two children. *Journal of Multilingual Communication Disorders, 1*, 184–193.

Pollock, K. E., & Yan, S. (2011, July). *Early and later language development in children adopted from China as infants/toddlers.* Paper presented at the International Association for the Study of Child Language (IASCL) as part of a symposium on language development in children adopted internationally, Montreal.

Powers, G., & Starr, C. D. (1974). The effects of muscle exercises on velopharyngeal gap and nasality. *Cleft Palate Journal, 11*, 28–35.

Price, J. R., Pollock, K. E., & Oller, D. K. (2006). Speech and language development in six infants adopted from China. *Journal of Multilingual Communication Disorders, 4*, 108–127.

Ray, J. (2002). Treating phonological disorders in a multilingual child: A case study. *American Journal of Speech-Language Pathology, 11*, 305–315.

Roberts, J., Pollock, K., Krakow, R., Price, J., Fulmer, K., & Wang, P. (2005). Language development in preschool-aged children adopted from China. *Journal of Speech-Language-Hearing Research, 48*, 93–107.

Rose, J. (2006). *Independent review into the teaching of early reading: Final report.* UK: Dept. of Education and Skills. Retrieved 26 September 2013 from https://www.education.gov.uk/publications/standard/publicationDetail/Page1/DFES-0201-2006.

Rosen, G. M., & Davidson, G. C. (2003). Psychology should list empirically supported principles of change (ESPs) and not credential trademarked therapies or other treatment packages. *Behavior Modification, 27*(3), 300–312.

Rowe, K., & National Inquiry into the Teaching of Literacy (Australia), "Teaching Reading" (2005). Retrieved 26 September 2013 from http://research.acer.edu.au/tll_misc/5.

Ruscello, D. M. (1982). A selected review of palatal training procedures. *Cleft Palate Journal, 18*, 181–193.

Ruscello, D. M., St. Louis, K. O., & Mason, N. (1991). School-aged children with phonologic disorders: Coexistence with other speech/language disorders. *Journal of Speech and Hearing Research, 34*, 236–242.

Rutter, M., & The English and Romanian Adoptees Study Team. (1998). Developmental catch-up and deficit following adoption after severe global early deprivation. *Journal of Child Psychology and Psychiatry, 39*, 465–476.

Scott, K., Roberts, J., & Krakow, R. (2008). Oral and written language development of children adopted from China. *American Journal of Speech-Language Pathology, 17*, 150–160.

Sell, D., & Harding-Bell, A. (2010). Cleft palate and velopharyngeal abnormalities. In: M. Kersner, & J. Wright (Eds.), *Speech and language therapy. The decision making process when working with children* (pp. 215–230). London: David Fulton Publishers.

Shprintzen, R. J. (1999). *The Velo-Cardio-Facial Syndrome Educational Foundation Clinical*

Database Project. Retrieved 10 April 2008 from http://www.vcfsef.org/pp/vcf_facts/index.htm

Shprintzen, R. J., & Croft, C. B. (1981). Abnormalities of the Eustachian tube orifice in individuals with cleft palate. *International Journal of Pediatric Otorhinolaryngology, 3*, 15–23.

Shprintzen, R. J., & Golding-Kushner, K. J. (2008). *Velo-cardio-facial syndrome: Volume 1*. San Diego, CA: Plural Publishing.

Shprintzen, R. J., & Golding-Kushner, K. J. (2012). International use of telepractice. *Perspectives on Telepractice, 12*, 16–25.

Shprintzen, R. J., Sher, A. E., & Croft, C. B. (1987). Hypernasal speech caused by hypertrophic tonsils. *International Journal of Pediatric Otorhinolaryngology, 14*, 45–56.

Snowling, M. J., Goulandris, N., & Stackhouse, J. (1994). Phonological constraints on learning to read: Evidence from single case studies of reading difficulty. In: C. Hulme, & M. Snowling (Eds.), *Reading development and dyslexia* (pp. 86–104). London: Whurr Publishers.

Snowling, M. J., & Hulme, C. (2012). Interventions for children's language and literacy difficulties. *International Journal of Language and Communication Disorders, 47*(1), 27–34.

So, L. K. H., & Dodd, B. (1995). The acquisition of phonology by Cantonese-speaking children. *Journal of Child Language, 22*, 473–495.

Spillers, C. (2007). An existential framework for understanding the counseling needs of clients. *American Journal of Speech-Language Pathology, 16*, 191–197.

Stackhouse, J. (1996). Speech, reading and spelling: Who is at risk, and why? In M. Snowling, & J. Stackhouse (Eds.), *Dyslexia, speech and language: A practitioner's handbook* (pp. 12–30). London: Whurr Publishers.

Stackhouse, J. (1997). Phonological awareness: Connecting speech and literacy problems. In: B. W. Hodson, & M. L. Edwards (Eds.), *Perspectives in applied phonology* (pp. 157–196). Gaithersburg, MD: Aspen.

Starr, C. D. (1990). Treatment by therapeutic exercises. In: J. Bardach, & H. L. Morris (Eds.), *Multidisciplinary management of cleft lip and palate* (pp. 792–798). Philadelphia, PA: W.B. Saunders Company.

Sweeney, T. J. (2009). *Adlerian counseling and psychotherapy: A practitioner's approach* (5th ed.). New York, NY: Routledge.

Takagi, S., & Yasuda, A. (1967). Seij_y_ji no k_onn_ryoku. *Sh_ni Hoken Igaku, 25*, 23–28.

Tindall, L., Cohn, E., Campbell, M., Golding-Kushner, K., & Christiana, D. (2012, November). *Special interest group 18 telepractice: today & tomorrow*. Poster session. American Speech-Language-Hearing Association Annual Convention, Atlanta, GA.

Toner, M. A., & Shadden, B. B. (2002). Counseling challenges: Working with older clients and caregivers. *Contemporary Issues in Communication Science and Disorders, 29*, 68–78.

Traquina, D., Golding-Kushner, K. J., Shprintzen, R. J. (1990, December). *Comparison of tonsil size based on oral and nasopharyngoscopic observation*. Paper presented at Society of Ear Nose and Throat Advances in Children, Washington, DC.

Tse, A. C. Y. (1991). *The acquisition process of Cantonese phonology: A case study* (Unpublished master's thesis). University of Hong Kong.

Tse, S. M. (1982). *The acquisition of Cantonese phonology* (Unpublished doctoral thesis). University of British Columbia, Canada.

Tyler, A. A. (2002). Language-based intervention for phonological disorders. *Seminars in Speech and Language, 23*, 69–82.

Tyler, A. A. (2010). Subgroups, comorbidity, and treatment implications. In: Paul, R., & Flipsen, P. (Eds.), *Speech sound disorders in children: In honor of Lawrence D. Shriberg* (pp. 71–92). San Diego, CA: Plural Publishing.

Tyler, A., & Watterson, K. (1991). Effects of phonological versus language intervention in preschoolers with both phonological and language impairment. *Child Language Teaching and Therapy, 7*, 141–160.

UN Millennium Project (2005). *Investing in development: A practical plan to achieve the millennium development goals*. Washington: Communication Developments Inc. Retrieved 19 September 2012 from http://www.unmillenniumproject.org/reports/fullreport.htm

Van Demark, D. R., & Hardin, M. A. (1990). Speech therapy for the child with cleft lip and palate. In: J. Bardach, & H. L. Morris (Eds.), *Multidisciplinary management of cleft lip and palate* (pp. 799–806). Philadelphia, PA: W.B Saunders Company.

Vellutino, F. R., Fletcher, J. M., Snowling, M. J., & Scanlon, D. M. (2004). Specific reading disability (dyslexia): What have we learned in the past four decades? *Journal of Child Psychology and Psychiatry, 45,* 2–40.

Von Almen, P., & Blair, J. (1989). Informational counseling for school-aged hearing-impaired students. *Language, Speech, and Hearing Services in Schools, 20,* 31–40.

Watts Pappas, N., McLeod, S., McAllister, L., & McKinnon, D. H. (2008). Parental involvement in speech intervention: A national survey. *Clinical Linguistics and Phonetics, 22*(4), 335–344.

Weatherby, A., & Prizant, B. (2002). *Communication and symbolic behavior scales – Developmental profile.* Baltimore, MD: Brookes Publishing Co.

Webster, R. J. (1977). *Counseling with parents of handicapped children.* San Diego, CA; College Hill Press.

WHO (2001). *ICF: International classification of functioning, disability and health.* Geneva: World Health Organization.

WHO (2007). World Health Organization (WHO Workgroup for development of version of ICF for Children. *International classification of functioning, disability and health – Version for children and youth: 2013-CY.* Geneva: World Health Organization.

Williams, A. L., & Miccio, A. W. (2010). Stimulability intervention. In: A. L. Williams, S. McLeod, & R. J. McCauley (Eds.), *Interventions for speech sound disorders in children* (pp. 179–202). Baltimore, MD: Brookes Publishing Co.

Williams, C. J., & McLeod, S. (2012). Speech-language pathologists' assessment and intervention practices with multilingual children. *International Journal of Speech-Language Pathology, 14*(3), 292–305.

Windsor, J., Glaze, L, Koga, S., & the Bucharest Early Intervention Project Core Group. (2007). Language acquisition with limited input: Romanian institution and foster care. *Journal of Speech-Language-Hearing Research, 50,* 1365–1381.

Wolf, M., Bowers, P. G., & Biddle, K. (2000). Naming-speech processes, timing, and reading: A conceptual review. *Journal of Learning Disabilities, 33*(4), 387–407.

Wolter, J., DiLollo, A., & Apel, K. (2006). A narrative therapy approach to counseling: A model for working with adolescents and adults with language-literacy deficits. *Language, Speech, and Hearing Services in Schools, 37,* 168–177.

Yavaş, M. (2013). Acquisition of #sC clusters: Universal grammar vs. language-specific grammar. *Letras de Hoje, Porto Alegre, 48*(3), 355–361.

Yavaş, M., & Goldstein, B. (1998). Phonological assessment and treatment of bilingual speakers. *American Journal of Speech-Language Pathology, 7,* 49–60.

Zajdó, K. (2002). *The acquisition of vowels in Hungarian-speaking children aged two to four years: A cross-sectional study* (Unpublished doctoral dissertation). University of Washington (Seattle), USA.

Zajdó, K. (2013). Cross-linguistic trends in the acquisition of speech sounds. In: B. Peter, & A. A. N. MacLeod (Eds.), *Comprehensive perspectives on speech sound development and disorders: Pathways from linguistic theory to clinical practice* (pp. 249–274). New York: Nova Science Publishers.

Zhu, H. (2002). *Phonological development in specific contexts.* Clevedon, UK: Multilingual Matters.

Zhu, H., & Dodd, B. (2000). The phonological acquisition of Putonghua (Modern Standard Chinese). *Journal of Child Language, 27*(1), 3–42.

Chapter 4

Intervention approaches

Evidence-based approaches to intervention with children with speech sound disorders (SSD) that *have* been covered elsewhere in this book are mentioned briefly in this chapter, along with more detailed accounts of those that have not. The reader is referred to Mirla Raz (A4) for information about an adaptation of traditional articulation therapy (Van Riper, 1978) she employs; to Barbara Hodson (A5) who describes the Cycles Phonological Patterns Approach (CPPA); and Karen Golding-Kushner (A17) and Dennis Ruscello (A48), both of whom share their expertise in managing resonance and speech difficulties, and compensatory errors in children with craniofacial anomalies, including clefts; Nicole Watts Pappas (A30) for a discussion of family-centred practice; and B. May Bernhardt and Angela Ullrich (A37) for an account of constraints-based non-linear phonology approaches. In Chapter 3, Karen Pollock (A18) clarifies the intervention needs of internationally adopted children, and Brian Goldstein (A19) advises on working with multilingual children who have SSD; information that is augmented by Krisztina Zajdó (A20)

writing about speech acquisition in languages other than English. In Chapter 7, where treatment approaches and techniques for childhood apraxia of speech (CAS) are presented, Edythe Strand (A45) explains Dynamic Assessment using the DEMSS and its relationship to Integral Stimulation, and, Dynamic Temporal and Tactile Cueing for Motor Speech Learning (DTTC); Pam Williams and Hilary Stephens (A46) describe the Nuffield Centre Dyspraxia Programme; and Patricia McCabe and Kirrie Ballard (A47) present the Rapid Syllable Transition Training (ReST) intervention for school-aged children with CAS. Each account contains enough information for clinicians to implement the methodologies and/or to locate relevant literature.

In *this* chapter, there is Stimulability Therapy (Miccio, A23); an account of Auditory Input Therapy by Gwen Lancaster (A24); Perceptually-based Interventions by Susan Rvachew (A25); a minimal pair approach, Multiple Oppositions intervention, presented by A. Lynn Williams (A26); the Stackhouse, Wells and colleagues' Psycholinguistic framework covered by Hilary

Children's Speech Sound Disorders, Second Edition. Caroline Bowen.
© 2015 John Wiley & Sons, Ltd. Published 2015 by John Wiley & Sons, Ltd.
Companion website: www.wiley.com/go/bowen/speechlanguagetherapy

Gardner (A27); Phoneme Awareness Therapy by Anne Hesketh (A28); and finally Vowel Therapy by Fiona Gibbon (A29). What a line-up!

Also in this chapter, are summaries of the phonetic, Grunwell and *Metaphon* approaches; three further minimal pair approaches: Weiner's Conventional Minimal Pairs, Gierut's Maximal Oppositions and Gierut's Empty Set; Klein's Imagery Therapy; the Whole Language Approach of Hoffman and Norris; and Dodd and co-workers' Core Vocabulary Approach. As noted above, interventions for CAS are in Chapter 7 along with Velleman's Phonotactic Therapy, which can be applicable to both phonological disorder and CAS. Parents and Children Together (PACT) which I developed, and ultimately evaluated under the supervision of Dr. Linda Cupples, for my doctoral research is detailed in Chapter 9.

Phonetic approaches

Phonetic approaches focus on discrimination and production of articulatory targets. Motor-skills learning techniques (Schmidt & Lee, 2011) are used to teach individual error phones to preset criteria. Therapy that targets the phonetic level has its roots in traditional articulation therapy, and as Van Riper (1978, p. 179) wrote, 'The hallmark of traditional therapy lies in its sequence of activities for: (1) identifying the standard sound, (2) discriminating it from its error through scanning and comparing, (3) varying and correcting the various productions until it is produced correctly, and finally, (4) strengthening and stabilizing it in all contexts and speaking situations.'

A phonetic approach or 'articulation therapy' is often used appropriately by SLPs/SLTs as a stand-alone intervention to address one or a few sound substitutions, omissions, distortions or additions in cases of functional articulation disorder, or persisting residual errors, where the client's difficulty with speech production is at the perceptual and/or phonetic level. That is, the client has a functional difficulty with producing the phone involved in terms of their ability to perceive the target, and articulate it with accurate place, man-

ner and voicing features. Furthermore, it can be the intervention of choice for children and youth whose articulation errors can be attributed to hearing impairment (e.g., those fitted with hearing aids or cochlear implants) or structural/anatomic differences (e.g., those with dental malocclusion or clefts). A sound-by-sound phonetic or articulatory approach is sometimes misapplied, however, by SLPs/SLTs when they use it as a stand-alone treatment for children with phonologically based difficulties, and in treating children with CAS.

Phonetic placement techniques are routinely incorporated into the treatment of children with SSD, whether they have a primary diagnosis of articulation disorder, or phonological disorder, or CAS, or structurally based speech impairment – or some permutation of these, with or without an auditory perceptual component. Target selection for children with articulation disorder is usually grounded in the eight traditional criteria displayed in Table 8.1, of (1) proceeding in typical developmental sequence, (2) favouring targets that are socially 'important' to the child or family, (3) prioritising phonemes that are readily stimulable in isolation, (4) using minimal feature contrasts, (5) selecting unfamiliar words as therapy targets, (6) giving preference to inconsistently erred sounds as treatment targets, (7) opting for sounds that have the most destructive effect on intelligibility and (8) addressing errors that are uncommon in typical development.

Co-occurring error types

It was indicated in the explanation for parents in Box 2.1 that the types, or levels, of difficulty that children with SSD have with their speech can co-occur in the *same* child. For example, a child with a clear diagnosis of CAS may have a motoric explanation for the majority of his or her speech production problems (hence the diagnosis), but the same child might *also* have, for example, a difficulty at the perceptual level in distinguishing /ʃ/ from /s/, as well as a phonemic level difficulty with phonological organisation, replacing /k, g/ with /t, d/, despite being able to produce the velar stops in CVs, VCs and CVCs. Similarly, a child with an unambiguous diagnosis of phonological disorder might have an articulatory (phonetic level) difficulty in producing the affricates /tʃ, dʒ/ and a perceptual level difficulty with distinguishing /ɹ/ from /w/. What this means is that children with SSD may have a predominant 'underlying cause' or explanation for their speech problems coupled with some combination of perceptual, phonetic (articulatory), phonological (phonemic) and motoric (as in CAS or one of the dysarthrias that can present in children) explanations.

In principle, separating phonetic approaches from phonemic approaches helps us think clearly about the level at which we are working. In practice, 'phonemic/phonological therapy', 'phonetic/articulation therapy', 'auditory discrimination training' (perceptual intervention) and 'Stimulability Therapy' are not always completely distinct. This means that in the intervention process the clinician sometimes has to stop and think, 'which level(s) am I addressing right now, and why?' For example, Stimulability Therapy, with its aim of phonetic inventory expansion, is rooted at the phonetic level and can be thought of as a form of pre-practice (see below). But in addressing a child's treatment goals, the clinician may combine it with auditory discrimination (perceptual) activities and group the child's targets systemically into sound classes and phonemic contrasts so that the stimulability intervention affects a phonological flavour.

Children with limited stimulability

The aim of stimulability assessment is to discover whether the production of an error sound or missing sound is enhanced or made possible when elicitation conditions are modified or simplified. Traditionally, in child speech *assessment*, a child was said to be stimulable for a sound if he or she could produce it in isolation when given auditory and visual models, encouragement and support while ensuring that distractions and linguistic demands on the child were minimal. Also

traditionally, developers of *treatment* approaches for child speech disorders have had no difficulty in persuading clinicians to focus on early developing and stimulable (in isolation) sounds first, on the basis that these sounds are easier for children to learn, and easier for the clinician to teach. As this made logical good sense, these rationales for treatment target selection remained unchallenged for decades; but eventually, dissenting voices were heard (Miccio, Elbert & Forrest, 1999; Powell & Miccio, 1996; Rvachew, Rafaat & Martin, 1999). The profession is now in a position to appreciate that stimulability data are of most interest in young children with severely restricted phonetic inventories, and of most use when they are collected for sounds absent from a child's inventory. What is the current understanding of the term 'stimulable'? In more recent speech *assessment* literature, 'stimulability' and 'true stimulability' have been used to mean that a child is stimulable for a consonant in at least two syllable positions, rather than simply being able to produce it imitatively in isolation. So, for example, a child would be considered stimulable for /k/ if able to produce it in isolation, and in the pre-vocalic and post-vocalic syllable positions (/k/, /ki/, /ak/); or in isolation, and in the pre-vocalic and inter-vocalic syllable positions (/k/, /ki/, /eɪki/). The child would not need to produce /k/ in a variety of vowel contexts (e.g., /ki/, /ku/, /kɔ/, /ka/; /ɪk/, /ɒk/, /ʌk/ and /æk/) in order to demonstrate 'true stimulability'; two syllable positions suffice.

Stimulability training, pre-practice and the SLP/SLT skill set

Schmidt and Lee (2011) define motor learning, discussed in more detail in Chapter 7, as 'a set of processes associated with practice or experience leading to relatively permanent changes in the capability for movement.' The precursors to motor learning are: (1) motivation, (2) focused attention and (3) pre-practice. In speech motor learning, pre-practice involves phonetic placement training prior to entering the practice phase; so, for many clients, it is inextricably bound up with stimulability training. Irrespective of speech diagnosis, for those clinicians who see their clients infrequently (e.g., on a sporadic consultative basis, or for brief therapy blocks of say, six consultations over six weeks), and for those who have virtually unlimited access to their clients, the modern notion of true stimulability for consonants has major implications.

Unfortunately – due to lack of personnel, funding and resources – in many clinical settings worldwide SLPs/SLTs see their clients with speech disorders infrequently. There are at least three common service delivery scenarios. First, some SLPs/SLTs working in consultative models may only see a given client once or twice a school term, and then only briefly. Second, other SLPs/SLTs see children for between 6 and 10 assessment/treatment sessions and then hand over the entire business of intervention to a parent in the form of a home program, or to a teacher, aide, assistant or other non-SLP/SLT as a school program, perhaps reviewing the child's progress at intervals, but possibly not. And third, and literally quite close to home for the me, children attending publicly funded (government) agencies are allocated, by legislation, a maximum of 10 SLP/SLT appointments. Not 10 per school term or 10 per year: 10 full stop! Against this background, we know that SLPs/SLTs are uniquely qualified to make non-stimulable sounds stimulable, whereas most non-SLPs/SLTs probably have to rely on luck to achieve success in this area!

Dr. Adele Miccio (1952–2009) explored the role of stimulability in the treatment of children with SSD in A23. When she wrote her essay, Dr. Miccio was Associate Professor of Communication Sciences and Disorders and Applied Linguistics and Co-Director of the Center for Language Science at Pennsylvania State University, where she taught courses in phonetics and phonology and conducted research on typical and atypical phonological acquisition, the relationship between bilingual phonological development and later literacy abilities, bilingual phonological assessment, and treatment efficacy. Formerly a clinical SLP in Colorado, she received her PhD in Speech and Hearing Sciences from Indiana University–Bloomington. She was an Associate Editor of the *American Journal of Speech-Language Pathology* and on the editorial board of *Clinical Linguistics & Phonetics*. Her contribution to scholarship in our field was immeasurable and she is sorely missed. Her contribution is included in the second edition of this book with the kind cooperation and permission of her children, Anthony and Claire Miccio.

Q23. Adele Miccio: Stimulability and phonetic inventory expansion

Should clinicians focus on stimulability training with infrequently seen 'home/school program' clients, and what should the parents' or other helpers' role be in this situation? In other situations, where the clinician has reasonably unfettered access to a client, how would you prioritise and implement work on stimulability?

A23. Adele Miccio: First things first: Stimulability Therapy for children with small phonetic repertoires

Stimulability has been defined a number of ways since the term first appeared in the speech pathology literature in the 1950s (Carter & Buck, 1958; Milisen, 1954), although Travis (1931) described the concept even earlier. Simply put, stimulability is a client's ability to immediately modify a speech production error when presented with an auditory and visual model (Lof, 1996; Powell & Miccio, 1996).

Stimulability assessment

Bain (1994) noted that stimulability testing determines the difference between a child's abilities during a highly supportive imitative condition and a typical spontaneous condition where the phonetic environment as well as lexical and syntactic issues may restrict articulatory abilities. To determine stimulability, target sounds are elicited in isolation, syllables and/or words (Carter & Buck, 1958). Earlier studies (Sommers, Leiss, Delp, Gerber, Fundrella, Smith, Revucky, Ellis & Haley, 1967) referred to a child's general stimulability or overall likelihood to self-correct. In other words, if a child's performance improves from that in spontaneous speech, a child is judged to have good stimulability skills – a positive prognosticator for future success in treatment. Thus, treatment is most important for children with poor stimulability skills.

Although more sophisticated phonological assessments that identify patterns of errors and illuminate a child's knowledge of the phonological system have been developed (Bernhardt & Stemberger, 2000; Elbert & Gierut, 1986; Ingram, 1981; Shriberg & Kwiatkowski, 1980; and see Stoel-Gammon, A9; Bernhardt and Ullrich, A37) and have increased our understanding of generalisation patterns, researchers have also documented a relationship between sound-specific stimulability and generalisation (Miccio, Elbert & Forrest, 1999; Powell, Elbert & Dinnsen, 1991). Consequently, stimulability continues to be used to prioritise caseloads. Children who are stimulable for consonants absent from their phonetic inventories will most likely acquire these sounds without treatment. Sounds absent from the child's inventory that are not stimulable are unlikely to be acquired without direct treatment.

Stimulability is also a consideration in treatment target selection. Treating non-stimulable sounds is most likely to result in the acquisition of both treated and non-treated sounds. Non-stimulable sounds tend to be more complex. Targeting more complex sounds promotes system-wide generalisation and increases the learnability of less complex sounds (Tyler & Figurski, 1994; Gierut, 2007; and see Baker, A13). Targeting both stimulable and non-stimulable sounds promotes early success (Edwards, 1983; Rvachew & Nowak, 2001).

Furthermore, stimulability testing may also be used to probe for learning during the course of treatment. Adaptations of Carter and Buck's (1958) protocols are still widely used for this purpose (Miccio, 2002; Powell & Miccio, 1996). Glaspey and Stoel-Gammon (2005, 2007) developed the Scaffolding Scale of Stimulability, a hierarchical scale of cues and linguistic environments, to monitor discrete changes in production in response to treatment. This scale also quantifies improved responses to cues as well as the change in the number of cues needed over time.

Targeting stimulability

Despite the positive aspects of using stimulability for assessment purposes, it has met with resistance, by clinicians, with regard to treatment target selection (Fey & Stalker, 1986; Hodson & Paden, 1991; Rvachew, 2005b). This generally relates to the difficulty of teaching non-stimulable sounds, the time involved in instruction or the increased frustration of children who have difficulty imitating sounds absent from their phonetic inventories. These concerns have motivated the development of treatment programs for young children with small phonetic inventories who are not stimulable for production of sounds missing from their inventories (Miccio & Elbert, 1996; Miccio, 2005; Powell & Miccio, 1996).

In order to target non-stimulable sounds and still achieve early success, Miccio and Elbert (1996) proposed teaching all consonants at once during every session (both stimulable and non-stimulable). The important components of this treatment strategy include directly targeting non-stimulable speech sounds, making targets the focus of joint attention, associating speech sounds with hand/body motions, associating the sounds with alliterative characters of interest to the child, encouraging vocal practice and ensuring successful communicative attempts.

Because the primary goal is to enhance stimulability, speech sounds are taught in isolation (e.g., [s::::::::::]) or in a CV context (e.g., [kʌ]). Each consonant is associated with a character and a hand or body motion. Details regarding the characters and their associated movements are shown in Table A23.1, and they are illustrated in Figure 4.1. Information on how stimulability probes are conducted and generalisation data are gathered across sessions may be found in Miccio (2005).

Case example

A typical treatment is described below for 'Fiona', age 4;3. Pre-treatment, Fiona's phonetic inventory consisted of [m n p b t d w j h]. None of the English consonants absent from her phonetic inventory were stimulable.

At the beginning of the session, following the administration of a brief stimulability probe, large 5 × 7-inch (13 cm × 18 cm) character cards were reviewed with the associated speech sound and motion. To focus Fiona's attention on each character, the cards were shown one at a time. Doing so ensured that Fiona understood the target sounds and their associated motions. Research on semantic development shows that children are more likely to spontaneously repeat the names

Table A23.1 Stimulus characters and associated motions

Manner	Consonant	Character	Associated motion
Stop	/p/	Putt-Putt Pig	Glide hands in a skating motion
	/b/	Baby Bear	Pantomime rocking a baby
	/t/	Talkie Turkey	Raise a pretend phone receiver to ear
	/d/	Dirty Dog	Make digging motion with hands
	/k/	Coughing Cow	Place hand near top of throat
	/g/	Goofy Goat	Roll eyes toward ceiling
Fricative	/f/	Fussy Fish	Fussily push hands away from body
	/v/	Viney Violet	Move arms up as a winding vine
	/θ/	Thinking Thumb	Move thumb in a circle
	/s/	Silly Snake	Move finger up arm
	/z/	Zippy Zebra	Zip coat
	/ʃ/	Shy Sheepy	Clutch hands together and push down
Affricate	/tʃ/	Cheeky Chick	Move hand sassily toward cheek
	/dʒ/	Giant Giraffe	Move hand upward in stair steps
Nasal	/m/	Munchie Mouse	Push lips together and rub tummy
	/n/	Naughty Newt	Shake finger in a scolding motion
Liquid	/l/	Lazy Lion	Stretch arms in 'L' shape
	/ɹ/	Rowdy Rooster	Rev motorcycle gears
Glide	/w/	Wiggly Worm	Shiver
	/j/	Yawning Yo-Yo	Yawn and move hand to suppress it
	/h/[a]	Happy Hippo	Laugh and shake shoulders

Source: Adapted from Miccio and Elbert (1996, Table 3). Reproduced with permission from Elsevier.
[a] From a phonological perspective, /h/ is considered a glide in English. It has no cognate and patterns as a glide (e.g., is not phonemic in coda position). Thus, all the sounds are listed from the front to the back and by sound class with stops, fricatives and affricates first, then the nasals, and finally, the liquids and glides. Because /h/ cannot be strictly continuous like the other fricatives, it has a CV motion, [ha].

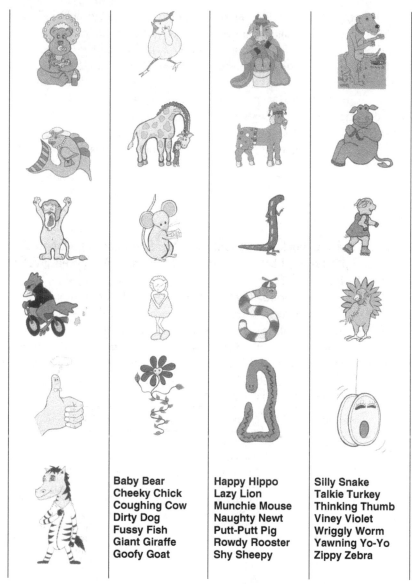

Baby Bear
Cheeky Chick
Coughing Cow
Dirty Dog
Fussy Fish
Giant Giraffe
Goofy Goat

Happy Hippo
Lazy Lion
Munchie Mouse
Naughty Newt
Putt-Putt Pig
Rowdy Rooster
Shy Sheepy

Silly Snake
Talkie Turkey
Thinking Thumb
Viney Violet
Wriggly Worm
Yawning Yo-Yo
Zippy Zebra

Figure 4.1 Miccio character cards

of objects that are the focus of joint attention and that were previously labelled for them (Baldwin & Markham, 1989). For this reason, speech sounds are associated with characters of interest to children.

The character cards, shown in greyscale in Figure 4.1, are freely available in colour at www.speech-language-therapy.com/pdf/miccio4s.pdf). The character for /z/, for example, is Zippy Zebra. Alliterative characters also provide an immediate opportunity to generalise new information to larger linguistic units and to facilitate phonological awareness (PA) and the alphabetic principle that are important for emerging literacy skills (Adams, Treiman & Pressley, 1998; Hesketh, A28; Neilson, A22). Each consonant is also associated with a motion. The motion for [z] is zipping up a coat. All fricatives are associated with continuous motions. All stop consonants, on the other hand, are associated with ballistic motions to draw a child's attention to these features of speech sounds. All consonants, including those that are present in the phonetic inventory, are reviewed (worked on), and associated body movements are always used concurrently with speech production. Fazio (1997) found that children with specific language impairment (SLI) remembered poems after a 2-day delay when the poem was learned with accompanying hand motions. The hand motions appeared to serve as retrieval cues. To learn new speech sounds, children must be able to retrieve the new articulatory information at a later date and to use the new sounds in words. Multimodal input increases the ability to remember new sounds (Rauscher, Krauss & Chen, 1996).

To facilitate speech sound production, treatment was embedded in play-like activities that provided Fiona with multiple opportunities to imitate consonants. Although direct imitation of the correct production of sounds in error is not required in this program, vocal practice is encouraged and children make verbal requests. For example, Fiona's favourite character was Happy Hippo. She would say, 'I'm happy like Happy Hippo. Ha Ha Ha! Are you happy, too?' Doing so is an important element for acquisition and generalisation to larger linguistic units (Powell, Elbert, Miccio et al. 1998; Saben & Ingham, 1991). In this program, children are encouraged to speak through turn-taking activities. A typical session utilises a maximum of three turn-taking activities that are designed specifically around the target speech sound characters. Both Fiona and the clinician were fully involved in turn-taking activities so that the clinician was constantly modelling the target sounds and Fiona had multiple opportunities to imitate them. Sometimes Fiona's parents participated in treatment activities. They also took turns and modelled the target sounds. Characters were printed on playing cards to easily facilitate sound production. Fiona's favourite activity was Go Fish. In this familiar game, everyone had a set of cards and took turns asking for a desired card. Because both stimulable and non-stimulable sounds were included, Fiona often failed to produce the intended sound when requesting a card. The associated movement, however, provided the clinician with the information needed to identify the intended sound. When Fiona produced [d] but mimed zipping up her coat, for example, the clinician knew the intended sound was [z]. Because the clinician handed Fiona a Zippy Zebra card, Fiona's communication attempt was successful. At the same time, the clinician provided feedback about how to produce [z] while miming zipping her coat: 'Let me see, do I have Zippy Zebra? Zippy Zebra says [z:::::::::]'. When Fiona requested Putt Putt Pig, a sound she knew, she said [pʌ pʌ] while making a skating motion with her hands (Putt Putt Pig is wearing roller skates). The clinician provided positive feedback, 'Great! You made the Putt Putt Pig sound, [pʌ pʌ]' while making the skating motion. Every time Fiona took a turn, she was free to request any character she wished.

Giving Fiona the freedom to choose any sound enabled immediate success. Successful communication, in turn, encouraged more verbalisation (Rescorla & Bernstein Ratner, 1996). Whenever the clinician took a turn, she requested a non-stimulable sound. In this way, Fiona was always assured of successful production attempts with stimulable sounds and had multiple opportunities to attempt non-stimulable sounds. In addition, the clinician had many opportunities to provide instruction without resorting to drill-like activities. Fiona was given an assertive role involving requesting and directing attention to sounds of interest. Because all characters are alliterative, multiple opportunities arose to indirectly target generalisation of newly learned sounds to lexical items and to use them spontaneously. Baby Bear, for example, has a bib and a bottle. Putt Putt Pig is pink and wears a purple dress. Fiona commented on these characteristics when she requested these characters and again received feedback about the sounds she made with accompanying motions. Fiona, as well as other young children, preferred simple games. Simple games also provide the most opportunities to attempt speech sounds. After playing Go Fish, Fiona played a game where she took turns requesting character cards to place in a space ship. At the end of the session, the space ship took off and a door opened with a sticker inside for Fiona to wear home. It is important to remember that Fiona was never required to imitate correct production after the clinician. The clinician identified the intended target by the associated motion even when it was produced incorrectly. The clinician drew attention to the correct production through modelling and phonetic placement cues. As Fiona became more comfortable with the clinician and had more successful communicative attempts, she also began to imitate the clinician more frequently and to attempt to correct herself. The treatment activities provided a supportive framework that encouraged speech production and enhanced Fiona's awareness of the properties of speech sounds. At the end of the session, a short probe of palindromes (dad, mom, pop, bob, etc.) was administered to assess generalisation to the coda position. Fiona's parents had a set of character cards at home. At the end of the session, we suggested a few sounds to work on at home. These are always stimulable sounds, for example, [n] and [d], and the parents were advised to always use the corresponding motions. Thus, the parents assisted with generalisation but did not force production of sounds that were difficult. At the end of the session, Fiona said, 'Mommy starts with the Munchy Mouse sound'. Fiona participated in this program twice weekly for 12 weeks. Sessions were 50 minutes in length. Post-treatment, she had added all fricatives, affricates and [ɹ] to her phonetic inventory and was stimulable for the production of [k ɡ l]. Pre-treatment, Fiona produced complete sentences, but with only stops, nasals and glides in her consonant inventory, and she was unintelligible to all but her immediate family. When she began treatment, she substituted [d] for velars, affricates and voiced fricatives, [h] for voiceless fricatives and [w] for liquids. Following 12 weeks of treatment to enhance stimulability, she was stimulable for all targeted sounds and produced many of them in simple words or used typical developmental substitutions in more difficult contexts. When Fiona returned to the clinic after a winter break of 4 weeks, she began a minimal pair treatment approach using *Maximal* Oppositions to directly target the contrastive nature of speech sounds and to continue to encourage generalisation across the phonological system.

Treatment research

This program to enhance stimulability for speech sound production is based on findings from treatment research. As noted above, non-stimulable sounds are least likely to change without treatment, and targeting non-stimulable sounds results in acquisition of the treated non-stimulable sounds as well as untreated stimulable sounds (Miccio, Elbert & Forrest 1999; Powell, Elbert & Dinnsen 1991). For children with small inventories, it is important to rapidly increase the size of the phonetic inventory for intelligibility reasons. This program is designed especially for young children with small phonetic inventories who are not stimulable for production of the speech sounds absent from their phonetic repertoires. Once children are stimulable for the majority of consonants, they move on to treatment using a contrastive approach or a combination of stimulability and phonological contrasts. In addition, children are ready for direct phonetic placement training if needed.

Auditory input

Several intervention approaches include the delivery of auditory input as key components. The rationale is the same for each, but the manner in which input is provided to children differs somewhat. The approaches are: CPPA with amplified auditory stimulation and focused auditory stimulation; PACT with listening lists and alliterative input delivered without amplification; Auditory Input Therapy described by Gwen Lancaster in A24; and Naturalistic Intervention (Camarata, 2010) in which multiple exemplars of target words are delivered as 'broad target recasts' to facilitate both increased sentence length and speech intelligibility.

Amplified auditory stimulation in CPPA[1]

Hodson and Paden (1983) incorporated amplified auditory stimulation, sometimes called 'amplified auditory input' at the beginning and ending of intervention sessions as a component of Cycles Therapy, also called the Cycles Phonological Remediation Approach (Prezas & Hodson, 2010). 'Cycles' has more recently come to be known as the *Cycles Phonological Patterns Approach (CPPA)* (Hodson, A5). Children listen to the clinician read 20 words with the week's target pattern. The words are amplified slightly. In the session described in Hodson and Paden (1991, pp. 107–109) Amplified auditory stimulation is but one important component, and it is stressed that most of the time in each intervention session is devoted to production-practice motivational activities (Hodson, personal correspondence, 2013). The child must produce the target pattern appropriately in order to 'take a turn'.

Amplified auditory stimulation

The small auditory input component involves children listening, through headphones for <30 seconds to 15–20 words, spoken by an adult, at the beginning and end of each session and once daily at home without amplification. Professor Hodson now prefers the terms 'amplified auditory stimulation' and 'focused auditory input' ('focused auditory stimulation') rather than 'auditory bombardment (AB)' because of concerns expressed by some caregivers and audiologists about possible

negative connotations of the word bombardment, in the sense that 'bombardment' suggests the procedure is damaging to the ears (it is not!). The terms 'focused auditory input' ('focused auditory stimulation') relate to a technique used in working with toddlers, described in the next section.

Hodson and Paden (1983) proposed that auditory stimulation helped develop 'auditory images', allowing the child to learn to monitor incorrect productions, while production practice helped children develop accurate kinaesthetic images, which also assisted in error monitoring. Commenting on this proposal, Ingram (1989), citing Pye, Ingram and List (1987) posited that a promising explanation for the apparent usefulness of AB might lie in preliminary data from cross-linguistic phonetic acquisition studies of phonological acquisition. The 1987 study by Pye et al. suggested that the acquisition of first sounds is influenced more by their linguistic prominence than by their assumed articulatory difficulty. For instance, /v/ is acquired early by monolingual French-speaking and late by monolingual English-speaking children. The incidence of /v/ in French is higher than in English. Accordingly, Ingram (1989) suggested that AB might facilitate phonological change by increasing the frequency of some targets.

Focused auditory input (focused auditory stimulation)

Professor Hodson describes a second procedure called focused auditory input (also known as focused auditory stimulation). It is intended for very young children who are unwilling or unable to participate in regular production practice activities when SLPs/SLTs first see them. In this case *no* production is requested. The clinician designs the environment to provide for lots of opportunities for the child to hear the target sound or pattern (Hodson, A5). The clinician essentially does language stimulation activities (following child's lead, talking about what the child is doing, and so on) and in the process the child is exposed to many examples of the target. Focused auditory input is only used for one 'cycle'.

Auditory input in PACT

In PACT intervention (Bowen & Cupples, 1999a), described in detail in Chapter 9, a variation of Hodson and Paden's (1983) 'original' AB appears as a constituent of the Multiple Exemplar Training component. Hodson and Paden used headphones *and* amplified AB, but in PACT neither is employed. Auditory input, or AB, without amplification, is used in PACT on the basis that phonological progress is sensitive to phonological input (Ingram, 1989). In practice there is overlap between the AB and the minimal pair games listed in Chapter 9. AB in the context of PACT sees the child:

- listening to words with common phonetic features (e.g., all starting with /ʃ/); or
- listening to minimally, or near-minimally contrasted words ('rhyming pairs') exemplifying a phonological process (e.g., the minimal pairs *ship–sip*, *shell–sell*, *shy–sigh*, etc., for palatal fronting; or the near minimal pairs *two–toot*, *tie–tight*, *toe–tote*, etc., for final consonant deletion; or the near minimal pairs *nip–snip*, *nail–snail*, *no–snow*, etc., for cluster reduction);
- hearing alliterative input in the context of games and stories (Bowen & Rippon, 2013); and
- engaging in Auditory Input Therapy (Lancaster, A24; Lancaster & Pope, 1989)/naturalistic intervention (Camarata, 2010).

Auditory Input Therapy (AIT)

Not to be confused with auditory integration training (also abbreviated AIT) (ASHA, 2004), Auditory Input Therapy (Lancaster & Pope, 1989; Flynn & Lancaster, 1996) has the advantage of being suitable for younger children and children with cognitive challenges, *and* it encourages the active participation of their caregivers (Lancaster, 1991). Camarata (2010) and co-workers use the

term 'Naturalistic Intervention' to refer to similar 'whole word' procedures to improve the overall intelligibility and sentence length of children with severe SSD, including children with Down syndrome, children with autism and children who stutter. The essence of both AIT and naturalistic intervention involves setting up interesting and attractive games and tasks, called 'thematic play' in some literature, during which the client is exposed to multiple 'repetitions' of particular sound or word targets, spoken by the adult, with no requirement for them to practice saying sounds or words. AIT incorporates Conventional Minimal Pair therapy and metalinguistic activities.

Mrs. Gwen Lancaster is a British SLT working for the London Borough of Merton. She was a lecturer at City University in London for 10 years, where she taught in the area of child speech at Master's level. Mrs. Lancaster is the surviving co-author of *Working with Children's Phonology* (Lancaster & Pope, 1989) and *Children's Phonology Sourcebook* (Flynn & Lancaster, 1996), and author of *Phoneme Factory: Developing Speech and Language Skills* (Lancaster, 2007), the companion book for the *Phoneme Factory* and *Phoneme Factory Sound Sorter* software (Roulstone, A8). She is involved in professional development teaching to SLT colleagues in the South West region of England, mentoring and providing second opinions. In A24 she talks about Auditory Input Therapy.

Q24.   Gwen Lancaster: Auditory Input Therapy

Has Auditory Input Therapy evolved since the first half of the 1990s? And, if so, what does it look like now? Can you outline the specifics of the planning approach to adopt in assessment, treatment goal setting, therapy delivery, caregiver training and outcome measurement with unintelligible 3 or 4 year olds? How is feedback about his/her performance provided to the child, and what does it comprise?

A24. Gwen Lancaster: Implementing Auditory Input Therapy

Developed in the mid-1980s in the United Kingdom, Auditory Input Therapy (AIT) evolved from clinical practice with children with speech impairments aged 3–6 years. AIT was inspired in part by the 'AB' component of the CPPA as delineated by Hodson and Paden (1983), and more recently called 'focused auditory input' (Hodson, 2007, 2010; Hodson, A5). AIT takes into account the unconscious or implicit level that is fundamental to learning first and additional languages (Velleman & Vihman, 2002). It focuses on the child listening to rather than producing speech, helping build up the information he or she needs about the speech sound system from repeated, intense auditory models delivered naturalistically. Similar to the suggestions of Ellis, Weismer and Robertson (2006), it is usually employed as a component of an eclectic approach to intervention for children's SSDs (Lancaster & Pope, 1989) and is not conceptualised as a total 'therapy package'.

Velleman and Vihman (2002) explain how typical language learners unconsciously register, and implicitly acquire, the features of their ambient language or languages. In keeping with this, the theory proposed for the effects of AIT is that at least some children with speech impairment benefit from receiving repeated exposure to carefully selected targets that are relevant for them. This intense exposure facilitates their acquisition of new syllable structures, speech sounds and contrastive phones. AIT activities are based around *topics* (e.g., things seen on a walk, such as *stick*, *rock* and *bike* to target /k/ SFWF), *semantic groups* (e.g., foods, such as *bean*, *burger* and *banana* to target /b/ SIWI) and *stories* (e.g., a story about a 'sad seal' to target /s/ SIWI) and can be used to address language and/or speech goals (Ellis,

Weismer, & Robertson, 2006). With regard to *speech* activities specifically, materials for most consonants are provided in Flynn and Lancaster (1996), but of course, ingenious clinicians and caregivers can invent novel activities to target consonants, vowels and syllable shapes according to the individual child's intervention needs and interests.

Individuals and groups

For an individual child, or for groups of up to six children, in the age range of 3–6 years, grouped by error type, the clinician selects games, activities and stories that will allow a particular speech sound or syllable structure to be repeated often by an adult for the children to hear. Treatment targets are selected relative to independent and relational analysis (Stoel-Gammon & Dunn, 1985; Stoel-Gammon, A9), including contrastive assessment (Grunwell, 1985a).

The activities are portrayed to the children as 'listening games', and while they are urged to listen, they are not actively encouraged to say the words. This means that AIT can sometimes be used with clients who are unwillingly to talk, or where compliance is difficult, including children who sit outside the therapy room door refusing to enter, and those who can't, won't or 'don't want to' co-operate. AIT can be incorporated into *any* appealing pursuit, so the creative adult is often in a position to follow the child's lead in the choice of materials and activities (Girolametto & Weitzman, 2006).

Implementing AIT

If, for example, a child's current target is /s/ SIWI, an appropriate game could be creating a collage with silver paper cut-outs of *scissors*, *saws* and *circles*. While making the collage, the SLP/SLT would produce utterances that included /s/ SIWI, frequently repeated but without hyperarticulation, such as 'Let's make some silver circles'. Another activity could be a story involving characters such as a *superhero, Sara* and *Surjeet,* who have favourite foods that are collected for them by the child in response to the therapist's input. The therapist might say, 'Sara wants some sauce', 'Give Surjeet a sandwich', and so on. The target sounds can be given *slight* additional emphasis, but the aim is for the child to hear natural sounding speech.

When using AIT with children of any age, it is necessary to include objects or items that can be easily illustrated (with pictures) or demonstrated by showing (e.g., for nouns and adjectives) or enactment (e.g., for verbs), so that unfamiliar vocabulary does not get in the way of enjoying the activities. The actual words used can include some that are unfamiliar to the child, potentially building their semantic knowledge. This suggests a possible additional reason for using AIT with preschoolers, since Rvachew (2006) concluded that maximising children's vocabulary and speech perception skills prior to school entry may be an important strategy for ensuring that children with SSDs start school with age-appropriate speech *and* PA abilities. Targets are *cycled,* in that a child, or children, grouped because they have similar error patterns, listen to a target (e.g., /s/ SIWI) in therapy sessions or at home, for 1 or 2 weeks, and then perhaps other initial or final fricative will be introduced. The same cycles may be repeated later in therapy, depending on progress. AIT activities provide a relatively easy way for many parents and caregivers, including education staff, to work with children. The clinician should make it clear to these adults that children involved in the activities are not expected to *say* the words themselves, and they may need demonstrations of how to play the games so that they do not feel self-conscious about the repetiveness of their input.

In the implementation of AIT, I follow the treatment principles of Grunwell (1985a, b) and Hodson and Paden (1991). Target selection is largely based on typical developmental expectations (e.g., those proposed by Dodd, Holm, Zhu et al. 2002), so that early sounds, such as /p/, /b/, and the nasals, are selected before later developing sounds, like the affricates. In acquisition of languages other than English, order of acquisition may differ (Goldstein, A19; Zajdó, A20) so appropriate normative expectations (McLeod, 2007) should be applied. I recommend that the activities be carried out daily at home or in educational settings for 5 or 10 minutes, once a day or more. Different people can play the games with the child, and siblings, friends and peers can be involved.

A comparative study

In my MSc research (Lancaster, 1991; Lancaster, Keusch, Levin, Pring & Martin, 2010), I compared the speech progress of groups of children receiving (1) parent-delivered AIT, (2) no treatment (the children in this control group later received therapy) and (3) clinician-delivered eclectic intervention with full parental participation. The research was conducted in a National Health Service (NHS) centre with 15 3- and 4-year-old clients on my caseload, referred by health or education professionals. The participants had moderate to severe speech impairments (Hodson & Paden, 1983) and were randomly assigned to the three groups. Intervention took place over 6 months and was followed by reassessment. The parents assigned to the parent-delivered AIT group received 2 hours of group training using materials later published in Flynn and Lancaster (1996). They were then supplied with materials to carry out AIT activities for 6 weeks. These addressed each child's speech targets determined via contrastive assessment (Grunwell, 1985a). At the end of each 6-week period, I met with each child's parent(s) to discuss their child's progress and set new therapy targets.

In order to evaluate the possible effectiveness of parental intervention alone, the child was not included in these meetings but was seen for reassessment after the 6-month treatment phase. It was found that the children in both intervention groups improved significantly more than those in the no-treatment control group, in terms of their percentage of occurrence of speech error patterns in a citation naming test of 55 single words: 41 from the *Edinburgh Articulation Test* (Anthony, Bogle, Ingram & McIsaac, 1971) plus 14 additional words. From the results of this and other studies, it appears, however, that therapy that directly involves both clinicians and parents or caregivers is the most effective therapy (Lancaster, Keusch, Levin et al. 2010).

Although intervention by caregivers alone may not be the most *effective* therapy, it can be used *efficiently*. My small study (Lancaster, 1991) demonstrated that the children who received AIT made significantly more progress than children who received no therapy, suggesting that AIT may provide a partial solution in situations where long waiting lists, unmanageable caseloads or gaps in provision exist. Between 1997 and 2000, clinicians working in a busy community clinic in Essex, UK, used AIT with all newly referred children with speech impairments. During the initial appointment, clinicians carried out a speech assessment and explained to caregivers how to conduct AIT. The clinician analysed the child's speech after the session and then mailed relevant AIT activities, including written instructions for how to carry out AIT, to the parents. This meant that, while waiting for 2–4 months for therapy, parents could start the intervention themselves.

Small groups in community settings

The following is a typical example of how I implement AIT in community settings. In 2007, I saw four boys aged from 3 to 4 years, in term-time for weekly therapy in their state nursery school in Bristol, UK, for 16 weeks. One of the boys received support from an adult who attended the groups and continued the activities throughout the week at nursery. Parents attended for at least 1 of the 16 group sessions and were provided weekly with homework activities. The children's needs differed, but there was overlap. For example, they all needed intervention for fricative targets. One deleted all fricatives, one was stopping, one replaced /f/ with [s] and the fourth boy replaced /s/ with [ʃ]. Their first cycle of AIT, conducted over 6 weeks (i.e., six treatment sessions), included voiceless fricatives SFWF and SIWI, changing phonemes each week: /f/, /s/ and /ʃ/ SFWF then /f/, /s/ and /ʃ/ SIWI. The boys' needs included increasing their awareness of velar stops, so in the ensuing 4 weeks, /k/ and /ʃ/ were the focus of therapy (four sessions in all) and caregiver-administered activities.

The duration of each session was 45 minutes and included three or four activities, at least one of which would be sent home. The first activity was usually a story. For example, when inputting /f/ SFWF, a story was told about 'Jeff the giraffe' (Flynn & Lancaster 1996, pp. 148–149) that included pictures of *Jeff* and his *wife, scarf, wolf, roof, knife* and *shelf*. The children took the pictures and the story home. A related game involved the objects *leaf, wolf, elf, knife, calf* and *giraffe*, which were covered in turn with a *scarf*. The support teacher whispered an instruction to a child like, 'Hide the knife under the scarf', putting the other items into a bag. The clinician then 'guessed', saying perhaps, 'I think the leaf is under the scarf', and a child took that object from the bag to indicate that the clinician's guess was incorrect. In these sorts of activities, the therapist seizes opportunities to say the objects' names repeatedly or to 'muse aloud' on what the object might be (e.g., *It can't be the leaf or calf, we only have elf, giraffe and wolf.*) to increase the children's exposure to the sound target in the particular syllable or word position. Another enjoyable game involved the clinician placing objects and toys for each sound target on a table for a beanbag-throwing game in which the adult told a child which object to aim for and knock to the floor. Alternatively, the adult hid something under an object and instructed the children, via a puppet, where to look for it (under the *leaf*, under the *knife*, etc.).

By week 6, other therapy methods were incorporated into the boys' sessions. Sets of minimal and near-minimal pair pictures and/or objects representing words that addressed speech input and output goals for *all* the children were introduced. One set of objects and pictures included *tea*, *key*, *sea*, *ski*, *eat*, *beat*, *feet*, *seat*, *wheat* and *sweet* to target several of the speech error patterns used by the boys (including fronting, stopping and deletion patterns). These were used for auditory *input* and then in auditory *discrimination* activities, where the children had to find objects named by an adult. Towards the end of 16 weeks, the children were able to say some of these words using newly emerging contrasts, so they were presented with opportunities to say the words more accurately using minimal contrast therapy (Weiner, 1981).

In AIT, as soon as any child achieves success in signalling a new contrast, he/she is encouraged to produce the particular target sound or structure in words. For some children, this happens faster than for others, so the short-term goals for each child in a group will not be the same and will change as they progress. For this reason, it is advisable to use a range of procedures and activities to address PA, auditory discrimination and speech production within the same session, especially in group work.

Perceptually based interventions

Dr. Susan Rvachew is a Professor in the School of Communication Sciences and Disorders at McGill University, Montreal, Canada. Her research interests are focused on phonological development and disorders with specific research topics, including the role of speech perception development in sound production learning, speech development in infancy, efficacy of interventions for phonological disorders and digital media applications in the treatment of phonological disorders. Current projects include an investigation of alternative approaches to the treatment of CAS, the generalisation of perceptually based interventions from the English to the French context and the impact of digital media on shared reading interactions. In A25, she discusses the role of speech perception development in sound production learning and the use of the Speech Assessment and Interactive Learning System (SAILS) software and other therapy tools in the remediation of categorical misperception (Rvachew, 2005a).

Q25.   Susan Rvachew: Speech perception training

'Children with expressive phonological delays often possess poor underlying perceptual knowledge of the sound system . . . ' (Rvachew, Nowak & Cloutier, 2004). What are the implications of this research finding for evidence-based clinical practice with children who have SSD? When would you introduce the SAILS computer game to improve children's speech perception skills? What low-tech approach alternatives to the SAILS program exist?

A25.   Susan Rvachew: Perceptually based interventions

Many studies have shown that a large proportion of children with SSD have difficulty with speech perception in comparison to children of the same age who do not have SSD. The speech perception difficulties may not be obvious to parents or other people who are talking with the child. However, these difficulties with speech perception have been found in studies using a large variety of assessment techniques and speech stimuli (Cohen & Diehl, 1963; Edwards, Fox & Rogers, 2002; Hoffman, Daniloff, Bengoa & Schuckers, 1985; Hoffman, Stager & Daniloff 1983; Munson, Baylis, Krause & Yim, 2006; Munson, Edwards & Beckman, 2005; Rvachew, 2007; Sherman & Geith, 1967; Shuster, 1998; Sutherland & Gillon, 2007). These findings imply that attention to children's speech perception abilities may be an important component of a speech therapy program, and indeed this hypothesis has been supported by intervention studies (Jamieson & Rvachew, 1992; Rvachew, 1994; Rvachew, Nowak & Cloutier, 2004; Rvachew, Rafaat & Martin, 1999). The SAILS is a computer-based tool that can be used to improve children's speech perception skills. SAILS targets commonly misarticulated consonant phonemes in the onset (initial) and coda (final) position of words. The program is based on recordings of naturally produced words. These words were recorded from English-speaking adult talkers with accurate speech, child talkers with accurate speech and child talkers with an SSD. The child's task is to listen to each word and indicate whether it is an exemplar of the target word or not an exemplar of the target word. The child responds by pointing to a picture of the target word or to an 'X'. Visual feedback is provided after the child's response. Typically, the child engages with the SAILS task for 5–10 minutes at the beginning or end of each therapy session. In Rvachew (1994), the SAILS program was used as part of a traditional speech therapy program in which phonetic placement, modelling and drill-play activities were used to help children master a single phoneme in syllables, words and sentences. In Rvachew, Rafaat and Martin (1999), SAILS was provided for three sessions concurrently with phonetic placement targeting three target phonemes, as a

prelude to a 9-week course of group phonological therapy using the 'Cycles approach' (Hodson & Paden, 1983). In Rvachew, Nowak and Cloutier (2004), the child's speech therapist decided whether to use a traditional or phonological approach, depending on her perception of the child's needs. The SAILS intervention was provided after each therapy session. In all of these studies, children who received the SAILS intervention showed twice as much progress toward the achievement of age-appropriate articulation accuracy than children whose intervention programs did not include a speech perception component.

What are the conditions under which the program has been shown to be effective?

In the studies mentioned above, the intervention was provided for only 5–10 minutes at the beginning or end of the child's therapy sessions. In these studies, a communication disorders assistant or undergraduate student research assistant provided the intervention. These individuals, who had access to a procedural manual if required, received about 1 hour of training in administering SAILS, all demonstrating that it can be provided very efficiently by non–SLPs/SLTs with minimal training. The children in all of these studies were 4–5 years of age with moderate or severe SSDs, as determined by a standardized test of articulation accuracy. Other groups of children are known to have difficulty with speech perception and thus may benefit from the intervention (e.g., older children who have residual distortion errors, second language learners and children with SLI or dyslexia). However, no studies have investigated the effectiveness of SAILS with these groups. I have found that children younger than 4 years of age have difficulty with the SAILS identification task. Finally, the program was developed for use with children who speak Canadian English. It would not be appropriate to use it with other dialect and language groups without first developing stimuli that represent the local dialect or language.

Are there alternatives to the SAILS program?

It is not known whether SAILS will improve the effectiveness of live-voice procedures for presenting good-quality speech input to children, such as focused stimulation or AIT. It is possible that these procedures are effective enough on their own. However, basic research on optimum procedures for perceptual training indicates that stimulus variability is very important. Therefore, SAILS includes multiple voices and a variety of good and poor exemplars of the target words. Thus, SAILS may be an effective adjunct to these live-voice procedures that usually involve the presentation of exaggerated speech models produced by one or two talkers (e.g., speech therapist and/or parent). If you do not have access to SAILS, you can still find ways to introduce multi-talker variability into your treatment. Many technologies exist that can be used to develop speech perception tasks for specific clients. For example, if you were working with a group of children who mis-articulate /ɹ/, you could use a computer with digital recording software to record the children's efforts to say words that contain this phoneme. If there is variability within the group and within children with respect to their production accuracy, you will have a perfect set of stimuli for teaching identification of correct and incorrect exemplars of the /ɹ/ phoneme. You can insert the recordings and pictures of the target words into power point slides for presentation to your students. Arrange the slides so that there is a random ordering of correct and incorrect exemplars and ask the children to identify the words that are pronounced correctly.

Case example

Kenny commenced speech therapy for treatment of a moderate SSD at age 3;8, when he presented with unintelligible speech despite above average receptive language abilities, age-appropriate expressive language skills and normal hearing and oral structure and function. His error patterns included backing of alveolar stops and nasals, backing of affricates, fronting of palatal fricatives and gliding of liquids. Initially, his SLP employed a traditional approach to target /l/ in word initial singleton and cluster contexts during weekly 1-hour individual speech therapy sessions. When Kenny was 4;3, he was enrolled in a randomized control trial (Rvachew, Nowak & Cloutier, 2004) and was assigned to receive the SAILS intervention in addition to his regular speech therapy program for 16 weeks. His SLP continued with weekly sessions, targeting /t/, /d/, /ʃ/ /tʃ/ using a traditional approach and a horizontal goal attack strategy. In addition to these sessions, he also received 15 minutes of the SAILS intervention, administered by his mother under the guidance of a student research assistant. Each week he learned to identify correct and incorrect versions of words that began or ended with a given phoneme, specifically /t p m k l ɹ f s/ in the word initial position for the first 8 weeks and in word final position for the second 8 weeks of the study (see the published research report for details of the phonemic perception and PA activities that were implemented by computer for these phonemes). All treatment was discontinued when he was 4;7, and he received no further treatment as a pre-schooler. It is not known whether he ever received speech therapy in elementary school.

His speech accuracy was assessed at enrolment to the study just as the SAILS intervention was about to begin (pre-treatment assessment), 6 months later (post-treatment assessment) and 12 months later (follow-up assessment). These assessments were conducted by an SLP who was blind to his assigned experimental treatment condition and who was not involved in the regular or experimental portion of his intervention. Obtained percentile rankings of 5, 10 and 32 on the Goldman–Fristoe Test of Articulation (Goldman & Fristoe, 2000) during the pre-treatment, post-treatment, and follow-up assessments, respectively, revealed excellent progress. When examining total number of errors on this test, his improvement between the pre- and post-treatment assessments was almost twice as great as the improvement that was observed on average for children in the control group who did not receive the SAILS intervention, mirroring the results obtained for the experimental group as a whole. The clinical importance of this outcome is highlighted by the fact that he began first grade with age-appropriate speech (w/ɹ substitutions being the only remaining speech error), an outcome enjoyed by comparatively few children in the control group. These improvements in speech accuracy were also reflected in significantly improved speech intelligibility, as illustrated in brief excerpts from speech samples that yield Percent Consonant Correct (PCC) scores of 65, 85 and 92 for the pre-treatment, post-treatment and follow-up assessments, respectively.

Pre-treatment Speech Sample Excerpt:
'Karl's putting her in there where is all fishes.'
[gɑɪz pʊgɪŋ hə ɪn gɛʌ wɛ ɪz ɑ fɪsəz]
Post-treatment Speech Sample Excerpt:
'He is putting the baby in there. In … tank. There's fishies.'
[hi ɪz pʊɾɪŋ ə bebi ɪn dɛʌ … ɪn … tæŋk … dɛɹz fɪʃiz]
Follow-up Speech Sample Excerpt:
'And then he takes the baby to the fishtank and the baby swimming in the fishtank.'
[æn ðɛn hi teks ə bebi tu ðə fɪʃtæŋk æn ðə bebi swɪmɪn ɪn ðə fɪʃtæŋk]

More information about the application of perceptually based approaches can be found in Rvachew and Brosseau-Lapré (2010; 2012). Contact susan.rvachew@mcgill.ca if you wish to create new stimuli appropriate to a different dialect or language group.

Phonemic intervention

Selecting targets for phonemic (phonological) intervention begins with describing the child's error patterns, and this can be done in at least two ways: by identifying phonological processes (phonological patterns) or by identifying phoneme collapses. Working from a natural processes perspective, the therapy targets are the correct productions; meaning that the correct adult form (the target) is contrasted with the sound the child usually produces (the error). For example, in working on velar fronting, with a child who replaces /ŋ/ with /n/, the therapist might choose *fan, run, pin, gone* and *thin* to contrast with *fang, rung, ping, gong* and *thing*, respectively. On the other hand, when working from the perspective of phoneme collapses, there are two steps. The first is to look for lost contrast, for example, *funny* → /tʌni/ *shell* → /tæw/ *cup* → /tʌp/ *cheese* → /tid/, where four phonemes have been collapsed into one: /t/. The second step is to decide how to present the minimal contrast in intervention: will the therapist choose a Minimal Opposition (as is usual but not binding in Conventional Minimal Pairs), Multiple Oppositions, a Maximal Opposition or an Empty Set (Unknown Set)? No matter how targets are selected, in minimal pair therapy, activities are designed to demonstrate to the child how changing sounds in words (e.g., from *back* to *bag*, or from *car* to *tar*), or how changing the structure of syllables (e.g., from *so* to *soap*, or from *tap* to *trap*), results in changes in word meaning, and that this affects communication. And, no matter which approach is chosen, feature contrasts are central to the child's learning.

Feature contrasts in English

Phonemes are not 'contrastive' but their features are. Featural distinctions serve to create 'opposition' between phonemes (see Table 2.5). The non-major class distinctions are in *place*: differentiating labial, coronal and dorsal consonants; *manner*: differentiating stops, fricatives, affricates, nasals, liquids, glides; and voice: differentiating the voiced–voiceless cognate pairs, /p b, t d, k g, f v, s z, ʃ ʒ, tʃ dʒ, θ ð/. Major class features distinguish between the main groupings of sounds in a language, namely, consonants versus vowels, glides versus consonants and obstruents (stops, fricatives, affricates) versus sonorants (nasals, liquids, glides, vowels). For example, *bake–make* illustrates a major class distinction between obstruents and sonorants; *make–wake* illustrates the major class distinction between consonants and glides. In the minimal pair *silly* versus *Billy*, the contrast is not *quite* maximal, but it is 'maximal enough' to be highly salient for a child receiving intervention. In *silly* versus *Billy* is labial /b/ versus coronal /s/, stop /b/ versus fricative /s/ and voiced /b/ versus voiceless /s/. It cuts across many featural dimensions, but as /s/ and /b/ are both obstruents there is no obstruent versus sonorant opposition (i.e., no major class feature distinction).

Recall that phonological (phonemic) approaches focus on teaching children the function of sounds, and all rest on the principle that, once it is introduced to a child's system, a featural contrast will show generalisation to other relevant phonemic pairs. Four stand-alone minimal pair therapies – Conventional Minimal Pairs, Multiple Oppositions, Maximal Oppositions and Empty Set (Unknown Set) – are described below. Other phonological approaches incorporate minimal pair therapy, and these include Grunwell's approach, *Metaphon*, Imagery Therapy, Auditory Input Therapy, CPPA, the Psycholinguistic Model and PACT, whereas minimal pair treatments are used in tandem with perceptually based interventions, such as SAILS (Rvachew, A25).

Grunwell's approach

Employing Stampe's natural phonology theory and identifying phonological processes in assessment (Grunwell, 1975, 1985a), British Linguist Pamela Grunwell proposed a treatment that was based around the principle that homophony motivates phonemic change, challenging the clinician to, 'Expose the child systematically to the dimensions of the target system absent from his or her speech in a way in which both their form and communicative functions are made evident' (Grunwell, 1989). Grunwell saw four main types of phonological change that could become the clinician's focus for target selection and intervention:

1. Stabilisation: the resolution of a variable pronunciation pattern into a stable pattern.
2. Destabilisation: the disruption of a stable pattern, resulting in variability.
3. Innovation: the introduction of a new pattern.
4. Generalisation: the transfer of a pronunciation pattern across four possible contexts: phonological, lexical, syntactic and socio-environmental.

In selecting targets, Grunwell advised therapists to work in developmental sequence where possible, giving priority to patterns most deviant from normal phonology and/or to those most destructive of communicative adequacy. Systemic feature contrasts were minimal (e.g., *fan* vs. *van*; *comb* vs. *cone*) and structural contrasts near minimal (e.g., *top* vs. *stop*; *Ben* vs. *bend*) on the basis that, with small feature difference between the target and the error, there was nothing else to get in the way. There was no attempt to increase the saliency of contrasts, and clinicians tended to accept, unquestioningly, the notion that something *might* 'get in the way' if there were more feature differences within a word pair. I am still thinking about that idea.

In Grunwell's approach, procedures are system based (metalinguistic) or word based (manipulative). Minimal pair therapy is a metalinguistic procedure, in Grunwell's terms, demonstrating to the child that sound differences signal meaning differences. A manipulative activity might involve listening to, and eventually saying in context, words that share common phonological features (e.g., all with fricatives in onset, or all ending with a final stop). The approach is suitable for children with mild to severe phonological disorder (or 'phonological disability' to use Grunwell's term), and procedures incorporate auditory discrimination, minimal pair and near-minimal pair games, homophony confrontation, phoneme–grapheme correspondences and metaphonological skills training. The far-reaching influence of Grunwell's pioneering research, pedagogy and her so called phonological principles can be seen in Auditory Input Therapy (A24), Multiple Oppositions Therapy (A26), Phoneme Awareness Therapy (A28) and the contrastive Vowel Therapy proposed by Gibbon (2013) [also see Gibbon (A29)], PACT (Bowen & Cupples, 1999a, b), and *Metaphon* (Dean, Howell, Waters & Reid, 1995).

Metaphon

Metaphon (Dean & Howell, 1986; Dean, Howell, Hill & Waters, 1990; Dean, Howell, Waters & Reid, 1995) is also based on the principle that homophony motivates phonemic change and its development was heavily influenced by Grunwell's work. Using the assessment materials in the *Metaphon Resource Pack* (now out of print) the SLP/SLT performs a phonological analysis on the child's production of single words in a picture-naming task, and errors are described in terms of phonological processes. Target versus substitute sound pairs are selected for treatment, as in Conventional Minimal Pair intervention (Weiner, 1981). For example, to eliminate palatal fronting, the target /ʃ/ might be contrasted with the substitute (error) [s] in word pairs such as *ship–sip, shine–sign, show–sew, shell–sell, shower–sour, push–puss, mesh–mess, gash–gas* and *ash–ass*. Feature contrasts are usually, but not necessarily, minimal or near minimal. *Metaphon* encompasses two overlapping treatment phases followed by a discrete final phase. Metaphonetic skills are trained to improve a child's 'cognitive awareness' of the properties of the sound system, whereas metalinguistic tasks are implemented

to develop communicative effectiveness through more successful use of repair strategies.

Metaphon Phase 1

In Phase 1, the child is taught that language is used to communicate and that language which is normally opaque can be made transparent or tangible. Phase 1 comprises Concept Level, Sound Level, Phoneme Level and Word Level. Phase 1 is considered by its developers to be the most important phase of *Metaphon*, and the one that in their view is most distinct from other published phonological intervention programs. The aim is to capture the child's interest in the phonology of the target language, to alert the child to the properties of sounds (in terms of place, manner and voice: PVM) and their contrastive potential, to show that contrasts between sounds convey meaning and to facilitate the child's knowledge that these features can be manipulated to increase the probability of being understood.

Concept Level

At Concept Level, individual speech sounds are *not* contrasted, and the child learns a conceptual vocabulary to use later for PVM awareness. Metaphors associated with voicing features are employed: for example, Mr. Noisy or Mr. Growly to denote voiced consonants and Mr. Whisper or Mr. Quiet for voiceless ones. Other concepts, such as long sound versus short sound (denoting fricative vs. stop) and back sound versus front sound (velar vs. alveolar) are introduced, with the aim of having children identify sounds by their properties with 100% accuracy. The *Metaphon* team reported that it might not take long for children to achieve this level of accuracy. The next step, Sound Level, is different depending whether substitution processes (e.g., fronting, stopping and gliding, where one sound replaces another) or syllable structure processes (e.g., cluster reduction, final consonant deletion or weak syllable deletion, where the structure of the syllable changes) are being targeted.

Substitution processes (Sound Level)

For *substitution processes* at Sound Level, the vocabulary the child has learned (Mr. Growly, Short Sound, etc.) is transferred to describing non-speech sounds: castanets, whistles, the therapist's vocalisations and animal and vehicle noises. The aim is to show the child those environmental sounds and vocalisations can be classified as long–short, front–back and noisy–whisper (growly–quiet). Then, at Phoneme Level, entire sound classes are contrasted, using visual cues. For example, all fricatives versus all stops are presented to the child, still referring to the sound properties (long–short, etc.). Next, the child enters Word Level, and minimally contrasted word pairs are introduced for *listening* (not production). The child judges whether a word has a long–short, front–back or noisy–whisper sound in it. Again, visual support is provided in the form of gesture cues and pictures.

Syllable structure processes (Sound Level)

For *syllable structure processes* at Sound Level, concepts such as 'beginning', as a preparation for working on initial consonant deletion, and 'end', in preparation for attacking final consonant deletion, are introduced, as well as imagery and concrete demonstrations. For example, for cluster reduction SIWI, imagery coupled with a concrete demonstration might involve a train with one locomotive (representing an initial consonant such as /ɹ/) versus a train with two locomotives (representing an initial two-element consonant cluster such as /tɹ/) in preparation for a near minimal pair such as *rip–trip* or *rap–trap*. At Syllable Level/Word Level, nonsense syllables and words are contrasted (e.g., *hot* has an engine, *ot* does not; *bin* has an engine, *in* does not).

Metaphon Phase 2

In Phase 2, metaphonological tasks involving minimal pairs (introduced in Phase 1) and homonymy confrontation are emphasised, and the focus shifts to developing communicative effectiveness by giving the child feedback about success or failure to convey meaning, through behavioural responses, prompting him/her to review output. Dean and Howell (1986) postulated that, in the short term, such feedback would improve production by triggering the use of repair strategies based on the new knowledge of sound contrasts learned in Phase 1, and that the long-term effect would be a change in central phonological processing. Phase 2 is concerned with developing phonological and communicative awareness, and the link between Phases 1 and 2 is achieved by incorporating Phase 1 activities into Phase 2. Phonological awareness and awareness of the properties of speech sounds must be well developed before the core activity of Phase 2 can be successful.

Core activity

In the *Metaphon* core activity, the clinician and child take turns to *produce* and *select* minimal pair words (e.g., *pin* vs. *fin*) pictured on cards or worksheets. If the child says a target word, such as *fin*, correctly: (1) The therapist selects the correct word; (2) feedback is given; and (3) guided discussion occurs; for example, 'Yes. That was a long sound. I guess you know lots of other long sounds'. If the child says the target word *incorrectly* (e.g., *bin* for *fin*): (1) The therapist selects the incorrect word (the one the child actually said); and (2) no feedback is given directly to the child, but the child's attention is drawn to the sound property; for example, 'That was a short sound. Should it have been a long sound?' The aim of the core activity is to have the child revise incorrect productions 'spontaneously'.

Metaphon final phase

In the final phase of *Metaphon*, minimal pair sentences are introduced. The therapist and child take turns, each instructing the other to, for example, 'Draw a *pin/fin* on the fish'; 'Draw a *pan/fan* in the box'; 'Draw a *pole/foal* in the stable'. Emphasis is still on guided discussion of sound properties ('I think that should have been a long sound') aimed at facilitating the spontaneous use of repair strategies.

Minimal pair approaches: Conventional Minimal Pairs

The Conventional Minimal Pair model (Weiner, 1981) rests on the principle that homonymy motivates phonemic change, and its foundation, according to Fey (1992), is to:

1. modify groups of sounds produced in error, in a patterned way;
2. highlight featural contrasts rather than accurate sound production; and
3. emphasise the use of sounds for communicative purposes.

Rewarding the use of contrast: (1) encourages a reduction in homophony, which (2) evokes an improvement in phonological organisation and (3) facilitates phonological restructuring. Selecting minimal pairs (e.g., *win* vs. *wing* for velar fronting) or near minimal pairs (e.g., *up* vs. *pup* for initial consonant deletion) is built on the idea that Grunwell (1989) shared, that of making the difference between the target and the error as small as possible so that there are no interfering featural factors ('nothing to get in the way'). Within intervention activities, a sound used in error (e.g., /v/) by the child is paired with its substitute (e.g., /b/). The approach may be suitable for children with mild and moderate phonological disorders. In the therapy activities, the child says the name of a picture or object, and the adult responds to what the child actually says. Only miscommunications (errors) attract feedback in the form of challenge or feigned listener confusion, and non-homophonous productions are rewarded by successful communication. For example, if the child says *bet* for target word *vet*, the therapist would hand over *bet* (listener confusion) or challenge it

('you take your puppy to the *bet*?'). If the child produced a different (non-target) voiced fricative in attempting *vet*, perhaps saying /zɛt/, then he or she would be rewarded by being handed the *vet* picture, because *bet–zet* is not homophonous and /v/ and /z/ are in the same sound class (fricatives) and are both voiced. Similarly, if the child said /fɛt/ for *vet*, then the non-homonymous production would be rewarded. In this way, the intervention is around homonymy, ambiguity, 'pretend' listener confusion and effective communication on the child's part ('making meaning' or 'making sense'). As a conceptual approach, phonetic manner and place cues and production drill do not occur in Conventional Minimal Pair intervention in its pure form, but in practice they are usually incorporated (see, for example, the video clips in Williams 2006a, and Williams, McLeod & McCauley, 2010).

Minimal pair approaches: Maximal Oppositions

The Maximal Oppositions approach (Gierut, 1989, 1992) is not based on homophony. Rather, the guiding principle is that heightened *saliency* of contrasts increases *learnability*, thereby facilitating phonemic change. The word pairs are still 'minimal pairs' in the sense that one sound changes, but the feature contrasts are 'maximal' or 'nearly maximal' (as in the 'nearly maximal' *silly* vs. *Billy* example used above). Gierut applies feature geometry in the explicit creation of pairs that are high and low on the feature tree. She called the contrastive pairs in Maximal Oppositions (and in its close relation, Empty Set or Unknown Set) 'non-proportional pairs'. Because non-proportional pairs do not share many features in common with other minimal pairs, they are highly perceptually salient, and, according to Gierut's findings, therefore more learnable. In Maximal Oppositions and Empty Set, the clinician aims to present a target and contrasting word that have many feature differences: in place, manner and voice; and major class. The contrasting sound is independent of the target sound, is produced correctly by the child and is maximally distinct.

As in the Conventional Minimal Pairs approach, only one contrast is presented at a time. Take for example my client Xing-Fu, 4;5 who was a monolingual Australian English speaker with a severe SSD. He exhibited velar fronting, replacing /k/ with /t/ in all contexts, whereas /ŋ/ was one of only eight consonants he produced correctly in all obligatory contexts. The voiced, velar nasal /ŋ/ differs from the voiceless, alveolar stop /k/ in place, manner, voice, major class (and markedness, for that matter), so when it came to contrasting a sound he knew with a sound he need to learn, /ŋ/ vs. /k/ was one obvious choice. The maximally opposed minimal pairs used in Xing-Fu's therapy included: *key–knee*, *cat–gnat*, *coat–note*, *cow–now*, and *cot–knot*. The Maximal Oppositions approach is suitable for children like Xing-Fu with severe phonological impairment, as is Empty Set.

Minimal pair approaches: Empty Set (Unknown Set)

Empty Set (Gierut, 1992) is a variation of Maximal Oppositions that also uses non-proportional pairs and is also *not* based on the idea of homophony motivating phonemic change. Again, the principle behind it is that heightened perceptual saliency of contrasts increases learnability, facilitating phonological restructuring. In Empty Set, two targets are addressed concurrently. An *error* the child has (the first target) is contrasted with *another* erred sound (the second target), and the two targets are maximally distinct from each other.

Probably the better name for this is 'Unknown Set' as it signals that the child 'knows' neither sound and is 'learning two *new* sounds'. So, error is contrasted with error – but not just any error pair! For example, my colleague's client Vaughan, 5;8 was from a monolingual South African English background, and was a recent migrant, with his family, to Australia. He had a severe SSD, and a PCC of 41%. Vaughan replaced /f/ with /b/ (stopping) and /ɹ/ with /w/ (gliding), and both /f/

and /ɹ/ were absent from his repertoire. Recognising the severity of his impairment, and wanting to use the Unknown Set approach, his speech–language pathologist needed to find a contrasting sound for his minimal-pair–maximally-opposed treatment set that was maximally distinct from /f/, remembering that the sound had not only to be maximally distinct but also *absent* from Vaughan's repertoire (representing least phonological knowledge: see Table 8.4). The /ɹ/ for which he was non-stimulable was a perfect choice. Accordingly, Vaughan's minimal word pairs (non-proportional and maximally contrasting) included *rind–find*, *reel–feel*, *red–fed*, and *rocks–fox*, which he produced at the outset of therapy as: [waɪnd-baɪnd, wil-bil, wɛd-bɛd, wɒks-bɒks]. As it happened, Vaughan's error productions were also maximally distinct (non-proportional), but not homonymous.

The procedures used in Empty Set are the same as for Conventional Minimal Pairs intervention and in the Maximal Oppositions approach and may include the provision of phonemic place and manner cues, suggestions and 'instructions' to the child.

Drawing on the results of several experiments, Gierut (1992) determined that therapy was most effective, promoting the greatest generalisation, if two new maximally opposed phonemes representing a major class feature difference were targeted, as in Vaughan's case. By contrast, targeting one new maximally opposed phoneme representing a non-major class distinction was effective, but less effective than the preceding option. Between these two were two further equally effective alternatives. The first was to target two new maximally opposed phonemes representing a non-major class distinction; and the second was to target one new maximally opposed phoneme representing a major class feature difference.

Minimal pair approaches: Multiple Oppositions

This systemic approach is geared to children whose intelligibility challenges fall at the higher end of the moderate range and in the severe range

(A. L. Williams, personal communication, 2013). Unlike the Conventional Minimal Pairs approach, in Multiple Oppositions Therapy it is not assumed that minimal or maximal *feature* contrasts will be formed, because, of course, the phoneme collapses (or homonymy) in which several targets are realised the same way determine which oppositions will be used.

In an intervention session, several targets are presented to the child at once, all contrasting simultaneously with what the child usually produces. For example, if a child collapsed the voiceless velar stop /k/, the voiceless alveolar fricative /s/, the voiceless affricate /tʃ/ and the consonant cluster /tɹ/ to /t/ so that *kick, sick, chick* and *trick* were all realised homophonously as [tɪk], his or her treatment sets (in the first two columns below) and their corresponding untreated set to use as a generalisation probe (shown in the third column) might look like this:

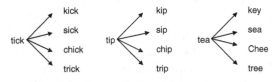

Any non-words would be made meaningful by using it as the name for a fictional person, fantasy creature or object, so you might have a picture of a person called *Chee* for the probe set above. Figure 4.2 displays examples of pictures that might be used in treatment sets and a probe set to address this phoneme collapse.

Two further examples of 'phoneme collapses', the term Williams uses to denote the simplified one-to-many correspondence between the child's customary (error) productions and targets, are: *lick, wick, rick* and *flick* all realised homophonously as [jɪk] and *beat, been, beak* and *beach* all produced as a CV [bi]. The collapse to [jɪk] is not amenable to description in terms of phonological processes or phonological patterns, while the second *could* be described as deletion of coda or final consonant deletion.

As noted above, in the Multiple Oppositions approach, it is *not* assumed that minimal or maximal feature contrasts will be formed. This is

Multiple Oppositions

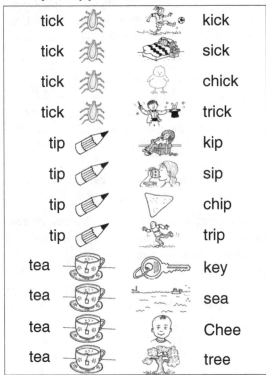

Figure 4.2 Multiple Opposition word pairs. Drawings by Helen Rippon, Speech and Language Therapist, www.blacksheeppress.co.uk

because the contrasts are based on a child's error relative to the adult target. A further difference between Multiple Oppositions and the Conventional Minimal Pairs paradigm is that it is not based on the assumption that a child's developing sound system can be adequately described in terms of phonological processes. A phoneme collapse portrays a child's phonological organisation more broadly, employing a child-based and systemic perspective. Hence, a phoneme collapse is considered as one rule, rather than several phonological processes. From this, it is clear that Multiple Oppositions is not only distinguished by having more targets in training than the other three minimal pair approaches, but also by the way in which those targets relate to each other as 'members' of one rule set.

So, multiple targets are treated simultaneously across a child's rule set. These multiple targets are contrasted one at a time with the child's error substitute, creating the so-called Multiple Oppositions. The activities themselves are as for Conventional Minimal Pair therapy. The intervention occurs in four phases.

1. Familiarisation + Production.
2. Contrasts + Naturalistic Play: Phase 2 begins at an imitative production level, and moves to spontaneous production by the child when the first training criterion of 70% accuracy is achieved.
3. Contrasts within Communicative Contexts.
4. Conversational Recasts.

With regard to production accuracy in connected speech, Williams uses a structured and systematic treatment paradigm to program for generalisation at all phases of intervention. She aims for high response rates in each treatment session (about 60–80 responses in a 30-minute session).

In the early phases of treatment, she commences a session with focused production practice of the contrasts and ends the session with a conversation-based naturalistic activity. She believes that this conversation-based activity provides a bridge to the focused practice and allows the child to hear and practice his or her sound(s) in a more naturalistic activity (in Phase 2). These brief naturalistic activities include sound-loaded conversational activities (cf. Bowen, 2010a; Camarata, 2010; Hodson, A5; Lancaster, A24) in which the child can hear and have opportunities to produce a large proportional frequency of his or her target sound(s). The approach is geared to children with severe phonological disorders and children whose difficulties are at the more severe end of the moderate range.

Sound contrasts in phonology

From the 1970s onwards, clinically applicable developments took place in Generative Phonology and Natural Phonology. Linguists turned their attention, in great detail for the first time, to the plight of children with speech impairment.

Although there were obvious clinical applications for this work (see for example, Grunwell's approach above), the hard task of converting it into intervention – that was ecologically valid, practical, efficient, effective and acceptable to practitioners and clients – required adequately funded, concentrated research effort from the SLP/SLT side.

I will not say she rode in on her white charger, but in an environment of often inefficient service delivery, and overstretched services within the SLP/SLT profession, with most clinicians only dimly aware of how the new knowledge from linguistics could inform practice, Lynn Williams responded by developing, implementing and successfully testing the efficacy of her Multiple Oppositions treatment approach. Knowing that it is all too likely for important clinical research to receive wide publication in the peer-reviewed literature (which it has) while remaining virtually undiscovered by grass roots practitioners, Williams devised ways of bringing her own and, quite remarkably, *other* evidence-based speech sound treatments (Conventional Minimal Pairs, Maximal Oppositions and Empty Set) to the world's workplace. A major outcome of her extraordinary endeavour has been the *Sound Contrasts in Phonology (SCIP)* intervention software (Williams, 2006a), currently in revision.

Commenting on the effects and efficiency of a Multiple Oppositions approach, Williams (2000a) wrote, 'The use of larger treatment sets in Multiple Oppositions may lead to several new phonemic contrasts being added to a child's system. Thus, Multiple Oppositions has a potential advantage over singular contrastive models of phonological intervention in terms of shortened length of treatment, improved intelligibility, and more efficient intervention.'

But implementing Multiple Oppositions through the use of *SCIP* is not just a question of client plus clinician plus software with a dash of homework! Whether it is done with the aid of the software or without, the success of the intervention rests on up to 2 hours of detailed assessment. Although Williams used a 245-item protocol for her clinical research, a clinician can base the analysis on a standardised test, such as the *GFTA-2* or the *DEAP*, and complete the analysis in much less time. Detailed assessment allows the clinician to map the child's sound system onto the adult system and determine the extent of the child's phonological knowledge and what he or she needs to learn. It is on the basis of such detailed assessment that the SLP/SLT can establish a treatment plan, with highly specified goals, aimed at expeditious restructuring of the child's disordered system in order for it to match age expectations.

Dr. Lynn Williams is Associate Director of the Center of Excellence in Early Childhood Learning and Development and Professor in the Department of Audiology and Speech-Language Pathology at East Tennessee State University (ETSU) in Johnson City, Tennessee, United States. She is a Fellow of the American Speech-Language-Hearing Association (ASHA), and she has served as an Associate Editor of *Language Speech and Hearing Services in the Schools* (2004–2007) and *American Journal of Speech-Language Pathology* (2009–present). Lynn is the author of *Speech Disorders Resource Guide for Preschool Children* (Williams, 2003), co-editor of *Interventions for Speech Sound Disorders in Children* (Williams, McLeod & McCauley, 2010), and she has published and presented extensively, nationally and internationally, on her research with children who have SSD. Lynn has received several grants from the National Institutes of Health in support of her translational research, resulting in the development of a software program called *SCIP* (Williams, 2006a). Embedded in *SCIP* is her own approach to speech therapy called *Multiple Oppositions*.

Q26. A. Lynn Williams: The Multiple Oppositions approach

The *SCIP* software includes clinical training videos that show, with helpful commentaries, snippets of four contrastive therapies in action, namely: Conventional Minimal Pairs, Multiple Oppositions, Maximal Oppositions and 'Empty' or Unknown Set. What assessment process is typical for a suitable candidate for Multiple Oppositions Therapy? And in terms of the intervention itself, can you give us a case example that demonstrates the aspects of the therapy not shown in the available videos (Williams, 2006a; 2010)? For example, how long are the treatment sessions, how frequent are they, are families involved in sessions or in homework, what procedures and activities are incorporated and at what stages of the child's progress are they introduced?

A26. A. Lynn Williams: Assessment and intervention from a systemic perspective

What assessment process is typical for a suitable candidate for this therapy?

In order to implement the systemic treatment approach of Multiple Oppositions, it is important to describe the child's speech disorder *systemically*. A systemic approach is a *system-based* approach that compares the child's system to the adult system by mapping the two sound systems to each other using phoneme collapses. For example, a child might produce [t] for several sounds in the adult target sounds, such as /s ʃ k tʃ st/. Systemically, this is viewed as one rule involving a phoneme collapse of voiceless obstruents and cluster (adult system) to the voiceless obstruent, [t] (child system). This broader system-to-system comparison provides a more holistic description of the child's speech than is possible with a sound-based approach that utilises a narrower sound-to-sound comparison of the child's production relative to an adult target. Using this example, a sound-to-sound comparison using phonological processes would describe the phoneme collapse as four separate and independent error patterns (i.e., stopping, fronting, deaffrication and cluster reduction).

In addition, a systemic analysis is *child based* rather than adult based, as is common in many traditional assessment approaches that are based on a pre-determined and finite number of rules (or processes) to describe the child's error patterns. As a consequence, the broader system-to-system comparison and child-based aspects of a systemic analysis allow the clinician to describe idiosyncratic errors that are common in unintelligible speech, as well as gain insight into the organisational structure the child has developed to compensate for a smaller sound system relative to the adult sound system. As Grunwell (1997) stated, we can discover the 'order in the disorder'.

To execute a systemic description of a child's speech, I administer the *Systemic Phonological Analysis of Child Speech (SPACS)* that provides information on the child's phonetic inventory (word initial and word final), distribution of English consonants relative to the ambient sound system and mapping of child : adult sound systems using phoneme collapses. For a more detailed description of the *SPACS* approach, readers can refer to Williams (2001, 2003, 2006b, 2010). In my clinical research, I use a 245-item single-word elicitation probe (*Systemic Phonological Protocol*, Williams, 2003) and a 15–20-minute conversational sample.

Clinically, however, this sample is likely to be too time consuming for SLPs/SLTs who have large caseloads and severe time constraints. Clinicians can complete a *SPACS* on smaller databases, such as the *Goldman–Fristoe Test of Articulation-2 (GFTA-2*; Goldman & Fristoe, 2000), or other sound inventory tests, that are commonly used. Phoneme collapses can be constructed *by initial and final word position* by mapping the adult sound targets that are replaced by the error production in the child's system. Using the *GFTA-2*, the clinician can look down the word-initial column on the response matrix to diagram phoneme collapses of frequently occurring error productions. For example, a case study of Adam indicated that he produced [g] for adult targets /b, d, f, v, ð, s, z, ʃ, tʃ, dʒ, dɹ, fɹ, gl, gɹ, kw, st, tɹ/ in word-initial position on the *GFTA-2*. This represents a 1:17 phoneme collapse between Adam's sound system and the adult sound system. A closer examination of the adult targets reveals that they are obstruents and clusters. Thus, Adam collapsed obstruents and clusters to [g], which is also an obstruent. This *SPACS* was completed easily and quickly and it represents Adam's logical and systemic organisation more clearly than if a phonological process analysis were completed on his *GFTA-2* responses.

What are the specific procedures involved in the Multiple Oppositions approach?

After the child's system has been described, a systemic intervention approach using Multiple Oppositions can be implemented in order to facilitate phonological restructuring with the greatest amount of change occurring in the least amount of time. I structure intervention using a treatment paradigm described in detail elsewhere (Williams, 2000a; 2003; 2005; 2010). There are four phases: All are data based with the exception of Phase 1, which is time based.

Basically, Phase 1 involves familiarisation (of the rule, the sounds and the vocabulary) + Production of the contrasts. This initial phase creates a meaningful context that lays a foundation for the feedback and work that will be carried out in the following treatment phases.

Phase 2 encompasses focused practice of the contrasts at an imitative level with a dense response rate (about 60–80 responses in a 30-minute individual session or 20–40 responses in a 30-minute small group session). Although the Multiple Oppositions paradigm has larger treatment sets of target sounds, the contrasts are practiced one at a time. For example, *tip–sip*; *tip–ship*; tip–*Kip*; *tip–trip*. The focused practice is followed by a short (5 minute) naturalistic play activity. These are brief, sound-loaded activities that bridge the focused practice that occurs on a narrow training set and the communicative use of the contrast within meaningful play activities. An example might be *I Spy* using objects or pictures of items that have the target sound in untrained words. The clinician and the child take turns giving hints for the other to guess the item. I typically use the naturalistic activity for one sound per session and generally choose the sound with which the child is having greatest difficulty. The focused practice continues at an imitative level until the child achieves training criterion (70% accuracy across two consecutive treatment sets; 1 treatment set = 20 responses). Once the criterion is met, Phase 2 continues with focused practice + naturalistic play, but at a spontaneous level of production. Intervention continues at the spontaneous level of Phase 2 until the second training criterion is met (90% accuracy across two consecutive treatment sets).

At that point, treatment moves to Phase 3: contrasts within naturalistic communicative contexts. This treatment phase integrates the focused practice and play so that the child plays games with the contrasts (such as, *Go Fish*). Although most children achieve the generalisation criterion (50% accuracy in conversational speech) in Phase 3, some children need additional intervention at a conversational level to attain generalisation (see Williams, 2000b for longitudinal data from an intervention study with 10 children). For those children who are doing well in Phase 3 at a spontaneous response level in communicative contexts, but not reaching generalisation, movement to Phase 4 occurs.

Phase 4 involves conversational recasts that encompass Stephen Camarata's *Naturalistic Speech Intelligibility Training* (cf., Camarata, 2010). In this phase, treatment switches from the contrasts in games to using the contrasts communicatively in conversational scenarios, such as ordering food at a restaurant that includes food items containing the target sounds. For example, for Adam with his 1:17 collapse to /g/, described above, words might include *deep dish pizza* and *dessert* for /d/; *fishfingers* and *fudge* for /f/; and *steak* and *stuffing* for /st/.

The treatment paradigm provides a structure, or blueprint, for intervention and the child's progression through the treatment phases. As noted earlier, the child is in the driver's seat, so to speak, and matriculation through the treatment phases is based on the child's performance data. The paradigm structures intervention to address two important aspects of phonological intervention: (1) the duality of sound learning: phonetic and phonemic aspects and (2) programming for generalisation.

In the early phases of treatment, greater emphasis and support are placed on helping the child learn the production aspects of the new contrast (the imitative response level, plus the focused practice with dense response rates). The early phases also control for extraneous distractors, such as playing board games, in order for the child to achieve the focused practice and dense response rates. Yet, I program for generalisation from the outset by pairing the focused practice with the bridging activities of naturalistic play involving the new contrast in sound-loaded activities. I want to quickly bring in the phonemic aspects of sound learning (moving from imitation to spontaneous with a lower training criterion level) and gradually and systematically re-introduce the distractors (playing games with the contrasts in Phase 3 or conversational recasts in Phase 4).

A summary of the treatment phases and activities is provided in Table A26.1. As you look at the treatment phases, activities and response levels, you will notice the systematic and gradual programming for generalisation, as well as the shift in intervention focus from phonetic learning to phonemic learning.

Table A26.1 Summary of Multiple Oppositions treatment phases

Treatment phase	Intervention focus	Response rate	Response level	Example of activities	Criterion
Phase 1: Familiarization + Production Example: 	Create a meaningful context that lays foundation of work the child will be doing	1 treatment set = 20 responses (5 contrastive word pairs of 4 target sounds = 20 responses)	Imitative	Familiarization of: Rules (long versus short [t~ s, ʃ]; front versus back [t ~ k]; buddy sounds [t ~ tɹ]) Sound (ticking clock sound versus flat tire sound and quiet lady sound; coughing man sound; sounds that go together) Vocabulary	First treatment session
Phase 2: Contrasts + naturalistic play	Initial focus is on the phonetic aspects of sound learning (imitative) and then moves to phonemic aspects (spontaneous)	60–80 responses (individual session); 20–40 responses (group session)	Imitative then spontaneous	Produce contrasts (5 contrastive word pairs) with imitative model (control distractors and get high response rate); give tokens for each response regardless of accuracy – when child gets 20 tokens, she/he has completed one treatment set and she/he gets a sticker; switch order of presentation of contrasts to prevent child developing articulatory set. Naturalistic play (e.g., I *Spy*)	70% accuracy across two consecutive treatment sets (move to Spontaneous); 90% accuracy across two consecutive treatment sets (move to Phase 3)
Phase 3: Contrasts within communicative contexts	Rule learning (phonemic)	60–80 responses (20–40 responses for group session)	Spontaneous	*Go Fish; Concentration; Memory; Teacher*	90% accuracy across two consecutive treatment sets (if generalization criterion of 50% accuracy in conversation speech not met, move to Phase 4)
Phase 4: Conversational recasts	Incorporate new contrast into conversational rule	60–80 responses (20–40 responses for group session)	Spontaneous	Communicative scenarios, such as a family restaurant	50% accuracy in conversational speech

Regarding the intervention 'dosage' a recent analysis of practice trials using Multiple Oppositions related to treatment outcomes revealed the following:

- A minimum dose of > 50 trials for a duration of 30 sessions is required for intervention to be effective.
- Greater intensity (70 trials for about 40 sessions) is required for children with more severe SSD.
- Quantitative changes in dose occur over the course of intervention with greater intensity at the beginning that decreases by about 20% during the second half of intervention on a specific goal.
- Qualitatively, focused practice and naturalistic play activities are implemented with a 2:1 ratio throughout intervention as the bridging activities are used to program for generalisation.

Engaging families in the intervention process is an important component of treatment and can take many different forms from active to passive involvement. The particular way that I involve families reflects my philosophy that (1) learning a sound system is similar to learning language – it involves communication and (2) parents are not trained therapists. As a consequence, I ask parents to leave the focused practice of facilitating new sound contrasts to me as the trained professional, and I ask them to extend the work the child and I are doing in the clinic at home through fun, play-based, sound-loaded activities that involve models and recasts.

I interview the parent(s) to find typical routines they share with their child through the week and then I develop naturalistic activities that they can implement within those routines. I know that many families live full and hectic lives with dual careers and frequent after school activities, so the naturalistic activities I send home have a greater chance of being completed (and enjoyed!) if I can ask them to do them within their normal routines. For example, at the grocery store, play a game to see who can identify the most items with the /k/ sound (*coffee, candy, cauliflower, carrots*, etc.). I teach the parents how to use set-ups, protests, models and recasts in the activity, such as identifying beans so the child can say a word that does not have their coughing man sound; or saying *torn* for *corn* to see if the child can correct them. I give the parents two to three activities each week, along with a questionnaire they complete about the number of times they used the activities, how well the activities worked, what questions they had, and so on. The questionnaire structures the home activities and communicates to the parents an expectation that they will carry out these activities on a regular basis. Occasionally, I give the parents a tape recorder to take home and record an activity that we will review together.

Imagery Therapy

In Imagery Therapy (Klein, 1996a, b), error and target are contrasted and the feature difference is usually minimal, so *Sue–zoo, sue–shoe*, or *Sue–soon* would be more usual oppositions for the therapist to introduce than more perceptually salient contrasts, like *Sue–moo* or *Sue–roo*. Labels and images of phonetic characteristics are used to aid the child's learning of new phonological rules, and once again, the rational for the approach is that homonymy motivates phonemic change. Klein (1996a) says that the approach is suitable

for 'children with one or many phonological processes' with mild to severe SSD. Therapy proceeds in three steps.

Step 1: Identification and production of the contrast in nonsense syllables

An imagery term or imagery label is assigned to the 'intruder' (Klein's term for error) and 'sound class' (target class). For example, if the child stops fricatives, the stops (intruders) may be called poppies, and fricatives (the target sound class) may be called windies. These are combined with vowels to make CVs, representing the intruders (e.g., *pah, pee, paw; tah, tee, taw*) and target sound classes (e.g., *fah, fee, faw; sah, see, saw*). The therapist produces a syllable (e.g., *paw*), and the child indicates the associated imagery term on a poppies poster or a windies poster (if the therapist has said *paw* then the child should choose the poppies poster). The child is then asked to produce a syllable containing a sound from each imagery class (e.g., *Give me a poppy sound or Give me a windy sound*). If the child is confused at this point, the therapist provides a choice, usually with the target produced first: 'which one is windy – *faw* or *paw*?' Printed captions accompany all picture-and-object stimuli to support literacy acquisition. Bear in mind that the child is required to produce CVs and not isolated phones.

Step 2: Identification, classification and production of the contrast in single words

Next, the therapist *shows* a picture or an object representing a real word containing either the intruder or the target, *says* the word and asks the child to indicate the imagery term associated with the word. For instance, the therapist says 'sail', and the child should respond correctly by placing the picture on the poster for 'windies' because he/she knows that /s/ is 'windy'. Then the therapist *silently* shows a picture or object with either the intruder or the target, and the child indicates the associated imagery term on one or other poster. By now, the clinician's production has been eliminated. The child is drawing on his/her own internal representation in order to make the classification, and each treatment word is classified thus.

Following classification of a word, the child is asked to *produce* the word, keeping in mind the classification. For example, the child is shown a picture of *sail* and classifies it as 'a windy'. The clinician responds, 'That's right. Now make it with a windy sound'. Note that the child is instructed to say the target word but *no model* is provided. The clinician responds to any errors in production by referring to the classification the child provided.

For example, if the child said *tail* for *sail*, the therapist might say, 'Tail? You said it was a windy word, but you made it with a poppy sound. Can you try it again and put in the windy sound that you said it should have?' Conventional Minimal Pair activities (Weiner, 1981) that include communicative consequences for using both the intruder and the target are *also* used at this level.

Throughout Step 1 and Step 2, isolated sounds are not elicited and the clinician does not overtly model how to say the treatment words. For example, when eliciting g-words, the therapist might say, proffering a picture, 'Can you say this one with your throatie?' Natural feedback is given if the child errs, perhaps by producing /d/ in place of /g/: 'But you said it was a throatie and you said it with a tippy. Try it again with your throatie?'

Step 3: Production in narratives and conversational speech

The procedures from this point on are quite 'traditional' and include activities such as story telling, games incorporating target sound classes and 'controlled conversation tasks'.

Whole Language Therapy

Whole Language Therapy (Hoffman, 1993; Hoffman & Norris, 2010; Tyler, 2002) is intended for children experiencing moderate to severe phonological issues and expressive language impairment concomitantly (McCauley, A12). A typical treatment session targets might include question forms, personal pronouns and /h/ SIWI. The clinician might read to the child a book such as *Are You My Mother?* from the Berenstain Bears series of children's books created by Stan and Jan Berenstain and continued by their son, Mike Berenstain, modelling the question form, pronouns and /h/ SIWI, especially in *he, his* and *her* that occur frequently in the story. Then the therapist would re-tell the story, starting with short utterances and gradually increasing their length. As the story is re-told, the child repeats each brief utterance and then, if able, tells the story again (perhaps to a puppet or doll). Intervention takes place via conversational interactions and story contexts, incorporating cues, cloze sentences, rebus stories, story reading (to the child) and story telling (to the child and by the child) with no picture- or object-naming *per se*.

Core Vocabulary Therapy

The Core Vocabulary Approach (Crosbie, Holm & Dodd, 2005; Crosbie, Pine, Holm & Dodd, 2006) is intended for children with inconsistent speech disorder (Broomfield & Dodd, 2004; Dodd, 2005) in Dodd's classification, described in Chapter 2. Hypothetically, the underlying deficit of inconsistent speech disorder is a phonological planning deficit, not a cognitive–linguistic deficit, and most affected children probably fall in the severe SSD range. The rationale for the approach is that different parts of the speech-processing chain respond differently to therapy targeting different processing skills, and that treatment that targets the speech-processing deficit underlying the child's speech disorder will result in system-wide change.

Following Independent and Relational Analysis, an Inconsistency Assessment (a component of the *DEAP* [Dodd, Zhu, Crosbie et al. 2002]) is administered. In this assessment, 25 pictures are named on three separate occasions *in one session*, ensuring that the same lexical items are elicited within an identical context. The productions are compared in order to calculate an inconsistency score. Children are deemed to have inconsistent speech disorder if 40% or more of the words are produced variably, and consistent speech disorder if they exhibit two or more atypical patterns and an inconsistency score below 40%.

The Core Vocabulary Therapy procedure begins with the child, parents and teacher selecting, with the therapist's help if required, 50 words that are functionally 'powerful' for the child and 'mean something' to him or her, such as names of family, friends, teacher, pets; places like school, library, a park, swimming, McDonalds; functional words like please, thank you, toilet; and favourite things like a sport, superheroes, games and characters. Ten words are selected from the list and best production is drilled in twice-weekly sessions. At the end of the week, the child produces the 10 words three times. Words produced consistently are removed from the list of 50 words. Words that are inconsistently produced remain on the list, from which the next week's 10 words are randomly chosen. Crosbie, Holm and Dodd (2005) reported that children with inconsistent speech disorder benefit most from Core Vocabulary Therapy in terms of increased consistency and PCC, whereas children with consistent speech disorder make the most change in PCC when error patterns are targeted. These results, for children aged 4;8 to 6;5, provide *support* for the hypothesis that the underlying deficit of inconsistent speech disorder is phonological planning and not a cognitive–linguistic deficit. By improving the child's ability to form or access phonological plans, the phonological system was self-corrected and operated successfully. An inexpensive resource CD that includes an explanatory video of a child and therapist engaged in Core Vocabulary Therapy is available from www.growwords.com.au/.

A psycholinguistic framework

'Comprehensive' and 'British' are the words that immediately occur when thinking of the psycholinguistic framework developed, and developing, in the hands of researchers and clinicians, particularly in the United Kingdom. The psycholinguistic approach (Stackhouse & Wells, 1997; Stackhouse, Wells, Pascoe & Rees, 2002; Stackhouse, Pascoe & Gardner, 2006) provides an inclusive means of investigating, describing and profiling children's speech and literacy difficulties through the application of a speech-processing model and a developmental phase model of speech and literacy. A child's spoken and written language skill strengths are identified and used as a foundation for selecting intervention targets that build on a child's existing abilities. For a child with speech processing and speech production difficulties, these targets are selected not only in relation to speech data but also in relation to linguistic, educational, medical and psychosocial factors, according to individual need, thereby optimising the prospect of across-the-board case management.

Dr. Hilary Gardner is a practising SLT and a senior lecturer and researcher in the Department of Human Communication Sciences at The University of Sheffield in England's north. Her research interests include conversation analysis of therapy interactions and other adult/communication-impaired-child dyads. Her findings have been directly applied to the training of other adults who support SLT work (Gardner, 2006a). Other strands include the nature of SLI, the interactional strategies of children affected by SLI and collaborative practice. Among her publications are two chapters on assessment (Gardner, 1997, 2006b). Dr. Gardner has been closely acquainted with the development of the psycholinguistic framework, and she discusses its practical implementation in A27.

Q27.   Hilary Gardner: Psycholinguistic profiling and intervention

Joffe and Pring (2008) reported that one of their UK clinical practice survey respondents said that she and other therapists she knew were 'terrified' by psycholinguistic models. Can you produce for the reader, who may not have heard of this approach before, what might be called an *unterrifying* Psycholinguistic Approach 101, emphasising its implementation in assessment and management of children with SSDs?

A27.   Hilary Gardner: Finding the psycholinguistic model in everyday practice

The 'psycholinguistic' model of assessment and intervention *can* seem a bit 'terrifying' as a therapist quoted in Joffe and Pring

(2008) suggested. Historically, there have been many variations in box and arrow processing models (Baker, Croot, McLeod & Paul, 2001) and the terminology perhaps made the whole concept seem complex and less intuitive, especially for the experienced clinician with established ways of working. Probably the most popular model for contemporary clinicians is that was first described by Stackhouse and Wells (1997, 2001). It certainly helped me understand what a 'psycholinguistic approach' meant in applied rather than purely theoretical terms. It will hopefully become apparent to those SLPs/SLTs who are fearful of the terminology that they are already being 'psycholinguistic' in their approach through the input and output tasks that they are performing on a daily basis with children with speech difficulties. The great thing is that the model can be applied when working with any type of speech disorder and across all languages.

What is a psycholinguistic model?

If you are interested in a theoretical perspective, then Baker et al. (2001) still stands as an excellent review of theory to practice, across a series of psycholinguistic speech processing models. Speech input and output abilities and deficits are mapped onto a speech chain from ear (input) through to the mouth (output). This can be seen quite literally displayed in Figure A27.1 (Stackhouse & Wells, 1997; Pascoe, Stackhouse & Wells, 2006). Underlying skills such as the ability to discriminate target sounds from other sounds, to imitate nonsense and real words or even to respond appropriately to their own errors are included. As I began to understand the model, it became less threatening: I could map on my own therapy techniques and come to grips with the whole concept.

In psycholinguistic terms a child perceives auditory and visual speech stimuli and then this information is analysed and stored as 'lexical representations' in the brain's word store or 'lexicon' (Stackhouse & Wells, 1997, p. 8). The stored information includes aspects of any word's meaning (semantics), its place in the sentence (grammar) and even written forms. Phonological information includes sound sequence (syllable structure), voice, place and manner of articulation. Information is then retrieved when the child wants to say a word.

When we implement tasks from a psycholinguistic perspective we are focussing on how a therapist can recognise the child's ability to process, store and retrieve lexical knowledge. Sound segments are consonants and vowels, combined according to the pattern of the language in question, in order to produce meaningful word contrasts. In other paradigms these sound segments would be called phones or phonetic realisations (Grunwell, 1997; Ingram, 1989). Stackhouse et al. (2007) emphasise that psycholinguistic profiling is based on the analysis of the child's behaviours throughout a period of intervention and using collected data, not undertaking a lengthy battery of 'tests'. They do however suggest 30 tasks that identify detail of the child's processing including connected speech as well as single words or sounds.

How does the 'psycholinguistic model reveal itself in the everyday work of an SLP/SLT?

Let us consider a child as he or she first comes to see a speech–language clinician. Even as we take the case history we are already attending to the child's psycholinguistic profile. For instance, we ask whether the child can hear well, whether they can distinguish speech in a noisy room or attend to environmental sounds. These are at the first level on the input side, that of peripheral hearing and perception. Also at the first level we may ask if they confuse similar words or have a good memory for new words.

Input processing

Having worked out what speech sound errors and immaturities the child has, we then start work on improving his or her intelligibility. Data from the child's responses to those tasks then contribute to ongoing assessment. Intervention may start with asking the child to listen and sort pictures that represent a range of meaningful word contrasts where saying the target sound makes meaning and saying the sound in error either does not make meaning, or makes an unintended meaning. By doing this, the SLP/SLT moves up the speech chain, increasing the degree of difficulty for the child in psycholinguistic terms. The child may be asked to perceive a target sound in isolation or in a nonsense word, so that he or she does not access his or her lexicon. Real word phonological knowledge, the most difficult level of the input chain, comes last.

Output processing

On the output side it is easier to see how processing difficulty equates to a traditional view of increasing task difficulty (see Raz, A4; Stone-Goldman, A44 and Williams & Stephens, A46). Routinely, the clinician may start by asking the child to say the sound in isolation, and/or in real words, starting with CVs, and progressing to more complex combinations, phrases and sentences, perhaps with the written form. Where a child has a phonological disorder many therapists use syllables or nonsense words as an interim stage in production (Meyer, 2004; Stackhouse, Vance, Pascoe & Wells, 2007). The child will probably find this easier as they can practise new sound combinations without getting muddled with habitual, faulty phonological patterns that are stored in the lexicon. This has nothing to do with an articulation difficulty *per se*. Therefore within a single task a child might imitate a word, without any recourse to stored knowledge, and say it correctly with the target sound in place, e.g., saying *fin* correctly when he or she typically replaces /f/ with [p]. Yet he or she may return to the stored incorrect version *pin*, when asked to produce the same word spontaneously.

The same production might have very different underlying deficits and 'psycholinguistic profiling' seeks to disentangle whether those processing errors lie in input and/or output. Think what it is like when, as an adult, you are about to greet a child's new teacher, Mr. Copperthwaite. His name is on the tip of your tongue and you know how many syllables it has, even some of the vowels and consonants but your initial perception of the name was poor and your memory of the name is fuzzy. So you say something rather approximate such as, 'Hello Mr. Potherway'. There is nothing wrong with your speech muscles or even your motor programming as you can say the necessary sound combinations in a different context. A young child however may not say it correctly because they cannot construct the motor program for the sounds /θw/, so, excusably, they correct you with 'No, it's Mr Copperpaite'!

Recognising children's processing skills 'online'

The child's abilities are revealed by his or her responses during the intervention process itself. It is the consummate skill of an experienced SLP/SLT that they can monitor the child's level of performance at each turn (Gardner, 2004) and this monitoring leads to subtle alterations of the task and targets, even the feedback to the child, based on this 'online' assessment of the child's processing skills. For instance, each time we respond to an error we are asking the child to think about sounds at a particular level of the speech chain, perhaps recognising their habitual error and matching it against the target, for example, the clinician says, 'Did you say *fin* or *pin*? (here, the target production is *fin*). The child cannot just parrot the answer

back but must process the error, *pin* (realising that in his lexical store it means something sharp, not part of a fish) and choose the contrasting form *fin*, finding the appropriate output program. Where a child has real difficulty in articulating a sound then the SLP/SLT helps him or her with instructions as to placement of the articulators, for example, 'That's it, put your teeth on your lip and say [f]'. This is at the lowest level of speech processing, literally at the mouth, with no recourse to the lexical store (until they are asked to produce it spontaneously, from memory). Thus the SLP/SLT has assessed different levels of speech processing simply by doing the tasks in the way they always have done.

I hope I have persuaded any 'scared' clinicians that they should take heart and be confident that they are already using a psycholinguistic approach in any interaction they have with a child with a speech difficulty or disorder. What might be good to develop is targeted assessment of the cognitive processes involved a little more explicitly. These skills are summarised in the Stackhouse and Wells (1997) speech-processing model displayed in Figure A27.1

Input

A. Tasks may simply require the child to discriminate between speech sounds in isolation, for instance pointing to one of two pictures representing two different sounds, for example, /f/ and /p/. As they are not in word or word-like contexts, simple perception or 'bottom up processing', without reference to lexical representations, is the skill being tested.

B. Here the child is asked to discriminate between a series of non-words or listen for rhyming syllables but does not need to access word knowledge (those lexical representations) as such.

D. Moving higher up the processing pathway requires the child to access the lexicon

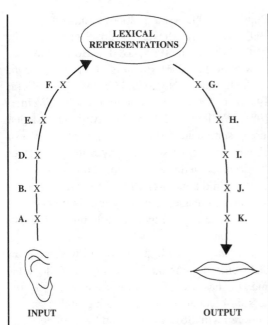

LEXICAL REPRESENTATIONS

F. X   X G.

E. X   X H.

D. X   X I.

B. X   X J.

A. X   X K.

INPUT   OUTPUT

Figure A27.1 Crosses A-K on the simple speech processing model mark levels at which tests cluster. Reproduced by kind permission of Wiley Publishers, from Stackhouse and Wells (1997)

(top down processing). One question is whether the child can discriminate between real spoken words. Does he or she recognise a segmental change, for example, from *pin* to *fin* as producing different meanings? Would he or she point to the same picture or respond at a chance level because no meaningful contrast is established?

E. A child has to detect whether the adult is saying a word correctly and spot any unusual variations as being 'incorrect'. Children with unclear storage of phonological information may respond to differences, for example, *poon* vs. *spoon* vs. *soon*, as if the words were interchangeable.

F. At the highest level children are able to manipulate sound segments in patterns that change the word and the meaning by generating the information required for themselves, for example, sorting pictures according to their phonological similarity, without hearing the words spoken by another person.

Output

G. At this level the child should be able to access accurate motor programs from the lexical store and name pictures spontaneously, without hearing another speaker give a model. He or she may be able to say sounds in nonsense words accurately, but cannot overcome habitual patterns to produce the correct version of a real word when accessing strongly established lexical representations.

H. and I. Here the child can manipulate or play around with sound segments. These levels relate to phonological output skills where the child has some ability to create novel rhymes or omit final consonants from a word he or she has just heard (consonant deletion). The child can imitate and articulate real words accurately, that is, with no motor difficulty without really thinking about the meaning of what they are saying (parroting is a term sometimes used!).

J. Here output tasks involve non-words, building or repeating syllables modelled by another person. Being non-words there is no recourse to the lexical store.

K. Physical or articulatory difficulties that prevent accurate production of the target are at this, the lowest level of processing.

Speech and literacy

As a profession we have also expanded the remit for our work and, as Stackhouse and Pascoe (2010) have stated, an understanding of speech processing also underlies our work in PA and literacy development. The link between oral and written skills further justifies the work of SLPs/SLTs with both pre- and school-age children. In the old days relating speech to literacy (even 'dyslexia') was 'out of bounds', with literacy seen as the educationalist's remit, within the UK system at least. Now speech and literacy are inextricably linked, with the latter more dependent on the former than first realised (see Neilson, A22; Hesketh, A28). SLPs/SLTs should be very confident that through psycholinguistic profiling they are targeting more than 'intelligible speech' and helping them achieve their educational potential. Tasks at the higher end of the speech chain have been added to the speech–language clinician's battery allowing a focus on tasks at the metalinguistic and even metacognitive level, helping the child to perceive and manipulate sound segments. This might sound quite sophisticated but of course refers to 'PA' tasks, the child recognising and creating rhymes, consonant deletions and even recognising jokes based on playing with word structure.

Conclusion

The psycholinguistic approach therefore explicates and enhances 'traditional' ways of working without replacing them. With growing confidence in newly discovered 'psycholinguistic' skills, clinicians may be tempted to read more about how this approach has been applied to intervention across settings. The fourth book in a series on the psycholinguistic approach by Professors Joy Stackhouse and Bill Wells with various colleagues (Stackhouse et al. 2007) offers a CD-ROM of materials for use in clinics and schools. To understand a little more about 'psycholinguistic' therapy in interaction read Gardner (2004, 2006a) and about Bowen and Cupples (1998) *Fixed- up-one routine*, displayed in Figure 9.4.

Phoneme Awareness Therapy

There are many reports in the literature of diverse, evidence-based therapies for SSD in children that incorporate metalinguistic techniques in general, and phonetic awareness and/or phonemic awareness in particular (e.g., Blache, 1982; Bowen &

Cupples, 1999a; Gillon, 2006; Grunwell, 1985b, 1992; Dean & Howell, 1986; Dean, Howell, Waters & Reid, 1995; Dodd, Holm, Crosbie & McIntosh, 2006; Flynn & Lancaster, 1996; Hesketh, Adams, Nightingale & Hall, 2000; Klein, 1996a, b; Moriarty and Gillon, 2006; Weiner, 1981; Williams, 2000a). To varying extents, these approaches specifically target and use *phoneme* awareness in therapy with pre-literate children, sometimes with the aim of improving the child's intelligibility and sometimes with the aim of enhancing literacy acquisition or pre-empting reading and spelling difficulties in at-risk populations.

Dr. Anne Hesketh qualified and worked as an SLT before joining the University of Manchester and now has over 30 years of experience encompassing clinical practice, teaching and research. Children with SSD are the main focus of her clinical work and teaching and her research includes both speech disorder and a broader interest in effective practice in speech and language therapy. In A28, she talks about Phoneme Awareness Therapy.

Q28. Anne Hesketh: Phonemic awareness, phonological representations and speech

You have said that, SLPs/SLTs 'can be confident about the early literacy achievement of most children with isolated speech disorder, but should undertake assessment of phonological awareness to identify those children whose phonological awareness skills after speech intervention continue to be low' (Hesketh, 2004). You have also shown (Hesketh, Dima & Nelson, 2007) that it is possible to stimulate change in at least some PA skills by direct intervention, but have since put more emphasis on the importance of underlying phonological representations (PRs), saying that they play an important role in all three areas of PA, speech and literacy (McNeill & Hesketh, 2010). Can you clarify the distinction between PRs and PA for the reader? How can SLPs/SLTs working in busy clinical settings identify the low PA or PR performers, and when and how should they step in? Can you provide a glimpse of what PA or PR intervention for these preschool children might entail, who should be implementing it and how clinicians can best integrate it into their therapy without compromising speech intelligibility progress or overloading the child?

A28. Anne Hesketh: Phoneme Awareness intervention for children with speech disorder: who, when and how?

Phonological awareness (PA) is an umbrella term for conscious knowledge about the sound structure of words, from syllables to phonemes. Phoneme awareness is a sub-type of PA, restricted to the awareness of individual phonemes within a word. It covers a range of levels of skills, for example, identification of the word onset, segmentation or movement of phonemes. Phonological representations (PRs) are the stored knowledge we have about the phonological form of words we know. If we can look (silently) at an object and know what sound its name begins with, that information has come from our representation of the word.

Development of PRs and Phonological Awareness

Walley, Metsala and Garlock (2003) propose that PRs of children's first words are holistic, underspecified units which only become more detailed as necessary, to distinguish among increasing vocabulary items. There will therefore be a good deal of development at the time of the early vocabulary spurt, but the gradual segmentation of rep-

resentations into smaller units continues into the early school years (McNeill & Hesketh, 2010; Claessen, Heath, Fletcher, Hogben & Leitão, 2009) with a likely boost when children become aware of letter–sound links. Before they are aware of phonemes, children may be using other features, or a concept of global similarity by which to index words (Carroll & Myers, 2011). It is difficult to know the status of a young child's PRs however, because of their limitations in metalinguistic PA: they cannot tell us explicitly what they know about words.

PA development is also gradual. The literature reports that many 4-year-old children have syllable awareness and the majority develop rhyme awareness during their fifth year, however, most children have only limited phoneme awareness before they start to read. Approximately half show some sensitivity to word-initial single consonants by 5 years but this is likely to vary with the exact nature of the task. Very few can deconstruct consonant clusters, or delete, add or move consonants in words at this age (Carroll, Snowling, Hulme & Stevenson, 2003).

Why are phonological representations important?

PRs are important in word learning, speech production and literacy development. We have to extract word-length units of information from the stream of speech and store them in a way that is flexible enough to allow their recognition in different forms (e.g., across accents and speakers), but stable and accurate enough to drive a consistent and recognisable spoken output.

Almost all researchers agree that Phoneme Level PA is important in the early stages of literacy development (Ehri et al., 2001; Hulme et al., 2002). In contrast, explicit PA is not necessary for typical speech development and we know little about the levels of PA necessary to elicit change in children with speech disorder.

What is the status of PA and PRs in children with speech disorder?

There is considerable evidence that children with SSD, as a group, show weakness in both PA (Carroll & Snowling, 2004; Anthony et al., 2011) and PRs (Anthony et al., 2011; Sutherland & Gillon, 2007). Weakness in establishing and accessing PRs may underlie the difficulties shown by children with speech disorder in both PA and early literacy. However, there is no correlation between judging the correctness of a specific word and being able to produce that word correctly, that is, the output form does not directly reflect the underlying representation. Claessen and Leitão (2012) specifically examined children's judgements of their own errors. Typically developing children were able to reject the majority of their own errors; children with specific language impairment (SLI) tended to do worse though they too rejected 50% of errors. This mirrors my clinical experience, where the large majority of children are amused by my production of their errors and quick to judge them as incorrect. However, when children are not able to distinguish correct and incorrect productions, it is a source of concern.

Assessment of PA and PR skills

It is vital to assess both skills, as, within the group of children with speech disorders, there are some whose PA and PR abilities are within normal limits and the prognosis for those children is different. Children with good PA tend to do better in speech intervention (Hesketh, Adams, Nightingale & Hall, 2000) and their early literacy performance matches their typically developing peers (Hesketh, 2004; Rvachew, 2007). For children with speech disorder, the assessment tasks should not require spoken output – otherwise speech errors can prevent valid interpretation of responses.

There exist a number of standardised assessments for phonological awareness. It is important that the standardisation sample is relevant to the specific child and context since different ages of school entry and exposure to literacy across countries can lead to different rates of PA development around 4–6 years. There is a considerable range of ability in PA in young typically developing children, as shown by the wide confidence intervals for standard scores, so it can be hard to know if there is actually a problem. Because speech intervention of whatever kind inherently involves PA and can trigger further PA development (Hesketh et al. 2000), I would be more confident diagnosing a significant PA problem based on the assessment of a five-year-old child at the end of therapy than I would for a four-year-old child prior to intervention.

The assessment of PRs is tricky as they are by nature implicit. Adults and older children can access their PRs to talk about the phonemic make-up of words, and assessment of PRs in older children can be via explicit, 'silent' PA tasks, such as silent deletion of phonemes (Claessen et al., 2010). However, young children do not have the explicit PA ability to think about and report on their implicit PRs and we need tasks that bypass conscious metalinguistic awareness in order to tap the underlying knowledge. The simplest of these is the mispronunciation detection task where a child sees a picture, hears the corresponding word and decides whether it 'sounds right' (Claessen et al., 2009; McNeill & Hesketh, 2010; Rvachew, Nowak & Cloutier, 2004). Aliens and puppets are often the inexperienced speakers who 'sometimes say words a bit wrong' and the task has been successfully utilised in children as young as 3;9.

Should we be targeting PA and PRs in our therapy?

PA is not a useful everyday skill in its own right; the reason for including it must be in the belief that it will help change speech and prevent literacy difficulties. Although there is a lack of strong evidence for the necessity of tackling PA for the purposes of speech change, most clinicians include PA in intervention to some extent. There is no clear answer to the question of when, how and whether to target PA; these decisions must depend on on-going assessment of the individual child's abilities.

There is evidence that working on PA does change PA itself; for example, two studies, Laing and Espeland (2005) and Hesketh, Dima and Nelson (2007), have both demonstrated gains in the PA of pre-school children following intervention. The highest level of skill achieved was isolation of word-initial consonants, that is, the earliest step into phoneme awareness.

The evidence for whether improvement in PA does, in turn, affect speech is mixed. However, Gillon (2000) showed that children aged 5;6–7;4 who received an integrated speech plus PA intervention made more improvement in both PA and early reading than children receiving a speech-focused regime. Gillon (2005) describes similar benefits for children aged 3;0–3;11 on study entry. In both studies, children made good progress in speech change too. The evidence for literacy is clearer (Ehri et al., 2001; Hulme, Bowyer-Crane, Carroll, Duff & Snowling, 2012), though neither of these references relate to speech and language therapy.

There is little research yet into therapy directed at underlying PRs. Rvachew et al. (2004) evaluated a training program involving mispronunciation detection alongside letter–sound and explicit PA (onset or rime matching) tasks. Children (41–59 months) in the experimental group made more progress in perception and in speech accuracy than the control group; however, more research specifically into PR-directed therapy is required.

What should PA/PR intervention be and who should be doing it?

My intervention principle, based on clinical experience and published research evidence, is to incorporate PA- and PR-type activities in support of speech change, using stimuli relevant to the child's speech targets, rather than seeing PA skills as a target in their own right. A typical intervention session will involve the child listening to, thinking about and producing sounds in words: but the balance between these three elements varies enormously across children and across sessions (Hesketh, 2010).

For PRs, where a child is having difficulty making mispronunciation decisions about their own errors (spoken by the therapist), I would regard the establishment of clearer representations as an essential part of therapy. Where PRs are adequate for a child easily to reject their own error, my focus will move to increasing self-monitoring and accuracy of production. For phonological awareness I start with a general expectation that PA work in my speech intervention will be directed at a small unit level (i.e., awareness of phonemes), though for many children this may be limited to awareness of the initial or final phoneme of a word. PA and speech work will be linked to graphemes or supported by sound symbol pictures as necessary, and all activities will focus on the child's specific current speech targets.

SLPs/SLTs should be responsible for planning the integration of PR and PA work into speech intervention, using the targets and contrasts relevant to the specific child. In order for me to understand the child's ability and gauge his or her needs, I find it necessary to implement the intervention myself; however, other people can be implementing it as well. Both parents and teaching support assistants are valuable allies in therapy, though great care must be taken to explain tasks clearly.

I have seen two children in my clinical practice recently with whom I have taken different approaches. Tim is just 5, a bright boy with a strong interest in learning to write. His current speech targets are /s/, /ʃ/ /tʃ/, all of which he replaces with /d/. Tim can easily categorise spoken words by their initial sounds and identify incorrect productions of words (using his own error), which he thinks sound very funny. PA and PR tasks are used for brief, fun reminders and feedback in therapy sessions which focus predominantly on the much harder task (for Tim) of producing the target sounds in words. His good letter knowledge is used to reinforce the need for a particular sound in a particular word. In contrast, Wesley (5;6) shows atypical speech with many consonant and vowel errors. His word attempts are also highly variable; he is not consistent at mispronunciation detection and he is finding it very difficult to grasp letter–sound links. Wesley has a broad, underlying phonological deficit that is affecting his ability to form accurate, stable phonological representations (for either speech recognition or production), to develop conscious phonological awareness of elements within words or to decode and encode written words. I liaise closely with his teaching support assistant to work on a very small vocabulary each week, all words beginning with the same letter/sound and taken from his current school spelling or reading targets. Sessions involve many opportunities to make mispronunciation decisions about the target words and require Wesley's best possible production of a word on all occasions. Where he varies from this, Wesley listens to me modelling both the correct version and the immediately preceding error, indicates which is best and imitates it after me to re-establish an acceptable production. Frequent reference is made to the word's written form.

How to integrate PA into speech work without compromising speech progress

Integration is the key word here. By embedding PA and PR work into sessions, which also include speech production practice, and by tailoring the tasks to highlight the concurrent speech targets, there should be no negative effect on speech progress. Gillon has successfully incorporated PA work (and has improved children's PA skills) without detriment to speech progress in two studies (Gillon, 2000, 2005), the latter with preschool children.

Summary

In summary, my approach is to integrate both PA and PRs into therapy in order to support speech change and literacy progress, according to the needs of the child. Phonological awareness and phonological representations have a close and reciprocal relationship with early literacy development, and the integration of speech work with literacy is an important element in the management of children with speech disorder as they enter school.

Vowel Therapy

Detailed case studies of child speech intervention are a comparatively rare find, and studies of vowel intervention even scarcer. It is delightful therefore, to encounter two case studies by Speake, Stackhouse and Pascoe (2012). They reported effective vowel targeted intervention (VTI), conducted over 6 months with a 6-week holiday break, involving intense production practice, for two quite different 10 year olds with severe and persisting speech difficulties. Speak et al. found that the principles that govern working on vowels or consonants are alike, in that 'production work is aided by discrimination and lexical work, and incorporating meta-skills are essential for progress' (citing Pascoe et al.,

2006). Cautioning that their findings could not be generalized to diverse populations of children with SSD, they said, 'Although ... vowels are established by the age of three in typically developing children, VTI is rarely carried out with young children who have developmental speech difficulties with no obvious cause such as hearing loss or cleft palate. If, as this study indicates, successful treatment of vowels can contribute towards intelligibility, there may be a case for suggesting that VTI could be incorporated earlier in intervention programmes for children with significant speech difficulties who present with atypical vowels' (p. 293). Fiona Gibbon has researched vowel disorders and intervention for many years and addresses these topics in A29.

Dr. Fiona E. Gibbon is a Professor and Head of Speech and Hearing Sciences at University College Cork, Ireland. Her research and clinical interests include the use of instrumentation to diagnose and treat speech disorders in children. She has published over 70 papers in professional/scientific journals and book chapters and has been awarded numerous research council and charity-funded grants. This research was awarded the Queen's Anniversary Prize for excellence in 2002. She is a Fellow of the Royal College of Speech and Language Therapists.

Q29. Fiona Gibbon: Vowel assessment and remediation

There is a commonly held SLP/SLT view that if you, 'work on the consonants, the vowels will take care of themselves'! You touched on this point in 2003 when you made an invited contribution to the 'Ask the Expert' column for the *Apraxia-Kids* Monthly Newsletter on the topic of vowel production (and possibly vowel perception) difficulties experienced by children with CAS. You wrote, 'At the moment there is a lack of research evidence to guide the SLP about the most efficacious therapy approach for vowel errors in CAS.' Can you expand on this, please? What is the current research

suggesting that clinicians do in terms of vowel assessment and intervention? Should we be giving consonants priority over vowels? Would you tackle vowel assessment and intervention differently for a child with CAS than you would with a highly unintelligible child of the same age with a phonological disorder?

A29. Fiona Gibbon: Vowel errors in children with speech disorders

It is undoubtedly true that SLPs/SLTs who work in clinical contexts tend to neglect vowels and focus primarily on identifying and remediating consonant errors in children's speech. However, as we will see in the sections that follow, it may be unwise to disregard vowels in the belief that errors affecting vowels will necessarily 'look after themselves'. Indeed, expert opinion suggests that the opposite is true, at least for children with CAS. Based on their extensive clinical experience, Hall, Jordan and Robin (1993) stated that 'some children self-correct vowel errors, but not many children ... have this experience' (p. 160).

The relative lack of attention to vowels is surprising when one considers what is now known about these types of errors. For example, children with CAS and children with moderate and severe phonological disorder (Flipsen Jr., A11) frequently experience difficulties producing vowels. Studies have shown that at least some vowel errors may occur in as many as 50% of children with these diagnoses (Eisenson & Ogilvie, 1963; Pollock, 2013). Vowel errors are also considered of diagnostic importance, with these errors posited as a potential diagnostic marker for CAS (Davis, Jakielski & Marquardt, 1998). Difficulties with vowels are additionally significant because they can have a detrimental impact on speech intelligibility (Stoel-Gammon & Pollock, 2008) and they often have serious consequences for consonant production, syllable structure and prosody. For these reasons, it is important that SLPs/SLTs are familiar with the types of vowel difficulties that occur in children's speech and are aware of different approaches to their remediation.

So why do clinicians and indeed researchers often ignore vowels? A combination of factors may explain this situation. Even skilled listeners, such as SLPs/SLTs, find vowel errors more difficult to detect through perceptual analysis compared to consonant errors. As a result, vowels are less reliably transcribed than consonants (Stoel-Gammon, 1990). Another important factor is that the normal dialectal differences that exist in vowel systems may make vowel errors difficult to identify perceptually. As a result, vowel errors can remain undetected in a transcription-based speech analysis. As well, more is known about patterns of abnormalities affecting the consonant system compared to the vowel system and consequently most standard assessment procedures are devised primarily to identify abnormal patterns of consonant production. Many assessment procedures therefore do not allow for a full range of vowels to be elicited, so vowel errors are not always recorded in routine clinical evaluations. Finally, even when vowel errors are identified as occurring in a child's speech, there remains little evidence about effective therapy approaches specifically for these types of difficulties (Gibbon, 2013). As Hall, Jordan and Robin (1993) stated, 'much has yet to be learned about strategies and techniques for vowel remediation' (p. 160).

Diagnosis and therapy for vowel errors

Despite the difficulties in identifying vowels outlined above, real progress has been made over the past 20 years in our understanding of normal and abnormal vowel systems in children's speech (see Jacks, Marquardt & Davis, 2013; Stoel-Gammon & Pollock, 2008; Ball & Gibbon, 2013). In relation to vowel errors, studies show that children can have complete or near complete vowel inventories, at least for nonrhotic monophthongs (e.g., Gibbon, Shockey & Reid, 1992). Furthermore, studies show that some vowels are more likely to be produced as errors than others, with diphthongs (e.g., /aɪ/, /ɔɪ/), rhotic vowels (e.g., /ɪɚ/, /ɝ/) and the midfront vowels /e/ and /a/ being particularly problematic. A number of recurring patterns of vowel difficulties, usually described in terms of phonological processes (e.g., lowering/raising, fronting/backing, diphthong reduction) have been documented by Reynolds (1990), Pollock and Hall (1991), Pollock (2013) and Bates, Watson and Scobbie (2013). It is now recognised that articulatory difficulties in positioning and sequencing of articulators, particularly the tongue and lips, affect vowel quality and accuracy. Timing difficulties also affect vowels, so that in some cases they may be excessively long. Vowels may also be distorted, for example partially voiced due to difficulties controlling vocal-fold vibration or with excessive nasality due to difficulties controlling velopharyngeal closure. These co-ordination difficulties are core features of CAS (Campbell, 2003; Hall et al. 1993; Rosenbek & Wertz, 1972) and often cause difficulties affecting vowels.

Unfortunately, advances in our knowledge about abnormal vowel systems are not mirrored in increased knowledge about therapy for these types of errors. Our understanding about therapy for abnormal vowels comes primarily from studies that focus on the remediation of abnormal consonants. SLPs/SLTs can apply to vowel intervention the same underlying principles of therapy approaches that were developed for remediating consonants. There is a remarkably wide selection of approaches available, however. Williams, McLeod and McCauley (2010) and Gibbon (2013) have described many therapy approaches that are currently used in clinical contexts. As well as having a wide choice of approaches, the evidence base for treating abnormal consonant systems in children with phonological disorder is strong and there is now a substantial literature demonstrating beneficial effects of phonological therapy (e.g., Gierut, 1998; Law, Garrett & Nye, 2003, 2004; Almost & Rosenbaum, 1998; Williams et al. 2010).

Therapy for vowels that has been adapted from an approach intended for consonants may prove useful but may also present with additional difficulties. Any therapy approach that requires a child to focus on his or her own articulatory activity is more difficult with vowels than it is with consonants. The high degree of vocal tract constriction involved in consonant production generally results in a high level of tactile feedback, which enhances speakers' awareness of articulatory placement. With the exception of close vowels, such as /i/ (as in *heat*) and /ɪ/ (as in *hit*), this tactile feedback is greatly decreased during vowel production. Furthermore, as Stoel-Gammon and Pollock (2008) point out, place of articulation for consonants tends to be discrete (e.g., labial, alveolar), as opposed to place features for vowels, which are continuous in terms of tongue height or advancement. As Hall et al. (1993) stated, these difficulties mean that for some SLPs/SLTs 'vowel therapy is elusive, frustrating, and often appears to be avoided' (p. 161).

Indirect versus direct focus on intervention targets

Despite good evidence that therapy is beneficial for abnormal consonant systems, it is not known whether therapy that focuses on improving the consonant system has an indirect, but equally beneficial, effect of improving the vowel system. Some support for the view that targeting consonants has an indirect and beneficial impact on vowel production comes from a study by Robb, Bleile and Yee (1999). They adopted an indirect approach to treating vowels in a 4-year-old girl with a phonological disorder that affected both consonants and vowels. Consonants were selected as targets in therapy and no emphasis was placed on accurate vowel production during the course of intervention. By the end of her therapy program, however, the size of her vowel inventory and overall vowel accuracy had improved. Robb et al. (1999) commented that although therapy did not focus on vowel accuracy, it was nevertheless possible that the activities undertaken in therapy facilitated improvements in both consonant and vowel production.

Early researchers into CAS recommended that vowels should be selected for direct remedial efforts because vowel errors have a detrimental effect on speech intelligibility (Chappell, 1973; Yoss & Darley, 1974). A handful of more recently published studies have reported therapy that directly focused on vowel error patterns in children with phonological disorder (for a review see Gibbon & Mackenzie Beck, 2002). The tentative conclusion that emerges is that direct therapy for vowels can have a positive outcome in some cases. The studies are limited, however, to reporting only small numbers of cases, so it is not possible to generalise the findings. Another limitation of these studies is that some did not report adequate baseline data, making it difficult to know whether the progress reported was a result of therapy or due to some other factor, such as spontaneous development.

Clinical implications

Turning now to the implications of current research, the finding that children with moderate to severe phonological disorders or CAS have a high risk of abnormal vowel systems means that it is important to screen all such children for vowel errors. There are various procedures that SLPs/SLTs can use for this purpose (e.g., the Quick Vowel Screener; Bowen, 2010b). Clinical assessment of vowels in CAS is usually based on phonetically transcribed speech samples, which SLPs/SLTs analyse and interpret vowel data alongside other routine clinical examinations. There are now readily available resources that SLPs/SLTs can use to assist in describing, transcribing and classifying normal and disordered vowel systems (Howard & Heselwood, 2013; Bates et al., 2013; Pollock, 2013; Watts, 2004). Speech samples usually include spontaneous and imitated speech consisting of single words/phrases of increasing phonetic complexity. Analysis of speech samples may involve identifying a child's vowel inventory, which in CAS may be restricted, with certain 'difficult to produce' vowels, such as diphthongs and rhotic vowels, absent.

An important component of an assessment of vowel systems is identification of error patterns of vowel substitutions, distortions and phonological processes. SLPs/SLTs are very familiar with phonological process analysis when applied to children's consonant systems. It is possible to apply this type of linguistic description to show how vowel errors are systematic and rule-governed, not separate, unrelated phenomena. Furthermore, it can be useful to conduct a vowel analysis in terms of vowel phoneme collapses where several vowels are collapsed to one (Gibbon, Shockey & Reid, 1992). Another feature of vowel systems that is relevant to assess is the nature and degree of variability in production, noting that in children with CAS, there is often a high degree of token-to-token variability. A final area to assess is the effect of surrounding consonants on vowel accuracy (Bates et al., 2013). Vowels may be produced correctly in some words, but not others, because the vowels are 'conditioned' by the surrounding consonants. The most frequently reported context-conditioned

error pattern in typically developing infants is the co-occurrence of alveolar stops /t/, /d/ and high front vowels, such as /i/, /ɪ/ and the co-occurrence of velar stops /k/, /g/ with high back vowels such as /u/ (Davis & MacNeilage, 1990). Bates et al. (2013) underline the importance of identifying such context-conditioned error patterns in children with speech disorders in order to focus therapy in the most effective way. For instance, accurate identification of such contexts will avoid wasting therapy time on practising targets in contexts that are unproblematic for the child. Bates et al. (2013) provide a comprehensive description of consonant–vowel interactions and how these can be assessed in clinical practice. These analyses will allow the SLP/SLT to make a diagnostic statement about a child's vowel production and to formulate goals of therapy in relation to any vowel difficulties highlighted during assessment.

In Gibbon (2013) I discuss general principles of Vowel Therapy and a range of therapy approaches that are of potential, although as yet unproven, value for increasing vowel production accuracy. In my view, a prerequisite for effective treatment is that clinicians should have good phonetic transcription skills to analyse vowels. SLP/SLPs also need to formulate therapy goals in light of a clear description of the adult target vowel system, that is, if and how the target system differs from standard systems (see Wells, 1982a, b, c, for detailed descriptions of how English vowels vary across the world). SLPs/SLTs should also consider children's overall speech and language processing skills (Stackhouse & Wells, 1997), as well as relevant information gathered as part of routine clinical assessment (see Gardner, A27). This profile will suggest the aspect or aspects of speech processing to focus on intervention and which approach is most likely to evoke improved speech intelligibility. Some children have demonstrable auditory perceptual deficits, for instance, whereas others have cognitive/linguistic deficits associated with the phonological structure of the language. A third possibility is that motoric/articulatory deficits, including dysarthria, affect the movements and co-ordination necessary for normal speech production. Gibbon (2013) describes a variety of approaches that focus on vowel errors in each category. In many cases, different approaches are not mutually exclusive, and the eclectic SLP/SLT will often select a combination of theoretically grounded multisensory techniques that will meet each child's specific needs.

Due to the lack of research evidence to guide the SLP/SLT about the most efficacious therapy approach for vowel errors, SLPs/SLTs need to select therapy techniques based on the most complementary matching between a child's specific speech difficulties and the strategies employed in a particular approach. SLPs/SLTs own vowel production skills are vital because they may need to model a full range of vowel qualities during therapy activities. Reid (2003) has developed a framework based on phonetic features of vowels, which also incorporates links to written vowels. This may be particularly useful for improving children's phonological awareness of vowels, for literacy teaching, as well as for targeting spoken vowel production difficulties. The framework has been specifically devised for the vowels of Scottish English, but it may be adapted for other varieties of English.

Implications for service delivery

The smorgasbord of intervention options described in this chapter carries with it serious implications for 'common', 'best' and evidence-based practice, the theme of the next chapter. In it, 11 contributors from around the world (Australia, Canada, Germany, New Zealand, the United Kingdom, the United States), reflect on pertinent issues in the transitions between theory and therapy, and research and ethical practice.

Note

1. This section on the CPPA was written in November 2013 with invaluable editorial input from Barbara Hodson.

References

Adams, M. J., Treiman, R., & Pressley, M. (1998). Reading, writing and literacy. In: I. Sigel, & A. Renninger (Eds.), *Handbook of child psychology, Volume 4: Child psychology in practice*. New York: Wiley.

Almost, D., & Rosenbaum, P. (1998). Effectiveness of speech intervention for phonological disorders: A randomized control trial. *Developmental Medicine and Child Neurology, 40*(5), 319–325.

Anthony, A., Bogle, D., Ingram, T. T. S., & McIsaac, M. W. (1971). *Edinburgh articulation test*. Edinburgh: Churchill Livingstone.

Anthony, J. L., Aghara, R. G., Dunkelberger, M. J., Anthony, T. I., Williams, J. M., & Zhang, Z. (2011). What factors place children with speech sound disorders at risk for reading problems? *American Journal of Speech-Language Pathology, 20*(2), 146–160.

ASHA (2004). *Auditory Integration Training* [Technical Report]. Retrieved 15 January 2014 from www.asha.org/policy

Bain, B. (1994). A framework for dynamic assessment in phonology: Stimulability revisited. *Clinics in Communication Disorders, 4*(1), 12–22.

Baker, E., Croot, K., McLeod, S., & Paul, R. (2001). Tutorial paper: Psycholinguistic models of speech development and their application to clinical practice. *Journal of Speech, Language, and Hearing Research, 44*, 685–702.

Baldwin, D. A., & Markham, E. M. (1989). Establishing word-object relations: A first step. *Child Development, 60*, 381–398.

Ball, M. J., & Gibbon, F. E. (Eds.) (2013). *Handbook of vowels and vowel disorders*. Psychology Press: Hove.

Bates, S. A. R., Watson, J. M. M., & Scobbie, J. M. (2013). Context-conditioned error patterns in disordered systems. In: M. J. Ball, & F. E. Gibbon (Eds), *Handbook of vowels and vowel disorders*, (pp. 288–325). Psychology Press: Hove.

Bernhardt, B., & Stemberger, J. P. (2000). *Workbook in nonlinear phonology for clinical application*. Austin, TX: Pro-Ed.

Blache, S. E. (1982). Minimal word pairs and distinctive feature training. In: M. Crary (Ed.), *Phonological intervention: Concepts and procedures*. San Diego, CA: College-Hill Press Inc.

Bowen, C. (2010a). Parents and children together (PACT) intervention for children with speech sound disorders. In: A. L. Williams, S. McLeod, & R. J. McCauley (Eds.), *Interventions for speech sound disorders in children* (pp. 407–426). Baltimore, MD: Paul H. Brookes Publishing Co.

Bowen, C. (2010b). *Child Speech Assessment Resources*. Retrieved 15 January 2014 from http://www.speech-language-therapy.com/index.php?Itemid=117

Bowen, C., & Cupples, L. (1998). A tested phonological therapy in practice. *Child Language Teaching and Therapy*, *14*(1), 29–50.

Bowen, C., & Cupples, L. (1999a). Parents and children together (PACT): A collaborative approach to phonological therapy. *International Journal of Language and Communication Disorders*, *34*(1), 35–55.

Bowen, C., & Cupples, L. (1999b). A phonological therapy in depth: a reply to commentaries. *International Journal of Language and Communication Disorders*, *34*(1), 65–83.

Bowen, C., & Rippon, H. (2013). *Consonant clusters: Alliterative stories and activities for phonological intervention*. Keighley: Black Sheep Press.

Broomfield, J., & Dodd, B. (2004). The nature of referred subtypes of primary speech disability. *Child Language Teaching and Therapy*, *20*, 135–151.

Camarata, S. M. (2010). Naturalistic intervention for speech intelligibility and speech accuracy. In: A. L. Williams, S. McLeod, & R. J. McCauley (Eds), *Interventions for speech sound disorders in children* (pp. 381–405). Baltimore, MD: Paul H. Brookes Publishing Co.

Campbell, T. F. (2003). Childhood apraxia of speech: Clinical symptoms and speech characteristics. In: L. D Shriberg, & T. F. Campbell (Eds.), *Proceedings of the 2002 childhood apraxia of speech research symposium* (pp. 37–47). Carlsbad, CA: Hendrix Foundation.

Carroll, J. M., & Myers, J. M. (2011). Spoken word classification in children and adults. *Journal of Speech Language and Hearing Research*, *54*(1), 127–147.

Carroll, J. M., & Snowling, M. J. (2004). Language and phonological skills in children at high risk of reading difficulties. *Journal of Child Psychology and Psychiatry*, *45*(3), 631–640.

Carroll, J. M., Snowling, M. J., Hulme, C., & Stevenson, J. (2003). The development of phonological awareness in preschool children. *Developmental Psychology*, *39*, 913–923.

Carter, E. T., & Buck, M. W. (1958). Prognostic testing for functional articulation disorders among children in the first grade. *Journal of Speech and Hearing Disorders*, *23*, 124–133.

Chappell, G. E. (1973). Childhood verbal apraxia and its treatment. *Journal of Speech and Hearing Disorders*, *38*, 362–368.

Claessen, M., Heath, S., Fletcher, J., Hogben, J., & Leitão, S. (2009). Quality of phonological representations: a window into the lexicon? *International Journal of Language & Communication Disorders*, *44*(2), 121–144.

Claessen, M., & Leitão, S. (2012). The relationship between stored phonological representations and speech output. *International Journal of Speech-Language Pathology*, *14*, 226–234.

Claessen, M., Leitão, S., & Barrett, N. (2010). Investigating children's ability to reflect on stored phonological representations: The Silent Deletion of Phonemes Task. *International Journal of Language & Communication Disorders*, *45*(4), 411–423.

Cohen, J. H., & Diehl, C. F. (1963). Relation of speech sound discrimination ability to articulation-type speech defects. *Journal of Speech and Hearing Disorders*, *28*, 187–190.

Crosbie, S., Holm, A., & Dodd, B. (2005). Intervention for children with severe speech disorder: A comparison of two approaches. *International Journal of Language and Communication Disorders*, *40*, 467–491.

Crosbie, S., Pine, C., Holm, A., & Dodd, B. (2006). Treating Jarrod: A core vocabulary approach. *Advances in Speech Language Pathology*, *8*(3), 316–321.

Davis, B., Jakielski, K., & Marquardt, T. (1998). Developmental apraxia of speech: Determiners of differential diagnosis. *Clinical Linguistics and Phonetics*, *12*(1), 25–45.

Davis, B. L., & MacNeilage, P. F. (1990). The acquisition of vowels: A case study. *Journal of Speech and Hearing Research*, *33*, 16–27.

Dean, E., & Howell, J. (1986). Developing linguistic awareness: A theoretically based approach to phonological disorders. *British Journal of Disorders of Communication*, *21*, 223–238.

Dean, E., Howell, J., Hill, A., & Waters, D. (1990). *Metaphon resource pack*. Windsor: NFER Nelson.

Dean, E. C., Howell, J., Waters, D., & Reid, J. (1995). *Metaphon*: A metalinguistic approach to the treatment of phonological disorder in children. *Clinical Linguistics and Phonetics*, *9*, 1–19.

Dodd, B. (2005). *Differential diagnosis and treatment of children with speech disorder* (2nd ed.). London: Whurr Publishers.

Dodd, B., Crosbie, S., Zhu, H., Holm, A., & Ozanne, A. (2002). *Diagnostic evaluation of articulation and phonology (DEAP)*. London: Psychological Corporation.

Dodd, B., Holm, A., Crosbie, S., & McIntosh, B. (2006). A core vocabulary approach for management of inconsistent speech disorder. *Advances in Speech-Language Pathology*, *8*(3), 220–230.

Edwards, J., Fox, R. A., & Rogers, C. L. (2002). Final consonant discrimination in children: Effects of phonological disorder, vocabulary size, and articulatory accuracy. *Journal of Speech, Language, and Hearing Research*, *45*, 231–242.

Edwards, M. L. (1983).Selection criteria for developing therapy goals. *Journal of Childhood Communication Disorders*, *7*, 36–45.

Ehri, L. C., Nunes, S. R., Willows, D. M., Schuster, B. V., Yaghoub-Zadeh, Z., & Shanahan, T. (2001). Phonemic awareness instruction helps children learn to read: Evidence from the National Reading Panel's meta-analysis. *Reading Research Quarterly*, *36*(3), 250–287.

Eisenson, J., & Ogilvie, M. (1963). *Speech correction in the schools*. New York: Macmillan.

Elbert, M., & Gierut, J. (1986). *Handbook of clinical phonology: Approaches to assessment and treatment*. San Diego, CA: College-Hill Press.

Ellis Weismer, S., & Robertson, S. (2006). Focused stimulation. In: R. J. McCauley, & M. E. Fey (Eds.), *Treatment of language disorders in children* (pp. 175–202). Baltimore, MD: Paul H. Brookes Publishing Co.

Fazio, B. B. (1997). Learning a new poem: Memory for connected speech and phonological awareness in low-income children with and without specific language impairment. *Journal of Speech, Language, and Hearing Research*, *40*, 1285–1297.

Fey, M. E. (1992). Phonological assessment and treatment. Articulation and phonology: An introduction. *Language Speech and Hearing Services in Schools*, *23*, 224.

Fey, M. E., & Stalker, C. (1986). A hypothesis testing approach to treatment of a child with an idiosyncratic (morpho)phonological system. *Journal of Speech and Hearing Disorders*, *41*, 324–336.

Flynn, L., & Lancaster, G. (1996). *Children's phonology sourcebook*. Oxford: Winslow Press.

Gardner, H. (1997). Assessment of developmental language disorders. In: C. Adams, M. Edwards, & B. Byers Brown (Eds.), *Developmental disorders of language* (2nd ed., pp. 135–160). London: Whurr Publishers.

Gardner, H. (2004). Doing being the therapist: A comparison of mothers and SLT therapists doing phonology therapy tasks. In: K. Richards, & P. Seedhouse (Eds.), *Applying conversation analysis*. Basingstoke: Palgrave Macmillan.

Gardner, H. (2006a). Training others in the art of therapy for speech sound disorders: An interactional approach. *Child Language Teaching and Therapy*, *22*(1), 27–46.

Gardner, H. (2006b). Assessing speech and language skills in the school-age child. In: Snowling, M.J. & Stackhouse, R. (Eds.), *Dyslexia, speech and language : A practitioners' handbook* (pp. 74–97). Chichester: Wiley.

Gibbon, F. (2013). Therapy for abnormal vowels in children with speech disorders. In: M. J. Ball, & F. E. Gibbon (Eds.), *Handbook of vowels and vowel disorders* (pp. 429–446). Hove: Psychology Press.

Gibbon, F. E., & Mackenzie Beck, J. (2002). Therapy for abnormal vowels in children with phonological impairment. In: M. J. Ball, & F. E. Gibbon (Eds.), *Vowel disorders* (pp. 217–248). Butterworth-Heinemann.

Gibbon F., Shockey, L., & Reid, J. (1992). Description and treatment of abnormal vowels in a phonologically disordered child. *Child Language Teaching and Therapy*, *8*, 30–59.

Gierut, J. (1989). Maximal opposition approach to phonological treatment. *Journal of Speech and Hearing Disorders*, *54*, 9–19.

Gierut, J. A. (1992). The conditions and course of clinically induced phonological change. *Journal of Speech and Hearing Research*, *35*, 1049–1063.

Gierut, J. A. (1998). Treatment efficacy: Functional phonological disorders in children. *Journal of Speech, Language and Hearing Research*, *41*, S85–S100.

Gierut, J. (2007). Phonological complexity and language learnability. *American Journal of Speech-Language Pathology*, *16*(1), 6–17.

Gillon, G. T. (2000). The efficacy of phonological awareness intervention for children with spoken language impairment, *Language, Speech, and Hearing Services in Schools*, *31*(2), 126–141.

Gillon, G. T. (2005). Facilitating phoneme awareness development in 3- and 4-year-old children with speech impairment. *Language Speech and Hearing Services in Schools*, *36*, 308–324.

Gillon, G. T. (2006). Phonological awareness: A preventative framework for preschool children with spoken language impairment. In: R. McCauley, & M. Fey (Eds), *Treatment of language disorders in children: Conventional and controversial approaches* (279–307). Baltimore, MD: Paul H. Brookes Publishing Co.

Girolametto, L., & Weitzman, E. (2006). It takes two to talk – The Hanen program for parents – Early language intervention through caregiver training. In: R. McCauley, & M. Fey (Eds.), *Treatment of language disorders in children* (pp. 77–104). Baltimore, MD: Paul H. Brookes Publishing Co.

Glaspey, A. M., & Stoel-Gammon, C. (2005). Dynamic assessment in phonological disorders: The scaffolding scale of stimulability. *Topics in Language Disorders: Clinical Perspectives on Speech Sound Disorders*, *25*(3), 220–230.

Glaspey, A. M., & Stoel-Gammon, C. (2007). A dynamic approach to phonological assessment. *International Journal of Speech-Language Pathology*, *9*, 286–296.

Goldman, R., & Fristoe, M. (2000). *Goldman-Fristoe test of articulation* (2nd ed.). Circle Pines, MN: American Guidance Service.

Grunwell, P. (1975). The phonological analysis of articulation disorders. *British Journal of Disorders of Communication*, *10*, 31–42.

Grunwell, P. (1985a). *Phonological assessment of child speech (PACS)*. Windsor: NFER-Nelson.

Grunwell, P. (1985b). Developing phonological skills. *Child Language Teaching and Therapy*, *1*, 65–72.

Grunwell, P. (1989). Developmental phonological disorders and normal speech development: A review and illustration. *Child Language Teaching and Therapy*, *5*, 304–319.

Grunwell, P. (1992). Process of phonological change in developmental speech disorders. *Clinical Linguistics and Phonetics*, *6*, 101–122.

Grunwell, P. (1997). Developmental phonological disability: Order in disorder. In: B. W. Hodson, & M. L. Edwards (Eds.), *Perspectives in applied phonology*. Gaithersburg, MD: Aspen Publications.

Hall, P. K., Jordan, L. S., & Robin, D. A. (1993). *Developmental apraxia of speech: Theory and clinical practice*. Austin, Texas: Pro-Ed.

Hesketh, A. (2004). Early literacy achievement of children with a history of speech problems. *International Journal of Language and Communication Disorders*, *39*, 453–468.

Hesketh, A. (2010). Metaphonological intervention. In: A. L. Williams, S. McLeod, & R. J. McCauley (Eds.), *Interventions for speech sound disorders in children* (pp. 247–274). Baltimore, MD: Paul H. Brookes Publishing Co.

Hesketh, A., Adams, C., Nightingale, C., & Hall, R. (2000). Phonological awareness therapy and articulatory training approaches for children with phonological disorders: A comparative outcome study. *International Journal of Language and Communication Disorders*, *35*, 337–354.

Hesketh, A., Dima, E., & Nelson, V. (2007). Teaching phoneme awareness to pre-literate children with speech disorder: A randomized controlled trial. *International Journal of Language and Communication Disorders*, *42*(3), 251–271.

Hodson, B. (2007, 2010). *Evaluating and enhancing children's phonological systems: Research and theory to practice*. Wichita, KS: PhonoComp Publishers.

Hodson, B. W., & Paden, E. P. (1983). *Targeting intelligible speech: A phonological approach to remediation*. San Diego, CA: College-Hill Press.

Hodson, B. W., & Paden, E. P. (1991). *Targeting intelligible speech: A phonological approach to remediation* (2nd ed.). Austin, TX: Pro-Ed.

Hoffman, P. R. (1993). A whole-language treatment perspective for phonological disorder. *Seminars in Speech and Language*, *14*, 142–151.

Hoffman, P. R., Daniloff, R. G., Bengoa, D., & Schuckers, G. (1985). Misarticulating and normally articulating children's identification and discrimination of synthetic [r] and [w]. *Journal of Speech and Hearing Disorders*, *50*, 46–53.

Hoffman, P. R., & Norris, J. A. (2010). Whole language (dynamical systems) phonological intervention. In: A. L. Williams, S. McLeod, & R. J. McCauley (Eds.), *Interventions for speech sound disorders* (pp. 347–382). Baltimore, MD: Paul H. Brookes Publishing Co.

Hoffman, P. R., Stager, S., & Daniloff, R. G. (1983). Perception and production of misarticulated /r. *Journal of Speech and Hearing Disorders*, *48*(2), 210–215.

Howard, S., & Heselwood, B. (2013). The contribution of phonetics to the study of vowel development and disorders. In: M. J. Ball, & F. E. Gibbon (Eds.),

Handbook of vowels and vowel disorders (pp. 61–112). Hove: Psychology Press.

Hulme, C., Bowyer-Crane, C., Carroll, J. M., Duff, F. J., & Snowling, M. J. (2012). The causal role of phoneme awareness and letter-sound knowledge in learning to read: Combining intervention studies with mediation analyses. *Psychological Science, 23*(6), 572–577.

Hulme, C., Hatcher, P. J., Nation, K., Brown, A., Adams, J., & Stuart, G. (2002). Phoneme awareness is a better predictor of early reading skill than onset-rime awareness. *Journal of Experimental Child Psychology, 82*, 2–28.

Ingram, D. (1981). *Procedures for the phonological analysis of children's language*. Baltimore, MD: University Park Press.

Ingram, D. (1989). *Phonological disability in children* (2nd ed.). London: Cole & Whurr Publishers.

Jacks, A., Marquardt, T. P., & Davis, B. (2013). Vowel production in childhood and acquired apraxia of speech. In: M. J. Ball, & F. E. Gibbon (Eds.), *Handbook of vowels and vowel disorders*, (pp. 326–346). Hove: Psychology Press.

Jamieson, D. G., & Rvachew, S. (1992). Remediation of speech production errors with sound identification training. *Journal of Speech-Language Pathology and Audiology, 16*, 201–210.

Joffe, V. L., & Pring, T. (2008). Children with phonological problems: A survey of clinical practice. *International Journal of Language and Communication Disorders, 43*(2), 154–164.

Klein, E. S. (1996a). Phonological/traditional approaches to articulation therapy: A retrospective group comparison. *Language, Speech and Hearing Services in Schools, 27*, 314–323.

Klein, E. S. (1996b). *Clinical phonology: Assessment and treatment of articulation disorders in children and adults*. San Diego, CA: Singular Publishing Group, Inc.

Laing, S. P., & Espeland, W. (2005). Low intensity phonological awareness training in a preschool classroom for children with communication impairments. *Journal of Communication Disorders, 38*, 65–82.

Lancaster, G. (1991). *The effectiveness of parent administered input training for children with phonological disorders* (Unpublished Master's thesis). City University, London.

Lancaster, G. (2007). *Developing speech and language skills*, London: David Fulton Publishers, Routledge.

Lancaster, G., Levin, A., Pring, T., & Martin, S. (2010). Treating children with phonological problems: Does an eclectic approach to therapy work? *International Journal of Language and Communication Disorders, 45*(2), 174–181.

Lancaster, G., & Pope, L. (1989). *Working with children's phonology*. Oxon: Winslow Press.

Law, J., Garrett, Z., & Nye, C. (2003). Speech and language therapy interventions for children with primary speech and language delay or disorder. *Cochrane Database of Systematic Reviews*, Issue 3, Art. No.: CD004110.

Law, J., Garrett, Z., & Nye, C. (2004). The efficacy of treatment for children with developmental speech and language delay/disorder: A meta-analysis. *Journal of Speech, Language and Hearing Research, 47*, 924–943.

Lof, G. L. (1996). Factors associated with speech-sound stimulability. *Journal of Communication Disorders, 29*, 255–278.

McLeod, S. (Ed.). (2007). *The international guide to speech acquisition*. Clifton Park, NY: Thomson Delmar Learning.

McNeill, B. C., & Hesketh, A. (2010). Developmental complexity of the stimuli included in mispronunciation detection tasks. *International Journal of Language & Communication Disorders, 45*(1), 72–82.

Meyer, S. M. (2004). *Survival guide for the beginning clinician* (2nd ed.). Austin, TX: Pro-ed.

Miccio, A. W. (2002). Clinical problem solving: Assessment of phonological disorders. *American Journal of Speech-Language Pathology, 11*, 221–229.

Miccio, A. W. (2005). A treatment program for enhancing stimulability. In: Kamhi, A. G., & Pollock, K. E. (Eds.), *Phonological disorders in children: Clinical decision making in assessment and intervention* (pp. 163–173). Baltimore, MD: Paul H. Brookes Publishing Co.

Miccio, A. W., & Elbert, M. (1996). Enhancing stimulability: A treatment program. *Journal of Communication Disorders, 29*, 335–352.

Miccio, A. W., Elbert, M., & Forrest, K. (1999). The relationship between stimulability and phonological acquisition in children with normally developing and disordered phonologies. *American Journal of Speech-Language Pathology, 8*, 347–363.

Milisen, R. (1954). A rationale for articulation disorders. *Journal of Speech and Hearing Disorders*. (Monograph supplement), *4*, 6–17.

Moriarty, B. C., & Gillon, G. T. (2006). Phonological awareness intervention for children with childhood apraxia of speech. *International Journal of*

Language and Communication Disorders, *41*, 713–734.

Munson, B., Baylis, A., Krause, M., & Yim, D-S. (2006). *Representation and access in phonological impairment.* Paper presented at the 10th conference on laboratory phonology, Paris, France, 30 June—2 July.

Munson, B., Edwards, J., & Beckman, M. E. (2005). Relationships between nonword repetition accuracy and other measures of linguistic development in children with phonological disorders. *Journal of Speech, Language, and Hearing Research, 48*, 61–78.

Pascoe, M., Stackhouse, J., & Wells, B. (2006). *Children's speech and literacy difficulties III: Persisting speech difficulties in children.* Chichester: John Wiley and Sons.

Pollock, K. E. (2013). The Memphis vowel project: Vowel errors in children with and without phonological disorders. In: M. J. Ball, & F. E. Gibbon (Eds.), *Handbook of vowels and vowel disorders* (pp. 260–287). Psychology Press: Hove.

Pollock, K. E., & Hall, P. K. (1991). An analysis of the vowel misarticulations of five children with developmental apraxia of speech. *Clinical Linguistics and Phonetics, 5*(3), 207–224.

Powell, T. W., Elbert, M., & Dinnsen, D. A. (1991). Stimulability as a factor in the phonological generalisation of misarticulating preschool children. *Journal of Speech and Hearing Research, 34*, 1318–1328.

Powell, T. W., Elbert, M., Miccio, A. W., Strike-Roussos, C., & Brasseur, J. (1998). Facilitating [s] production in young children: An experimental evaluation of motoric and conceptual treatment approaches. *Clinical Linguistics and Phonetics, 12*, 127–146.

Powell, T. W., & Miccio, A. W. (1996). Stimulability: A useful clinical tool. *Journal of Communication Disorders, 29*, 237–253.

Prezas, R. F., & Hodson, B. W. (2010). The cycles phonological remediation approach. In: A. L. Williams, S. McLeod, & R. J. McCauley (Eds.), *Interventions for speech sound disorders in children* (pp. 137–157). Baltimore, MD: Paul H. Brookes Publishing Co.

Pye, C., Ingram, D., & List, H. (1987). A comparison of initial consonant acquisition in English and Quiche. In: K. E. Nelson, & A. Van Kleek (Eds.), *Children's language.* Hillsdale, NJ: Erlbaum.

Rauscher, F. B., Krauss, R. M., & Chen, Y. (1996). Gesture, speech and lexical access: The role of lexical movements in speech production. *Psychological Science, 7*, 226–231.

Reid, J. (2003). The vowel house: A cognitive approach to vowels for literacy and speech. *Child Language Teaching and Therapy, 19*, 152–180.

Rescorla, L., & Bernstein Ratner, N. (1996). Phonetic profiles of typically developing and language-delayed toddlers. *Journal of Speech and Hearing Research, 39*, 153–165.

Reynolds, J. (1990). Abnormal vowel patterns in phonological disorder: Some data and a hypothesis. *British Journal of Disorders of Communication, 25*, 115–148.

Robb, M. P., Bleile, K. M., & Yee, S. S. L. (1999). A phonetic analysis of vowel errors during the course of treatment. *Clinical Linguistics and Phonetics, 13*(4), 309–321.

Rosenbek, J. C., & Wertz, R. T. (1972). A review of 50 cases of developmental apraxia of speech. *Language, Speech, and Hearing Services in Schools, 3*, 23–33.

Rvachew, S. (1994). Speech perception training can facilitate sound production learning. *Journal of Speech and Hearing Research, 37*, 347–357.

Rvachew, S. (2005a). The importance of phonetic factors in phonological intervention. In: A. G. Kamhi, & K. E. Pollock (Eds.), *Phonological disorders in children: Clinical decision making in assessment and intervention* (pp. 175–187). Baltimore, MD: Paul H. Brookes Publishing Co.

Rvachew, S. (2005b). Stimulability and treatment success. *Topics in Language Disorders, 25*(3), 207–219.

Rvachew, S. (2006). Longitudinal predictors of implicit phonological awareness skills. *American Journal of Speech-Language Pathology, 15*, 165–176.

Rvachew, S. (2007). Phonological processing and reading in children with speech sound disorders. *American Journal of Speech-Language Pathology, 16*, 260–270.

Rvachew, S., & Brosseau-Lapré, F. (2010). Speech perception intervention. In: A. L. Williams, S. McLeod, & R. McCauley (Eds.), *Treatment of speech sound disorders in children* (pp. 295–314). Baltimore, MD: Paul H. Brookes Publishing Co.

Rvachew, S., & Brosseau-Lapré, F. (2012). *Developmental phonological disorders: Foundations of clinical practice.* San Diego, CA: Plural Publishing.

Rvachew, S., & Nowak, M. (2001). The effect of target-selection strategy of phonological learning. *Journal of Speech, Language and Hearing Research, 44*, 610–623.

Rvachew, S., Nowak, M., & Cloutier, G. (2004). Effect of phonemic perception training on the speech production and phonological awareness skills of children with expressive phonological delay. *American Journal of Speech-Language Pathology, 13*, 250–263.

Rvachew, S., Rafaat, S., & Martin, M. (1999). Stimulability, speech perception and the treatment of phonological disorders. *American Journal of Speech-Language Pathology, 8*, 33–43.

Saben, C.B., & Ingham, J.C. (1991). The effects of minimal pairs treatment on the speech-sound production of two children with phonologic disorders. *Journal of Speech and Hearing Research, 34*, 1023–1040.

Schmidt, R. A., & Lee, T. D. (2011). *Motor control and learning: A behavioural emphasis* (5th ed.). Champaign, IL: Human Kinetics.

Sherman, D., & Geith, A. (1967). Speech sound discrimination and articulation skill. *Journal of Speech and Hearing Research, 10*, 277–280.

Shriberg, L. D., & Kwiatkowski, J. (1980). *Natural Process Analysis* New York: Academic Press.

Shuster, L. I. (1998). The perception of correctly and incorrectly produced /r/. *Journal of Speech, Language, and Hearing Research, 41*, 941–950.

Sommers, R. K., Leiss, R. H., Delp, M., Gerber, A., Fundrella, D., Smith, R., Revucky, M., Ellis, D., & Haley, V. (1967). Factors related to the effectiveness of articulation therapy for kindergarten, first and second grade children. *Journal of Speech and Hearing Research, 13*, 428–437.

Speake, J., Stackhouse, J., & Pascoe, M. (2012). Vowel targeted intervention for children with persisting speech difficulties: Impact on intelligibility. *Child Language Teaching and Therapy, 28*(3), 277–295.

Stackhouse, J., & Pascoe, M. (2010). Psycholinguistic intervention. In: A. L. Williams, S. McLeod, & R. J. McCauley (Eds.), *Interventions for speech sound disorders in children* (pp. 219–246). Paul H. Brookes Publishing Co.

Stackhouse, J., Pascoe, M., & Gardner, H. (2006). Intervention for a child with persisting speech and literacy difficulties: A psycholinguistic approach. *Advances in Speech-Language Pathology, 8*(3), 231–244.

Stackhouse, J., Vance, M., Pascoe, M., & Wells, B. (2007). *Children's speech and literacy difficulties IV: Compendium of auditory and speech tasks.* Chichester: John Wiley and Sons.

Stackhouse, J., & Wells, B. (1997). *Children's speech and literacy difficulties I: A psycholinguistic framework.* London: Whurr Publishers.

Stackhouse, J., & Wells, B. (2001). *Children's speech and literacy difficulties II: Identification and intervention.* London: Whurr Publishers.

Stackhouse, J., Wells, B., Pascoe, M., & Rees, R. (2002). From phonological therapy to phonological awareness. *Seminars in Speech and Language, 23*(1), 27–42.

Stoel-Gammon, C. (1990). Issues in phonological development and disorders. In: J. Miller (Ed.), *Progress in research on child language disorders.* Austin, TX: PRO-ED.

Stoel-Gammon, C., & Dunn, C. (1985). *Normal and disordered phonology in children.* Baltimore, MD: University Park Press.

Stoel-Gammon, C., & Pollock, K.E. (2008). Vowel development and disorders. In: M. Ball, M. Perkins, N. Müller, & S. Howard (Eds.), *Handbook of clinical linguistics.* Oxford: Blackwell Publishers.

Sutherland, D., & Gillon, G. T. (2007). The development of phonological representations and phonological awareness in children with speech impairment. *International Journal of Language and Communication Disorders, 42*(2), 229–250.

Travis, L. E. (1931). *Speech pathology: A dynamic neurological treatment of normal speech and speech deviations.* New York: D. Appleton Co.

Tyler, A. A. (2002). Language-based intervention for phonological disorders. *Seminars in Speech and Language, 23*, 69–82.

Tyler, A. A., & Figurski, G. R. (1994). Phonetic inventory changes after treating distinctions along an implicational hierarchy. *Clinical Linguistics & Phonetics, 8*, 91–107.

Van Riper, C. (1978). *Speech correction: Principles and methods* (6th ed.). Englewood Cliffs, NJ: Prentice-Hall.

Velleman, S. L., & Vihman, M. M. (2002). Whole-word phonology and templates: Trap, bootstrap, or some of each? *Language, Speech, and Hearing Services in the Schools, 33*, 9–23.

Walley, A. C., Metsala, J. L., & Garlock, V. M. (2003). Spoken vocabulary growth: Its role in the development of phoneme awareness and early reading ability. *Reading and Writing, 16*, 5–20.

Watts, N. (2004). Assessment of vowels summary. *ACQuiring Knowledge in Speech, Language and Hearing, Speech Pathology Australia, 6*(1), 22–25.

Weiner, F. (1981). Treatment of phonological disability using the method of meaningful contrast: Two case studies. *Journal of Speech and Hearing Disorders*, *46*, 97–103.

Wells, J. C. (1982a). *Accents of English 1: An introduction*. Cambridge: Cambridge University Press.

Wells, J. C. (1982b). *Accents of English 2: The British Isles*. Cambridge: Cambridge University Press.

Wells, J. C. (1982c). *Accents of English 3: Beyond the British Isles*. Cambridge: Cambridge University Press.

Williams, A. L. (2000a). Multiple oppositions: Theoretical foundations for an alternative contrastive intervention approach. *American Journal of Speech-Language Pathology*, *9*, 282–288.

Williams, A. L. (2000b). Multiple oppositions: Case Studies of variables in Phonological intervention. *American Journal of Speech-Language Pathology*, *9*, 289–299.

Williams, A. L. (2001). Phonological assessment of child speech. In: D. M. Ruscello (Ed.), *Tests and measurements in speech-language pathology* (pp. 31–76). Woburn, MA: Butterworth-Heinemann.

Williams, A. L. (2003). *Speech disorders: Resource guide for preschool children*. Clifton Park, NY: Thomson Delmar Learning.

Williams, A. L. (2005). From developmental norms to distance metrics: Past, present, and future directions for target selection practices. In: A. G. Kamhi, & K. E. Pollock (Eds.), *Phonological disorders in children: Clinical decision making in assessment and intervention* (pp. 101–108). Baltimore: MD: Paul. H. Brookes Publishing.

Williams, A. L. (2006a). *Sound contrasts in phonology (SCIP)*. Greenville, SC: Super Duper.

Williams, A. L. (2006b). A systemic perspective for assessment and intervention: A case study. *Advances in Speech-Language Pathology*, *8*(3), 245–256.

Williams, A. L. (2010). Multiple oppositions intervention. In: A. L. Williams, S. McLeod, & R. J. McCauley (Eds.), *Interventions for speech sound disorders in children* (pp. 73–94). Baltimore, MD: Paul H. Brookes Publishing Co.

Williams, A. L., McLeod, S., & McCauley, R. J. (2010). (Eds.) *Interventions for speech sound disorders in children*. Baltimore, MD: Paul H. Brookes Publishing Co.

Yoss, K. A., & Darley, F. L. (1974). Developmental apraxia of speech in children with defective articulation. *Journal of Speech and Hearing Research*, *17*, 399–416.

Chapter 5

'Common', 'best' and evidence-based practice

In Chapter 5, contributors working in Australia, Canada, Germany, New Zealand, the United Kingdom and the United States present information, opinions and reflections on clinical 'common', 'best' and evidence-based practice (EBP). The questions that are put to them vary considerably, covering diverse issues and canvassing a range of views. In A30, Nicole Watts Pappas appraises several studies of SLP/SLT clinical 'common practice' in child speech, with an emphasis on family-centred practice in Australia. Megan Hodge (A31) follows with insights into clinical practice gained from a survey of Canadian SLPs' opinions and experience using non-speech oral motor exercises (NS-OME) in children's speech therapy. Next, Gail Gillon (A32) discusses effective practice and positive and enduring partnerships between SLT and Education in New Zealand. Kylie Toynton (A33), a speech pathologist in private practice in an Australian rural setting broaches the issues that arise when SLPs/SLTs use (largely nonevidence-based) software applications (Apps) in working with children with speech sound disorders (SSD). Drawing on the results of a survey of clinicians, Victoria Joffe (A34) examines minimalist assessment practices in the United Kingdom. Echoing Hodge (A31), Gregory Lof (A35) then talks about the puzzling situation wherein large numbers of north American SLPs, who have been steeped, at Master's level, in scientific method and critical analysis of the evidence base, continue to implement a therapy methodology with children with SSD that is anything *but* scientific (McCauley, Strand, Lof, Schooling & Frymark, 2009). These six contributions are followed by discussion of four related issues. Karen McComas (A36) reflects on the transformation from student to ethical practitioner that occurs when a student *participates* in integrated, educative experiences (Palmer & Zajonc, 2010); B. May Bernhardt and Angela Ullrich (A37) review the role of linguistic theory, particularly non-linear phonology, in clinical problem solving; Karen Froud (A38) has interesting things to add about reading and critically evaluating the literature around the so-called 'terrifying therapies' (Gardner, A27; Joffe, A34) and the research-practice gap; and Thomas Powell (A39) presents a multifaceted model for ethical practices.

Children's Speech Sound Disorders, Second Edition. Caroline Bowen.
© 2015 John Wiley & Sons, Ltd. Published 2015 by John Wiley & Sons, Ltd.
Companion website: www.wiley.com/go/bowen/speechlanguagetherapy

Speech acquisition and the family

Some years ago I had the pleasure of joining Nicole Watts Pappas and seventy other contributors to Sharynne McLeod's remarkable 2007 book, *The International Guide to Speech Acquisition*. In our chapter on speech acquisition and the family (Watts Pappas & Bowen, 2007, p 89) we wrote the following.

> *Part of the expertise of the competent SLP is to be sensitive and open to families' beliefs and practices around development, child rearing, and customary interaction with infants and youngsters growing up, because all of these important factors vary. In a shrinking world, it is also incumbent upon speech and language professionals to recognise, accommodate and respect the differing roles, expectations, and speech assessment and intervention practices of SLP colleagues, in their family, work and community contexts, internationally. Occurring through a gradual, dynamic, and multifaceted process of genetic endowment, instinct, discovery and learning, speech acquisition is inevitably the product of elements residing in the child, within the family, shaped by their unique cultural, social and linguistic milieu.*

Dr. Nicole Watts Pappas is actively engaged in research, publication and SLP clinical practice in a community clinic in Brisbane, Australia, where she endeavours to use family-centred approaches in her work with young children and their families. In her PhD research, she explored the involvement of families in SLP/SLT intervention for speech impairment.

Q30.   Nicole Watts Pappas: Family-centred speech intervention in Australia

The distinction between involving parents in their own children's speech intervention, and involving them as collaborative partners in the assessment, intervention and management process, is not always clear to the parties concerned: child, parent, therapist and policy maker. Against a background of common practice (McLeod & Baker, 2004), the nexus between therapists' beliefs and practice (Watts Pappas, McLeod, McAllister & Daniel, 2006), and what the evidence-base would encourage us to do (Baker & McLeod, 2011a, b), what is the Australian experience of family-centred practice in the area of children's SSD?

A30.   Nicole Watts Pappas: The Australian experience of family-centred practice in intervention for speech impairment

History of parental and family involvement in speech intervention

What is considered 'best practice' in working with parents and families in paediatric intervention has undergone significant changes over time. Traditionally, parents were given limited opportunity to be involved in their child's speech intervention with services planned and delivered by the SLP/SLT in a therapist-centred approach to management (Crais, 1991). In the late 1970s and 1980s, SLPs/SLTs and other allied health professionals were encouraged to increase parents' participation in intervention, primarily by requesting them to complete home activities with their child (Bazyk, 1989). However, parental involvement in these activities tended to be expected rather than optional and parents continued to have limited involvement in service planning and decision-making.

More recently, a new philosophy of working with parents and families, family-centred service, has been recommended as best practice (Rosenbaum, King, Law, King & Evans, 1998). Family-centred practice promotes the formation of collaborative parent/

professional partnerships and acknowledges parents and families as the primary decision-makers regarding their child's intervention (Bailey, McWilliam & Winton, 1992). In addition, based on the theory that change to one family member will affect all other family members, family-centred practice considers the whole family as client rather than just the child.

Typical practice of parental involvement in speech intervention

While recommended models for working with parents and families in SLP/SLT practice have changed, the practices of clinicians may not have undergone a corresponding transformation. The well-documented researcher/practice gap highlights the fact that clinicians may take time to incorporate new models of service into their clinical practice (McLeod & Baker, 2004). Three Australian studies have investigated how SLP clinicians involve parents in intervention for speech impairment. A survey conducted by McLeod and Baker (2004) of the speech intervention practices of 270 SLPs found that 88.2% of respondents reported they involved parents in their intervention for speech impairment. However, this involvement appeared to occur predominantly in intervention provision rather than planning – when asked about factors they considered when selecting treatment targets only 49.6% of respondents indicated they considered parental preference as a high priority.

In a more comprehensive study, Watts Pappas, McLeod, McAllister and McKinnon (2008) surveyed 277 SLPs regarding their beliefs and practices of parental involvement in speech intervention. The results of the survey indicated that the vast majority of respondents involved parents in some way in their intervention for speech impairment. The most common form of involvement was the provi-

sion of home activities with 95% of respondents indicating they always or usually provided home activities to parents. Other typical forms of involvement included parental attendance at assessment (84%) and intervention (80%) sessions. The SLPs reported using family-centred practices such as considering parents' time and priorities when providing home activities (94%). However, the respondents did not use other family-centred practices as frequently. For example, only 44% of the SLPs indicated they allowed parents to choose the extent of their involvement in the intervention and only 17% always or usually gave parents an option regarding the service delivery format provided to their child. Parental involvement in intervention planning occurred less frequently than some other forms of involvement; 67% of the SLPs reported they involved parents in goal-setting; however, only 38% always or usually allowed parents to make the *final* decisions about intervention goals and activities.

A more recent study of parental involvement in speech intervention investigated the frequency and nature of parental involvement from the perspectives of the parents. Ruggero, McCabe, Ballard and Munro (2012) explored, through the use of an online survey, the experiences of 154 parents accessing speech pathology services for their child. Fifty-four percent of the children of the parents in the study were identified as receiving intervention for an SSD. The results indicated that while 76% of parents were asked to do homework activities with their child, only 43% were involved in goal-setting.

The results of these studies of the typical practice of SLPs indicate that although parents are usually involved in speech intervention services, the SLP retains primary control over the direction of the intervention, in a therapist-centred rather than a family-centred approach to management. However, a gap may be present between SLPs' typical practice and their beliefs about what constitutes ideal practice, especially if barriers to using ideal practice exist.

SLPs' beliefs regarding parent and family involvement in speech intervention

Two studies have investigated Australian SLPs' beliefs regarding parental and family involvement in intervention for speech impairment. The previously described study conducted by Watts Pappas and colleagues (2007) also investigated the SLPs' beliefs with regards to parental involvement. We found in this study that the overwhelming majority of respondents (98%) agreed or strongly agreed that parental involvement is essential for speech intervention to be effective. The SLPs also believed that parents should be present at (78%) and participate (97%) in intervention sessions. However, 40% of respondents indicated they were not happy with the level of parental participation in their service or aspects of their service. In open-ended questions the SLPs reported the presence of various barriers that they believed prevented them from giving what they considered 'ideal' services to the parents they worked with. These included workplace barriers (such as working in a school setting), parent barriers (such as parent time, skills and inclination to be involved) and personal barriers (such as a lack of knowledge and confidence in working with parents in intervention for speech impairment).

Similar to the findings of other studies of professionals' perceptions of working with families (Bruce et al., 2002; Litchfield & MacDougall, 2002; Minke & Scott, 1995), although the SLPs held a strong belief in the importance of parental involvement in intervention *provision*, they generally supported a more therapist-centred (as opposed to a family-centred) approach to management in the area of intervention *planning* and decision-making. For example,

only 42% of the SLPs indicated that they agreed that parents should have the final say on the content of intervention goals and activities.

Why did the SLPs' reported beliefs and practice support a more traditional approach to working with parents and families than is recommended by the literature? A second, more in depth study of the beliefs and practices of Australian SLPs addressed this issue. Watts Pappas and McLeod (2008b) conducted a focus group of six SLPs working with children with speech impairment. The focus group discussion centred on parental and family involvement in speech intervention and parent/professional relationships. The findings of the analysis of the group interview indicated that the SLP participants believed strongly in the importance of parental involvement in speech intervention and attempted to engage parents and families in their child's intervention as much as possible. They also believed in providing respectful and supportive service to families. However, similar to the results from the survey, although the SLPs felt that parental involvement in intervention was critical, they also held a strong belief that the professional should make the final decisions regarding intervention planning and provision.

Several factors may have contributed to this belief. The SLPs considered themselves as the specialists in intervention for speech impairment. As the specialists they felt it was their role and responsibility to take the lead in the management of speech intervention. In addition, the participants in the focus group believed that parents both wanted and needed guidance from their SLP. Considering the complexity of intervention for speech impairment, the SLPs felt that parents did not have the skills to have the final say about intervention. Indeed, adopting parents' choices for goals was postulated as an ethical issue if parents requested goals or activities that were contraindicated for the child.

With the current focus on efficiency and accountability in paediatric intervention services, SLPs are under pressure to ensure their intervention is evidence-based and effective (Reilly, 2004; Roddam & Skeat, 2010). Most evidence-based speech intervention approaches require specific choices regarding treatment targets or intervention activities (Baker, 2006). These approaches may be difficult to provide if parents insist on alternative goals and activities. The literature and policy makers have promoted family-centred practice as best practice in intervention for young children (Crais, Poston Roy & Free, 2006), but there is little evidence of its impact on speech intervention outcomes or its acceptability to parents is available. Only one study to date has investigated the effectiveness of a family-centred versus a therapist-centred approach to intervention for SSDs. McKean, Phillips and Thompson (2012) conducted a study of 20 children receiving intervention for speech impairment. Ten of the children received intervention incorporating family-centred principles; the remaining ten children received what was termed as 'usual practice'. The outcomes of the study indicated that the family-centred condition did not lead to greater treatment gains. Considering the lack of evidence for family-centred practice, SLPs/SLTs may be reluctant to use this approach when it contravenes other demands of their workplace such as providing service that is evidence-based and efficacious.

Parents' beliefs regarding parent and family involvement in speech intervention

Contrary to the recommendations of best practice, the studies that have investigated parental involvement in speech intervention in Australia have indicated that SLPs' beliefs and practice are not supportive of a truly family-centred model of service, particularly in relation to decision-making. However, a progressive in-depth study of the views of seven parents accessing speech intervention for their child (Watts Pappas & McLeod, 2008a) indicated that Australian parents might not necessarily want a family-centred approach to intervention for their child with speech impairment. The analysis of the interviews indicated that the parents believed that it was a SLP's role and responsibility to both work with their child in the intervention sessions and to provide guidance about intervention goals and activities. If the parent trusted their SLP they felt the best thing they could do for their child was to follow the SLP's lead in the intervention process. Comparably, Ruggero et al. (2012) found that involvement in goal-setting was not a contributing factor in parental satisfaction with intervention. Similar beliefs and expectations about parent/professional roles have been reported in other studies of parents' perceptions of paediatric allied health intervention (Glogowska & Campbell, 2000; Leiter, 2004; MacKean, Thurston & Scott, 2005; Mirabito & Armstrong, 2004; Thompson, 1998). While the parents felt that their involvement in their child's intervention (particularly the provision of home activities) was important, they wanted their SLP to take the lead role in intervention provision and planning and preferred intervention to focus on their child rather than their family.

Summary

SLPs/SLTs believe strongly in parental participation in speech intervention and, within a background of various barriers to family involvement, strategise to engage families as much as possible in the process. They also attempt to provide respectful and supportive care to families and consider their needs and wishes in intervention planning. Allowing parents to take the lead in intervention planning and delivery however poses a dilemma for SLPs/SLTs, especially when parents' wishes are at odds with the demands of EBP. While SLPs/SLTs consider the child within the context of their family, it appears that clinicians, as well as parents prefer an approach to intervention for speech impairment that is SLP/SLT-led and also predominantly child focused.

A Canadian survey

In a survey of SLPs (Hodge, Salonka & Kollias, 2005), clinicians in Alberta, Canada were asked about their use, and the roles and benefits as they saw them, of NS-OME in the treatment of children with speech disorders. Like Lof and Watson (2008), who analysed survey responses from 537 US SLPs and found that 85% used NS-OME to target speech, the Canadian researchers found that 85% of 535 Albertan respondents used NS-OME for the purpose of changing speech sound production.

Dr. Megan Hodge is an SLP and professor emerita in the Department of Speech Pathology and Audiology at the University of Alberta, where she directs the Children's Speech Intelligibility Research and Education (CSPIRE) laboratory. She has taught in the areas of anatomy and physiology of the speech mechanism, speech science and motor speech disorders. Her research interests include developmental aspects of normal and disordered speech production, perceptual-acoustic correlates of speech intelligibility and linking theory with practice in evaluating and treating children with motor speech disorders. Currently she is engaged in several collaborative projects with community partners to create care pathways to improve services and outcomes for children with complex speech disorders. In her response to Q31, Dr. Hodge discusses the survey results and their implications, providing an informed view of common practice in at least one Canadian province, and effective practice as it is taught in Canadian universities.

Q31.   Megan M. Hodge: A Canadian perspective on oral motor exercises

What insights do the results of the 2004 survey of Albertan SLPs' use of NS-OME in children's speech therapy reveal about common clinical practice, compared with effective practice as taught in Canadian universities?

A31.   Megan M. Hodge: What can we learn about clinical practice from SLPs' experiences using NS-OME in children's speech therapy?

Information about the survey conducted by Sophie Kollias and Robin Lester (2004) under my supervision is followed by conclusions from our research. After each conclusion, I comment on (a) what it might reveal about clinical practice for childhood SSDs, (b) how this relates to my knowledge about effective practice as taught in Canadian universities and (c) what I see as the implications to address the evidence-to-practice gap for SLPs serving Canadian children with SSD.

The survey results represented responses from approximately 28% of SLPs registered with the Alberta College of Speech-Language Pathologists and Audiologists (ACSLPA) who provided speech therapy to children (0–16 years of age) during June 2004. The survey collected information about respondents' opinions and experiences using NS-OME. We do not know how representative the sample is of Albertan or Canadian SLPs who use NS-OME so these results cannot be generalised to all SLPs. However, they represent a range of responses from a substantial sample of SLPs. It is also important to understand that the purpose of this survey was *not* to describe common practice for children with SSD; rather, it addressed use of NS-OME in children's speech therapy. Eighty percent of survey respondents served children between birth and 8 years; 30% worked in schools, 25% in community health centres, 18% in private practice, 16% in early education settings, 8% in hospitals and 3% in other settings. The majority of respondents (67%) had more than 5 years of clinical work experience.

Conclusion 1

For the 85% of respondents who reported using NS-OME with at least one child between 1999 and 2004, the most common practice was to use NS-OME in therapy as warm-up activities, as part of a speech goal, and/or assigned for home practice. The three most common therapy objectives identified for using NS-OME were to increase articulator strength and coordination, facilitate stimulability for consonants and vowels and improve speech intelligibility. Respondents' reasons for using NS-OME were their beliefs that NS-OME were effective or that no other intervention had worked. When NS-OME were used, 56% of SLPs reported spending from 5 to 15 minutes performing these exercises in therapy, while 31% spent less than 5 minutes. However, some SLPs reported using NS-OME for an entire treatment session and, in a few cases, not as part of a speech goal (e.g., to decrease drooling, improve feeding skills, strengthen muscle groups unrelated to a specific articulation goal).

Comment

'Warm-up' activities in speech therapy sessions, assigning NS-OME as home practice activities and training articulator strength are not presented as EBPs for childhood SSD in Canadian university training programs. Clark (2010) concluded that 'much more extensive and higher quality treatment literature is needed to determine the conditions under which OMEs are most beneficial as well as the therapeutic mechanisms underlying their effectiveness' (p. 579). Information that is available in NS-OME materials appears useful to SLPs in stimulating production of difficult to elicit sounds. Scholarly publications such as Secord, Boyce, Donohue, Fox & Shine's (2007) *Eliciting Sounds: Techniques and Strategies for Clinicians* are useful resources for students and clinicians. In some cases, this may involve using tools such as bite blocks to stabilise the jaw, allowing the child to experience articulatory movements of the tongue and lips that are independent of the jaw (Hodge, 2010).

Conclusion 2

In general, developers of NS-OME advocate their use for improving speech intelligibility in individuals with various communication disorders (e.g., Chapman Bahr, 2001; Rosenfeld-Johnson, 2001, 2010). Published peer-reviewed original research does not exist currently to substantiate or unequivocally discredit these claims (Clark, 2010). Not surprisingly, survey respondents reported using NS-OME most often for children with phonology/articulation delay/disorder (37%), suspected childhood apraxia of speech or CAS (33%) and dysarthria (15%). Answers to open-ended survey questions suggested that (a) respondents have children on their caseloads with these diagnoses that are challenging to treat and NS-OME seem to be helpful in some cases, and (b) the prescriptive treatment offered by NS-OME allow SLPs to be 'time efficient'. Many clinicians stated that they use whatever technique works for them (including NS-OME), or that NS-OME are a place to start when they do not know what else to do. NS-OME appeared to be used most commonly for clients with syndromes and medical conditions that typically result in concomitant difficulties producing intelligible speech, such as Down syndrome and cerebral palsy. Possible reasons for the higher frequency of NS-OME with these syndromes and conditions include (a) developers of NS-OME often 'market' their use for these children, (b) NS-OME provide a step-by-step approach for children with more complex speech disorders and challenging speech intelligibility problems and (c) intuitively it may make sense to use motor exercises in therapy because children with these conditions have difficulty controlling the oral musculature as part of their impairment (see Clark, 2003; 2010, for discussion about why this 'intuition' needs careful examination).

Comment

SLPs appear most likely to use NS-OME in treatment for children who (a) appear to have a motor component to their speech disorder and do not benefit from traditional articulation therapy approaches, and/or (b) present with a severe and complex SSD. Canadian university training programs are heterogeneous in how they teach students to diagnose and treat children with SSD that have a suspected or known motor component (i.e., CAS, dysarthria, mixed CAS-dysarthria). ASHA's (2007) position statement standardises basic information about CAS for students and professionals, provides guidelines for treatment that explicitly exclude NS-OME, and highlights the need for treatment research. As an alternative to NS-OME, Davis and Velleman (2008) proposed a 'means, motive and opportunity' conceptual framework to establish a speech repertoire in children with severe speech delay. Their framework focuses on stimulation of meaningful vocalisations for functional communication, which is validated by the early language development literature. There is a very small but growing body of research about effectiveness of speech-based interventions for children with dysarthria (e.g., Pennington, Miller, Robson & Steen, 2010; Pennington et al.,

2012). My experience is that most Canadian universities currently provide minimal information about speech therapy practice for this population of children. Development and dissemination of current best practice guidelines and development and evaluation of therapy programs for children with motor speech disorders, which include clinicians as collaborators, are obvious needs in Canada. The care pathway for managing pre-school children with suspected CAS presented by the Ontario Ministry of Children and Youth 2010 Working Group for Children with Suspected Motor Speech Difficulties (OMCY-2010WG) (April, 2011) is an example of an initiative that addresses this need. Based on the lack of research support and questionable theoretical constructs for using NS-OME for children with speech difficulties, the Working Group also recommended that NS-OME be considered an alternative treatment approach, governed by the College of Audiologists and Speech-Language Pathologists of Ontario's position statement for Alternative Approaches to Intervention (B. R. Gaines, personal communication. April 19, 2013.) This requires that clinicians who intend to use NS-OME obtain informed consent from parents.

Conclusion 3

Users of NS-OME indicated that they were influenced by the high degree of exposure to NS-OME products and materials (e.g., products marketed by Rosenfeld-Johnson, 2001, Super Duper Publications, LinguiSystems and www.pammarshalla.com), and clinical success (self and reported by colleagues).

Comment

SLPs' responses reveal the weight put on knowledge of products gained through 'marketing' exposure and that of their own and colleagues' experience in influencing their practice. All Canadian training programs aspire to graduate SLP professionals who can think independently and critically. Concerted, focused efforts are needed to foster and develop these skills in coursework and clinical placements so that graduates are informed, judicious consumers of products in the marketplace and colleagues' advice. As noted in the comments for Conclusion 2, many survey respondents who used NS-OME reported using them with children suspected to have a motor speech disorder and/or presenting with a severe and complex SSD. We need to increase the number of graduates who are knowledgeable and confident about practice for these subgroups of children. There also appears to be a disconnect between what is presented as effective practice in Canadian training programs and what information is presented by invited speakers and marketed by exhibitors at professional conferences and professional development events. Sara Rosenfeld-Johnson has been an invited speaker at several conferences hosted by professional associations in Canada. Greater communication and collaboration between Canadian academic training programs and national and regional professional conference committees to promote and debate best practices in SSD appear warranted.

Conclusion 4

Survey respondents were asked if they have seen significant changes in clients' speech because of NS-OME and, if so, to describe the changes observed. Those who answered 'yes' typically stated that NS-OME improved the strength/coordination of articulators as well as overall speech intelligibility or resulted in stimulability of speech sounds and improved production of particular sounds classes (i.e., rhotics and sibilants). Respondents who reported variable results stated that NS-OME helped with stimulability/awareness

or strength/coordination of the articulators, but were ineffective with certain children and that some NS-OME programs were not as effective as others. A strong theme that emerged was that NS-OME are useful with certain children but they are not meant for everyone. Many respondents explained that NS-OME have a small role in a therapy session, and are not the sole treatment strategy. Other treatment approaches mentioned were traditional articulation therapy, Hodson's cycles, phonological processes, minimal pairs, phonetic placement, auditory discrimination, visual feedback, multiple opposition, maximal opposition, non-linear, PROMPT, rate reduction, whole language and total communication that incorporates some form of AAC. However, a small subgroup of respondents appeared to use NS-OME for many clients and disorders and believed that NS-OME produce effective changes in multiple areas. The majority of respondents rated the evidence base for NS-OME as minimal or non-existent (64%). Surprisingly, 36% of the 137 respondents rated the evidence as adequate or extensive. While only 36% of respondents thought there was evidence to support NS-OME in SSD, 50% claimed that NS-OME have an important role in children's speech therapy. Obviously, some clinicians who do not think there is evidence to support the use of NS-OME believe that they have an important role in speech therapy. Many respondents commented that they would like to see research investigating the benefits of NS-OME.

Comment

The survey results revealed that Canadian SLPs are heterogeneous in their beliefs and practices about using NS-OME for treating children with SSD and use an eclectic and pragmatic approach to speech therapy. Experience/exposure, training and available resources were common responses for why

SLPs do or do not use NS-OME. Some SLPs firmly believe that NS-OME are effective in improving children's speech based on their clinical experience. Other SLPs do not see any benefit from NS-OME and will not use them without research-based evidence. The majority of SLPs surveyed fell between these two positions.

Summary

In summary, the role of NS-OME in children's speech therapy is an example of a complicated issue for which SLPs need and desire clearer guidance. Clark (2010) encouraged clinicians who use NS-OME to contribute well-designed single subject studies that use measures of both speech ability and the physiological mechanisms addressed by the NS-OME used (e.g., strength).

Although these survey results were obtained in 2004, they still provide several hypotheses to test in research about clinical use of NS-OME in SSD. For example, 'Do NS-OME improve strength and coordination of the articulators and do these improvements increase speech intelligibility?' and 'Are NS-OME more effective at increasing speech intelligibility than treatment approaches where NS-OME are not used?'

The results of this project also revealed gaps in knowledge that Canadian SLPs have about treating certain children with SSD. However progress is being made. Canadian academics and clinical researchers are generating and disseminating research evidence (e.g., Rvachew & Brosseau-Lapré, 2012), helping SLPs to locate and translate evidence to practice for children with SSD (Johnson, 2006) and influencing policies for services for children with SSD (Hodge, November, 2011; OMCY-2010WG, April, 2011). Our training programs and professional associations advocate and support EBP and SLP managers and policy makers are expressing their desire to do so (e.g., Robertson, 2007). Major continuing challenges in the Canadian context include scarce research dollars for treatment research for SSD and limitations on public funding for clinical services.

SLT and education in New Zealand

With a population of fewer than 4.5 million inhabitants New Zealand is a young and remarkable country that consistently punches above its weight in areas as diverse as adventure tourism, film and television, human rights, science and speech-language therapy.

Dr. Gail Gillon (Ngāi Tahu iwi) (ASHA Fellow) is Pro-Vice-Chancellor of the College of Education at the University of Canterbury in Christchurch, New Zealand. A professor in speech-language therapy, Dr. Gillon has been involved in writing best practice documents relating to speech and language therapy services for school-aged children for the New Zealand Ministry of Education. Her own research work has focused on enhancing the literacy success of children with speech and language impairment in the New Zealand pre-school and primary school educational context. Professor Gillon discusses effective practice within a New Zealand context and issues facing new graduates from SLT university programs as they blend into the reality of the education workplace.

Q32.   Gail T. Gillon: New Zealand Speech-Language Therapy and Education

What is the relationship between the SLT academic community and education community in New Zealand given the profession's historical development from an educational context? What are some of the challenges facing SLTs working in educational contexts in New Zealand in terms of meeting 'best practice', and how may these challenges best be addressed?

A32. Gail T. Gillon: New Zealand SLT: partnerships between the academic and educational community

The successful management of childhood speech and language disorders has been a dominant theme in the history of speech and language therapy within New Zealand. The education of New Zealand SLTs grew from a teacher education context. Christchurch Teacher's College established the first tertiary education course for SLTs in 1942, with a 1-year intensive diploma course that followed a 2-year training program in teacher education.

Over time, the education of SLTs in New Zealand expanded to reflect the increasing scope of practice in the discipline and to ensure that graduates could serve the needs of both adults and children with communication and swallowing disorders. The University of Canterbury in Christchurch first offered a 4-year Bachelor of Speech and Language Therapy degree in 1989 and continues to offer this degree alongside Master's and PhD research degrees in speech-language therapy. In 2003, Massey University began a 4-year Bachelor of Speech-Language Therapy degree program at its Auckland Campus and the University of Auckland now offers a 2-year Master's Degree in Speech and Language Therapy Practice.

All three providers of SLT education in New Zealand are committed to ensuring that graduates are well qualified to manage communication and swallowing difficulties across the lifespan, and their graduates readily gain employment with a variety of employers in the health, education and private sectors. However, the relationship with the Education sector and the profession of SLT and, in particular, the New Zealand Ministry of Education continues to be robust.

The Ministry of Education is one of the main employers of SLTs in New Zealand.

Through its Special Education Division, its SLT services concentrate on children who have significant communication impairments. In its endeavours to ensure that this population is well served, the Ministry commissioned a 'best practice' report of SLT assessment and treatment practices for children aged 5–8 years with speech and language disorders in 1998 and commissioned updates in 2001 and 2006 (Gillon & Schwarz, 1998, 2001a; Gillon, Moriarty & Schwarz, 2006). Policy makers and budget holders in education rightly asked fundamental questions about the delivery of SLT services for children in New Zealand Schools, including:

- What are the most valid and reliable assessment methods for identifying children who are in need of SLT services?
- What is the best method to treat a particular type of childhood speech and language disorder?
- How much treatment time is required to resolve a particular disorder?
- What are the most cost effective methods to address the needs of young children with communication disorders?
- How can the needs of young Māori (New Zealand indigenous population) be best met, particularly for those children with speech-language needs who are being educated in Māori immersion education environments?

Addressing the last question has been particularly emphasised in recent years. To respond to the academic underachievement identified for Māori children in the education system, the New Zealand Ministry of Education introduced, in 2008, *Ka Hikitia*; a strategy aimed at ensuring Māori students enjoy education success as Māori. Phase 2 of this strategy, Ka Hikitia: Accelerating Success 2013–2017, has recently been released (Ministry of Education, 2013). In 2009, over 28,000 Māori students were being educated in Māori medium education programs (i.e., either all or some curriculum subjects were taught in the Māori language) and statistical forecasts for the New Zealand population show that by 2030 the proportion of school-aged children who are Māori is likely to increase to around 30%. It is important for SLTs working in New Zealand to understand culturally responsive practices in working with Māori children, their teachers and their families.

Answering questions regarding best practices, cost efficient practices and culturally appropriate practices is not straightforward (Goldstein, A19; Zajdó, A20). The complexities of communication development and cultural influences from diverse populations result in there being no single assessment tool or intervention program that is recognised as universally effective for all children with speech or language impairment. Rather, SLTs must use a range of assessment measures and plan intervention that is specific to a child's needs, including educational needs, and is sensitive to the child's cultural and family environment (Watts Pappas, A30). The intervention approach selected needs to be appropriate to the type and level of severity of the child's communication impairment and must foster both spoken and written language abilities and the prerequisite skills for successful reading and writing development.

Understanding effective or best practices for children based on research evidence is of fundamental importance to the advancement of the SLT profession. The claim made by some practitioners that an intervention method is adopted clinically 'because it works' has been challenged (Gruber, Lowery, Seung & Deal, 2003). More powerful justification for an intervention decision than clinical perception is required (Hodge, A31; Powell, A39). The many confounding variables that influence the perception of intervention effectiveness necessitate the use of well-designed research studies to demonstrate an intervention method is causing the positive changes observed in children's communication development.

Thus, the profession of SLT is being challenged to be more accountable for the services provided to children with communication impairment and to ensure services are educationally relevant and culturally and linguistically appropriate. Service providers need to have confidence that assessment and treatment methods implemented with children are grounded in research and theory, validating their use. Therapists need to demonstrate the effectiveness of their services for diverse populations, and within a limited resourcing funding model for SLT, the cost efficiency of the services must also be considered.

The challenges of providing effective, cost-efficient services for children with communication impairment occur in a context of increasing demand for services. The need for childhood SLT services in New Zealand is undeniably high. The New Zealand Government's educational strategy places a strong emphasis on enhancing literacy success and improving academic achievement for all New Zealanders. A core element of literacy and academic success is proficient reading ability. Although New Zealand continues to enjoy an above average overall reading standard at an international level, there are areas of significant concern that warrant urgent attention. For example, children in New Zealand who enter school at 5 years of age with low 'literate cultural capital' (low levels of phonological awareness (PA), grammatical sensitivity, receptive vocabulary, and letter knowledge), frequently children from low socioeconomic areas, continue to demonstrate poor reading achievement in year 7 (Tunmer, Chapman & Prochnow, 2006). Tunmer et al. concluded from their longitudinal study, which followed 76 children from 5 to 11 years of age, that the current language curriculum and standard reading interventions provided in New Zealand schools do not adequately address the needs of children who enter school with low language abilities. This suggests that either the curriculum or the methods of reading instruction require modification or new interventions need to be implemented to enhance these children's development in the early school years. SLTs' expertise and scope of practice suggest that they have a critical role in supporting and collaborating with teachers to ensure that the language needs of young children are being enhanced within their classroom learning (Neilson, A22).

Of fundamental importance to literacy and academic success is strong oral language development. Gillon and Schwarz (2001b) developed and administered a screening test to explore critical spoken language skills for academic success in 6-year-old children in New Zealand. The screening test measures articulation, receptive and expressive language and PA. A total of 952 children were screened across the country, with children with any type of diagnosed disorder that would influence speech or language development excluded from the study. The results indicated that as many as 18% of the children warranted in-depth assessment of their spoken language skills. Consistent with Tunmer, et al.'s (2006) findings, the study indicted those children from schools in low socioeconomic areas and Māori children were overrepresented in the at-risk group.

Provision of SLT services needs to expand to ensure adequate resourcing for SLTs to work with educators in early intervention and preventative roles. Subsequent reading and writing difficulties experienced by young New Zealand children identified as being at risk due to delayed or disordered spoken language development can be prevented with appropriate intensity levels of intervention and intervention focused on building underlying skills critical for literacy success (Carson, Gillon & Boustead, 2013; Gillon, 2000, 2002, 2005). Funding of SLT services must be at a sufficient level to ensure that research-based interventions can be implemented when appropriate to meet individual children's needs.

A further challenge for the educational community is raising literacy achievement for boys. A recent international literacy study documenting reading comprehension performance of fourth-grade children (average age 9;6) in 45 countries (Progress in International Reading Literacy Study, PIRLS, 2011; Mullis, Martin, Foy & Drucker, 2012) indicated that boys are achieving significantly lower than girls in literacy at an international level. In nearly all of the countries, girls outperformed boys, and there has been little reduction in the reading achievement gender gap over the last decade. In New Zealand, the difference between boys' and girls' reading comprehension performance was more marked than in many other countries such as Italy, France, Germany, USA and Canada, but similar to the difference between boys and girls reading comprehension abilities in Australia, England and Finland. Mirroring these data clinically, SLTs typically have many more boys on their caseloads than girls, and the relationship between early speech and language difficulties observed in boys and their academic achievement needs to be further explored.

Challenges are frequently best addressed through collaborative efforts. The current challenges in meeting the needs of children with speech and language impairments require enhanced meaningful relationships between various communities. Partnerships between universities (or the providers of SLT and teacher education), school and family communities, government bodies in policy and funding services and appropriate cultural and ethnic groups need to be well established. Such collaborations must be directed towards a common goal of ensuring that every child meets his or her educational, social and cultural potential to contribute to their society in positive ways.

The New Zealand education system provides a strong context for collaborative efforts between SLTs and teachers to flourish.

The PIRLS 2011 study (Mullis et al., 2012) also investigated teaching contexts and how teachers work together. Teachers in the middle schools years frequently favour collaborative teaching practices and in New Zealand primary school children are more likely to have been taught by 'very collaborative' teachers than many other countries.

Maintaining meaningful partnerships between universities and the education community is an area of particular importance. In New Zealand, all providers of SLT training are in universities that have a strong research orientation. Academics teaching in SLT education programs are expected to conduct research in areas of relevance and importance to their discipline. Robust, scientific models of research using both quantitative and/or qualitative designs are embraced. Effective partnerships between the academic communities of SLT (as well as other relevant academic disciplines, such as audiology, education, linguistics and psychology) will help facilitate the transfer of knowledge from research to the practice of SLT.

As with all good partnerships, trust and respect between the academic communities of SLT and the educational community are vital. The knowledge of the researcher and the knowledge of the practitioner need to be understood and equally respected. Ethical responsibilities in conducting human research must be of paramount importance, yet a balance between protecting children, families and school communities and potentially restricting most forms of science-based research needs to be reached. The practitioners must trust the researcher to act in an ethically responsible manner and adopt methodological procedures approved via robust ethical clearance processes. The researchers need to trust practitioners involved in research studies to implement research protocols as agreed, to maintain confidentiality, and to adhere to standard research procedures. Developing vigorous partnerships in research where both practitioners and researchers in SLT and teacher education contribute to the advancement of knowledge is essential, to address the challenges faced by our profession.

Through partnerships, the practical implications of the research can be more adequately addressed. Consideration of a number of factors is important in deciding whether it is appropriate for the latest research findings to be immediately integrated into clinical or teaching practice (Ingram, 1998). The depth of the research body, the quality of the research methodologies employed and treatment fidelity measures, the relevance of the findings to a specific clinical population, the practicalities of implementing an assessment or intervention technique explored under ideal research conditions into a school setting and the appropriateness of the intervention to a child's cultural, family and educational environment all influence the transfer of research knowledge to practice.

The small population base and geographical size of New Zealand is conducive to facilitating relationships at regional and national levels. Indeed, historically, there have always been strong and close affiliations between the academic and professional community in SLT and New Zealand educational communities both from a teaching and research perspective. Maintaining and further enhancing these partnerships will be critical as we move forward in the 21st century in successfully addressing the needs of individuals with communication impairments.

Technology, tablet computers and Apps

In A4, Mirla Raz, an SLP clinician in Arizona with over 40 years' experience in private practice and school settings, was cautiously optimistic about the potential for tablet computers and application software (Apps) to enhance the delivery of speech assessment and intervention. At the same time, she pointed to a number of technical shortcomings that currently limit their usefulness as clinical tools. By contrast, when I first heard the next contributor talk about information and communication technology (ICT), tablet computers and Apps it was apparent that, as a speech and language clinician, she embraced their use more wholeheartedly than Raz. Indeed, she wrote, 'the use of Apps and technology has revolutionised how I can and do provide intervention' (Kylie Toynton, personal communication, 2013).

Mrs. Kylie Toynton graduated as a speech pathologist in 2000, and was awarded a Master's degree in Gerontology in 2012. After 12 years in the public sector, Mrs. Toynton is engaged in private practice in a rural Australian location near the small country town of Coonabarabran, NSW. She provides SLP/SLT services to a general paediatric caseload in settings that include early intervention Aboriginal children's services, pre-schools, schools, special education and early education. Her professional interests include the classroom use of technology, access to SLP/SLT services for rural and remote clients, the suitability of Apps and other technology for indigenous Australian and low-income populations, parent and community education regarding technology options and access to ICT in urban centres.

Q33.   Kylie Toynton: A rural Australian view of ICT and Apps in SSD

Technology and speech-language pathology are frequent bedfellows. But, for the SLP/SLT who is interested in EBP the bed *can* be a little uncomfortable. Numerous developers of downloadable worksheets, Apps, online games and other technological offerings have quickly risen to the challenge of developing attractive, inexpensive resources for clinicians to use when working with children with SSD. In this rapidly expanding niche market, some are marketed primarily to clinicians who have welcomed

them with enthusiasm. As well, many if not most are presented as useful tools for parents and teachers to purchase too, to use as well as or instead of SLP/SLT intervention, for children with articulation disorders, phonological disorders and CAS. Unrelenting social media recommendations, online discussion and advertising of Apps and devices mean that clients will often come with questions about them, including questions about their effectiveness. As an ethical SLP in a rural setting, how do you make sense of all of this and guide clients and colleagues towards productive choices? How do you utilise child speech related technology, and what might the future hold?

A33.   Kylie Toynton: Technology and SSD: navigating new pathways, keeping best practice

The vast array of ICT available to SLPs/SLTs may offer the potential to allow us to work more efficiently and at a greater geographical distance from our clients. SLPs/SLTs have embraced ICT even though the rapid increase in technological development has not been associated with a corresponding increase in an evidence base to support its application in clinical settings. This gap creates a difficulty for the clinician pursuing the ideal of evidence-based practice (E³BP, Dollaghan, 2007). While many SLPs/SLTs and consumers are aware of the range of technology available, we need to educate others and ourselves on how best to implement what is on offer to meet our clients' goals (Meredith, Firmin & McAllister, 2013).

ICT affords more service delivery options in the form of telehealth and computer aided intervention. It has created stronger professional connections that allow national and international communication and knowledge sharing, between new and more seasoned colleagues, through the use of Skype,

Twitter and other social media (Davis, 2013). Two questions arise regarding children's SSD: Does ICT help in their assessment and treatment, and do tablet computers and their Apps enhance intervention outcomes?

Assessment Apps may be useful to reduce time spent analysing assessment data. Although this may be an attractive feature for overstretched SLPs/SLTs, speech assessments need to be valid and reliable (Joffe, A34, Skahan, Watson & Lof, 2007, p. 252). The *Sunny Articulation Phonology Test*[1] (Smarty Ears LLC, 2010), the *Bilingual Articulation Phonology Assessment: English/Spanish* (Smarty Ears LLC, 2012) and *Articulation Screener Pro* (Synapse Apps LLC, 2012) make provision for calculating percentage consonants correct (PCC), doing an intelligibility rating, recording the error-types substitution, omission, distortion and additions and phonological process analysis covering backing, cluster reduction, consonant deletion, devoicing, fronting, gliding and stopping. Only one of the few Apps currently available for child speech assessment the *LinguiSystems Articulation Test* (LinguiSystems Inc., 2012) is standardised. It has associated reliability and validity data, and results can be expressed as standard scores, percentile ranks and age equivalents. This is obviously problematic because it is not possible to create articulation tests with 'more difficult words' as the child's age increases. This means that the bell curve that you can have in language testing where test items increase in difficulty, is impossible with articulation tests.

---

[1] All the Apps mentioned in A33 were available in the iTunes App Store (www.apple.com/itunes) at the time of writing: Articulation Station (Little Bee Speech, 2007), ArtikPix (Expressive Solutions LLC, 2010), GoodReader (Selukoff, 2010), EverNote (EverNote, 2012), Speech Sounds on Cue (Bishop, 2011), Speech Tutor (Synapse Apps LLC, 2011), Pocket Artic (Synapse Apps LLC, 2012), PhonoPix (Expressive Solutions LLC, 2010), PocketPairs (Synapse Apps LLC, 2012), SLP Minimal Pairs (SLP Tech Tools, 2012), ApraxiaCards (LinguiSystems Inc., 2012).

A growing number of Apps address intervention for articulation disorders, phonological disorders and CAS. *Articulation Station*, *ArtikPix*, *Speech Sounds on Cue*, *Speech Tutor* and *Pocket Artic*, are designed for traditional articulation therapy (Van Riper, 1978). Apps that incorporate minimal pair activities for children with phonological disorder include *PhonoPix*, *PocketPairs* and *SLP Minimal Pairs*. An App intended for drill practice for children with CAS is *ApraxiaCards*. All of the Apps mentioned have useful features to support intervention for children with SSD, but no one app can support all the activities an SLP/SLT might want to implement in a treatment session. Judicious selection of an App, or a combination of Apps, in conjunction with paper- or game-based activities can potentially meet both clinician and client needs.

Guiding parents

In my clinical experience, parents want support and advice regarding purchase of tablet computers and Apps for their child with SSD. Apps can create an enjoyable learning environment for the child, potentially increasing the likelihood that they will engage in home practice (Toki & Pange, 2012, p. 278). I approach the role of a 'technology advisor' keeping in mind families' different expectations, budgets and knowledge of ICT as exemplified when I was asked by the mother of Sasha, 6;0 to provide advice on the Apps to buy to complete home practice for /s/ and /ɹ/. She wished to buy no more than three, and I suggested *Speech Tutor*, *Speech Sounds on Cue* and *Articulation Station* all cited above. *Speech Tutor* provides lateral cross-sectional and frontal views of the production of individual phonemes only, appealing to children from 4 years of age to adolescents, and those struggling to visualise correct production. The client's sound production can be recorded and the playback speed can be adjusted to facilitate phonetic transcription. This App is valuable only in the phonetic placement (isolated sound stimulability) aspect of intervention. *Speech Sounds on Cue* provides videos of productions of sounds in isolation, words and short phrases, multiple cues for prompting correct production of the target and is available in a US English, a UK English and General Australian English (Cox, 2012). Whilst this App was developed for both adults and children, it is particularly suitable for use in the paediatric population with clear verbal prompts for sound production of individual phonemes and target phonemes in initial position in words with the accompanying visual cues and multiple presentations of the target. Although the child's productions can be recorded and replayed during intervention, audio cannot be stored and there is no provision to record and keep client data within the App. This App is particularly useful in phonetic production training. *Articulation Station* offers photo flashcards to elicit production of consonants in all positions in words at word, sentence and story level suitable for children aged 4;0 and above. Individual and group data can be stored, as can audio data that has been recorded during therapy. The App allows for custom words and images to be uploaded to create personalised word lists. Verbal prompts are presented in Standard American English only, so families who are speakers of other varieties of English need to mute the device and present the cues 'live' to the child in homework sessions.

For the family of Thomas, 4;11 with a phonological disorder, Apps were not a homework option, as they did not own a tablet. However, his pre-school was equipped an iPad, a full-time aide to support the implementation of a speech program and a small fund for purchasing Apps. The pre-school asked me to recommend an App that might help him, and other children with speech difficulties. I recommended the purchase of *PocketPairs* that employs minimal pairs, with listening and production tasks, intended to target 12 developmental processes. The App offers diagrams of the oral cavity for placement, the capacity to store and graph client data and an across venue communication option using comment boxes. It can be used with individuals or groups with children 4;0 and above.

The Tomarakos (2012) *App Review Rating Scale* is a means of scoring and assigning a 1–5 star rating to speech, language and education Apps and users can elect to enter their rating on the App's product page in the iTunes store. I used this tool to evaluate *PocketPairs*, giving it a 4-star rating (15/20).

My use of technology

In my view, the use of Apps and other technology enhances my practice. That being the case, I use a tablet computer in every therapy session I conduct with children with SSD. I utilise technology to access information, and therapy tools and materials from multiple sources, with targets presented in multiple modalities. This enables me to conduct sessions that are motivating for child and parent, and evidence based. My practice is also enhanced through the use of Facebook, Twitter, Pinterest (a pin board style, photo sharing website), YouTube, and web-based resources such as *LessonPix*, and *Tar Heel Reader*.

I use Apps in a variety of other ways. I take advantage of timesaving tools like chronological age calculators, and torch Apps for oral examinations, voice recording Apps, popular game Apps for eliciting production of targets at sentence and conversational level. (Clausen, 2013). I also use document storage Apps like *GoodReader* and *EverNote* for PDF's of therapy materials.

Social media, used for professional purposes provides opportunities to network colleagues and experts worldwide in a way never possible before (Davis, 2013, p. 28). SLPs/SLTs specialising in SSD, organisations supporting children with SSD such as Child-hood Apraxia of Speech Association of North America (Gretz, A7) and some professional journals have Twitter and Facebook accounts linking to information gateways. Online discussion such as phonological therapy group (Bowen, 2001) provides opportunities to ask questions and post information relevant to SSD. Finally, Pinterest is useful for finding, storing and organising ideas for therapy sessions and YouTube for 'how to' videos for new Apps or online programs. Web-based resources such as *LessonPix* allow quick and efficient creation of visuals for use in therapy sessions that can also be emailed to parents for home practice.

The range and immediacy of all these forms of information access help me to feel connected to a much larger community: a very important thing for a rural sole therapist. As well, it connects me to the evidence via professional learning communities (PLCs). PLCs created through social media sites allow SLPs/SLTs to seek the advice of experienced therapists (Davis, 2013, p. 13) and be directed to quality evidence in SSD by their colleagues.

Conclusion

By the time A33 is published there will have been another wave of technological development. I believe that ICT will change our practice in the field of SSD in the areas of service delivery, intervention and professional development. Telehealth will become a familiar service delivery option as the technology that supports its advances. Online virtual worlds could become a method for training parents in SSD therapy techniques (Meredith et al., 2013 p. 45) while waiting for service or to supplement individual therapy (Ruggero, McCabe, Ballard & Munro, 2012). There will be increased availability of standardised articulation and phonology assessments and informal assessments to suit mobile devices

(Limbrick, McCormack & McLeod, 2013, p. 306), and more intervention Apps. Specialty Apps that measure speech acoustics and allow for phonetic transcriptions of speech samples will become more refined. I believe that professional development opportunities will increase with the growth of PLCs via social media, and wider availability of webinars on demand filmed at live events and conferences.

Whether child-speech-related technology enhances intervention outcomes for children with SSD has not yet been studied. However, in my opinion ICT can increase participation and access to appropriate therapy for geographically or socially isolated clients; assist in engaging the 'hard to reach' child in intervention activities through motivating, varied presentation of therapy targets; and improve uptake of home programs by parents due to the universality of the computer/tablet platform. The choice and implementation of technology for each individual child, family and professional will always need to be based on a thorough assessment and the thoughtful selection of targets and goals. The onus of responsibility to do so will always come down to individual clinicians and their commitment to keeping up to date with the new developments and evidence.

Child speech assessment and intervention practices in UK

Dr. Victoria Joffe is a specialist speech and language therapist and professor in developmental speech, language and communication impairments in the Department of Language and Communication Science at City University, London. She is program director of an MSc degree in *Joint Professional Practice: Language and Communication* run in conjunction with the Institute of Education, London (www.talklink.org). Victoria obtained her DPhil degree in the Department of Experimental Psychology, The University of

Oxford, exploring the relationship between oral language ability, metalinguistic awareness and literacy in language-impaired children. Her areas of clinical and research interest include specific language impairment, speech disorder, the interface between education and SLT, the relationship between language and literacy, narrative therapy and language impairment in secondary school age children. Victoria is currently involved in a large-scale intervention project funded by the Nuffield Foundation on enhancing language and communication in secondary school age children with language impairments (http://www.elciss.com).

In research with a colleague at City University (Joffe & Pring, 2008), Dr. Joffe investigated the methods of assessment and remediation of 'phonological problems' used by therapists working in the United Kingdom. The surveyed therapists comprised 9 who were in their first year of practice, 25 with 1–3 years, 13 with 4–6 years, 13 with 7–10 years and 38 with more than 10 years of experience. These SLTs reported using a variety of therapies: auditory discrimination, minimal contrast therapy and phonological awareness were the most popular and were often used in combination. Most respondents reported involving parents, and, in planning therapy, clinicians were more influenced by children's language and cognitive abilities and the motivation of parents than by the nature of the impairment. Probably the most striking outcome of this research was the information about assessment practices. Dr. Joffe talks about this in her response to Q34.

Q34. Victoria Joffe: Common practice in speech sound disorders in UK

Reporting on a survey of child speech practice in the United Kingdom (Joffe & Pring, 2008), you wrote: 'Constraints upon clinicians make it difficult for them to convert research findings to practice. In particular, assessments that allow more individualised and targeted interventions appear little used. Clinicians are aware of research but there is

a danger that clinical practice and research are diverging.' Of your 98 respondents, 83 (85%) used the South Tyneside Assessment of Phonology (STAP; Armstrong & Ainley, 1988) as a primary data source for planning speech intervention. Assessment with the STAP would provide only one small, non-standardised fraction of the relational analysis component of phonological assessment (Baker, 2004; Stoel-Gammon & Dunn, 1985), sufficient for intervention planning. Nonetheless, 77% of the respondents rated themselves 'very confident' or 'confident' in their ability to select therapies. A later survey (Pring, Flood, Dodd & Joffe, 2012) revealed similar practices and beliefs. Can you comment on these remarkable findings and reflect on the possible barriers, in the British context, between pedagogy, research findings and EBP?

A34. Victoria Joffe: Surveys of clinical practice in UK

Around $6\frac{1}{2}$ percent of all UK children have an SSD in the absence of any other cognitive, sensory or physical impairment (Broomfield & Dodd, 2004a). Such children typically dominate SLP/SLT paediatric caseloads (Gierut, 1998), and in Britain most receive treatment in community clinics or schools. Except for anecdotal accounts, little information exists about the practices of SLTs, and a dearth of information around the relationship between practice and outcomes constitutes a serious gap (Kamhi, 2006b). In Joffe, 2009, I provided information on a survey undertaken in 2007 through a carefully constructed questionnaire involving paediatric SLT clinicians across the United Kingdom (Joffe & Pring, 2008). It sought to build a detailed picture of routine practices, experiences and opinions around SSD. In 2010, another national survey was conducted of working practices and clinical experiences of paediatric SLTs (Pring et al., 2012). In A34, I report the findings from both surveys.

The 2007 and 2010 respondents

The 2007 respondents comprised a representative sample of 98 clinicians from the health, education and private sectors. The proportion of children with SSD ranged from 40% or more of their caseloads (44% of participants) to 70% or more (10% of participants). The respondents' clinical experience extended from 1 to 3 years (35%), 4 to 10 years (26%) and over 10 years (39%). Only 7% specialised exclusively in SSD, whereas 42% identified it as one of several specialist areas.

Data from the 2010 study were obtained online via Survey Monkey in three sections, Section A focused on the therapists' level and type of expertise, work settings and work practices; Section B included information on assessment, treatment and management and Section C canvassed SLT's views on changes in healthcare and the benefits to children with speech, language and communication needs (see Pring et al., 2012 for further details of the second study). Approximately 7.5% of paediatric SLTs in the United Kingdom; $n = 516$) responded to the new survey. They appeared broadly representative of paediatric therapists and their workplaces were UK wide. Most respondents worked in the National Health Services (87.6%) with 7.1% in private practice. Years of clinical experience ranged from 0 to 2 years (17.3%); 3 to 5 years (20.3%); 6 to 10 years (19.9%) and over 10 years (42.5%). Respondents were asked to identify the age groups of children with whom they worked classified across five levels: infants (<3 years), pre-school (3–4 years), junior primary (5–7 years), senior primary (8–11 years) and secondary (11–18 years). Most worked with more than one age group, with an average number of age groups across SLTs being 3.33. One hundred and ten

(21.7%) SLTs worked across all 5 age-bands, and only 35 (6.9%) worked in only one. The main work setting for most respondents was mainstream schools (67.4%) and community clinics (52.3%) with some working in special schools (25.4%) and specialist language units (23.5%). The average number of settings for SLTs was 2.34, with some seeing children in five or six different settings.

Generic versus specialist SLTs working in SSD

The respondents were asked to indicate, using five broad categories, the time they spent on specific areas of clinical practice: none; 1–25%; 26–50%; 51–75% and 76–100%. Of the 516 respondents, 428 (82.9%) worked with children with SSD. This high percentage reflects the dominance of SSD in routine clinical practice of paediatric SLTs in the United Kingdom. Of the 428, only 9 (2.1%) reported working in this area for over 75% of their time. Thirty-nine (9.1%) worked with SSD between 51% and 75% of the time, 113 (26.4%) worked in this area between 26% and 50%, with the majority, 268 SLTs (62.6%) working between 0% and 25% of the time with this client group. It appears that an overwhelming majority of paediatric SLTs work with SSD in addition to a range of other difficulties within their expertise. Not all the SLTs working more than 50% of the time with children with SSD perceive themselves as specialists in SSD. Indeed, only 23 of the 48 SLTs (47.9%) working with this client group over 50% did so; whilst 110 of the 381 SLTs (28.8%) working with this client group for less than 50% of their time viewed themselves as specialists in this area. This indicates that most SLTs working with children with SSD are not specialists in the field, and that many affected children are seen by non-specialist SLTs. This is a similar finding across all types of paediatric speech and language disorders, except for paediatric dysphagia, where specialists see most clients (Pring et al., 2012). These data reflect the respondents' comments. One-fifth of them (20.5%) said their caseload did not utilise their specialist skills. Critical that the structure of their service required them to be generalists, respondents expressed frustration at their inability to use or establish their specialist areas. They identified heavy caseloads, with insufficient time for reading, training and mentoring less experienced clinicians as a main reason why they could not develop their specialist areas. This worrying trend of SLTs being restricted by their managers (frequently non clinicians) in attending training and other CPD has been identified by the RCSLT. It is being addressed by the College through several initiatives, for example, the creation of RCSLT regional hubs to encourage greater collaboration across SLTs and higher education institutions (Gadhok, 2013), and the name change for specialist groups, from 'Specific Interest Groups' to 'Clinical Excellence Networks' to highlight the importance of training in achieving clinical excellence (Harulow, 2013).

A day in the life of a paediatric SLT

In the 2010 survey we explored participants' time management, asking them to quantify the time they spent on assessment, intervention (direct and indirect), on report writing, attending meetings and administration. As a whole group, 22.4% reported to be involved in direct intervention, with 27.5% involved in indirect intervention (14.8% training other professionals and 12.7% training parents). Conducting and analysing assessments took a further 13.2% of time with the remainder on some combination of administration, meetings and report writing. Thus, less than 25% of their time is devoted to direct intervention. Over 40% of SLTs (44.7%) felt their workload and distribution did not make the best use of their time. When asked what their ideal

work distribution would be, the percentage of time increased for intervention to 64.5%, with 28.3% of time for direct intervention. Time allocated for all other activities, including assessment, were reduced (Pring et al., 2012). Twenty-five percent of SLTs working with SSD reported to undertake direct speech intervention more than 50% of their time with only 5.8% and 3.9% conducting indirect therapy with the training of other professionals and parents over 50% of their time, respectively.

Whilst the survey did not have a category for keeping current with the literature or undertaking research or research-related activities, there was an open category, 'other'. No participant mentioned research or any research-related activity in this category.

Assessment

In our first survey, the participants identified 21 assessments, between them, that they used most frequently to identify and assess SSD, with majority (85%) nominating the *South Tyneside Assessment of Phonology: STAP* (Armstrong & Ainley, 1988; 1992). A picture emerged of clinicians choosing this quick screening tool, supplemented by other non-standardised assessments, including personally designed assessments and informal observation. The picture remained similar in 2010 among the 221 therapists who worked mainly with children with SSD. Fifteen assessments were identified between all 221, with most identifying the *STAP* as their assessment of choice (27.6%), compared with the *Diagnostic Evaluation of Articulation of Phonology (DEAP)* (11.3%) (Dodd, Zhu, Crosbie, Holm & Ozanne, 2002), the *CLEAR Phonology Screening Assessment* (9.5%) (Keeling & Keeling, 2006) and the *Nuffield Dyspraxia Program Assessment* (8.5%) (in Williams & Stephens, 2004). Sixteen percent identified 'informal assessment' as their assessment of choice, with 9%

identifying the Renfrew Action Picture Test (RAPT) (Renfrew, 2010). The top reasons for their choices were: test availability speed and ease of administration, scoring and analysis; and test familiarity. The specific reason for including the RAPT was to quickly gain an overview of language ability together with speech in context.

The popularity of the inexpensive, small, easily transportable *STAP* and *CLEAR* with their quick administration and scoring, plus informal observations is somewhat understandable. Regrettably, they are unlikely to provide sufficient detail to permit adequate description, diagnosis or optimal therapy planning. Moreover, there is a danger that incomplete or insufficient assessment protocols will seriously limit intervention practices (Bernhardt & Holdgrafer, 2001a, b). It is pleasing, therefore, that the *DEAP* was more prominent in the 2010 survey and second to STAP in popularity, albeit with much less frequency.

Alternative, detailed linguistic analyses such as psycholinguistic profiling (Stack-house & Wells, 1997) and non-linear analysis (Bernhardt & Stemberger, 2000) enable more precise identification of the nature and levels of speech impairment (see Bernhardt & Ullrich, A37; Gardner, A27; Froud, A38). These analyses take more time than STAP-type measures, and perhaps more time than many clinicians might have. This is reflected in the second survey with only one therapist mentioning the psycholinguistic framework and none mentioning non-linear analysis. They also require specialist knowledge, sometimes necessitating additional training. The financial climate has, if anything worsened since the first survey and clinicians are increasingly restricted in the CPD/CEU events they can attend, exacerbating a situation in which the 2010 respondents identified heavy caseloads and insufficient time for reading as major barriers to developing specialisms. Additionally and anecdotally, UK SLTs fear implementing in-depth speech anal-

yses, sometimes acknowledging their own lack of expertise, like one 2007 respondent who claimed she and some of her colleagues were 'terrified' by psycholinguistic models (Gardner, A27 provides reassurance!). The few references to psycholinguistic profiling in the 2010 survey suggest this fear and uncertainty persists.

The 2007 and 2010 respondents noted dissatisfaction with their limited assessment options, and were often unable to extend their choices due to financial restrictions. We found that some workplaces could afford just one copy of an assessment, obviating its routine use throughout a service. For example, the *DEAP* costs over £300, so most clinic budgets can only extend to purchasing one or two. Clinicians using screening measures rather than comprehensive phonological analysis mean they gain insufficient information for selecting the most appropriate intervention *and* treatment targets for an individual child.

Therapy, clinician confidence and evidence

Our first survey suggested that SLTs were aware of research, and that this awareness reinforced their confidence in choosing between therapies, but this was not necessarily so. Some respondents expressed confidence although unimpressed by or unaware of the evidence, whereas some *were* aware of the evidence but reported a lack of confidence. In the analysis, confidence was particularly high, especially among experienced clinicians, with 79% of all respondents confident or very confident in their ability to select an appropriate therapy. Only 3 of the 98 rated themselves as 'not very' or 'not at all' confident. Asked whether they felt there was sufficient evidence for the effectiveness of therapy for SSD, 72% agreed or strongly agreed that strong evidence supported their clinical practice.

Confidence and knowledge of the evidence appear closely related. While 60% agreed or strongly agreed that sufficient evidence existed, and were confident or very confident about selecting a therapy, a substantial minority disagreed, with 19% of respondents confident in their therapy choice but ambivalent about the evidence for its effectiveness, and 11% agreeing that there was sufficient evidence while reporting low confidence in choosing a therapy. So, very intriguingly, on one hand, therapists appear to know about available research evidence and this knowledge improved their confidence in selecting a therapy, but on the other hand, a sizable minority, who expressed confidence, were either unimpressed by or unaware of the evidence. This suggests that their confidence emanated from clinical experience rather than from their reading of research findings, exemplifying the research-practice gap (Duchan, 2001; Joffe, 2008; McLeod & Baker, 2004).

This notion of confidence emanating from the therapists' own clinical experience is supported by the 2010 findings. Participants were asked to identify whether the following options influenced their interventions, 'a lot', 'a little' or 'not at all'. The options included (1) own experience of working with this client group; (2) experience passed on by other therapists; (3) treatment protocols set by the workplace; (4) theoretical research on the client group; or (5) research evidence underpinning the intervention. Seventy-six percent reported that their intervention choices were influenced 'a lot' by their own clinical experiences, with just over half of them (54.2%) influenced a lot by other therapists, and only 21% being influenced a lot by set protocols. Thirty-four percent and 35.7% of respondents said they were influenced 'a lot' by theoretical research on the client group and the evidence underpinning the intervention, respectively. Just over half of respondents were influenced 'a little' by the theoretical research on the client

group (52%) and evidence of the effectiveness of the intervention (52%), with 2.7% and 3.6% not influenced at all by either, respectively. It appears that the main influence of treatment options is the therapists' own clinical experience and judgement and that most use the literature and research evidence 'a little'. Therapists do not appear to be engaging with the research or drawing on research evidence to inform intervention practices.

Therapy selection

The first survey explored the factors that drove the SLTs' therapy choices. They appeared most concerned about general factors that might affect therapy, particularly the child's age (57%) and parental 'attitude' (56%), including the parents' motivation, awareness of the problem and level of concern. Then, they were interested in general indicators of children's ability, specifically: attention and listening (30%), language performance (21%) and cognitive ability (17%). The child's own awareness of his or her problem was important to 15% of respondents. The child's phonological characteristics were given far less prominence than the considerations itemised above. Here, the severity of the disorder was the *only* frequently mentioned factor (40%) followed by information about delay/disorder (16%) and stimulability (11%). Strikingly, and undoubtedly due to time and expertise constraints, few therapists said they would conduct more detailed phonological analyses or investigate phonological knowledge as a basis for choosing a therapy.

Drawing on 14 readily identifiable therapies from published sources, the 2007 participants reported their frequency of use as: just over 2 therapies all the time, 4–5 most of the time and 8–9 sometimes, indicating SLTs' eclecticism in choosing and combining approaches across clients and SSD types.

They also had clear favourites: with 50% always or often using *auditory discrimination*, *minimal contrast therapy* and *phonological awareness*, and 84% employing all three at least some of the time. Apparently, therapists combine them as a core (or 'standard package') method of treatment, targeting different levels of input and output processing (Pascoe, Stackhouse & Wells, 2005). These findings are supported, to some extent, in the second survey, where therapists were asked to list the interventions they used. The same three favourites from 2007 were named the most by therapists in 2010: auditory discrimination, minimal contrast therapy and phonological awareness. Interestingly, this triad were the most frequent interventions mentioned in a more recent survey of 536 UK paediatric SLTs (Roulstone, Wren, Bakopoulou, Goodlad & Lindsay, 2012).

Several therapists referred to using 'an eclectic approach' and both traditional articulation therapy and phonological intervention were listed as treatment options. The published treatment approach named the most by therapists was the *Nuffield Dyspraxia Program* (39 citations) (Williams & Stephens, 2004), compared with *Metaphon* (16 citations) (Dean, Howell, Waters & Reid, 1995), and *Core Vocabulary* (16 citations) (Crosbie, Holm & Dodd, 2005). Five therapists mentioned using psycholinguistic profiling to underpin their intervention and seven referred to oro-motor work. Other therapies named included Cued Articulation (5 citations) (Passy, 1993); Talk Tools (4 citations), (Rosenfeld-Johnson, 2001); Jolly Phonics (4 citations) (Lloyd & Wernham, 1992; Signalong) (3 citations) (Kennard, 1997); Cycles Approach (1 citation) (Hodson & Paden, 1991) and PROMPT (1 citation) (Hayden, 1984).

The popularity of the conventional minimal pair approach (Weiner, 1981), one of the most commonly cited SSD interventions (Joffe & Serry, 2004) is confirmed by McLeod and Baker (2004). The prevalent use of phonological awareness (PA) activities was unsurprising given PA's prominence in the SLP/SLT, psychology and education literature (Hatcher, Hulme & Ellis, 1994; Hulme et al., 2002). Reports of the effectiveness of PA training in remediating speech disorders are equivocal (Hesketh, Adams, Nightingale & Hall, 2000; Gillon, 2000; Denne, Langdown, Pring & Roy, 2005) and its customary adoption with all speech-disordered children should be viewed cautiously (Dodd & Gillon, 2001). The inclusion of auditory discrimination is quite remarkable, as some children with SSD have robust auditory discrimination skills alongside severe output difficulties (Stackhouse & Wells, 1997), and for them, work on auditory discrimination may be redundant, time wasting and unjustifiable. The inclusion of oro-motor work is also surprising, considering the absence of evidence supporting its use (Hodge, A31; Lof, A35; Powell, A39). The occurrence, albeit small, of psycholinguistic profiling, in assessment and treatment, in the second survey, may indicate growing confidence in using psycholinguistic processing models.

Parents and intervention

Three quarters of respondents in the first survey reported always or often involving parents in therapy, with 43% in the 'always' category, whilst respondents in the second survey spent 12.7% of their time undertaking indirect intervention with parents. Seeing parents as a useful resource in SSD management may have been encouraged by research accounts of their use (e.g., Bowen & Cupples, 1999a, b, 2004; Lancaster, Keusch, Levin, Pring & Martin, 2010). It is difficult to determine the expectations SLTs have of parents, and whether they select their treatments with parental involvement in mind (Watts Pappas, A30). Parents' variability in their ability to assist their own children may affect therapy outcomes unpredictably. In fact, it may be a *concern* if SLTs are so accustomed to engaging them routinely as 'co-therapists' that they are reluctant to treat children whose parents are unable, unavailable or unwilling to participate in therapy sessions or homework. There is a hint that this may *indeed* be the case with over 50% of the 2007 respondents emphasising the importance of parental attitude or motivation in making decisions about treatment. Therapists' preference for including parents in their intervention remains strong, as seen from survey two, where, when asked for their ideal distribution of their time, therapists increased the existing time they spent working with parents from 12% to 17%.

Eclecticism

Curiously, therapists are both confident in selecting therapies and convinced they work. Support for the view that 'therapies work' comes from research demonstrating various therapy approaches are effective for a substantial number of children with SSD (e.g., Allen, 2013; Gillon, 2000; Hesketh et al., 2000; Rvachew, Nowak & Cloutier, 2004; Rvachew, Ohberg, Grawburg & Heyding, 2003). But this evidence may confuse practitioners wanting to apply it clinically, and little advice exists to tell them which therapies to use for what and with whom! These different therapies may all appear effective because of careful research-subject selection and because they each constitute an optimal approach for certain children (or certain SSDs). If this holds, then even greater gains may be achieved if clinicians eschew eclecticism, incorporating into their practices explicitly principled, evidence-based matching between children and therapies.

Alarmingly, the eclecticism that, from our studies, appears *usual* in UK clinical practice is unsupported by recent SSD research, which more typically examines the effects of specific therapies, for example, phonologi-

cal awareness (Gillon, 2000; Hesketh et al., 2000) and core vocabulary (Crosbie, Holm & Dodd, 2005; Dodd, Holm, Crosbie & McIntosh, 2006). While the therapies in the evidence-base for SSD treatment foster optimism, they are not the therapies of choice for our representative UK clinicians across both surveys, and little is known about the effectiveness of their preferred (auditory discrimination plus minimal contrast therapy plus phonological awareness) eclectic approach.

By the same token, eclecticism seems reasonable in relation to the heterogeneity of children with SSD (Dodd, 2005). The chances are relatively good that one area of focus of a 'catch all' eclectic approach will meet the needs of particular individual clients. At least one small-n study (Lancaster et al., 2010) shows promising outcomes from an eclectic therapeutic approach. An eclectic approach may work because it targets a variety of levels, and therefore may benefit a wide range of children. But although *effective*, such an approach may not be the most *efficient* and, as discussed above more powerful *effects* may be achieved by matching specific therapies to different types of SSD. This continues to be the challenge for researchers and clinicians working with SSD.

Implications of the surveys

Our surveys, despite being 3 years apart, and having different areas of focus, report greater similarity of findings than differences, and provide a unified, clear direction for researchers and therapists. There is a continuing need to address questions of which specific therapy, or therapy mix, is most effective for which group of children with SSD, rather than simply asking whether a therapy is effective for SSD. In addition, ways must be identified for clinicians to incorporate detailed phonological analyses into their customary assessment protocols. Our second survey shows that therapists continue to use quick screening tools as their assessment of choice, with negligible psycholinguistic profiling or in-depth speech analysis reported in routine clinical practice. The extent of training in SSD provided to student SLTs during graduate training, and the subsequent availability of CPD and training in SSD for graduate SLTs demand further reflection, considering that the majority of paediatric SLTs work with SSD, whether as specialists or non-specialists. This has important resource implications and discussions must involve SLTs, SLT managers, national health and education managers, policy makers and professional bodies. Furthermore, researchers and therapists must cooperate in diminishing the research-practice gap. Once clinical researchers have investigated the efficacy of specific treatments, SLTs should be encouraged to evaluate their effectiveness and fidelity in 'real' clinical contexts, as part of routine clinical practice. Researchers should be encouraged to increase their focus on issues that directly reflect, and influence, clinical practice, like the differential impact of service delivery models (including dose, schedule and agent of therapy) on outcome (Cirrin & Gillam, 2008; Kamhi, 2006a). As work partners, researchers and therapists can succeed in identifying the most effective, efficient and efficacious therapies for this client group.

Non-speech oral motor exercises

In the same vein as Dr. Megan Hodge in Canada (A31), our next author has investigated the extent of the use of NS-OME by speech-language clinicians in the United States, and the reasons they are employed. In doing so, he has searched for possible explanations for the enduring popularity of these practices despite their having to compete with interventions for SSD that, unlike NS-OME, have empirical support (Baker & McLeod, 2011a,

2011b; Muttiah, Georges & Brackenbury, 2011; Tyler, 2008).

Dr. Gregory Lof is a Professor and the Chair of the Department of Communication Sciences and Disorders at the MGH institute of Health Professions, a graduate school founded by the Massachusetts General Hospital in Boston, Massachusetts. His research, teaching and clinical work primarily involve children with SSD. He is also interested in professional issues, specifically the use of science and pseudoscience in speech-language pathology. Recent research, writings and lectures have been in the area of the lack of efficacy of using NS-OME to change speech sound productions. Dr. Lof was the 2004 and 2009 topic coordinator for SSD for the ASHA conventions and served on the 1995, 1998, 2002, 2007 and 2008 ASHA Convention Program Committees. He is or has been an editorial consultant for the journals *Journal of Speech, Language, Hearing Research, American Journal of Speech-Language Pathology, Contemporary Issues in Communication Sciences and Disorders* and *Language, Speech, and Hearing Services in Schools*. He was a member on ASHA's Center for Evidence-Based Practice in Communication Disorders that conducted evidence-based systematic reviews of oral motor exercises. He has published numerous articles and has presented over 50 peer-reviewed and 70 invited presentations and workshops at ASHA conventions, universities, school districts and state and international association conventions. He was a keynote speaker at the annual convention of the Speech Pathology Australia (2010), the Velo-Cardio-Facial Syndrome international conference (2011) and at the Oyer Distinguished Lecturer Series (2013) at Michigan State University. He became an ASHA Fellow in 2012.

Q35.   Gregory L. Lof: NS-OME in North America under the microscope

Controversy surrounds the range of therapy activities and techniques categorised as NS-OME or 'oral motor activities' that are implemented in an effort to address speech sound production problems. Nevertheless, they are commonly used by SLPs in North America, often in conjunction with 'tools and toys', including bite blocks, straws and tubes, horns and other toy wind instruments, chewable objects such as 'chewy tubes' and thickened drinks. What exercises are used and why? What is the evidence and logic against using these exercises? Is there evidence and logic in their favour? Why do clinicians continue to use them? What is the responsibility of ASHA and other continuing education providers and sponsors in ensuring that therapy techniques that are presented to CEU/CPD participants adhere to the principles of EBP?

A35. Gregory L. Lof: The NS-OME phenomenon in speech pathology practice

It is puzzling to think that the controversial therapy technique of NS-OME to change speech sound production problems is in common practice among SLPs. In North America, NS-OME is used by approximately 85% of SLPs in the United States (Lof & Watson, 2008) and Canada (Hodge et al., 2005); there are reports that these exercises are frequently used in other parts of the world, as well (Mackenzie, Muir & Allen, 2010). Why 'puzzling'? Because convincing evidence for their use is lacking and motor and linguistic theories do not support them. My exploration of the issues surrounding NS-OME begins with a series of questions. How can NS-OME be defined? What exercises are used and why? What is the logic and evidence against using these exercises? Why do clinicians continue to use them? How can we ensure that clinicians are using therapy techniques that adhere to the principles of EBP?

One of several possible definitions of NS-OME is any technique that does not require the child to produce a speech sound but is used to influence the development of speaking abilities (Lof & Watson, 2008; see also McCauley et al., 2009; Ruscello, 2008). The term 'oral motor' relates to movements and placements of the oral musculature. While the existence and importance of the oral motor aspects of speech production are not in dispute, the use of NS-OME is controversial. Such exercises, aimed at directly changing the performance of the articulators for speech production, typically include blowing horns, whistles and cotton balls; tongue wags, curls and push-ups; tongue-to-nose-to-chin, pucker-smile and big-smile movements; puffing cheeks out; and blowing kisses (Lof & Watson, 2008). SLPs who use them believe their clients' speech will benefit relative to enhanced tongue elevation and lateralisation; better oral-kinaesthetic awareness; stronger tongues, lips and sucking; and improved jaw stabilisation, lip/tongue protrusion, control of drooling and velopharyngeal competence (Lof & Watson, 2008).

Theoretical issues

Many scholars and clinicians have questioned the use of NS-OME on theoretical grounds (Clark, 2003, 2005, 2010; Forrest, 2002; Lof, 2003; Lof, 2008; Lof & Watson, 2008, 2010; Ruscello, 2008; Watson & Lof, 2008), raising issues of (1) part–whole training and transfer, (2) strengthening of the articulators, (3) task specificity, (4) relevancy and (5) awareness.

Part–whole training and transfer

Part–whole training and transfer imply that breaking a task (in this instance, speaking) into smaller components will have an on production of the whole task; for example, working on isolated sounds rather than linguistic units. Researchers and clinicians have demonstrated repeatedly that segmental production will not transfer to the syllable or word levels (e.g., Bernhardt & Stemberger, 2000; Hodson, 2007, 2010; Ingram & Ingram, 2001). But curiously, NS-OME breaks the speaking task into even smaller gestures than sounds-in-isolation, when, for example, tongue tip-to-alveolar ridge movement gestures are practised to teach alveolar stops, or lip puckers are elicited repeatedly in hopes of enhancing lip rounding for vowel productions. Criticising this compartmentalisation, Forrest (2002, pp. 18–19) noted, '... tasks that comprise highly organized or integrated movements will not be enhanced by learning the constituent parts; rather training on parts of these organized behaviors will diminish learning'. She reminds us that, 'Fractionating a behavior that is composed of interrelated parts is not likely to provide relevant information for the appropriate development of neural substrates'. Applying this reasoning, it appears there is inadequate theoretical justification for training disconnected, small 'component' parts of the speech gestures on the assumption that it will transfer to the whole, namely speech.

Strengthening of the articulators

The supposed need for strength is a frequently stated reason for conducting NS-OME (Lof & Watson, 2008), raising four pertinent questions (1) How do clinicians verify that oral musculature strength is diminished in children with SSD? (2) How much strength does speaking require? (3) Do NS-OME increase articulator strength? (4) Do children with SSD have weak articulators? Clinicians typically measure articulator strength subjectively, for example, by feeling the force of the tongue pushing against a tongue depressor, gloved finger, or cheek, or by simply 'observing' weakness (Solomon & Munson, 2004). But seasoned clinicians are even less accurate in their 'guesstimations' of reduced strength than are student clinicians (Clark,

Hensen, Barber, Stierwalt & Sherrill, 2003). This means that SLPs/SLTs probably cannot initially verify whether strength is diminished so they also cannot then report an increase in strength following an NS-OME regimen. But how much strength is needed for speaking? The answer: 'not much', prompted Wenke, Goozee, Murdoch & LaPointe (2006 p. 15) to state, '... caution should be taken when directly associating tongue strength to speech'. For example, lip muscle-force for speaking is only about 10–20% of the maximal capabilities for lip-force, and the jaws use only about 11–15% of their potential force (Bunton & Weismer, 1994; Forrest, 2002).

Even if strengthening were necessary, the question remains, 'Do NS-OME really increase articulator strength?' Answer: 'probably not.' To strengthen any muscle, exercises must be done repeatedly, against resistance, to the point of fatigue... again and again. This standard and empirically supported muscle-strengthening paradigm, relevant to all muscle groups, is used whenever someone adheres to a weight-training program (Clark, 2008; Clark, O'Brien, Calleja & Corrie, 2009). Armed with this indisputable evidence, let's pose a three-part question about a commonly used NS-OME. How many tongue-wag repetitions do most clinicians require clients to perform, how often and are the wags done against resistance? If the answers are 'not many', 'not often' and 'seldom,' respectively – probably *no* lasting strength gains accrue from these exercises. And when strengthening does occur due to extensive exercise drills, not only are the articulator strength gains not maintained over time, but they also do not improve speech (Sjögreena, Tuliniusb, Kiliaridisc & Lohmanderd, 2010). Finally, do children with SSD have oral weakness? Definitely not, according to Sudbery, Wilson, Broaddus and Potter (2006) who demonstrated objectively that pre-school-aged children with SSD had *stronger* articulators than their peers with age-typical speech (see also Dworkin & Culatta, 1980).

Task specificity

Addressing the topic of task specificity leads us to the truism: 'speech is special' (Kent, 2004; Liberman, 1996). The anatomical structures used for speaking and other mouth tasks, like swallowing, sucking and breathing, function in different ways, each mediated by different parts of the brain (Bunton, 2008; Wilson, Green, Yunusova & Moore, 2008). In other words, although identical structures are involved, organisation of movements within the nervous system is not the same for speech gestures as it is for non-speech gestures; and the neural bases of motor control are different for speech and non-speech oral movements. An example of this can be observed in patients with dysphagia, whose swallowing function (non-speech) is compromised while the same structures function adequately for speech (Ziegler, 2003). Weismer (2006) summarises 11 studies showing that speech and non-speech neuromotor movements are different for numerous structures, including facial muscles, the maxilla, mandible, tongue, lips and palate. Furthermore, Bonilha, Moser, Rorden, Bylis and Fredriksson (2006) used functional magnetic resonance imaging (fMRI) to demonstrate that non-speech movements activated different parts of the brain than did speech movements. Evidence from task specificity studies therefore indicates that working on non-speech activities will fail to change speech (Ludlow et al., 2008; Schulz, Dingwall & Ludlow, 1999).

Relevance

NS-OME usually lack relevance. Because isolated articulator movements do not constitute or even resemble the actual gestures used for the production of any sounds in English, their value in improving phonetic production is highly questionable. It seems ridiculous to contemplate, but no speech sounds require tongue-tip elevation towards the nose, puffed-out cheeks, blowing, or tongue wagging! Oral movements that are irrelevant to speech movements will not be effective as speech therapy techniques.

Awareness

Some NS-OME programs centre on a 'meta-mouth' assumption of children developing, via the exercises, metacognitive awareness of articulatory place, manner and movement, alongside a process of 'waking up' or 'warming up' the speech musculature (Lof & Watson, 2008). Muscle warm-up may be appropriate prior to exercise regimens, like distance running or weight training, designed to maximally tax the system (Pollock et al., 1998). Conversely, muscle warm-up is superfluous for less strenuous tasks that are below the maximum, like walking, handwriting or lifting a spoon-to-mouth. Because speaking does not even approach the oral muscular maximum, warm-up is unnecessary. Besides, children up to and including 7-year olds are probably unable to use the mouth cues provided by NS-OME to make themselves more aware of their oral structures (Klein, Lederer & Cortese, 1991; Koegel, Koegel & Ingham, 1986). Because of this lack of 'metamouth' awareness, no transfer to speech occurs from the NS-OME movements and mouth awareness cues.

The research evidence

The *theoretical* underpinnings for using NS-OME to improve children's speech are not strong, but might a literature search reveal *research* supporting their widespread use by clinicians who want their practices to be guided by the principles of EBP? Answer: 'no'. Exhaustive systematic reviews of available published data have been conducted, only to report that no studies exist showing that NS-OME for speech are or are not beneficial (Lee & Gibbon, 2011; McCauley et al., 2009). This confusing conclusion is due to the shortage of published well-designed research studies. On the other hand, several unpublished research studies that have been presented at peer-reviewed ASHA national conventions (e.g., Abrahamsen & Flack, 2002; Bush, Stager, Mann-Kahris & Insalaco, 2004; Colone & Forrest, 2000; Occhino & McCann, 2001; Roehrig, Suiter & Pierce, 2004) and in other forums (Forrest & Iuzzini, 2008; Guisti & Cascella, 2005) report that NS-OME are ineffective in bringing about changes in speech sound productions. Only one presentation (Fields & Polmanteer, 2002) shows any positive effects of NS-OME, and that study has fatal methodological flaws. The available evidence overwhelming demonstrates no benefits from using NS-OME either alone or in combination with proven therapy techniques.

Research has been conducted on the popular horn hierarchy (Talk Tools®) to determine the progression of blowing difficulty over a series of 10 prescribed horns. Proposed reasons for using this horn program are to ' . . . normalise oral musculature, correct articulation errors, improve abdominal grading and speech clarity . . . ' (Talk-Tools, 2013). Purportedly, this horn blowing strengthens targeted muscle groups in a 'measured progression' (Rosenfeld-Johnson, 1999). Jones and colleagues (Jones, Hardin-Jones & Brown, 2011; Ogg, Jones & Hardin-Jones, 2012) tested the horns by using a compressed air tank to determine the aerodynamic thresholds required to produce sound, as well as measuring intraoral pressures from typically developing children using the same horns. Not only was it determined that the horns were not at all representative of typical speech production, but also that the intraoral pressures required to blow the horns did not increase systematically from horns to horn up the hierarchy. This calls into question the

basic premise of the blowing exercise kit. At the time of writing, similar claims for the straw hierarchy have not been evaluated.

Clinicians' and associations' responsibilities

Given the weak theoretical underpinnings and the absence of evidence supporting the use of NS-OME, why do clinicians persist in using this technique? Muttiah et al. (2011) were interested in this question in their qualitative study where they interviewed 11 SLPs who used NS-OME and 11 researchers who do not. The main conclusion was that these two groups use different forms of 'evidence' to make clinical decisions: researchers rely on published research and sound theoretical concepts while clinicians rely on observations of perceived effectiveness. SLPs/SLTs probably continue to use NS-OME for a range of reasons: the procedures constitute an easy 'cookbook' approach that can be followed in a step-by-step fashion; the exercises give the appearance that something tangible is being 'done' in therapy; various techniques and tools have been heavily and attractively promoted in self-published materials and workshops; many practicing clinicians do not read the peer-reviewed professional literature; occupational and physical therapists on multidisciplinary teams encourage exercises; and frequently other clinicians persuade their colleagues to use these techniques (Lof & Watson, 2008). This final reason reminds me of Kamhi (2004, p. 110), who said, ' . . . no human being is immune to hearing a not-so-good idea and passing it on to someone else'.

Professional organisations and universities can play a role in fostering scientific environments that enable clinicians to become more knowledgeable consumers of new, innovative and controversial treatments (Watson & Lof, 2009). But ultimately the SLP/SLT him- or herself must be able to critically evaluate the logic used and the evidence claimed because it is only through adherence to scientific methodologies that our field can progress (Kamhi, 2004; Lof, 2011). As stated by Mackenzie et al. (2010), we must be willing to give up the 'folklore' of our profession that has been handed down by word of mouth for generations so we can move forward with the adoption of scientifically valid procedures.

While it would be most advantageous to have one efficient, effective treatment procedure like NS-OME to correct all types of problems, it must be conceded that the likelihood of the existence of such a magical procedure is improbable. One of the reasons for EBP is not only to promote the use of proven effective treatments, but also to delay the adoption of unproven ones (ASHA, 2004). At this time, it seems that this delay in using NS-OME is most prudent.

The student experience

In their clinical placements for child speech, student clinicians may encounter practices that they have never heard of in class. Conversely, they may learn of therapy methodologies in lectures and in their readings that they never encounter in clinics. When given appropriate support and guidance during the progression of easing into professional practice roles, students absorb and embrace the language, literature, issues and modes and methods of enquiry of their chosen discipline. The support comes from people: peers, instructors, mentors, and clinical supervisors, and formal guidance comes from documents: codes of ethics, standards of practice, and expected competencies. Throughout the process, students are encouraged to think, evaluate, question, challenge, know, understand, and make sensible connections between what they are taught as best practice and what they observe to be common practice in formal clinical placements, in anecdotal discussion list offerings, and of course on various websites that promise client and clinician the earth.

Speech-Language Pathologist Dr. Karen McComas is a Professor of Communication Disorders and the Assistant Director of the Center for Teaching and Learning at Marshall University in Huntington, West Virginia, USA. She holds the ASHA Certificate of Clinical Competence in Speech-Language Pathology and Audiology. McComas is a founding member of a community of research practice (CoRP) and she leads a narrative, collaborative ethnographic research study focusing on the faculty/student community. Additional research interests include narrative studies about identity development in women researchers, the experiences and lives of caregivers and disabled persons in Appalachia, and Appalachian discourse. Her book (McComas, 2014) focuses on the relationship between imagination and the development of research identities in women. McComas' response to Q36 emphasises the ways in which educational programs can facilitate the transfer from being a student in training to an ethical practitioner.

Q36. Karen McComas: Shaping professional identities in a US context

How can the socialisation experience of being a member of a disciplinary community help the transformation from student to ethical practitioner?

A36. Karen McComas: Communities of practice in CSD: facilitating transformational learning

In the first edition of this text I responded to a question about how communication science and disorders (CSD) programs could remain viable and relevant in a world where information is generated – and replaced – at an incredible pace. I suggested that programs should decrease their emphasis on transmitting information, increase their emphasis on the processes of learning and 'require students to ask questions; collect, select and analyse resources; and publish their findings' (McComas, 2009, p. 189). Furthermore, I argued that academic programs should actively socialise students into the culture of the discipline, a process that 'fosters the development of a professional identity in learners as they acquire and refine the habits of mind and practice that will be required of them throughout their professional careers' (p. 186). Essentially, I claimed that change at the programmatic level could facilitate transformations at the student level. However, my recommendations were theoretical with little practical advice, a void I intend to fill in this edition of *Children's Speech Sound Disorders*.

Transformations from students to ethical practitioners occur when students *participate* in integrated, educative experiences (Palmer & Zajonc, 2010). These kinds of experiences engage 'students in the systematic exploration of the relationship between their studies of the "objective" world and the purpose, meaning, limits and aspirations of their lives' and are grounded in a communal reality; promote social and experiential knowing; require teaching strategies that promote change; and, lead to ethical ways of thinking and being (Palmer & Zajonc, 2010, p. 10). Students want to participate in communities and solve challenging problems; their transformations begin when we invite them into our professional communities, to work alongside us and experience *being* a member of a disciplinary community.

Participation

Students participate in countless academic experiences that have prescribed ways of learning (curricula). All too frequently, student participation is passive (e.g., when instructors transmit information to students), or unrelated to the practice of the discipline

(e.g., taking multiple choice examinations). This approach is a *teaching curriculum* and limits what students might learn about practice (Lave & Wenger, 1991). Instead, student learning is 'mediated through an instructor's participation (in practice), by an external view of what knowing is about' (Lave & Wenger, p. 97). Of greater value to students would be a *learning curriculum*, which features 'situated opportunities ... for the improvisational development of new practice ... a field of learning resources in everyday practice *viewed from the perspective of learners*' (Lave & Wenger, p. 97). A learning curriculum 'evolves out of participation in a specific community of practice engendered by pedagogical relations and by a prescriptive view of the target practice as the subject matter' (Lave & Wenger, p. 97).

Lave and Wenger (1991) posit that community participation is 'a way of learning – of both absorbing and being absorbed in – the "culture of practice"' (p. 95). Indeed, of five communities of practice examined in one study, they found that 'there was very little observable teaching; the more basic phenomenon is learning' (Lave & Wenger, p. 92). In other words, by participating in a community of practice individuals learn content and skills.

Communities of Practice

Communities of practice promote a learning curriculum where participants engage in practice; thus, mediation by others (e.g., instructors) is unnecessary. They invite 'participation in an activity system about which participants share understandings concerning what they are doing and what that means in their lives' (Lave & Wenger, 1991, p. 98). These communities are natural hosts for integrative, educative experiences that eventually lead to ethical ways of thinking and being (Palmer & Zajonc, 2010). In addition, they have observable ways of being (ontology), knowing (episte-mology), teaching (pedagogy), and living (ethics) (Palmer & Zajonc, 2010). Coherence among these four increases the understanding and meaning individuals derive from community participation. In short, participation in a coherent community enables learning.

I participate in a faculty and student community of practice – CoRP – at my institution. Our 'activity system' is research and our members

> *meet because they find value in their interactions.... They help each other solve problems. They ponder common issues, explore ideas, and act as sounding boards.... However they accumulate knowledge, they become informally bound by the value that they find in learning together*
>
> (Wenger, McDermott & Snyder, 2002, pp. 4–5).

Participating in this community of practice promotes content learning (research topic) and skill development (research process). As a model, we can see that CoRP is characterised by ways of being which support particular ways of knowing which, in turn, suggest certain ways of teaching which lead to ethical ways of practicing and living. As an experience, a community of practice like CoRP prompted one student to say, 'I love CoRP – I love it! It has become the high point of my collegiate experience!'

Community of Research Practice

The experiences students have in CoRP are integrated and educative, two pre-requisites for transformation (Palmer & Zajonc, 2010). CoRP began September of 2008 and is composed of faculty members, graduate students and undergraduate students. In addition to various studies about particular content areas, a study of the community is completed each year by a team of faculty and student researchers. For our fourth study, a qualitative, narrative study, we explored the concept of research as pedagogy. We interviewed seven graduate students who had participated in CoRP for at least two semesters and had authored and presented research at a state or national conference.

These interviews revealed portrayals of CSD students who were transforming into ethical practitioners; transformations they associated with their experiences in CoRP. Inductive analyses revealed a single dominant theme – with multiple sub-themes: relationships with processes (e.g., the research process), relationships with external worlds (e.g., content or people), and relationships with internal worlds (e.g., self and identity). More specifically, their stories told about changes, or transformations, in relationships; changes that Palmer and Zajonc (2010) predicted will occur when individuals participate in communities with coherence in how to be, know, teacher and learn, and live. Examining CoRP in the context of these four aspects of the community provided insight into the transformations experienced by our students.

Ontologically, to 'be' in CoRP is to be in communal, not competitive, relationships. One student said, 'I don't want to fight for my spot somewhere. I don't want to feel like I have to beat this other person because I need to be better than them. In class it is like that. In CoRP it is not like that'. In addition to the communal ontology, one student described CoRP as a 'safe place and a sanctuary for research'. Indeed, several students commented that the community made it easier for them to take risks, as they sought to develop their professional identities.

At the same time as students characterised CoRP as communal, they made distinctions about how specific individuals related to the community. One student described herself as a member of the community, saying,

'I'm an active member who contributes and engages with other people's ideas and projects'. For her and others, being a member of the community means being present and being actively engaged in the community. Describing the relationship between CoRP and individuals who are active in research but infrequent participants in CoRP, another student said, 'She's associated with CoRP, but she's not associated with the community'. These observations support the idea that CoRP has a communal ontology.

Epistemologically, to 'know' in CoRP is both a social and an experiential process. Socially, students value the relationships they develop with other students and faculty mentors. One student observed that being in CoRP has 'helped relationships with other students because it is a different kind of curriculum. We are still learning but we are learning from each other'. Numerous students described their relationships with faculty as 'being on the same level' or 'being on a level playing field'. In this equitable environment, students interact freely in the community. One student said, 'I love it that any idea you have in CoRP is not a wrong one or ever shut out'. Because the community is built on social interactions concerning a wide range of research topics, participant learning is diverse. 'I pretty much know what everyone else is doing', said one student. This social epistemology promotes a way of knowing that resonates strongly with our students. 'CoRP is so beneficial to me, my studies, and [my] learning', another student reported.

Experientially, students described ways of knowing that were both external, such as engaging with others on a research project or with the literature, and internal, such as accepting self, challenging self and imagining self as other. One student told us that she was 'a very independent, determined, driven person who learns from her mistakes'. 'Failure', she continued, 'is not the end for me; it's the start of learning.'

Pedagogically, to 'teach' in CoRP is to create an environment where change can happen. This environment included, for our students, experiences that were personally relevant (with emotional connections), divergent, metacognitive and collaborative. These kinds of experiences articulate well with a communal ontology and social and experiential epistemology. Our students want to have relationships in community, to learn from meaningful experiences, and to share those experiences *with* their mentors. In other words, they want the integrated, educative experiences that lead to ethical ways of living.

Ethically, to 'live' (professionally and personally) is a function of the ontology, epistemology and pedagogy of the community (Palmer & Zajonc, 2010). The epistemology of CoRP is 'rooted … in a particular ontology, and manifesting … in a particular pedagogy. [It] has an impact on the ethical formation of learners' (Palmer & Zajonc, 2010, p. 32). Ethical ways of living are not just aspirational. Instead, they are the product of conscious choices. Our students are learning to live as evidence-based practitioners and making connections between ASHA's code of ethics and their personal ethics. One participant explained how understanding ethics develops from an external concept to an internalised way of living:

I think CoRP does a really good job of honing in on evidence-based practice. You hear about it in class but you really don't know much about it. First, you learn it as a term … and learn it for the vocabulary section on your test. Then they say you have to do it because we have an obligation to our clients and you can relate it to the code of ethics, which has been read 17,000 times. Then when you start practicing it's more real. You know you can't take [just] anything into your clients because they want to get back to doing what they love to do. You have to have something to back it up. I wouldn't want somebody to just bring some half-planned treatment plan to my dad when he was sick. I want to see where you are getting it and how you know it's effective.

Discussion

In this brief essay, I set out to fill the void I left in the first edition by suggesting that we invite students into our communities, to work alongside us and experience *being* a member of the discipline. I described a community of research practice, providing one model for facilitating the transformation of students to ethical practitioners.

Central to our research community is our shared practice, a test of community rarely achieved in classrooms or practicum placements. In classrooms, teachers engage in multiple practices, such as lecturing, facilitating discussions, organising and supervising learning activities, and assessing and evaluating students' performances. Simultaneously, students are likely listening, taking notes, discussing or completing assessments. These mismatches of practice continue, albeit to a lesser extent, in clinical placements where supervisors observe, assess and evaluate the supervised, while the supervised engage in diagnostic and therapeutic activities with clients.

Clinical problem solving

In the first edition of this book, Nunes (2009) wrote, 'suspiciousness of theory opens the door

to subjectivism, easily mistaken for the right to believe what one wants', positing that 'this can allow false claims, such as those put forward by the proponents of non-speech oral motor therapies [treatments] (NS-OMT), to become the cornerstones of therapy modalities'. It probably goes without saying that certain linguistic principles can help us in devising evidence-based therapies that are conducive to treatment efficacy, but many SLPs/SLTs tend to shy away from gaining a deeper understanding of linguistics terminology and theory (Ingram, A6; Froud, A38) and establishing a regular discipline of reading published research (Highman, A41). Their preference is often to 'share tips' via social media, and participate in continuing professional development with a 'how to', 'hands on' and an atheoretical focus. May Bernhardt and Angela Ullrich, discuss this topic, relative to non-linear phonology, in A37.

Dr. B. May Bernhardt has been a clinical SLP since 1972 and is a professor at the University of British Columbia in Vancouver, Canada. Her major areas of research are in phonological and phonetic development, assessment, and intervention. Other interests include general language impairment in children and implications of First Nations English dialects for SLP.

Dr. Angela Ullrich worked as a research associate at the University of Cologne in Germany from 2005 to 2011 and as a clinical SLP in a private clinic, mainly with children with protracted phonological development (PPD). In her PhD thesis, under the co-supervision of Dr. Roswitha Romonath and Dr. B. May Bernhardt, she developed a phonological assessment tool for German-speaking children (NILPOD), based on constraint-based non-linear phonological theories. She continues to pursue her interest in child phonology as an independent scholar.

Q37.   B. May Bernhardt and Angela Ullrich: A German–Canadian connection with non-linear phonology

A striking finding that arose from non-linear phonological intervention studies in British Columbia (Major & Bernhardt, 1998; Bernhardt, Brooke & Major, 2003) was the relationship between therapists' academic preparation and children's speech production outcomes. An analysis of factors such as educational background, years of experience, confidence level in the non-linear approaches, and general treatment style (drill, play or both) revealed that therapists with undergraduate linguistics degrees achieved superior results to therapists with SLP Master's degrees and no linguistics undergraduate training. As Bernhardt (2004) points out, there is much yet to learn about practitioner training and intervention outcomes. What in particular would you both encourage SLPs/SLTs who do not have a strong linguistics background to pursue in their CPD/CEU endeavours, and how can goal-setting based on constraints-based non-linear phonological analyses expedite intelligibility gains?

A37.   B. May Bernhardt and Angela Ullrich: Constraints-based non-linear phonology: why and how to start

Primary sources of CE for SLPs/SLTs are on-the-job training from other SLPs/SLTs, workshops, conferences and readings, the majority of which are focused directly on the clinical practice of SLP. Given an option between a workshop demonstrating some new clinical procedure and a conference on the latest developments in linguistics or psychology, the vast majority of SLPs/SLTs will choose to attend the former educational opportunity. The gap between research in psychology and linguistics and therapy with 'Susie' at 10 AM on Friday may seem insurmountable for clinicians without a strong university preparation in psychology or linguistics. Yet, as noted in the preamble to this question, one small study (Bernhardt, 2004) has suggested that there may be a good reason for clinicians to be well informed in linguistics. Goal-setting based on constraints-based non-linear phonological analyses may expedite gains in intelligibility. The following section provides an overview of studies supporting that perspective, before we return to the question of CE for SLTs/SLPs.

Constraints-based non-linear phonological theories have arisen over the last three decades in linguistics. Many of the basic tenets of the theories are assumed currently: that there are many levels of phonological form, from the phrase to the word to the syllable to the consonant or vowel to the feature, and that, in terms of phonological patterns, these levels can act independently ('constraints on pronunciation' affecting specific features or syllable positions) or interactively ('constraints' affecting features in specific contexts only). A description of current phonological theories is beyond the scope of this contribution, but the following short overview of clinical studies may provide some motivation for readers to learn more about these theories.

Table A37.1 lists the major British Columbia studies of non-linear phonological intervention for children with moderately-to-severely PPD. Each single-subject design study included from 2 to 20 children, with durations of 16–18 weeks.

Although there was considerable variation in how the projects were implemented, four types of goals were generally targeted (see Table A37.2) that addressed word structure or segments (consonants and vowels) as either 'new' elements or elements in new combinations. SLPs/SLTs used both familiar activities and new ones that fitted the particular words for treatment (which did not include words for test probes). Caregivers were involved in the sessions and conducted home activities.

Two major results pertain particularly to this question. The first concerns the goal type, and the second, clinician effectiveness. Concerning goal type, it was found that word shape goals (CVC, CVCV, CCV, etc.) were attained significantly faster than segmental goals in the first half of each study. Although intelligibility studies were not conducted, it is clear that an increase in use of within-word and word-final consonants and clusters would have an immediate positive effect on intelligibility.

Table A37.1 Field studies conducted in non-linear phonological intervention in British Columbia

Year	Investigators	Type	Number, ages of children	Project Duration
1990	Bernhardt (1990)	Dissertation	6: 3–6 years	18 weeks, 3x/week
	Von Bremen (1990)	Master's thesis	Twin boys: 5 years	18 weeks, 3x/week
1993–1994	Field SLPs across BC B. M. Bernhardt – Introductory workshop – Rigid design direction (Bernhardt & Major, 2005; Major & Bernhardt, 1998)	Quasi-experimental alternating conditions, rigid single subject design	20: 3–5 years	16 weeks, 3x/week
1995	Edwards (1995)	Flexible single-subject design	2: 4 years	16 weeks, 2x/week
1997–to date	Field SLPs Bernhardt, Major, Edwards – Introductory workshop – Minimal direction (Bernhardt et al., 2003)	Flexible single-subject design	17: 3–6 years	16 weeks, 2x/week

Table A37.2 Types of goals addressed in non-linear phonological intervention studies

Phonological level in the hierarchy	New Form	New Combinations or Interactions of Existing Form
Phrase and word structures	New word shapes, e.g., CVC	Establishing an existing segment (consonant or vowel) in (a) an established word position new to that segment, or (b) in a new sequence by word position
Segments (consonants or vowels) and their features	New features, e.g., [Dorsal] (velar)	New combinations of features already in the system, e.g., combining the 'fricative' features of an existing [f] with the coronal (alveolar) features of a /t/ to target [s]

The second result concerns clinician effectiveness. The 1994 and 1997 studies differed in that, for the former, Bernhardt did the analyses, chose goals and provided stimuli and treatment strategies for the clinicians. In the 1997 study, clinicians were given the transcripts of the assessment tapes. In accordance with what they had learned in a workshop, they did their own data analyses and goal-setting (which were briefly confirmed by the investigator). Principles of goal-setting and sequence were the same, but there was more flexibility, with the treatment being individualised. Another difference was that the 1997 study had twice-weekly therapy compared with thrice weekly for the 1994 study. In terms of overall gains in Percent Consonant Match (PCM), there was no significant difference between the studies across children: a 16.4% gain in 1994 and 18.6% in 1997. These outcomes demonstrate that clinicians can learn to implement new ideas in treatment with minimal supervision. Comparing the results with other studies not based on non-linear phonology, Tyler and Lewis (2005) reported PCM gains of 7–20% for a longer (24-week) study, and Erickson (2007) a 7% mean gain for a 12–16 week study. Thus, non-linear phonological intervention for English has had observable benefits for clients in clinical field research studies of 16–18 weeks' duration. But what can be expected after single-weekend workshops? We turn now to a project by Angela Ullrich on this topic.

Non-linear phonological theories in clinical assessment have been mainly applied in Anglo-American countries. For Angela Ullrich's dissertation project, a non-linear phonological assessment tool (Nichtlineare phonologische Diagnostik, NILPOD; Ullrich 2007) was developed for German-speaking children. NILPOD is conceptually based on Bernhardt and Stemberger's (2000) non-linear scan analysis in its application of constraint-based non-linear phonological theories (as shown in Table A37.2).

To evaluate effectiveness and clinical applicability of NILPOD, and also importantly, the effectiveness of knowledge transfer concerning a complex linguistic theory like non-linear phonology, an evaluation study was conducted in Cologne. Fifty-seven clinicians were trained in a 3-day weekend workshop to apply the assessment tool NILPOD. The group included German SLPs and logopedists with a range of 2–35 years of clinical practice experience. The linguistics background of most participating clinicians was rather limited, because linguistics coursework has been under-represented in the SLP curriculum in Germany. The first and second days of the workshop thus outlined basic concepts of phonetics and constraint-based non-linear phonology before the demonstration of phonological analyses using NILPOD. On the third day, a hands-on session was conducted, in which participants were given a transcribed dataset of a child with PPD. They performed a non-linear analysis of the data alone or in groups, including identification of therapy goals. Ullrich assisted them as required and reviewed results at the end of the day.

At the end of the workshop, clinicians were asked to complete an evaluation form covering questions about their professional background, the structure and content of the workshop, and how the knowledge gained about non-linear phonology might affect their assessment and treatment of phonological impairment. Every clinician also received background information and transcribed data from four German-speaking children with PPD for home practice and NILPOD evaluation. Clinicians were asked to analyse the data by using the NILPOD analysis and select three short-term therapy goals. Clinicians were also asked to complete a final questionnaire, which included rating scales concerning the analysis sheets, the applicability and the efficiency of analysis, and the relevance of therapy goals, plus a set of open-ended questions inviting their suggestions for improvements to NILPOD.

The workshop evaluation form showed that 86% of the clinicians wanted to learn more about non-linear phonology and NILPOD; 70% stated that they understood the theoretical background; and 67% found the workshop, including the linguistic theory, relevant for their clinical practice. A lower percentage (39%) indicated that the workshop clearly changed their perception of phonological impairment. A number of key themes arose in response to an open-ended question set (1) the importance of word structure for work in phonological intervention, (2) the importance of considering strengths and needs of the phonological system in goal selection, and (3) the relevance of the concept of phonological hierarchy for understanding phonological difficulties. After performing the four NILPOD analyses at home, similar results were observed in the 30 clinicians who returned the analyses. In addition, 67% found that NILPOD gave detailed information to derive useful therapy goals. A lower percentage (29%) stated that they realised the necessity of doing detailed phonological analyses that are based on complex linguistic theories. Five clinicians wrote explicitly that they had already noticed the positive effects of the workshop training in their clinical work. As a negative open-ended comment, 42% noted that the analysis was both too time-consuming and complex in its current (workshop) version. Others stated that they did not feel confident enough yet to implement NILPOD themselves. Clinician's suggestions are being incorporated in the final (pre-publication) revision of NILPOD, especially ideas to improve time efficiency, avoid redundancy of analysis steps, and streamline and clarify analysis sheets. The comments regarding the NILPOD resonate with many of those offered in evaluation forms for Bernhardt's workshops on non-linear phonology: 'I'll never look at an artic test the same way again'; 'I will pay far more attention to word structure than I ever did before' (very frequent comment); 'The idea of identifying both strengths and needs of the phonological system makes sense'; or 'The concept of "default" was useful and interesting'. Overall results show that a workshop can improve a clinician's basic understanding of phonological impairment and positively influence his or her clinical practice, through application of some of the major principles of constraint-based non-linear phonology, that is, taking phonological hierarchy into account, paying attention to word structure, considering strengths and needs of the phonological system when choosing therapy goals and using constraints to explain underlying phonological difficulties.

The results of the studies in Canada and Germany suggest that clinicians can learn to incorporate more current versions of phonological analyses into practice with short-term training. If there are no available workshops or university courses in the clinician's immediate area, however, what options are there for CE? A book or journal club may be a useful solution, perhaps starting with the readings recommended below. Another suggestion might be for a clinical agency to form a partnership with a university linguistics program. Through ongoing case study, readings and dialogue, the linguists could provide current theoretical perspectives, and the clinicians could provide data for the linguists to consider when developing theories. The Bernhardt studies suggest a more formal possibility: university researchers and students are often looking for clinicians to participate in evaluation studies of assessment or therapy approaches. Such partnerships can help close the gap between research and practice and, in so doing, enhance outcomes for the clients: one of the main objectives of CE.

Recommended readings

For English, an introductory article that may be easy to locate is Bernhardt and Stoel-Gammon (1994). For German, Ullrich and Bernhardt (2005) includes an introduction to non-linear phonology. For more in-depth learning, the Bernhardt and Stemberger (2000) *Workbook in Non-linear Phonology for Clinical Application* has exercises for practice, case examples and treatment method suggestions. This workbook is no longer in print, but a free electronic version is available on a secure website and access can be arranged by emailing may.bernhardt@audiospeech.ubc.ca. Other case-based articles provide more examples of analysis and goal-setting, for example, Bernhardt (1992a, b), Bernhardt and Gilbert (1992), Baker and Bernhardt (2004), Bernhardt (2005) and Bernhardt, Stemberger and Major (2006). Advanced readings include Bernhardt and Stemberger (1998, 2007), Bernhardt, Gilbert and Ingram (1996) and Dinnsen and Gierut (2008).

For SLP/SLT readers who want to begin their own clinical application of non-linear phonology, Bernhardt and Holdgrafer (2001a, b) give information on word list construction for speech samples that facilitate non-linear analyses. Computer programs that provide quantitative support for non-linear analyses are Masterson and Bernhardt's (2001) Computerised Articulation and Phonology Evaluation System (CAPES) available as a free electronic download from the authors (may.bernhardt@audiospeech.ubc.ca and JulieMasterson@missouristate.edu), and Computerised Profiling (Long, 2007).

Embracing change

Assuming that the reader had covered phonological theory 101, and no more, Bernhardt and Stemberger (1998) provided an introduction to non-linear phonology and to its constraint-based implementation in Optimality Theory, explaining how this framework can describe and explain data on protracted phonological development (PPD), and the interface of their work with speech processing and connectionism. Then, helpfully switching focus to address SLP/SLT clinicians, Bernhardt and Stemberger (1998) produced a plain-English workbook in non-linear phonology for clinical application. These publications were predated by accessible tutorial articles for clinicians, for example, Bernhardt and Stoel-Gammon (1994), and Stemberger and Bernhardt (1997), and followed by case-based accounts, such as Baker and Bernhardt (2004). Rather than regularly turning to these works and others like them for elucidation and help with difficult phonologies, clinicians recoil (Bernhardt & Ullrich, A37), regarding non-linear approaches in general as something new and difficult. Similarly, the author has seen many experienced, committed clinicians in CPD/CEU events tune out at the sight of syllable trees in the context of phonotactic therapy (Velleman, 2002), and as mentioned previously Joffe and Pring (2008) even report that one of their respondents said that she and other therapists she knew were 'terrified' by psycholinguistic models (Gardner, A27; Joffe, A34; Stackhouse & Wells, 1997).

Q38 is addressed to Dr. Karen Froud, the director of the Neurocognition of Language Lab, and Associate Professor of Speech-Language Pathology in the Department of Biobehavioral Sciences at Teachers College, Columbia University, in New York. She holds a PhD in Linguistics from University College London, and her research is concerned with the neurological underpinnings of linguistic processing and representation in normal and disordered language. She teaches Neuroscience, Adult Language Disorders, and Language Development to graduate students in the SLP program at TC, while maintaining a wide range of collaborative research projects in linguistics and the neurosciences, including work on the neural correlates of child speech disorders.

Q38.   Karen Froud: An international aspect of SSD: the theory to practice gap

There is an immediate and striking applicability to our understanding of children's phonological disorders, and approaches to their assessment and treatment, of non-linear models and psycholinguistic frameworks. Why do you think it is that clinicians around the world are apparently unambitious in tackling the research literature, and so conservative in applying and evaluating for themselves new, and not so new, theories and findings?

A38.   Karen Froud: Understanding and addressing the theory-to-practice divide in clinical training and practice

Why do we need theoretical models and frameworks? It has long been understood that there is a kind of 'disconnect' between sensory percepts (e.g., acoustic signals) and mental representations (e.g., the mental image of an object or a situation in the world). In the domain of speech and language, this disconnect is particularly evident. There is nothing in the properties of an acoustic signal which requires that signal to be interpreted by the human mind as having referential properties; for example, auditory coding of frequency, intensity and phase in the cochlea is not directly related to retrieving the semantic properties of a real-life object or situation (although it seems likely that cochlear coding mechanisms may have adapted to selectively maximise speech sound processing; Smith & Lewicki, 2006). The relationship between mental representations and speech signals is quite opaque, yet our profession works exactly at this interface: between speech and language, receptive and expressive modalities, perception and production, sensorimotor and cognitive processes.

One way to yield greater understanding of the interfaces between sensory and cognitive phenomena has been to develop models that help to identify separate sub-processes involved in relating sensory phenomena (e.g., sounds) to mental representations (e.g., concepts). Such models are useful because they permit a breakdown of the ways in which complex mental operations may occur, at the same time as abstracting away from complicating factors like individual differences, contextual effects or psychological states. Developing models which provide step-by-step breakdowns of the sub-processes and different levels of representation involved in speech and language processing has been very informative for clinicians and has led to the development and testing of various approaches to assessment and treatment. For example, Hodson and Paden (1981), in their well-known *Cycles Phonological Pattern Approach* (*CPPA*; Hodson, A5), take the view that stimulability (and hence perception) for a particular speech sound should be in place *before* that sound is targeted for production. This theory-based treatment approach demonstrates how interdisciplinary advances can be made when talented clinicians engage with theoretical frameworks.

Models that represent speech and language processing in a step-by-step manner can be thought of as linear, in the sense that they depict a series of processes that succeed each other in a predictable sequence. We are used to thinking of speech and language in a linear way, largely because the first step in any kind of fine-grained analysis is to chop up the signal into segments of information, to better examine each segment independently of other factors. This is a standard approach in all kinds of linguistic (and speech sound) analyses and was detailed very early in the history of generative linguistics (e.g., Harris, 1951). However, it is clear that speech and language are not really linear at all: these complex signals are multi-dimensional in nature, and different aspects of the speech stream overlap one another in processing and representation (Goldsmith, 1972). Especially since it has become stan-

dard to examine cognitive operations from the perspective of their neural correlates, in experimental investigations utilising EEG, fMRI and other brain imaging techniques, it has become ever more apparent that the mapping between sensory stimuli and mental representations is complex, multi-layered and not sequential in nature. Distinctions have been drawn between basic processes (e.g., sensory and motor processing), specialisations that arise from functional integration between distributed systems, and reverberations between feedback and feedforward mechanisms at both cortical and subcortical levels (e.g.,Davis & Johnsrude, 2007; Dhanjal, Handunnetthi, Patel & Wise, 2008; Hickok & Poeppel, 2004; Hickok, Houde & Rong, 2011; Kotz & Schwartze, 2010; Londei et al., 2010). Activations overlap in time and in space, and even on an intuitive level we 'know' that we do not wait to build the syntactic structure of a whole phrase – or the phonological structure of a whole word, or the metrical structure of a whole syllable – before we begin to engage other systems, such as those required to identify semantic or pragmatic or prosodic properties of the same incoming signal. Even in the acoustic signal itself, the lowest-level sensory input, there is no discreteness of phonemes, syllables or words; instead, these units overlap and are not perceived independently of one another (Fowler, 1995). Rather than simplifying everything into a series of linearly associated representations, it seems more appropriate to take a non-linear approach, to take account of multiple levels of processing and representation that are occurring simultaneously (e.g., Goldsmith, 1972; Liberman & Prince, 1977; McCarthy, 1988). Non-linear theories of speech and language, then, allow us to delineate hierarchical relationships between cognitive processes, while at the same time permitting understanding of the highly interactive and integrative organisation of these complex systems (e.g., Price, 2012).

Given this situation, what is it that makes current theoretical frameworks so apparently unappealing to those of us working in clinical professions? Is it just that the non-linear theoretical frameworks are somehow too 'difficult' for us, so we prefer not to concern ourselves with them and work instead within the 'simpler', linear approaches? This argument cannot really hold, since linear approaches are not necessarily 'simpler'. New theoretical developments are typically aimed at simplifying the amount of theoretical machinery required to gain the same (or a greater) degree of empirical coverage as earlier versions, and the shift from linear to non-linear approaches in models of speech and language processing, like the move towards a Minimalist framework for syntax (Chomsky, 1995), shares this goal. Most recent developments in relating linguistic theory to speech-language pathology have been motivated by simplification, too. For instance, before distinctive feature theory (Chomsky & Halle, 1968) was widely accepted, the typical approach to remediation of phonological or articulation disorders was to take each 'error' individually, classify it as substitution, omission, distortion or addition (Van Riper, 1978), and treat it separately from any other errors with no expectation of generalisation (Bernhardt & Stoel-Gammon, 1994). With the widespread acceptance of phonological features (rather than segments) as the units of analysis and treatment, generalisation within classes of sounds was expected and documented (e.g., Costello & Onstine, 1976). Theoretical advances, far from being complications, actually resulted in simplification of remediation approaches *and* in greater generalisation of therapeutic gains.

It has been argued that non-linear approaches have the potential to do the same. For instance, feature geometry clearly outlines how change at one level could be expected to filter throughout the entire system for speech sound representation. Feature geometries (e.g., Bernhardt & Stemberger, 1998; McCarthy, 1988) attempt to show how the relations between phonological features are hierarchically organised. Targeting speech sound intervention at higher levels in such a hierarchy is predicted to result in 'trickle-down' effects, meaning that careful targeting of intervention can have widespread effects on the child's representation of many speech sounds. Supporting evidence has even been provided, in the form of several studies that have examined children's phonological disorders within non-linear frameworks, developed intervention strategies based on constructs of such frameworks, and evaluated the efficacy of these strategies in clinical cases (e.g., Bernhardt, 1992a; Bernhardt & Stoel-Gammon, 1994; Gierut, 1989). Examples are proliferating: within the field of SSD, theoretically motivated interventions based on non-linear frameworks include minimal contrast approaches (e.g., *PACT*: Bowen & Cupples, 1999a, b), maximal oppositions (Gierut, 1992), and approaches designed to increase metaphonological awareness (*Metaphon*: Howell & Dean, 1994).

So, it's not apparent that linear approaches are 'simpler' than more current non-linear frameworks. It is not true that the non-linear approaches have no applicability in the field. It is not even the case that we have no evidence for the efficacy and generalisability of non-linear approaches to speech sound remediation. So what is going on? Why is there such resistance in our profession to staying abreast of theoretical advances that have great potential to enhance our understanding and remediation of speech and language disorders?

This situation seems rather circular in nature. At least in part, it arises because clinicians are too busy, and lacking in the necessary background, to read and critically evaluate the research literature. Most students still do not encounter the newer theoretical approaches during their academic training, and most clinicians (there are notable exceptions, of course) do not use any recognisable theoretical framework to inform their interventions. The direct effect of this is that even students who do care about theoretical frameworks and their utility in clinical investigations will have, at best, only limited opportunities to explore these, in or out of the classroom – yielding another generation of clinicians who lack the confidence and background to implement shifts in thinking about representation and process in speech and language. The frustration gets compounded on all sides: clinicians feel that the research is lagging way behind their own intuitive thinking for treatment planning and implementation, and researchers think that clinicians simply ignore or do not use the work that goes into elucidating questions with deep relevance for clinical practice.

We all carry responsibility for this state of affairs. As educators, we are obligated to provide students with the tools to approach the relevant research independently, and critically; and to instil into them that reading the literature is not just another commitment to fit in around field placements and caseloads. This means teaching rigorous courses in research design, evaluation of research, statistics and even philosophy of science. For instance, the processes of hypothesis formation and testing within a rigorous and evidence-based theoretical framework should be basic, consciously available tools in the repertoire of *every* clinician. Furthermore, it seems to me essential that every SLP/SLT program provide a fair degree of training in linguistics. SSDs are not just articulatory disorders; we are speech and *language* pathologists, and the training should support this duality. This is the first step in taking theory into practice: we must provide the theoretical frameworks, the evidence on which they are based, and the tools for critical evaluation of both theory and evidence.

Clinicians and supervisors can shift their mindsets and their practices; they can assimilate new theoretical developments and discuss these with colleagues; they can develop and implement strategies for assessment and intervention that have a firm theoretical grounding. Our professional regulatory bodies can explicitly acknowledge the reality that informed and ethical clinical practice is much more than 'knee-to-knee time'. By doing so, not only do we stand to provide better training for our students and better care for our clients, we also stand to contribute data and experience that can guide the development of ever more fine-grained theories of the mental representations and processes involved in speech and language.

In summary, theoretical frameworks serve a purpose: they are there to help us understand complex processes at a level of abstraction that renders the complexities at least somewhat transparent. In clinical fields like SLP/SLT, this should have the advantage of permitting a more detailed understanding of the mechanisms underlying a disorder, thereby motivating approaches to assessment and intervention. In linguistics, there have been exponential advances in recent years in our understanding of linguistic rules and representations at every level, from speech sounds to mapping between language and cognition. Better understanding leads to better approaches to assessment and remediation.

The challenge to our field, then, is to keep abreast of theoretical advances and to incorporate them into our practice. This is a necessary step for everyone – from students to clinical fellows, clinical supervisors, senior professionals, researchers, the professors providing the academic training, and the regulators who determine standards for professional practice and certification – to maintain ethical, efficacious, well-motivated approaches to assessment and remediation in our field.

Recommended resource

The *Workbook in Non-linear Phonology for Clinical Application* (Bernhardt & Stemberger, 2000) is recommended. As mentioned, it is out of print. For a free electronic version readers may request access to a secure website courtesy of may.bernhardt@audiospeech.ubc.ca.

A model for ethical practices

The starting point for research in clinical linguistics and phonetics is always going to be a person with impaired language or speech, whether he or she is a participant in a group study, or a single "case." While ethical conduct is of course a prerequisite of all good research, working with vulnerable populations such as children or people with a variety of impairments of communication and cognition imposes particularly stringent requirements.

(Muller & Ball, 2013, p. 5)

Some of the early 19th-century therapies used by public school clinicians have gone out of fashion. These include stuttering therapy methods to "educate the emotions" and methods involving visual and auditory imagery. Other methods, such as those involving exercises and drills, are still in common use. Exercise therapies then and now include practice in breath control, exercising the speech articulators (called speech gymnastics by our ancestors), relaxation therapies, practicing slow articulation, and working with speech rhythms (Nemoy & Davis, 1937; Schoolfield, 1937). Today, the oral-motor therapies designed to exercise the speech musculature (e.g., Rosenfeld-Johnson, 2001) have come under scrutiny. That is, they have been criticized because they are not passing the historically new standards arising from evidence-based research (e.g., Lass & Pannbacker, 2008).

Rather than making therapy choices based on research, these early school therapists were creating and choosing their approaches using their clinical logic and intuition.'

(Duchan, 2010, p. 156)

Dr. Thomas W. Powell is Professor of Speech-Language Pathology in the Department of Rehabilitation Sciences at Louisiana State University Health Sciences Center in Shreveport. He serves as a co-editor of the international journal *Clinical Linguistics and Phonetics*. His professional interests include phonological disorders, aphasia, clinical phonetics, multilingualism and ethics. In A39 he explores the ethical issues associated with the vexed question of many SLPs'/SLTs' persistent love affair with NS-OME.

Q39.   Thomas W. Powell: International, multidisciplinary codes of ethics and NS-OME

In a nationwide survey of 537 SLPs in the United States, Lof and Watson (2004) determined that 85% used NS-OME to change speech sound productions, and a similar study of 535 SLPs across Canada by Hodge et al. (2005) yielded exactly the same finding (Hodge, A31; Lof, A35). Your multi-faceted Model for Ethical Practices in Clinical Phonetics and Linguistics, presented at the 11th Symposium of the International Clinical Phonetics and Linguistics Association (ICPLA) in Dubrovnik, Croatia, in 2006, delineates six ethical domains. They are: beneficence, non-maleficence, competence, compliance, integrity and respect; and they apply across four levels of interaction with peers, students, participants and the general public. Can you provide the reader with an account of the model, and explain how it could be applied to the decision-making process of to be or not to be an oral motor therapist?

A39.   Thomas W. Powell: NS-OME: an ethical challenge

As speech and language professionals, we enjoy certain benefits and privileges. We make decisions and provide services that impact the lives of others. In return, we receive compensation for our expertise, as well as the satisfaction that results from helping another human to communicate more effectively. As professionals, we also share a responsibility for providing the highest possible quality of service and for protecting our clients from exploitation. Ethical codes empower us to monitor and evaluate our own conduct; they help us to maintain professional autonomy and reduce the need for external regulation (Irwin, Pannbacker, Powell & Vekovius, 2007).

The model of ethics in Figure A39.1 is adapted from previous work (Powell, 2007, 2013). It was inspired by an international sample of ethical codes from professional associations for speech and language professionals, as well as codes from related disciplines (i.e., linguistics, forensic phonetics and acoustics).

Several common principles were identified during this review process:

- **Beneficence:** We seek to do good by acting in the best interest in others.
- **Non-maleficence:** We pledge to do no harm and to minimise risks to others.
- **Respect:** We agree to respect differences, as well as the rights of others.

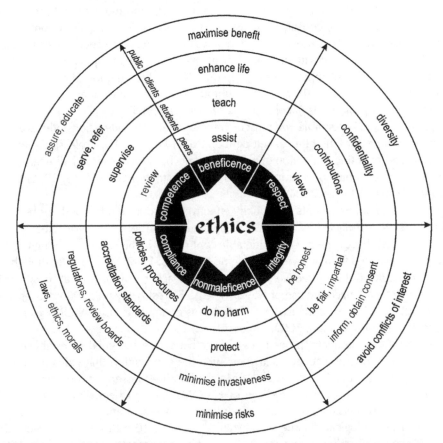

Figure A39.1 A six-factor model for ethical practice in SLP/SLT

- **Integrity:** We promise to be honest and to avoid conflicts of interest.
- **Compliance:** We agree to work within established rules and laws.
- **Competence:** We accept responsibility for ensuring a high quality of service, including appropriate delegation and referral.

Most ethical standards for professional and scientific associations are linked to one or more of these six principles.

Principles of ethical behaviour may have somewhat different implications as we interact with different groups. This model differentiates among four levels of interaction: with other professionals (peers), with students and/or assistants (subordinates), with clients and with the general public. Here, we will focus on an ethical challenge that impacts the clinician–client relationship.

Our ethical imperative to act in the best interest of our clients includes the responsibility for selection of appropriate treatment approaches (i.e., beneficence). Accordingly, we avoid treatments that carry a degree of risk (non-maleficence). We are respectful of differences and affirm others' right to privacy (respect). We seek to be honest and to provide information accurately and impartially (integrity). We recognise the limits of our knowledge and skills, and we refer appropriately (competence). Finally, we agree to observe and obey relevant policies, procedures, guidelines and laws (compliance).

I believe that the resourcefulness and creativity of speech and language clinicians is strength of our profession. Our education encourages critical thinking and independent problem solving (McAllister & Lincoln, 2004); consequently, we tend to be sceptical of generic 'one size fits all' treatments. Instead, we tend to value intervention plans that address the specific needs of our clients (Kamhi, 2006a, b). When faced with difficult clinical challenges, we may put on our 'thinking caps' and develop novel treatment approaches to help our clients. But are good intentions sufficient in an ethical sense? Sadly, history shows many dubious treatments developed by well-intentioned people in the helping professions (Jacobson, Foxx & Mulick, 2005).

Although innovation is desirable, we must be mindful of our ethical responsibilities as we introduce novel treatments into the clinical setting (Lof, 2011; Lum, 2002). Professional associations advocate unbiased scientific evaluation of new treatments before widespread clinical application, and currently the most commonly employed framework is that of EBP (ASHA, 2005; Dollaghan, 2007; Reilly, Douglas & Oates, 2004; Taylor-Goh, 2005).

Unfortunately, not all treatments are equally effective, and our field has perhaps been less systematic in assessing treatment efficacy than one might wish (Tharpe, 1998). Non-speech oral-motor treatments (NS-OMT) have generated considerable controversy in this regard. Although non-speech exercises have been used for many years (cf. Nemoy & Davis, 1937; Swift, 1918), there have been few controlled studies of their effectiveness (Lass & Pannbacker, 2008). Several prospective treatment studies have challenged the use of NS-OMT (e.g., Forrest & Iuzzini, 2008; Hayes, Savinelli, Roberts & Caldito, 2007); nevertheless, many clinicians continue to use NS-OMT as part of their treatment regimen (Lof & Watson, 2008; Muttiah et al., 2011).

In theory, NS-OMT products, procedures and activities are designed to establish improved articulator control during non-speech activities, with the expectation that gains in oral function will enhance speech production (Bahr, 2001; Marshalla, 2004; Rosenfeld-Johnson, 2001; Strode & Chamberlain, 1997). In practice, the use of NS-OMT has not been limited to motor-based speech movement disorders (i.e., dysarthria). Proponents have recommended oral-motor exercises for treatment of phonological disorders (Marshalla, 2004, p. 109; Rosenfeld-Johnson, 2001, p. 1), as well as speech disorders associated with hearing impairment (Loncar-Belding, 1998, p. 5; Orr, 1998, p. 1). The diversity of presenting diagnoses is perhaps most strikingly illustrated in a retrospective study by Beckman et al. (2004), who described the use of NS-OMT with children representing more than 75 different diagnoses, including Trisomy 21, ankyloglossia, cleft lip and palate, ear infections, heart problems, spina bifida and bruxism. Larroudé (2004, p. 139) described the use of oral-motor exercises within a multicultural–multilingual group program designed to improve functional communication. Clearly, NS-OMT interventions are being used to treat a wide range of conditions, aside from primary motor speech disorders.

Although many speech and language clinicians employ NS-OMT approaches, there has been considerable controversy regarding the adequacy of the underlying theory (Lof, 2003; Ruscello, 2008), as well as a disconcerting lack of experimental evidence (Bowen, 2005; Clark, 2010; Forrest, 2002). Several systematic reviews have been initiated to assess the efficacy of NS-OMT for children with developmental SSDs within an EBP framework (Lass & Pannbacker, 2008; Lee & Gibbon, 2011; McCauley et al., 2009; also see Ruscello, 2010, for commentary). In addition, concerns about the widespread adoption of such methods have been voiced by many authorities on SSDs in children (Baker & Bernhardt, 2004; Bernthal, Bankson & Flipsen, 2013; Bowen, 2005; Camarata, 2010; Clark, 2003, 2010; Davis & Velleman, 2000; Forrest, 2002; Hodge, 2002, A31; Kamhi, 2006b; Lof, 2002, 2003, A35; Lof and Watson, 2008; Powell, 2008a; Ruscello, 2008, A48; Rvachew, 2005, Shelton, 2005; Shriberg, 2003; Tyler, 2005; Weismer, 1997; Williams, 2003a,b).

Ethical principles can help one evaluate treatment decisions and other professional dilemmas (Kenny, Lincoln & Balandin, 2010). This process is especially important when one considers a controversial approach such as NS-OMT. The principle of beneficence leads us to consider treatment options critically and to adopt procedures that are appropriate for the individual client. Factors to be considered include the nature of the disorder, the client's capability and focus, the clinician's knowledge and skills, the nature and basis of the treatment, as well as logistical considerations such as scheduling frequency (Baker & Bernhardt, 2004; Kwiatkowski & Shriberg, 1998; Powell, 2008b).

Although the use of controversial or experimental treatments is not prohibited by most codes of professional ethics, certain conditions should be met to ensure their ethical use. First, treatment methods and outcome measures must be clearly defined, and these procedures must be evaluated and approved by an institutional ethical review board (compliance). Treatment should be provided only if the clinician possesses the appropriate knowledge and skills (competence). Potential contraindications and safety issues (e.g., infection control) should be considered carefully (non-maleficence). In addition, we have an obligation to provide the client (or responsible adult, in the case of minors) with honest information about the procedure, including potential risks and cost-to-benefit ratios (integrity). Informed consent must be obtained (compliance). To experiment on a client who is unaware of the controversial nature of the treatment would represent a serious infraction of basic ethical standards (Irwin et al., 2007).

Although ethical models provide guidelines for ethical problem solving, ultimately professionals are faced with the difficult task of making clinical decisions on the basis of incomplete and conflicting information (Muttiah et al., 2011). Duchan, Calculator, Sonnenmeier, Diehl and Cumley (2001) provided a useful framework for clinicians who elect to provide controversial treatments (such as NS-OMT). This framework encourages a thorough understanding of controversial practices, including how they relate to more accepted treatment options. Procedures for obtaining informed consent should be developed, as well as for adapting treatment procedures to reflect the needs of individual clients. Clinicians are well advised to be scrupulous in their documentation (Duchan et al., 2001). The use of single-subject methodologies, for example, can be an effective means of demonstrating accountability (Lum, 2002). Finally, it is important to anticipate professional and/or legal challenges and to be prepared to resolve them (Duchan et al., 2001).

In summary, although NS-OMTs are widely used, they continue to generate considerable controversy. Carefully designed studies are needed to evaluate NS-OMT practices systematically across target populations; however, such studies must comply with generally accepted ethical practices, including informed consent. Until such data become available, speech and language clinicians are encouraged to utilise treatments with stronger scientific support (Forrest, 2002; Gierut, 1998). Aggressive marketing, at any rate, should never be mistaken for scientific evidence.

The last say

Best practice guidelines for SLP/SLT services require clinicians to act in accordance with the evidence and ethics of their own profession while keeping a larger framework of knowledge, principles, philosophies and beliefs in mind (see Leitão, A53 and Powell, A39 for discussion). The bigger-picture framework grew out of years of collective research, practice, and client-and-family experiences across disciplines, settings, and cultures. Reflecting on the big picture, Bernstein Ratner (2006, p. 257) wrote:

> *EBP is a valuable construct in ensuring quality of care. However, bridging between research evidence and clinical practice may require us to confront potentially difficult issues and establish thoughtful dialogue about best practices in fostering EBP itself.*

Bernstein Ratner stresses the necessity for us to establish robust communication at all points, from laboratory to clinic. That is, between the funding bodies and researchers who develop the evidence, the academics who spread the word, the administrators who regulate change, the employers charged with maintaining beneficial workplaces, the practitioners who implement the evidence, and the client who, in egalitarian speech intervention in everyday practice, may have the last say.

References

ASHA. (2004). Preferred practice patterns for the profession of speech-language pathology. [Preferred Practice Patterns]. Available at www.asha.org/policy.

ASHA. (2005). *Evidence-based practice in communication disorders* [Position Statement]. Retrieved 15 January 2014 from www.asha.org/policy/PS2005-00221.htm

ASHA (2007). *Childhood Apraxia of Speech [Technical Report]*. Retrieved 15 January 2014 from www.asha.org/docs/html/TR2007-00278.html

Abrahamsen, E., & Flack, L. (2002). Do sensory and motor techniques improve accurate phoneme production? Paper presented at the annual convention of the American Speech-Language-Hearing Association, Atlanta, GA.

Allen, M. M. (2013). Intervention efficacy and intensity for children with speech sound disorder. *Journal of Speech, Language and Hearing Research*, 56(3), 865–877.

Armstrong, S., & Ainley, M. (1988). *The South Tyneside assessment of phonology*. Northumberland: Stass Publications.

Armstrong, S., & Ainley, M. (1992). *The South Tyneside assessment of phonology* (2nd ed.). Northumberland: Stass Publications.

Bahr, D. C. (2001). *Oral motor assessment and treatment: Ages and stages*. Boston, MA: Allyn and Bacon.

Bailey, D. B., McWilliam, P., & Winton, P. J. (1992). Building family-centred practices in early intervention: A team-based model for change. *Infants and Young Children*, 5(1), 73–82.

Baker, E. (2004). Phonological analysis, summary and management plan. *ACQuiring Knowledge in Speech, Language and Hearing*, 6(1), 14–21.

Baker, E. (2006). Management of speech impairment in children: The journey so far and the road ahead. *Advances in Speech-Language Pathology*, 8(3), 156–163.

Baker, E., & Bernhardt, B. (2004). From hindsight to foresight: working around barriers to success in phonological intervention. *Child Language Teaching and Therapy*, 20(3), 287–318.

Baker, E., & McLeod, S. (2011a). Evidence-based practice for children with speech sound disorders: Part 1 narrative review, *Language, Speech, and Hearing Services in Schools, 42*(2), 102–139.

Baker, E., & McLeod, S. (2011b). Evidence-based practice for children with speech sound disorders: Part 2 application to clinical practice, *Language, Speech, and Hearing Services in Schools, 42*(2), 140–141.

Bazyk, S. (1989). Changes in attitudes and beliefs regarding parent participation and home programs: An update. *The American Journal of Occupational Therapy, 43*(11), 723–728.

Beckman, D. A., Neal, C. D., Phirsichbaum, J. L., Stratton, L. J., Taylor, V. D., & Ratusnik, D. (2004). Range of movement and strength in oral motor therapy: A retrospective study. *Florida Journal of Communication Disorders, 21*, 7–14.

Bernhardt, B. (1990). *Application of nonlinear phonological theory to intervention with six phonologically disordered children*. Unpublished doctoral dissertation, University of British Columbia.

Bernhardt, B. (1992a). The application of nonlinear phonological theory to intervention with one phonologically disordered child. *Clinical Linguistics and Phonetics, 6*, 283–316.

Bernhardt, B. (1992b). Developmental implications of nonlinear phonological theory. *Clinical Linguistics and Phonetics, 6*, 259–282.

Bernhardt, B. (2004). Introduction to the Issue: Maximizing success in phonological intervention. *Child Language Teaching and Therapy, 20*, 195–198.

Bernhardt, B. (2005). Selection of phonological goals and targets: Not just an exercise in phonological analysis. In: A. Kamhi, & K. Pollock (Eds.), *Phonological disorders in children: Clinical decision-making in assessment and intervention* (pp. 109–120). Baltimore, MD: Paul H. Brookes Publishing Co.

Bernhardt, B., Brooke, M., & Major, E. (2003). Acquisition of structure versus features in nonlinear phonological intervention. Poster presented at the *Child Phonology Conference*, UBC, July 2003, Vancouver, BC, Canada.

Bernhardt, B., & Gilbert, J. (1992). Applying linguistic theory to speech-language pathology: the case for nonlinear phonology. *Clinical Linguistics and Phonetics, 6*, 123–145.

Bernhardt, B., Gilbert, J., & Ingram, D. (1996). *Proceedings of the UBC International Conference on Phonological Acquisition*. Boston, MA: Cascadilla Press.

Bernhardt, B., & Holdgrafer, G. (2001a). Beyond the Basics I: The need for strategic sampling for in-depth phonological analysis. *Language, Speech, and Hearing Services in Schools, 32*, 18–27.

Bernhardt, B., & Holdgrafer, G. (2001b). Beyond the Basics II: Supplemental sampling for in-depth phonological analysis. *Language, Speech, and Hearing Services in Schools, 32*, 28–37.

Bernhardt, B., & Major, E. (2005). Speech, language and literacy skills 3 years later: a follow-up study of early phonological and metaphonological intervention. *International Journal of Language and Communication Disorders, 40*(1), 1–27.

Bernhardt, B. H., & Stemberger, J. P. (1998). *Handbook of Phonological Development: From a nonlinear constraints-based perspective*. San Diego: Academic Press.

Bernhardt, B., & Stemberger, J. P. (2000). *Workbook in nonlinear phonology for clinical application*. Austin, TX: Pro-Ed.

Bernhardt, B. H., & Stemberger, J. P. (2007). Phonological impairment. In: P. Lacy (Ed.), *Handbook of Phonology* (pp. 575–593) Cambridge, UK: Cambridge University Press.

Bernhardt, B., Stemberger, J., & Major, E. (2006). General and nonlinear phonological intervention perspectives for a child with a resistant phonological impairment. *Advances in Speech-Language Pathology, 8*, 190–206.

Bernhardt, B., & Stoel-Gammon, C. (1994). Nonlinear phonology: Introduction and clinical application, *Journal of Speech and Hearing Research, 37*, 123–143.

Bernstein Ratner, N. (2006). Evidence-based practice: An examination of its ramifications for the practice of speech-language pathology. *Language, Speech & Hearing Services in Schools, 37*, 257–267.

Bernthal, J. E., Bankson, N. W., & Flipsen, P., Jr. (2013). *Articulation and Phonological Disorders* (7th d.). Boston, MA: Pearson Education.

Bonilha, L, Moser, D., Rorden, C., Bylis, G., & Fridriksson, J. (2006). Speech apraxia without oral apraxia: Can normal brain function explain the physiopathology? *Brain Imaging, 17*(10), 1027–1031.

Bowen, C. (2001). *Children's speech sound disorders (phonologicaltherapy) discussion group*. Retrieved 15 January 2014 from http://groups.yahoo.com/neo/groups/phonologicaltherapy/info

Bowen, C. (2005). What is the evidence for . . . ? Oral motor therapy. *ACQuiring Knowledge in Speech, Language, and Hearing, 7*, 144–147.

Bowen, C., & Cupples, L. (1999a). Parents and children together (PACT): A collaborative approach to phonological therapy. *International Journal of Language and Communication Disorders, 34*(1), 35–55.

Bowen, C., & Cupples, L. (1999b). A phonological therapy in depth: a reply to commentaries. *International Journal of Language and Communication Disorders, 34*(1), 65–83.

Bowen, C., & Cupples, L. (2004). The role of families in optimizing phonological therapy outcomes, *Child Language Teaching and Therapy, 20*, 245–260.

Broomfield, J., & Dodd, B. (2004a). The nature of referred subtypes of primary speech disability. *Child Language Teaching and Therapy, 20*, 135–151.

Bruce, B., Letourneau, N., Ritchie, J., Larocque, S., Dennis, C., & Elliott, M. R. (2002). A multi-site study of health professionals' perceptions and practices of family-centred care. *Journal of Family Nursing, 8*, 408–429.

Bunton, K. (2008). Speech versus nonspeech: Different tasks, different neural organization. *Seminars in Speech and Language, 29*(4), 267–275.

Bunton, K., & Weismer, G. (1994). Evaluation of a reiterant force-impulse task in the tongue, *Journal of Speech and Hearing Research, 37*, 1020–1031.

Bush, C., Steger, M., Mann-Kahris, S., & Insalaco, D. (2004). *Equivocal results of oral motor treatment on a child's articulation.* Poster presented at the annual meeting of the American Speech-Language-Hearing Association, Philadelphia, PA.

Camarata, S. M. (2010). Naturalistic intervention for speech intelligibility and speech accuracy. In: A. L. Williams, S. McLeod, and R. J. McCauley (Eds.), *Interventions for speech sound disorders in children* (pp. 381–405). Baltimore, MD: Paul H. Brookes Publishing Co.

Carson, K., Gillon, G., & Boustead, T. (2013). 'Classroom phonological awareness instruction and literacy outcomes in the first year of school', *Language Speech, and Hearing Services in Schools, 44*(2), 147–160.

Chapman Bahr, D. (2001). *Oral motor assessment and treatment: Ages and stages.* Boston: Allyn & Bacon.

Chomsky, N. (1995). *The minimalist program.* Cambridge, MA: MIT Press.

Chomsky, N., & Halle, M. (1968). *The sound pattern of English.* New York, NY: Harper and Row.

Cirrin, F., & Gillam, R. (2008). Language intervention practices for school-age children with spoken language disorders: A systematic review. *Language, Speech and Hearing Services in Schools, 39*, S110–S137.

Clark, H. M. (2003). Neuromuscular treatments for speech and swallowing: A tutorial. *American Journal of Speech Language Pathology, 12*(4), 400–415.

Clark, H. (2005). Clinical decision making and oral motor treatments. *The ASHA Leader, 10*(8), 8–9.

Clark, H. (2008). The role of strength training in speech sound disorders. *Seminars in Speech and Language, 29*(4), 276–283.

Clark, H. M. (2010). Nonspeech oral motor intervention. In: A. L. Williams, S. McLeod S., & R. J. McCauley (Eds.), *Interventions for Speech Sound Disorders in Children* (pp. 579–599). Baltimore, MD: Paul H. Brookes Publishing Co.

Clark, H., Hensen, P., Barber, W., Stierwalt, J., & Sherrill, M. (2003). Relationships among subjective and objective measures of tongue strength and oral phase swallowing impairments. *American Journal of Speech and Language Pathology, 12*, 40–50.

Clark, H., O'Brien, K., Calleja, A., & Corrie, S. (2009). Effects of directional exercise on lingual strength. *Journal of Speech, Language and Hearing Research, 52*, 1034–1047.

Clausen, R. (2013). School matters: Tech tools for schools. *The ASHA Leader.* Retrieved 1 January 2013 from http://www.asha.org/Publications/leader/2013/130101/School-Matters–Tech-Tools-for-Schools.htm

Colone, E., & Forrest, K. (2000). Comparison of treatment efficacy for persistent speech sound disorders. Poster presented at the *Annual Convention of the American Speech-Language-Hearing Association, Washington, DC.*

Costello, J., & Onstine, J. (1976). The modification of multiple articulation errors based on distinctive feature theory. *Journal of Speech and Hearing Disorders, 41*, 199–215.

Cox, F., (2012). *Australian English: Pronunciation and Transcription.* Cambridge University Press.

Crais, E. (1991). Moving from "parent involvement" to family-centred services. *American Journal of Speech-Language Pathology, 1*(1), 5–8. 29.

Crais, E., Poston Roy, V., & Free, K. (2006). Parents' and professionals' perceptions of family-centered practices: What are actual practices vs. what are ideal practices? *American Journal of Speech-Language Pathology, 15*, 365–377.

Crosbie, S., Holm, A., & Dodd, B. (2005). Intervention for children with severe speech disorder: A comparison of two approaches. *International Journal of Language and Communication Disorders*, *40*, 467–491.

Davis, B. L., & Velleman, S. L. (2000). Differential diagnosis and treatment of developmental apraxia of speech in infants and toddlers. *Infant-Toddler Intervention*, *10*(3), 177–192.

Davis, B., & Velleman, S. (2008). Establishing a basic repertoire without using NS-OME: Means, motive and opportunity. *Seminars in Speech and Language*, *29*(4), 312–319.

Davis, K. J. (2013). Exploring virtual PLCs. *Perspectives on School Based Issues*, *14*(2), 28–32.

Davis, M. H., & Johnsrude, I. S. (2007). Hearing speech sounds: top-down influences on the interface between audition and speech perception, *Journal of Hearing Research*, *229*, 132–147.

Dean, E. C., Howell, J., Waters, D., & Reid, J. (1995). *Metaphon*: A metalinguistic approach to the treatment of phonological disorder in children. *Clinical Linguistics and Phonetics*, *9*, 1–19.

Denne, M., Langdown, N., Pring, T., & Roy, P. (2005). Treating children with expressive phonological disorders: does phonological awareness therapy work in the clinic? *International Journal of Language and Communication Disorders*, *40*(4), 493–504.

Dhanjal, N. S., Handunnetthi, L., Patel, M. C., & Wise, R. J. (2008). Perceptual systems controlling speech production. *Journal of Neuroscience*, *28*, 9969–9975.

Dinnsen, D. A., & Gierut, J. (2008). *Optimality theory, phonological acquisition and disorders*. London, UK: Equinox.

Dodd, B. (2005). *Differential diagnosis and treatment of children with speech disorder* (2nd ed.). London, UK: Whurr Publishers.

Dodd, B., Crosbie, S., Zhu, H., Holm, A., & Ozanne, A. (2002). *Diagnostic evaluation of articulation and phonology (DEAP)*. London, UK: Psychological Corporation.

Dodd, B., & Gillon, G. (2001). Exploring the relationship between phonological awareness, speech impairment and literacy. *Advances in Speech Language Pathology*, *3*(2), 139–147.

Dodd, B., Holm, A., Crosbie, S., & McIntosh, B. (2006). A core vocabulary approach for management of inconsistent speech disorder. *Advances in Speech-Language Pathology*, *8*(3), 220–230.

Dollaghan, C. A. (2007). *The handbook for evidence-based practice in communication disorders*. Baltimore, MD: Paul H. Brookes Publishing Co.

Duchan, J. F. (2001). *History of Speech-Language Pathology in America*. Retrieved 15 January 2014 from http://www.acsu.buffalo.edu/~duchan/history.html

Duchan, J. F. (2010). The Early Years of Language, Speech, and Hearing Services in U.S. Schools. *Language, Speech, and Hearing Services in Schools*, *41*(2), 152–160.

Duchan, J. F., Calculator, S., Sonnenmeier, R., Diehl, S., & Cumley, G. (2001). A framework for managing controversial practices. *Language Speech and Hearing Services in Schools*, *32*, 133–141.

Dworkin, J., & Cullatta, R., (1980). Tongue strength: its relationship to tongue thrusting, open-bite, and articulatory proficiency. *Journal of Speech and Hearing Disorders*, *45*, 277–282.

Edwards, S. M. (1995). *Optimizing outcomes of nonlinear phonological intervention*. Unpublished Master's thesis, University of British Columbia.

Erickson, K. (2007). Children with atypical phonological development: Assessment profiles and rates of change. Unpublished Master's thesis, University of British Columbia.

Fields, D., & Polmanteer, K. (2002). Effectiveness of oral motor techniques in articulation and phonology treatment. Poster presented at the annual convention of the American Speech-Language-Hearing Association, Atlanta, GA.

Forrest, K. (2002). Are oral-motor exercises useful in the treatment of phonological/articulatory disorders? *Seminars in Speech and Language*, *23*, 15–25.

Forrest, K., & Iuzzini, J. (2008). A comparison of oral motor and production training for children with speech sound disorders. *Seminars in Speech and Language*, *29*(4), 304–311.

Fowler, C. A. (1995). Speech production. In: J. L. Miller, & P. D. Eimas (Eds.), *Handbook of perception and cognition: Speech, language and communication* (pp. 29–61). San Diego, CA: Academic Press.

Gadhok, K. (2013). Making friends and influencing people. *RCSLT Bulletin*.

Gierut, J. (1989). Maximal opposition approach to phonological treatment. *Journal of Speech and Hearing Disorders*, *54*, 9–19.

Gierut, J. A. (1992). The conditions and course of clinically induced phonological change. *Journal of Speech and Hearing Research*, *35*, 1049–1063.

Gierut, J. A. (1998). Treatment efficacy: Functional phonological disorders in children. *Journal of Speech, Language and Hearing Research, 41*, S85–S100.

Gillon, G. T. (2000). The efficacy of phonological awareness intervention for children with spoken language impairment, *Language, Speech, and Hearing Services in Schools, 31*(2), 126–141.

Gillon, G. T. (2002). Follow-up study investigating benefits of phonological awareness intervention for children with spoken language impairment. *International Journal of Language and Communication Disorders, 37*(4), 381–400.

Gillon, G. T. (2005). Facilitating phoneme awareness development in 3- and 4-year-old children with speech impairment, *Language Speech and Hearing Services in Schools, 36*, 308–324.

Gillon, G. T., Moriarty, B., & Schwarz, I. (2006). *Evidence based practice: An update of best practices in Speech-Language Therapy*. Wellington: Ministry of Education.

Gillon, G. T., & Schwarz, I. E. (1998). *An international literature review of best practices in speech and language therapy for preschool and school aged children*. Wellington: Ministry of Education.

Gillon, G. T., & Schwarz, I. E. (2001a). An international literature review of best practices in speech and language therapy: 2001 update. Wellington: Ministry of Education.

Gillon, G. T., & Schwarz, I. (2001b). Screening Spoken Language Skills for Academic Success. *Paper presented at the Proceedings of the 2001 Speech Pathology Australia National Conference: Evidence and Innovation*, Melbourne.

Glogowska, M., & Campbell, R. (2000). Investigating parental views of involvement in pre-school speech and language therapy. *International Journal of Language and Communication Disorders, 35*(3), 391–405.

Goldsmith, J. A. (1972). *Autosegmental phonology*. MIT doctoral dissertation.

Gruber, F. A., Lowery, S. D., Seung, H-K., & Deal, R. (2003). Approaches to speech/language intervention and the true believer. *Journal of Medical Speech-Language Pathology, 11*(2), 95–104.

Guisti Braislin, M., & Cascella, P. (2005). A preliminary investigation of the efficacy of oral motor exercises for children with mild articulation disorders. *International Journal of Rehabilitation Research, 28*, 263–266.

Harris, Z. (1951). *Methods in structural linguistics*. Chicago, IL: Chicago University Press.

Harulow, S. (2013). RCSLT SIGs: the names they are a changing. *RCSLT Bulletin*.

Hatcher, P. J., Hulme, C., & Ellis, A. W. (1994). Ameliorating early reading failure by integrating the teaching of reading and phonological skills: The phonological linkage hypothesis. *Child Development, 65*, 41–57.

Hayden, D. (1984). The PROMPT system of therapy: Theoretical framework and applications for developmental apraxia of speech. *Seminars in Speech and Language, 5*(2), 139–155.

Hayes, S., Savinelli, S., Roberts, E., & Caldito, G. (2007). Use of nonspeech oral motor treatment for functional articulation disorders. *Early Childhood Services: An Interdisciplinary Journal of Effectiveness, 1*(4), 261–281.

Hesketh, A., Adams, C., Nightingale, C., & Hall, R. (2000). Phonological awareness therapy and articulatory training approaches for children with phonological disorders: a comparative outcome study. *International Journal of Language and Communication Disorders, 35*, 337–354.

Hickok, G., & Poeppel, D. (2004). Dorsal and ventral streams: a framework for understanding aspects of the functional anatomy of language. *Cognition, 92*, 67–99.

Hickok, G., Houde, J., & Rong, F. (2011). Sensorimotor integration in speech processing: computational basis and neural organization. *Neuron, 69*, 407–422.

Hodge, M. (2002). Nonspeech oral motor treatment approaches for dysarthria: Perspectives on a controversial clinical practice. *Perspectives on Neurophysiology and Neurogenic Speech and Language Disorders, 12*(4), 22–28.

Hodge, M. (2010). Intervention for developmental dysarthria. In: A. L. Williams, S. McLeod, & R. J. McCauley (Eds.), *Interventions for speech sound disorders in children* (pp. 557–578). Baltimore, MD: Paul H. Brookes Publishing Co.

Hodge, M. (2011). University-community collaboration to advance practice and improve outcomes in complex childhood speech disorders. Paper presented at the Alberta Rehabilitation Conference, Edmonton, Canada.

Hodge, M., Salonka, R., & Kollias, S. (2005). Use of nonspeech oral-motor exercises in children's speech therapy. Poster presented at the *American Speech-Language-Hearing Association Convention*, San Diego, CA.

Hodson, B. (2007, 2010). *Evaluating and enhancing children's phonological systems: Research and theory to practice*. Wichita, KS: PhonoComp Publishers.

Hodson, B. W., & Paden, E. P. (1981). Phonological processes which characterize unintelligible and unintelligible speech in early childhood. *Journal of Speech and Hearing Disorders, 46*, 369–373.

Hodson, B. W., & Paden, E. P. (1991). *Targeting intelligible speech: A phonological approach to remediation* (2nd ed.). Austin, TX: Pro-Ed.

Howell, J., & Dean. E. (1994). *Treating phonological disorders in children: Metaphon theory to practice*. London: Whurr Publishers.

Hulme, C., Hatcher, P. J., Nation, K., Brown, A., Adams, J., & Stuart, G. (2002). Phoneme awareness is a better predictor of early reading skill than onset-rime awareness. *Journal of Experimental Child Psychology, 82*, 2–28.

Ingram, D. (1998). Research-practice relationships in speech-language pathology. *Topics in Language Disorders, 18*, 2, 1–9.

Ingram, D., & Ingram, K. (2001). A whole word approach to phonological intervention. *Language, Speech and Hearing Services in Schools, 32*, 271–283.

Irwin, D., Pannbacker, M., Powell, T. W., & Vekovius, G. T. (2007). *Ethics for speech-language pathologists and audiologists: An illustrative casebook*. Clifton Park, NY: Thomson Delmar Learning.

Jacobson, J. W., Foxx, R. M., & Mulick, J. A. (2005). *Controversial therapies for developmental disabilities: Fad fashion and science in professional practice*. Mahwah, NJ: Lawrence Erlbaum Associates.

Joffe, V. L. (2008). Minding the gap between research and practice in developmental language disorders. In: V. L. Joffe, M. Cruice, & S. Chiat (Eds), *Language disorders in children and adults: New issues in research and practice*. London, UK: John Wiley.

Joffe, V. L. (2009). A survey of clinical practice in the UK. In C. Bowen, *Children's speech sound disorders*. (pp. 175–179). Oxford: Wiley-Blackwell.

Joffe, B., & Serry, T. (2004). The evidence base for the treatment of articulation and phonological disorders in children. In: S. Reilly, J. Douglas, & J. Oates (Eds.), *Evidence based practice in speech pathology*. London, UK: Whurr Publishers.

Joffe, V. L., & Pring, T. (2008). Children with phonological problems: A survey of clinical practice. *International Journal of Language and Communication Disorders. 43*(2), 154–164.

Johnson, C. J. (2006). Getting started in evidence-based practice for childhood speech-language disorders. *American Journal of Speech-Language Pathology, 15*(1), 20–35.

Jones, D. L., Hardin-Jones, M. A., & Brown, C. (2011). Aerodynamic requirements for blowing novelty horns. Poster presented at the annual convention of the American Speech-Language-Hearing Association, San Diego, CA.

Kamhi, A. (2004). A meme's eye view of speech-language pathology. *Language, Speech, and Hearing in the Schools, 35*, 105–111.

Kahmi, A. G. (2006a). Prologue: Combining research and reason to make treatment decisions. *Language Speech and Hearing Services in Schools, 37*(4), 255–257.

Kamhi, A. G. (2006b). Treatment decisions for children with speech-sound disorders. *Language, Speech, and Hearing Services in Schools, 37*(4), 271–279.

Keeling, M., & Keeling, K. J. (2006). *CLEAR phonology screening assessment*. (2nd ed.). Spilsby, Lincolnshire: CLEAR Resources.

Kennard, G. (1997). *Signalong: Basic vocabulary. Phase 1*. London, UK: Signalong Group.

Kenny, B., Lincoln, M., & Balandin, S. (2010). Experienced speech-language pathologists' responses to ethical dilemmas: An integrated approach to ethical reasoning. *American Journal of Speech-Language Pathology, 19*, 121–134.

Kent, R. (2004). The uniqueness of speech among motor systems. *Clinical Linguistics & Phonetics, 18*, 495–505.

Klein, H., Lederer, S., & Cortese, E. (1991). Children's knowledge of auditory/articulator correspondences: Phonologic and metaphonologic. *Journal of Speech and Hearing Research, 34*, 559–564.

Koegel, L., Koegel, R., & Ingham, J. (1986). Programming rapid generalization of correct articulation through self-monitoring procedures. *Journal of Speech and Hearing Disorders, 51*, 24–32.

Kollias, S., & Lester, R. (2004). *Nonspeech oral motor exercises in children's speech therapy: Clinicians' opinions and experiences*. Edmonton, AB: Unpublished manuscript. University of Alberta.

Kotz, S. A., & Schwartze, M. (2010). Cortical speech processing unplugged: a timely subcortico-cortical framework. *Trends in Cognitive Sciences, 14*, 392–399.

Kwiatkowski, J., & Shriberg, L. D. (1998). The capability-focus treatment framework for child speech disorders. *American Journal of Speech-Language Pathology*, 7, 27–38.

Lancaster, G. S., Levin, A., Pring, T., & Martin, S. (2010). Treating children with phonological problems: Does an eclectic approach to therapy work? *International Journal of Language and Communication Disorders* 45(2), 174–181.

Larroudé, B. (2004). Multicultural-multilingual group sessions: Development of functional communication. *Topics in language disorders*, *24*, 137–140.

Lass, N. J., & Pannbacker, M. (2008). The application of evidence-based practice to oral motor treatment. *Language, Speech, and Hearing Services in Schools*, 39(3), 408–421.

Lave, J., & Wenger, E. (1991). *Situated learning: Legitimate peripheral participation*. New York, NY: Cambridge University Press.

Lee, A. S-Y., & Gibbon, F. E. (2011). 'Non-speech oral motor treatment for developmental speech sound disorders in children (Protocol)'. *Cochrane Database of Systematic Reviews 2011*, (10). Art. No.: CD009383.

Leiter, V. (2004). Dilemmas in sharing care: maternal provision of professionally driven therapy for children with disabilities. *Social Science & Medicine*, *58*, 837–849.

Liberman, A. M. (1996). *Speech: A special code*. Cambridge, MA: MIT Press.

Liberman, M., & Prince, A. (1977). On stress and linguistic rhythm. *Linguistic Inquiry*, 8, 249–336.

Limbrick, N., McCormack, S., & McLeod, S. (2013). Designs and decisions: The creation of informal measures for assessing speech production in children. *International Journal of Speech-Language Pathology*, *15*(3), 296–311.

Litchfield, R., & MacDougall, C. (2002). Professional issues for physiotherapists in family-centred and community-based settings. *Australian Journal of Physiotherapy*, *48*, 105–112.

Lloyd, S., & Wernham, S. (1992). *The Phonics Handbook, (1994 onwards) Jolly Phonics*. Chigwell, Essex, UK: Jolly Learning Ltd.

Lof, G. L. (2002). Special forum on phonology: Two comments on this assessment series. *American Journal of Speech-Language Pathology*, *11*, 255–256.

Lof, G. L. (2003). Oral motor exercises and treatment outcomes. *Perspectives on Language, Learning and Education*, *10*(1), 7–12.

Lof, G. L. (2008). Introduction to controversies about the use of nonspeech oral motor exercises. *Seminars in Speech and Language*, *29*(4), 253–256.

Lof, G. L. (2011). Science-based practice and the speech-language pathologist. *International Journal of Speech-Language Pathology*, *13*(3), 189–196.

Lof, G. L., & Watson, M. M. (2004). Speech-language pathologists' use of nonspeech oral-motor drills: National survey results. Poster presented at the *American Speech-Language-Hearing Association Convention*, Philadelphia, PA.

Lof, G. L., & Watson, M. M. (2008). A nationwide survey of non-speech oral motor exercise use: Implications for evidence-based practice. *Language, Speech, and Hearing in Schools*, 39(3), 392–407.

Lof, G. L., & Watson, M. (2010). Five reasons why nonspeech oral-motor exercises do not work. *Perspectives in Language and Learning*, *11*, 109–117.

Loncar-Belding, L. (1998). *Take Home™ Oral-motor exercises*. East Moline, IL: LinguiSystems.

Londei, A., D'Ausilio, A., Basso, D., Sestieri, C., Gratta, C. D., Romani, G. L., & Belardinelli, M. O. (2010). Sensory-motor brain network connectivity for speech comprehension. *Human Brain Mapping*, *31*, 567–580.

Long, S. H. (2007). Computerized Profiling (Version 9.7.0) [Computer software]. Arcata, CA: Author. Retrieved 15 January 2014 from www.computerizedprofiling.org.

Ludlow, C., Hoit, J., Kent, R., Ramig, L., Shrivastav, R., Strand, E., Yorkston, K., & Sapienza, C. (2008). Translating principles of neural plasticity into research on speech motor control recovery and rehabilitation. *Journal of Speech, Language, and Hearing Research*, *51*, S240–S258.

Lum, C. (2002). *Scientific thinking in speech and language therapy*. Mahwah, NJ: Lawrence Erlbaum Associates.

MacKean, G., Thurston, W., & Scott, C. (2005). Bridging the divide between families and health professionals' perspectives on family-centred care. *Health Expectations*, 8, 74–85.

Mackenzie, C., Muir, M., & Allen, C. (2010). Non-speech oro-motor exercise use in acquire dysarthria management: Regimes and rationales. *International Journal of Language and Communication Disorders*, *45*, 617–629.

Major, E., & Bernhardt, B. (1998). Metaphonological skills of children with phonological disorders before and after phonological and metaphonological intervention. *International Journal of Language and Communication Disorders*, *33*, 413–444.

Marshalla, P. (2004). Oral-motor techniques in articulation and phonological therapy (Millennium Edn, revised 2000). Kirkland, WA: Marshalla Speech and Language.

Masterson, J., & Bernhardt, B. (2001). *Computerized articulation and evaluation phonology system (CAPES)*. San Antonio, TX: The Psychological Corporation.

McAllister, L., & Lincoln, M. (2004). *Clinical education in speech-language pathology*. London, UK: Whurr Publishers.

McCarthy, J. (1988). Feature geometry and dependency: a review. *Phonetica, 43*, 84–108.

McCauley, R. J., Strand, E., Lof, G. L., Schooling, T., & Frymark, T. (2009). Evidence-based systematic review: Effects of nonspeech oral motor exercises on speech, *American Journal of Speech-Language Pathology, 18*, 343–360.

McComas, K. L. (2009). Developing professional identities: A goal for educational programs. In: Bowen, C. *Children's speech sound disorders* (pp. 185–189). Oxford: Wiley-Blackwell.

McComas, K. L. (2014). *Dig in Your Heels and Fight: How Women Become Researchers in Communication Sciences and Disorders*. Guildford: J & R Press.

McKean, K., Phillips, B., & Thompson, A. (2012). A family-centred model of care in paediatric speech-language pathology. *International Journal of Speech-Language Pathology, 14*(3), 235–246.

McLeod, S., & Baker, E. (2004). Current clinical practice for children with speech impairment. In: B. E. Murdoch, J. Goozee, B. M. Whelan, & K. Docking (Eds.), *Proceedings of the 26th World Congress of the International Association of logopedics and phoniatrics*. Brisbane: University of Queensland.

Meredith, G., Firmin, S., & McAllister, L. (2013). Digital possibilities and ethical considerations: Speech language pathologists and the web. *Journal of Clinical Practice in Speech-Language Pathology, 15*(1), 44–47.

Minke, K., & Scott, M. (1995). Parent-professional relationships in early intervention: A qualitative investigation. *Topics in Early Childhood Special Education, 15*(3), 335–352.

Mirabito, K., & Armstrong, E. (2005, May). *Parent reactions to speech therapy involvement*. Paper presented at the Speech Pathology Australia National Conference, Canberra.

Mullis I., Martin M., Foy P., & Drucker K. (2012). Progress in International Literacy Study (PIRLS, 2011). Amsterdam, the Netherlands: International Association for the Evaluation of Educational Achievement (IEA) Available from http://timss.bc.edu/pirls2011/downloads/P11_IR_FullBook.pdf.

Muttiah, N., Georges, K., & Brackenbury, T. (2011). Clinical and research perspectives on nonspeech oral motor treatments and evidence-based practice. *American Journal of Speech-Language Pathology, 20*, 47–59.

Nemoy, E., & Davis, S. (1937). *The correction of defective consonant sounds*. Boston: Expression Company.

Nunes, A. (2009). A legacy lost. In: C. Bowen, *Children's speech sound disorders* (pp. 4–7). Oxford: Wiley-Blackwell.

Occhino, C., & McCann, J. (2001). *Do oral motor exercise affect articulation?* Poster presented at the annual meeting of the American Speech-Language-Hearing Association, New Orleans, LA.

Ogg, K., Jones, D. L., & Hardin-Jones, M. (2012). Oral pressure requirements for common blow toys. Poster presented at the annual meeting of the American Speech-Language-Hearing Association, Atlanta, GA.

Orr, C. (1998). *Mouth madness: Oral motor activities for children*. San Antonio, TX: Therapy Skill Builders.

Palmer, P. J., & Zajonc, A. (2010). *The heart of higher education: A call to renewal*. San Francisco, CA: Jossey-Bass.

Pascoe, M., Stackhouse, J., & Wells, B. (2005). Phonological therapy within a psycholinguistic framework: promoting change in a child with persisting speech difficulties. *International Journal of Language and Communication Disorders, 40*(2), 189–220.

Passy, J. (1993). *Cued articulation*. Ponteland, Northumberland: STASS Publications.

Pennington, L., Miller, N., Robson, S., & Steen, N. (2010). Intensive speech and language therapy for older children with cerebral palsy: A systems approach. *Developmental Medicine and Child Neurology, 52*(4), 337–344.

Pennington, L., Roelant, E., Thompson, V., Robson, S., Steen, N., & Miller, N. (2012). Intensive dysarthria therapy for younger children with cerebral palsy. *Developmental Medicine and Child Neurology, 55*(4), 464–471.

Pollock, M., Gaesser, G., Butcher, J., Despres, J., Dishman, R., Franklin, B., & Ewing Garber, C. (1998). The recommended quantity and quality of exercise for developing and maintaining cardiorespiratory and muscular fitness, and flexibility in healthy adults. *Medicine & Science in Sports & Exercise, 30*, 975–991.

Powell, T. W. (2007). A model for ethical practices in clinical phonetics and linguistics. *Clinical Linguistics & Phonetics, 21*, 851–857.

Powell, T. W. (2008a). The use of nonspeech oral motor treatments for developmental speech sound production disorders: Interventions and interactions. *Language, Speech, and Hearing Services in Schools, 39*(3), 374–379.

Powell, T. W. (2008b). An integrated evaluation of nonspeech oral-motor treatments. *Language, Speech, and Hearing Services in Schools, 39*(3), 422–427.

Powell, T. W. (2013). Research ethics. In: N. Müller, & M. J. Ball (Eds.), *Research methods in clinical linguistics and phonetics: A practical guide* (pp. 10–27). Malden, MA: Wiley-Blackwell.

Price, C. J. (2012). A review and synthesis of the first 20 years of PET and fMRI studies of heard speech, spoken language and reading. *NeuroImage, 62*, 816–847.

Pring, T., Flood, E., Dodd, B., & Joffe, V. (2012). The working practices and clinical experiences of paediatric speech and language therapists: A national UK survey. *International Journal of Language and Communication Disorders, 47*, 6, 696–708.

Reilly, S. (2004). The move to evidence-based practice within speech pathology. In: S. Reilly, J. Douglas, & J. Oates (Eds.), *Evidence-based practice in speech pathology* (pp. 3–17). London: Whurr Publishers.

Reilly, S., Douglas, J., & Oates, J. (Eds.) (2004). *Evidence-based practice in speech pathology*. London: Whurr Publishers.

Renfrew, C. (2010). *Renfrew action picture test*. Milton Keynes, UK: Speechmark Publishing.

Robertson, M. (2007). Speech sound disorders: Comments on Prezas and Hodson, *Encyclopedia of Language and Literacy Development* (pp. 1–7). London, ON: Canadian Language and Literacy Research Network. Retrieved 28 September 2013 from www.literacyencyclopedia.ca/pdfs/topic.php?topld=37

Roddam, H., & Skeat, J. (2010). *Embedding evidence-based practice in speech and language therapy: International examples*. London, UK: Wiley-Blackwell.

Roehrig, S., Suiter, D., & Pierce, T. (2004). An examination of the effectiveness of passive oral-motor exercises. Poster presented at the *Annual Convention of the American Speech-Language-Hearing Association, Philadelphia, PA.*

Rosenbaum, P., King, S., Law, M., King, G., & Evans, J. (1998). Family-centred service: A conceptual framework and research review. *Physical & Occupational Therapy in Pediatrics, 18*, 1–20.

Rosenfeld-Johnson, S. (1999). *Oral motor exercises for speech clarity*. Tucson, AZ: Ravenhawk.

Rosenfeld-Johnson, S. (2001). *Oral-motor exercises for speech clarity*. Tucson, AZ: Innovative Therapists International.

Rosenfeld-Johnson, S. (2010). Muscle placement and movement patterns for speech clarity and feeding safety. *Workshop presented at the Annual Conference of the Canadian Association of Speech-Language Pathologists and Audiologists,* Whitehorse, Canada.

Roulstone, S., Wren, Y., Bakopoulou, I., Goodlad, S., Lindsay, G. (2012). *Exploring interventions for children and young people with speech, language and communication needs: A study of practice*. London, UK: Department for Education.

Ruggero, L., McCabe, P., Ballard, K. J., & Munro, N. (2012). Paediatric speech language pathology service delivery: An exploratory survey of Australian parents. *International Journal of Speech-Language Pathology, 14*(4), 338–350.

Ruscello, D. M. (2008). Oral motor treatment issues related to children with developmental speech sound disorders. *Language, Speech, and Hearing Services in Schools, 39*(3), 380–391.

Ruscello, D. M. (2010). Collective findings neither support nor refute the use of oral motor exercises as a treatment for speech sound disorders. *Evidence-based Communication Assessment and Intervention, 4*, 65–72.

Rvachew, S. (2005). The importance of phonetic factors in phonological intervention. In: A. G. Kamhi, & K. E. Pollock (Eds.), *Phonological disorders in children: Clinical decision making in assessment and intervention* (pp. 175–187). Baltimore, MD: Paul H. Brookes Publishing Co.

Rvachew, S., & Brosseau-Lapré, F. (2012). *Developmental phonological disorders: Foundations of clinical practice*. San Diego, CA: Plural Publishing.

Rvachew, S., Nowak, M., & Cloutier, G. (2004). Effect of phonemic perception training on the speech production and phonological awareness skills of children with expressive phonological delay. *American Journal of Speech-Language Pathology, 13*, 250–263.

Rvachew, S., Ohberg, A., Grawburg, M., & Heyding, J. (2003). Phonological awareness and phonemic perception in 4-year-old children with delayed expressive phonology skills. *American Journal of Speech-Language Pathology, 12,* 463–471.

Schoolfield, L. (1937). *Better speech and better reading.* Boston, MA: Expression.

Schulz, G., Dingwall, W., & Ludlow, C. (1999). Speech and oral motor learning in individuals with cerebellar atrophy. *Journal of Speech, Language, and Hearing Research, 42,* 1157–1175.

Secord, W., Boyce, S. Donohue, J., Fox, R., & Shine R. (2007). *Eliciting Sounds: Techniques and Strategies for Clinicians* (2nd ed.). Clifton Park, NY: Thompson Delmar Learning.

Shelton, R. L. (2005). Oral motor treatments [letter to the editor]. *ASHA Leader, 10*(12), 36.

Shriberg, L. D. (2003). Diagnostic markers for child speech-sound disorders: Introductory comments. *Clinical Linguistics and Phonetics, 17,* 501–505.

Sjögreena, L., Tuliniusb, M., Kiliaridisc, S., & Lohmanderd, A. (2010). The effect of lip strengthening exercises in children and adolescents with myotonic dystrophy type 1. *International Journal of Pediatric Otorhinolaryngology, 74*(10), 1126–1134.

Skahan, S. M., Watson, M., & Lof, G. L. (2007). Speech language pathologist assessment practices for children with suspected speech sound disorders: Results of a national survey. *American Journal of Speech-Language Pathology, 16,* 246–259.

Smith, E. C., & Lewicki, M. S. (2006). Efficient auditory coding. *Nature, 439,* 978–982.

Solomon, N., & Munson, B. (2004). The effect of jaw position on measures of tongue strength and endurance. *Journal of Speech, Language, and Hearing Research, 47,* 584–594.

Stackhouse, J., & Wells, B. (1997). *Children's speech and literacy difficulties I: A psycholinguistic framework.* London, UK: Whurr Publishers.

Stemberger, J. P., & Bernhardt, B. (1997). Optimality theory. In: M. Ball, & R. Kent (Eds.) *The new phonologies.* (pp. 211–245). San Diego, CA: Singular Press.

Stoel-Gammon, C., & Dunn, C. (1985). *Normal and disordered phonology in children.* Baltimore, MD: University Park Press.

Strode, R., & Chamberlain, C. (1997). *Easy does it*™ *for articulation: An oral-motor approach.* E. Moline, IL: LinguiSystems.

Sudbery, A., Wilson, E, Broaddus, T., & Potter, N. (2006). Tongue strength in preschool children: Measures, implications, and revelations. Poster pre-

sented at the annual convention of the American Speech-Language-Hearing Association, Miami Beach, FL.

Swift, W. B. (1918). *Speech defects in school children and how to treat them.* Boston, MA: Houghton Mifflin.

TalkTools (2013). Original horn kit. Retrieved 15 January 2014 from www.talktools.com/original-horn-kit/.

Taylor-Goh, S. (2005). *royal college of speech and language therapists: Clinical guidelines.* Brackley: Speechmark Publishing.

Tharpe, A. M. (1998). Treatment fads versus evidence-based practice. In: F. H. Bess (Ed.), *Children with hearing impairment: Contemporary trends* (pp. 179–188). Nashville, TN: Vanderbilt Bill Wilkerson Press.

Thompson, K. (1998). Early intervention services in daily family life: mothers' perceptions of 'ideal' versus 'actual' service provision. *Occupational Therapy International, 5*(3), 206–221.

Toki, E.I., & Pange, J. (2012). E-learning activities for articulation in speech-language therapy and learning for preschool children. *Procedia Social and Behavioural Sciences, 2,* 4274–4278.

Tomarakos, D. (2012). App Review Rating Scale. Retrieved 10 October 2013 from http://www.speechgadget.com

Tunmer, W., Chapman, J., & Prochnow, J. (2006). Literate cultural capital at school entry predicts later reading achievement: A seven year longitudinal study. *New Zealand Journal of Educational Studies.*

Tyler, A. A. (2005). Planning and monitoring intervention programs. In: A. G. Kamhi, & K. E. Pollock (Eds.), *Phonological disorders in children: Clinical decision making in assessment and intervention* (pp. 123–137). Baltimore, MD: Paul H. Brookes Publishing Co.

Tyler, A. A. (2008). What works: evidence-based intervention for children with speech sound disorders. *Seminars in Speech and Language, 29*(4), 320–330.

Tyler, A. A. & Lewis, K.E. (2005). Relationships among consistency/variability and other phonological measures over time. *Topics in Language Disorder: Clinical Perspectives on Speech Sound Disorders, 25*(3), 243–253.

Ullrich, A. (2007). *Nichtlineare phonologische Diagnostik, NILPOD.* Unpublished manuscript. [Nonlinear phonological assessment].

Ullrich, A., & Bernhardt, B. (2005). Neue Perspektiven der phonologischen Analyse - Implikationen für die

Untersuchungphonologischer Entwicklungsstörungen. *Die Sprachheilarbeit, 5,* 221–233. [New perspectives in phonological analysis – Implications for the investigation of developmental phonological impairments.]

Van Riper, C. (1978). *Speech correction: Principles and methods* (6th ed.). Englewood Cliffs, NJ: Prentice-Hall.

Velleman, S. (2002). Phonotactic therapy. *Seminars in Speech and Language, 23,* 43–57.

Von Bremen, V. (1990). *A nonlinear phonological approach to intervention with severely phonologically disordered twins.* Unpublished Master's thesis, University of British Columbia.

Watts Pappas, N., & Bowen, C. (2007). Speech Acquisition and the Family. In: McLeod, S. (Ed.), *The International guide to speech acquisition.* Clifton Park, NY: Thomson Delmar Learning.

Watts Pappas, N., & McLeod, S. (2008a). Parents' perceptions of their involvement in paediatric allied health intervention. In: N. Watts Pappas, & S. McLeod (Eds.), *Working with families in speech-language pathology.* San Diego, CA: Plural Publishing.

Watts Pappas, N., & McLeod, S. (2008b). Speech-language pathologists' and other allied health professionals' perceptions of working with parents and families. In: N. Watts Pappas, & S. McLeod (Eds.), *Working with families in speech-language pathology.* San Diego, CA: Plural Publishing.

Watts Pappas, N., McLeod, S., McAllister, L., & Daniel, G. (2006). Parental involvement in phonological intervention. Paper presented to *International Clinical Linguistics and Phonetics Association Conference,* Dubrovnik, Croatia, May 31–June 3.

Watts Pappas, N., McLeod, S., McAllister, L., & Mc-Kinnon, D. H. (2008). Parental involvement in speech intervention: A national survey. *Clinical Linguistics and Phonetics, 22*(4), 335–344.

Watson, M., & Lof, G. L. (2008). What we know about nonspeech oral motor exercises. *Seminars in Speech and Language, 29*(4), 320–330.

Watson, M., & Lof, G. L. (2009). A survey of university professors teaching speech sound disorders: Nonspeech oral motor exercise and other topics. *Language, Speech and Hearing Services in the Schools, 40,* 256–270.

Weiner, F. (1981). Treatment of phonological disability using the method of meaningful contrast: Two case studies. *Journal of Speech and Hearing Disorders, 46,* 97–103.

Weismer, G. (1997). *Assessment of oromotor, nonspeech gestures in speech-language pathology: A critical review* (Videotape recording Telerounds 35). Tucson, AX: National Center for Neurologic Communication Disorders.

Weismer, G. (2006). Philosophy of research in motor speech disorders. *Clinical Linguistics & Phonetics, 20,* 315–349.

Wenger, E., McDermott, R., & Snyder, W. M. (2002). *A guide to managing knowledge: Cultivating communities of practice.* Boston, MA: Harvard Business School Press.

Wenke, R., Goozee, J., Murdoch, B., & LaPointe, L. (2006). Dynamic assessment of articulation during lingual fatigue in myasthenia gravis. *Journal of Medical Speech-Language Pathology, 14,* 13–32.

Williams, A. L. (2003a). Target selection and treatment outcomes. *Perspectives on Language Learning and Education, 10,* 1, 12–16.

Williams, A. L. (2003b). *Speech disorders: Resource guide for preschool children.* Clifton Park, NY: Thomson Delmar Learning.

Williams, P. & Stephens, H. (2004). *Nuffield centre dyspraxia programme* (3rd ed.) Windsor, UK: The Miracle Factory.

Wilson, E., Green, J., Yunusova, Y., & Moore, C. (2008). Task specificity in early oral motor development. *Seminars in Speech and Language, 29*(4), 257–266.

Ziegler, W. (2003). Speech motor control is task-specific: Evidence from dysarthria and apraxia of speech. *Aphasiology, 17,* 3–36.

Part II

Speech intervention in everyday practice

Introduction

In A15 in Part I of this book, family therapist and professor of family counselling James Bitter presented systemic interventions that SLPs/SLTs working in treatment teams can use with the families of children with speech sound disorders whose behaviour is difficult. In a related essay, A16, SLPs Megan Overby and John Bernthal reviewed the literature associated with counselling in communication sciences generally, and in SSD specifically, and pointed to the signs that might prompt the speech–language clinician to refer a family and/or their child to a professional counsellor. In both of these essays there was a sense that the SLP/SLT could call on an expert (counsellor) if the demands of the situation exceeded their capabilities. In some situations, however, calling in outside counselling help may not be a possibility, and, even if it is an available option, it may not be the *best* one.

Information sharing and parent and/or client counselling often overlap in SLP/SLT practice, and both can occur expectedly or unpredictably. They can be prompted, for example by a mother's impulsive query about prognosis that must be considered and carefully answered if possible; a father's unanticipated revelation of relevant family history that needs sensitive tracking through; a spontaneous emotional response on a parent's part that requires proper acknowledgement; an extended family members' confusion about inaccurate information about a child's SSD, perhaps provided by either an SLP/SLT colleague or by a non-SLP/SLT, that necessitates clarification; or a child with a speech sound disorder suddenly asking, 'Why me?' Mostly, calling in a professional counsellor is not indicated when questions and situations such as these arise, and the counselling role falls most appropriately to the SLP/SLT who knows the family, the child, the presenting issues and the range of pertinent, obtainable supports that might be helpful for them.

SLPs/SLTs as counsellors

Despite relevant academic and clinical preparation, and/or clinical experience, our counselling and information-sharing capacities are

Children's Speech Sound Disorders, Second Edition. Caroline Bowen.
© 2015 John Wiley & Sons, Ltd. Published 2015 by John Wiley & Sons, Ltd.
Companion website: www.wiley.com/go/bowen/speechlanguagetherapy

often tested when issues of severity of involvement and complex comorbidities arise, and Dr. Ruth Stoeckel has thought about this deeply. Dr. Stoeckel is an SLP engaged in clinical and research work. For her PhD at the University of Minnesota, she investigated development of phonological knowledge in young children. She is employed at the Mayo Clinic in Rochester, Minnesota, where she evaluates and treats young children with a range of speech–language difficulties, including motor speech disorders. She presents her work at professional conference and CEU events locally and nationally in the United States and is strongly identified with CASANA (Gretz, A7) through advisory board, workshop and other contributions. Dr. Stoeckel is known for her theoretically unassailable and evidence-based postings to the Apraxia-KIDS listserv, and for her skill as a writer in e-mail and message board discussion in expressing complex, technical and potentially disquieting information unambiguously and supportively. It may be that the empathy she brings to these, sometimes delicate, exchanges is a product not only of her professional experience but also of her personal insight as a parent of a young adult struggling with aspects of speech–language processing, and with the way she is perceived.

Q40.   Ruth Stoeckel: Counselling families of children with SSD plus

For SLPs/SLTs, fundamental aspects of child-centred dynamic assessment (Stone-Goldman, A44; Strand, A45) and therapy delivery within family-centred practice frameworks (Watts Pappas, A30) are the provision of accurate and timely information. There is also an obligation for us to communicate empathically in a manner that 'fits' with the needs, capacities, cultures, value systems and beliefs, levels of acceptance and emotional landscapes of the family and their significant others. In each unique and changing situation that arises around minimally verbal or highly unintelligible children with major SSD, such as

severe CAS, we have both an educative and a counselling role. Many of our families, endlessly striving to do the best they can for their children, are influenced by information about the nature and management of their children's issues that is variously unscientific, misleading, time-wasting, worrying, or downright dangerous.

This is of particular concern in cases of children who may indeed have CAS, and for whom its treatment becomes a *raison d'etre* for their parents, but who have a range of other challenges impacting progress. It is also of concern with regard to parents of severely communicatively impaired children who do not have, and may never have, a definite speech–language disorder or other diagnosis. Misinformation can come from the immediate and wider circle of family and friends, where inevitably there will be a self-styled, often critical or denying, child development expert at hand! It can also come from our SLP/SLT and other professional colleagues and friends, and from faceless but ostensibly authoritative Internet 'experts' and 'e-friends'. There are no easy answers, but how would you educate the educators and counsel the counsellors charged with these important and demanding SLP/SLT educative and counselling tasks?

A40.   Ruth Stoeckel: Discussing appropriate treatment options for children with SSD and comorbid conditions

Mrs. Smith's 4-year-old son, Bobby, runs around the room, opens every door and drawer, impulsively picks up then drops toys, and produces a constant stream of unintelligible jargon. He does not look at you or his mother, even when you are trying to get his attention so that you can begin the evaluation. Attempts to have him sit quietly for a moment result in screaming and resisting.

Mrs. Smith reports that Bobby has diagnoses of delayed language, verbal apraxia and sensory issues. His progress in speech therapy has been slow. You are being asked for a second opinion about diagnosis and appropriate treatment strategies. Mrs. Smith expresses an expectation that if Bobby can communicate more effectively, his behaviour will be much improved as well. Do you agree with Mrs. Smith? How would you approach concerns about Bobby's behaviour with her?

A 5-year-old girl with Down syndrome named Precious comes for evaluation with her father, Mr. Sanchez. Precious has 15 recognisable word approximations and can produce most speech sounds in isolation. She expresses herself through a combination of vocalizations and signing. Her sign-language vocabulary includes 50 single signs, used to label objects and to make requests. Her only two-sign combinations consist of 'want' plus a noun. She follows one-step directions easily, but needs help to follow two-step directions. Precious can identify several letters of the alphabet and tries to count along with her teacher. Mr. Sanchez has heard about childhood apraxia of speech (CAS) from the parent of another child in his daughter's preschool program, and wants to know if that is the reason his daughter is not talking. He wonders if her delay in language is a result of difficulty saying words clearly. How would you explain the relative contribution of cognitive issues, language impairment and speech impairment to Mr. Sanchez? What goals would you suggest to facilitate Precious' ability to communicate?

Sigrid is the 27-month-old daughter of Mr. and Mrs. Happel. She was born nearly 6 weeks premature, and has been slow to achieve developmental milestones. Sigrid began walking at 19 months. She had difficulty sucking as an infant and now chokes easily on foods other than thickened cereal. Babbling is limited to 'ah' alone or repeated in syllable strings. Sigrid is just beginning to point to objects and to manipulate toys rather than put them in her mouth. Her parents realise that she is delayed in several areas and have been searching the Internet for answers. They tell you that Sigrid 'fits all the signs' of CAS that they found at one site and want to know if you can begin intensive speech therapy immediately to help their daughter overcome this disorder. They are looking for someone to do *demosthenic rock therapy* (DRT) because they have read testimonials suggesting that correct use of the special rocks sold by the developer of this therapy will result in dramatic improvements in the speech of children with a range of developmental challenges. How will you help the family to evaluate this unproven treatment and make your own reasoned decision about whether to provide it? How will you counsel the parents about their child's communication in the context of her overall presentation?

Ten-year-old Abdi was given a diagnosis of CAS by his paediatrician when he was 3 years old because he was unintelligible. He is now speaking clearly, except for a mild distortion of /r/, for which he continues in speech therapy. Abdi has struggled with learning to read. Other children are reading at a much higher level, while Abdi is still working hard to read books designed for beginning readers. Abdi does well in other academic areas but struggles to grasp information that he has read or to sound out words that he does not already know. His parents are frustrated and ask you to intensify your efforts to 'fix his apraxia' in hopes that this will facilitate improvements in reading. How could you include support for literacy skills in your work with Abdi? How would you explain to Abdi's parents that while his history of speech impairment is a risk factor for later literacy issues, his current difficulty might need to be treated as a related, but separate, area of need?

What the above scenarios have in common is the likelihood that there are developmental issues in addition to speech sound impairment. Some parents recognise their child's speech disorder as just one of multiple challenges. Others may be focused on speech as the core problem, which, when treated, they hope will result in improvements in other areas. Our job as clinicians is to not only evaluate and treat a child's speech and language disorder, but also to help parents understand the relative contribution of speech and language problems within the context of the 'whole child'. In terms of the preceding examples, that means identifying to what extent each child's problem with communication may reflect the effects of, or interaction with, a more general developmental disorder.

Whether or not comorbid problems exist, it is important for clinicians to be empathetic listeners who are sensitive to what parents are ready to hear (Luterman, 2008). It can be helpful to invite parents to work *with* us in discovering their child's strengths as well as their needs (Hennessy & Hennessy, 2013). In some cases, intervention will need to address a child's other areas of need as the priority. Clinicians can describe specifically how a proposed intervention will address the child's current communication needs and how it will be modified in the future based on the child's progress. A study by Miron (2012) reported that for parents of children with speech disorders, parenting stress appears to be influenced significantly by external factors such as misdiagnosis, lack of adequate insurance coverage, or inadequate services and that positive encounters with providers appear to facilitate positive adaptation. This underlines the importance of providing competent service and developing a professional relationship in which parents have confidence in the services being provided to their child.

Even when parents and clinicians share a common understanding of diagnosis and intervention, perspectives about desired outcomes for treatment may be different. Thomas-Stonell, Oddson, Robertson and Rosenbaum (2009) used the World Health Organization's (WHO) International Classification of Functioning, Disability and Health—Child and Youth Version (ICF-CY) to ask parents and clinicians to classify expectations and outcomes of therapy. They found that clinicians tended to focus on treatment of Body Function and Activities/Capacities, which is in keeping with the 'medical' model and behavioural emphasis in training programs, parents were more likely to express concern about Participation Restrictions or Personal Factors (e.g., shyness, behaviour problems). McCormack, McLeod, Harrison and McAllister (2010) similarly found that while clinicians and parents agreed that verbal communication was an area of impact for children with speech impairment, there were differences in perceived priority of other factors, such as social relationships and learning. To address these larger goals, clinicians may need to consider a broad-based treatment approach that includes work on improved attention, participation in play or learning tasks, and socialisation as they work to improve communication skills. This broad perspective facilitates intervention that incorporates a variety of factors that influence communication at home and in the community as opposed to a narrow focus on speech sound accuracy or acquisition of vocabulary.

Parents can find a wealth of information about speech–language disorders through a variety of sources, including seminars, stories in the popular press, and Internet sites that run the gamut from general information to product advertisements. This ease of access can facilitate their ability to learn more about their child's disorder and more actively participate in the process of assessment and treatment. However, critical evaluation of this information to recognise content that may be incomplete, incorrect or even irresponsible is essential. As clinicians, we have a responsibility to guide parents to the best available information.

Clinicians can help parents understand speech–language problems by sharing information based on our own knowledge and experience and be supportive if there is a request for second opinion. We can demonstrate a sense of mutual respect and shared power for decision-making (Stone & Olswang, 1989) by facilitating parents' efforts to learn more about their child's difficulties. We encourage parents to become our partners when we respond to questions with explanations based on the best available evidence and keep an open mind about ideas that may be new to us. Parents may realise that something is 'too good to be true', but when they are desperately seeking answers it can be hard for them to set aside the desire to try unproven interventions. The emotional aspects of dealing with a child's special needs should not be underestimated; we need to acknowledge parents' concerns while trying to guide them towards choices that are most likely to benefit the child. The ASHA (n.d.) brochure *Heard About a New Product or Treatment: Ask These Questions Before Deciding What to Do* and the book *Beyond Baby Talk* are examples of materials that can be helpful for facilitating discussion about treatment options. Resources such as the Apraxia-KIDS website (www.apraxia-kids.org) offer both a network of support and credible information for parents to review at their own pace. We can combine face-to-face education with directing parents to credible resources (print and electronic media or other professionals). This will not only help parents to be prepared to work with us more effectively, but also to be confident enough in their knowledge to handle well-meaning but misguided advice or awkward questions from friends or relatives. Educating parents should not be considered a one-time event, completed at the time of evaluation or as a prelude to initiation of therapy. It should be an ongoing, reciprocal process between clinician and parents, in which both parties come to appreciate and build on the child's strengths as well as addressing areas of need.

Parents need to understand that SLPs/SLTs are the professionals with the particular knowledge and expertise to diagnose speech and language problems. Other professionals, such as physicians, educators, and occupational or physical therapists, may contribute important observations and information, but it is within our scope of practice to evaluate and treat disorders of speech and language (e.g., ASHA, 2007). In the sample cases of the children above, there would certainly be a need to include other professionals in the child's care to assure appropriate intervention for all their areas of need. Ethical practice requires us to operate within our scope of practice and make referrals as needed.

Clinicians can provide parents with a variety of resources, help them evaluate information that they obtain under our guidance or on their own, and be supportive and respectful in our interactions. We can listen carefully for concerns that are difficult for parents to express, and make a genuine effort to learn about this child and his or her place in the family, so we can be effective in our educational and intervention efforts. Bobby, Precious, Sigrid and Abdi are counting on us to help their parents understand that learning to speak clearly may not be all that is required to help them achieve their fullest potential, but that we are ready to help them seek answers while we work to help them communicate more effectively.

New and potentially better ideas

Building on the theory and evidence presented in Part I, the emphasis in Part II is the clinical reality of day-to-day assessment and treatment of children for their speech sound disorders and associated issues. Before moving on to this, the reader is invited to reflect on three quotations. First:

> *For some diagnostic categories, the research literature in speech language pathology does not provide any usable data concerning the best treatment approach. For many clients, the research literature may be contradictory,*

offering evidence for the usefulness of different treatment approaches. Given the lack of definitive evidence, and the heterogeneous nature of the population served by speech language pathologists, there is a need for reliance on clinical expertise and building the knowledge base by recording the outcome of intervention.

(Dodd, 2007, p. 125)

Clinicians do not have to look far for advice on *reading* the literature (Highman, A41), but what Dodd (2007) is suggesting is that we clinicians have an important role to play in *writing* it. By contributing clinical case studies (Horner et al., 2005; Vance & Clegg, 2012), outcome studies (Olswang, 1998) and other accounts of our day-to-day work to the peer reviewed scholarly journals, we clinicians can play several important roles (Apel, 2009).

First, we can help close the theory–therapy gap or the research–practice gap (Duchan, 2001), potentially improving communication and collaboration between the clinic and the academe.

Second, we can demonstrate the clinical utility (or not) of an intervention that looked good on paper when it was delivered in idealised conditions to carefully selected participants, and present potential modifications to help it work with a general clinical population exhibiting the usual range of complicating factors, comorbidities and confounds (Apel, 1999). How, for example might clinicians customise Core Vocabulary Intervention (Crosbie, Pine, Holm & Dodd, 2006) for a child with an intellectual disability; or multiple oppositions intervention (Williams, 2010) for a multilingual child with SSD; or the Cycles Phonological Pattern Approach (Hodson, 2007, 2010) for a child fitted with a cochlear implant?

And third, we can initiate exploration and evaluation of new treatments and techniques which currently lack empirical support, but which are theoretically strong and intuitively appealing. Which leads back to the 'two questions' discussed in the Introduction to Part I, and the next quotation:

... EBP encompasses varied forms of evidence, including theoretical grounding and clinical expertise, and does not preclude use of experimental interventions. However, EBP dictates that we be aware of what evidence does or does not exist for our practices and that we give thought to why certain strategies and techniques might be successful. Without an understanding of why something works, there is always the danger that it will be misapplied, and we will be left unable to build on the strategy to form new and potentially better ideas.

(DeThorne, Johnson, Walder & Mahurin-Smith, 2009, p. 134)

There are echoes here of Clark (2003), mentioned in the introduction to Part I. The reader will recall that Clark discussed two strategies SLPs/SLTs can employ when selecting an intervention. She suggested that the clinician can start with the question '*Does* this therapy work; is it evidence-based?' and seek answers via a literature search. If the literature search fails to reveal evidence for the therapy the clinician can ask a second, different question: '*Should* this therapy work; is it theoretically sound?' and seek an understanding of how the nonevidence-based intervention is *supposed* to work, developing an account of the mechanism underpinning the intervention. If that too proves unsatisfactory, then in most cases the treatment will not be selected. After all, we do not knowingly embark on an intervention path unless we believe that it is likely to work in the client's favour, culminating in intelligible speech and discharge. But of course, the two do not always coincide and the experience is not always positive, as the final quotation reveals:

The experience of discharging children and their families from phonological intervention can be both rewarding and disheartening. As Hersh (2010) points out, there is a pressing need to better understand this complex yet understudied issue. Given the potential for children with a phonological impairment to be discharged with intelligible speech, it would be important that this research consider the impact of the discharge experience on SLPs, the children and the families they work in both ideal and less than ideal situations. It would also be worthwhile knowing how SLPs can be best equipped to cope with discharge dilemmas. What is more, it would be valuable to determine the ideal intensity of intervention needed to make unintelligible speech intelligible, so as to help SLPs navigate a course of phonological intervention for a child and his or her family towards a happy ending.

(Baker, 2010, p. 328)

References

Apel, K. (1999). Checks and balances: Keeping the science in our profession. *American Journal of Speech-Language Pathology, 30*, 98–107.

Apel, K. (2009). Editorial: Can clinicians be scientists? *Language, Speech, and Hearing Services in the Schools, 40*, 3–4.

ASHA. (2007). Scope of practice in speech-language pathology [Scope of Practice]. Retrieved 30 April 2014 from www.asha.org/policy

ASHA (n.d.). *Heard about a new product or treatment? Ask these questions before deciding what to do.* Retrieved 3 November 2013 from www.asha.org/public/speech/consumerqa/

Baker, E. (2010). The experience of discharging children from phonological intervention. *International Journal of Speech-Language Pathology, 12*(4), 325–328.

Clark, H. M. (2003). Neuromuscular treatments for speech and swallowing: A tutorial. *American Journal of Speech Language Pathology, 12*(4), 400–415.

Crosbie, S., Pine, C., Holm, A., & Dodd, B. (2006). Treating Jarrod: A core vocabulary approach. *Advances in Speech Language Pathology, 8*(3), 316–321.

De Thorne, L. S., Johnson, C. J., Walder, L., & Mahurin-Smith, J. (2009). When 'Simon Says' doesn't work: Alternative to imitation for facilitating early speech development. *American Journal of Speech-Language Pathology, 18*, 133–145.

Dodd, B. (2007). Evidence-based practice and speech-language pathology: Strengths, weaknesses, opportunities and threats. *Folia Phoniatrica et Logopaedica, 59*,118–129.

Duchan, J. F. (2001). *History of speech-language pathology in America.* Retrieved 15 January 2014 from http://www.acsu.buffalo.edu/~duchan/history.html

Hennessy, K., & Hennessy, K. (2013). *Anything but silent: Our family's journey through childhood apraxia of speech.* Tarentum, PA: Word Association Publishers.

Hersh, D. (2010). I can't sleep at night with discharging this lady: The personal impact of ending therapy on speech-language pathologists. *International Journal of Speech-Language Pathology, 12*(4), 283–291.

Hodson, B. (2007, 2010). *Evaluating and enhancing children's phonological systems: Research and theory to practice.* Wichita, KS: PhonoComp Publishers.

Horner, R. H., Carr, E. G., Halle, J., McGee, G., Odom, S., & Wolery, M. (2005). The use of single-subject research to identify evidence-based practice in special education. *Exceptional Children, 71*: 65–180. Retrieved 30 November 2013 from http://www.freewebs.com/lowvisionstuff/Single_Subject.pdf

Luterman, D. M. (2008). *Counseling persons with communication disorders and their families* (5th ed.). Austin, TX: Pro-Ed.

McCormack, J., McLeod, S., Harrison, L. J., & McAllister, L. (2010). The impact of speech impairment in early childhood: Investigating parents' and speech-language pathologists' perspectives using the ICF-CY. *Journal of Communication Disorders, 43*(5), 378–396.

Miron, C. (2012). The parent experience: When a child is diagnosed with childhood apraxia of speech. *Communication Disorders Quarterly, 33*(2), 96–110.

Olswang, L. B. (1998). Treatment efficacy research. In: C. M. Frattali (Ed.), *Measuring outcomes in speech-language pathology* (pp. 134–150). New York: Thieme.

Stone, J., & Olswang, L. (1989). The hidden challenge in counseling. *American speech language hearing association* (pp. 27–31).

Thomas-Stonell, N., Oddson, B., Robertson, B., & Rosenbaum, P. (2009). Predicted and observed outcomes in preschool children following speech and language treatment: Parent and clinician perspectives. *Journal of Communication Disorders, 42*, 29–42.

Vance, M., & Clegg, J. (2012). Editorial: Use of single case study research in child speech, language and communication interventions. *Child Language Teaching & Therapy, 28*(3), 255–258.

Williams, A. L. (2010). Multiple oppositions intervention. In: A. L. Williams, S. McLeod, & R. J. McCauley (Eds.), *Interventions for speech sound disorders in children* (pp. 73–94). MD: Paul H. Brookes Publishing Co.

Chapter 6

Phonological disorder and CAS: Characteristics, goals and treatment

Chapter 6 addresses a range of practical issues in the dynamic assessment, and differential diagnosis of children with moderate and severe SSD, including childhood apraxia of speech (CAS) or suspected CAS, sometimes abbreviated as sCAS. The chapter also contains suggestions for and discussion of intervention goals, approaches and techniques for these children. It starts with the proposition (Velleman, 2005) that phonological disorder and CAS have at least six inter-related characteristics in common that, when it gets right down to it in everyday practice, we find ourselves treating symptomatically, while still taking the primary diagnosis into account. In this sense, we 'treat the symptoms and not the label'.

The four contributors to this chapter are Chantelle Highman (A41) on staying in touch with the juried literature, Karen Froud and Reem Khamis-Dakwar (A42) on the neural underpinnings of CAS, and Amy E. Skinder-Meredith (A43) on rating a child's speech characteristics.

Treat the symptoms, not the label

As a motor speech disorder, CAS is a discrete diagnostic subtype of childhood (paediatric) SSD. There is a conservative consensus view that it is best characterised as a symptom complex rather than as a unitary disorder and that it may affect, to varying degrees, some combination of: non-speech motor behaviours; speech motor behaviours; production of speech sounds and structures (word and syllable shapes); prosody; language; metalinguistic/phonemic awareness; and literacy (ASHA, 2007b). Maassen (2002) reflected on a finding of Shriberg, Aram, and Kwiatkowski (1997c) that, whereas late onset of speech and slow development are usual in CAS, neither a typical phonological developmental pathway nor a characteristic phonological profile for children with sCAS has been found, and that CAS has no phonological characteristics that are uniquely its own.

It is also generally agreed that many 'CAS characteristics' can be found in children with other subtypes of SSD, and that CAS and phonological disorder can co-occur in an individual child. Little wonder then, that Velleman and Strand (1994) declared that this, 'may result in a variety of motor, phonologic, linguistic or neurologic signs or symptoms and in fact inconsistency among symptoms may be expected as typical'.

Children's Speech Sound Disorders, Second Edition. Caroline Bowen.
© 2015 John Wiley & Sons, Ltd. Published 2015 by John Wiley & Sons, Ltd.
Companion website: www.wiley.com/go/bowen/speechlanguagetherapy

Box 6.1 Testing for and observations of phonological disorder

Characteristics	Testing for Phonological Disorder
1. Static speech sound system	Test: Relational Analysis. Look for stable PCC and stable percentage of occurrence of processes over time (6–12 weeks should do).
2. Variability without gradual improvement	Test: Inconsistency Assessment: What <u>kind</u> of inconsistency? DEAP Inconsistency Assessment (Dodd et al., 2002) uses single words, *also* observe CS.
3. Persisting phonological processes	Test: Relational Analysis (study the norms). Look for phonological processes/patterns that 'should have been' eliminated.
4. Chronological mismatch	Test: Study inventories for later sounds and absent earlier sounds.
5. Idiosyncratic rules	Test: Relational Analysis. Look for atypical patterns.
6. Restricted use of contrast	Test: Contrastive Assessment; Phoneme Collapses.
7. Puzzle phenomenon	Test: Look at phonetic mastery relative to phonemic organization.
8. Unusual errors	Test: Observations of Conversational Speech (CS) if possible. Look for unusual error-types: systematic sound preference – 'favourite sound'/'favourite place'/'favourite manner' of articulation.
9. Marking	Test: Look for marking with *nasality* and marking with *vowel length*.
10. Stimulability	Test: Stimulability testing to 2 syllable positions.

(Items 7–10 are bracketed under the vertical label: DIAGNOSTIC SIGNS)

Current thinking in academia, and in the clinical field, tends towards a focus on the overlap of symptoms, and the overlap of treatment methodologies, for children with CAS and children with moderate through to severe phonological disorder. A common-sense (to some) symptomatic approach to treatment has emerged. Velleman (2005) wrote: 'CAS is different from "regular" phonological disorders, but there are still patterns to be found and treated. There is a great deal of overlap in the symptoms of CAS and the symptoms of other phonological disorders, so it is often difficult to decide whether a diagnosis of CAS is appropriate. But, in a sense, that does not matter. Treat the symptoms, not the label. But then, in an area that enjoys its spirited controversies, this idea does not appeal to all!

Six characteristics CAS and phonological disorder may have in common

The characteristics that can be evident in either disorder, or that may be present when CAS and phonological disorder co-occur in the same child, are

1. consonant (C), vowel (V) and phonotactic inventory constraints (i.e., consonants, vowels and syllable-word shapes are missing from the respective inventories);

2. omissions of segments and structures: that is, omissions of consonants, vowels and syllable shapes that are already present in the child's repertoire;

3. vowel errors including vowel replacements and vowel distortions;

4. altered suprasegmentals: that is, atypical prosody;

5. increased errors with utterance length and/or complexity; and,

6. the use of simple, but not complex, syllable and word shapes.

In Box 6.1, the characteristics and signs of phonological disorder are listed in the left column and suggestions for how to test and what to look for are listed in the right column. Similarly, Box 6.2 shows the characteristics of CAS, how to test, and observations to be made.

Intervention goals that are common to phonological disorder and CAS

The six characteristics are listed in the left column of Table 6.1. Reading across Row 1, we see that the first characteristic is consonant and vowel

Box 6.2 Testing for and observations of Childhood Apraxia of Speech

Characteristics	Testing for childhood apraxia of speech Use DEMSS very young children with low volubility and for children with severe CAS/sCAS.
Receptive–expressive gap	Administer any language test procedure(s) the child can manage. Formal testing may not be possible for some children (too difficult). Assessment may range from a list of the child's words and/or word approximations, to a Structural Analysis, right up to demanding standardised language batteries.
Delayed syllable/word structure development	Use a process analysis (e.g., DEAP (Dodd et al., 2002), HAPP-3 (Hodson, 2004), The Quick Screener (QS) (Bowen, 1996)) and/or a Conversation Sample. Look for syllable structure processes, phonotactic constraints.
Deviant syllable structures and word structures	Use DEAP, HAPP-3, QS, SPACS (Williams, 2006) and/or a Process Analysis of a Speech Sample. Look for deviant syllable structure errors (especially Initial Consonant Deletion and schwa insertion/addition, and replacing a consonant with a diphthong).
Sequencing difficulties	Use motor speech examination; DEAP, NDP-3 (Williams & Stephens, 2004); or make informal observations of 'long words' of >2 syllables (e.g., Debbie's clinically useful words in Figure 6.1). Families frequently recount 'big words' and the word combinations their child often has difficulty sequencing. Look for metathesis (pasketti), word reversals (mat door) and unusual sequencing: muesli pronounced as yoomsli/yoombleese; Open up it.
Word stress errors; syllable stress errors	Look for excessive and equal stress and Weak Syllable Deletion. Make a syllable stress patterns inventory. Consider an informal long words task.
Vowel constraints; vowel deviations	Look for vowel replacements that do not match adult targets. List vowel inventory/constraints and calculate Percentage of Vowels Correct (PVC) if applicable. Do vowels 'wander'? Use the Quick Vowel Screener (Bowen, 2010) and Speech Characteristics Rating (Table A43.1).
Prosodic differences	Use the Speech Characteristics Rating. Does prosody affect intelligibility (Flipsen, 2006; Klopfenstein, 2009)? Does it affect the child's presentation/'image'.
Phonological awareness difficulties – school-aged children	Use PA Tests, e.g., SPAT-R (Neilson, 2003). Note rhyme awareness, syllable awareness, blending. https://shop.acer.edu.au/acer-shop/group/SPT. Look for literacy issues generally (Zaretsky, Velleman & Curro, 2010).

inventory constraints, or in other words, missing vowels and consonants. In phonological disorder, this manifests as systemic simplifications (substitution processes), such as stopping, gliding

client Costa, 5;8, with CAS referred to 'Henry the green engine' which has 10 consonants, as ['dʒɛndˌɹi vɜ 'dʒɹ ʷind 'ɛnˌdʒɹənd] which has 15. Other examples of his 'complexification' were:

jump	dʒɹʌːmpə	blackout	'vəɹakˌʒout	real	bəɹiʊ ʷdə
twin	tʃəɹɪnᵈ	kilometer	'klɹləˌməməˈlitlə	fishing	'tʃɹˌtʃɹŋ
fastest	tʃəˈɹatˌsɪst	Mrs. Oates	'mɪtʃˌʌz ˌout'ʃəz	creepy-crawley	'kəlibˌɹiˈglɔˌɹid

and fronting where one sound replaces another (see Table 2.4 for consumer-friendly descriptions and examples these error-types and more).

In CAS, consonant and vowel inventory constraints manifest as the same sorts of *simplification* errors that are found in phonological disorder, but in addition to these, errors that involve increased phonetic *complexity* are found. For example, my

Costa's complexity errors included schwa addition and insertion (both occurred in *real*), affricates replacing stops, for example, *top* pronounced as [dʒɒbə] or [dzɒptə]; clusters replacing singletons, for example, *rabbit* pronounced as [bɹæbɪt] or [dɹæbɪt]; and diphthongs replacing vowels, for example, *bed* pronounced as [baɪd] or [biːəd].

Table 6.1 Phonological disorder and childhood apraxia of speech: Characteristics and goals in common

Phonological disorder (PD) and childhood apraxia of speech (CAS)	Phonological disorder	Childhood apraxia of speech	Phonological disorder and CAS
Characteristics in common	**Typical errors**	**Typical errors**	**Typical goals**
(1) Consonant inventory constraints; vowel inventory constraints; and phonotactic inventory constraints.	Simplifications in the form of systemic or substitution processes, e.g., stopping, gliding; simplifications of syllable structures, e.g., FCD, CR, WSD	Simplifications AND increased segmental complexity: e.g., affricates replacing stops; clusters replacing singletons; diphthongs replacing vowels	1. Consonant inventory expansion. 2. Vowel inventory expansion. 3. Phonotactic inventory expansion.
(2) Omissions of consonants, vowels and syllable shapes that are already in the inventory.	Simplifications in the form of syllable structure processes and phonotactic errors: e.g., ICD, FCD, CR, WSD	Simplification AND increased structural complexity, e.g., epenthesis (schwa insertion) /səked/ for 'scared'.	4. Syllable shape inventory expansion. 5. Word shape inventory expansion. 6. Increased accuracy of production of target structures.
(3) Vowel errors.	Vowel errors are less common in children who don't have CAS	Vowel errors are more common, and more persistent in CAS	7. More complete vowel repertoire. 8. More accurate vowel production.
(4) Altered suprasegmentals.	Weak syllable deletion	Excessive and equal stress	9. Production of strong and weak syllables. 10. Differentiation of strong and weak syllables.
(5) More errors with longer and/or more complex utterances, including the so-called 'SODA' errors of substitution, omission, distortion and addition.	SODA, process errors, and segmental complexity errors increase as contexts become more difficult, reducing intelligibility.	SODA, process errors, and segmental complexity errors increase as contexts become more difficult. This is even more obvious in children with CAS.	11. Generalisation of new consonants and vowels, syllable structures, and word structures, to more challenging contexts.
(6) Use of simple, but not complex, syllable shapes and word shapes.	Syllable structure processes: ICD, FCD, CR, WSD and reduplication	Syllable structure processes are more prevalent and persistent, even when phonetic repertoire is apparently adequate.	12. More complete phonotactic repertoire. 13. More varied use of phonotactic range within syllables and words. 14. Improved accuracy.

In the right column of Row 1, we see that the typical therapy goals in common are consonant and vowel inventory expansion to give the child 'more to work with'. The same format is used in the following five rows of Table 6.1. The clinician then has to determine how best to address these goals given the child's overall presenting picture.

This question of 'how' is addressed towards the end of this chapter, and the reader who cannot stand the suspense is referred to Table 6.4!

A difficulty associated with this commonality of characteristics is that, when families who do not have a background in SLP/SLT seek out information without professional guidance, suspecting or even convinced that their child has CAS, they will often recognise enough 'features' of CAS to be certain that they 'know' what their child's speech problem is. Clinical experience suggests that they often do this without realising that those same symptoms are *far* more likely to signal phonological disorder, given the low incidence of CAS.

Compounding this problem, when lay people turn to the Internet for elucidation, they find a disproportionately high number of websites dealing with CAS, the less frequent speech sound disorder, and these may contain inaccurate information. Some of the misleading sites present unsubstantiated opinion and supposition as fact to sell products (e.g., dietary supplements and complementary treatments) and services (e.g., online treatment). By contrast, few sites deal explicitly and accurately with phonological disorder, the more common SSD. It may not be obvious to lay people that SSD affects about 7 children in every 100, with approximately 86% of *these* children having articulation and phonological difficulties (if we combine SD-GEN and SD-OME), or 98% if we combine SD-GEN, SD-OME and SD-DPI, whereas the CAS-affected children (SD-AOS) represent a miniscule <1% of the SSD population (as discussed in Chapter 2, and see Shriberg et al. (2010)).

An exemplary Internet source of trustworthy CAS information for consumers and clinicians is the Apraxia-KIDS website (Gretz, A7). A positive effect of the growth of Apraxia-KIDS and CASANA has been increased accuracy of information about speech development and disorders circulating on the Web, and with it enhanced communication concerning CAS between consumers and professionals. For some clinicians, this has enabled a 'more equal' relationship with clients and a sharper appreciation of the effects of communication disorders on affected individuals and their families, perhaps with the added benefit of improving their skills both as counsellors, and of knowing when to refer to a professional counsellor (Bitter, A15; Overby & Bernthal, A16; Stoeckel, A40).

Among the issues and concerns that arise in parent and family counselling, and in counselling

'older' children and youth with persisting SSD, are the potential long-term consequences of these conditions. Gierut (1998) provides a concise summary of likely repercussions, indicating that some individuals can expect lifetime challenges in terms of their retrieval, manipulation and comprehension of linguistic information; their expressive language capabilities; and their education and work choices. Discussing these ramifications, Gierut, p. S87, takes the view that, 'research calls for both retrospective and prospective studies of the etiology of phonological disorders and the identification of integrated causal relationships and their outcome on a speaker's daily life'. Such implications impact the assessment and intervention process, right from the opening moments of the initial consultation or case history interview.

Case history interview

Table 6.2 provides 'assessment prompt' notes, developed over many years, that clinicians can use, and potentially modify, for case history-taking when they suspect that a child has CAS. Procedures and observations will vary with the child's age and stage; there is overlap between the 10 sections, and not every section will be needed for every child. If they feel it may facilitate communication, information sharing and insight building, the clinician may wish to provide parents with the prompt, without the footnotes, prior to, or at the beginning of the case history and assessment process. This is not to suggest that it be used as a questionnaire, but rather as a general indication to parents of the territory to be covered in the process of conducting the initial assessment and working towards a provisional diagnosis or diagnosis.

Motor speech examination worksheet

In working through the motor speech examination worksheet, displayed in Table 6.3, the tasks chosen and the order or presentation depend on the severity of the particular child's difficulties and any predictions the clinician makes

Table 6.2 A 10-point CAS Assessment Prompt

Procedures and observations vary with the child's age and stage. Note that there is overlap between the 10 sections.

1. Hearing	Audiology report		Hearing history
2. Development	**Perinatal history** **Milestones** **Motor development**	**Cognition** see point 4 below Psychometric/Paediatric report. Be mindful that that speakers with CAS have speech processing deficits in encoding, memory and transcoding (Shriberg, Lohmeier, Strand & Jakielski, 2012).	**Social development** Wants to communicate; solitary; aloof; 'separation issues'; clingy, why? Play: who with? Nature of play? Persistent personality? Reactive personality? Ask about teasing/bullying (Hennessy & Hennessy, 2013, pp. 119–122).
	Feeding Latching issues, fighting the breast, sucking, lactation consultant, other intervention re: feeding (and/or sleep pattern), drinking from cup, chewing, gag reflex, vomiting, reflux, failure to thrive, holding food in the mouth, breast or bottle, diet, mouth as a sensor, mouth stuffing, variety of foods.	**Health/Wellbeing** Illnesses, 'always at the doctor's office', accidents, injuries, ear infections, seizures, 'separation', hospital, operations, tires easily, sleep pattern; always 'on the go'.	**Intelligibility** Ask parents: can you put a percentage on it? Who understands? Does another child 'interpret'? Does the other child make mistakes in interpreting? Does the child's intelligibility vary? Worse when tired? Worse/better in certain situations? Worse with longer utterances? Uses signs or actions to help get the message across. Aware?
	Babble Quiet baby, no babbling, late babbling; lots of babbling, lots of vocal play (gurgling/ raspberries); undifferentiated babbling (all sounded the same); few or no consonants in babbled utterances; 'babble' mainly squeals and grunts (i.e., not true babbling).	**Sounds/Words** Can say words that are not used in every day speech. How many intelligible words; how many approximations; first words (when?), low vocabulary for age (parents' judgement), comparison with other children in the family and/or age-peers; one word for many meanings ('big' for all machines/vehicles).	**Gesture/Grunts** Uses gesture instead of words; uses vowels and grunts instead of words. Creative use of gesture.
	Imitation Tries hard to imitate all the time; Little attempt to imitate sounds; disinterested in imitating words; refusal to imitate words; upset if asked to imitate words. Does/does not imitate play.	Only says words at home. Won't attempt certain words. Can't say own name. Plays remarkably quietly. Low volubility at home (parents' judgement).	**Frustration** Frustrated when not understood (or passive, or unhappy), or 'resigned' or 'adjusted' to not being a talker?
	Lost sounds/words Says a word and it is never heard again, keeps a word for a while then 'loses' it; words come and go. Sounds come and go.	**Comprehension**[a] Ask parents for example of how well the child comprehends spoken language. Is there a receptive–expressive gap (comprehension higher than output would suggest)?	**Theories? History?** Ask parents what they think the problem might be (or might be 'called'). Have you wondered about a 'label', searched the web and joined a discussion group, received advice or 'suggestions' from family, friends and others? Thought about family history? What brought you here?
	Groping/Struggle Mouthing words? Silent posturing?		

(continued)

Table 6.2 (*Continued*)

---

3. Language
Ask parents; formal tests

---

4. Cognition
Ask parents; formal tests

---

5. PA/Literacy
Ask parents; formal tests. Story time? Consider offering ONE piece of advice.[b]

---

6. Neuromuscular examination	Posture (sitting/W-sitting?) Muscle Tone Coordination Reflexes	Gait	Sensory function Involuntary movements (if yes, query dysarthria) Physiotherapist or OT reports?

---

7. Motor speech examination (Table 6.3)

---

8. Speech and non-speech characteristics – note the general agreement between ASHA (2007a,b) and Davis, Jakielski and Marquardt (1998)

Non-speech characteristics speech (Davis et al., 1998; see also Teverovsky, Bickel & Feldman, 2009 for parents' perception of the functional characteristics of children with CAS within the ICF-CY framework)

(1) Impaired volitional oral movements
(2) Reduced expressive compared to receptive language skills (receptive–expressive gap)
(3) Reduced diadochokinetic rates

Speech characteristics (Davis et al., 1998)

1. Limited consonant repertoire
2. Limited vowel repertoire
3. Frequent omissions
4. High incidence of vowel errors
5. Inconsistent articulation errors (Token-to-Token)
6. Altered suprasegmentals (prosody)
7. Increased errors with output length/complexity
8. Difficulty in imitation (groping or refusal)
9. Use of simple syllable shapes

> Three core features of CAS (ASHA, 2007a,b)
> **SEGMENTAL**
> Sound production inconsistency
> **STRUCTURAL**
> Difficulty with transition between syllables
> **SUPRASEGMENTAL**
> Inconsistent realisation of Lexical stress/ Prosody; nasality

---

9. Speech assessment
Standardised Articulation and Phonology Test (e.g., DEAP, HAPP-3)
Independent and Relational Analysis
Inconsistency Assessment
Compare Single Word and Conversational Speech PCC and PVC
Intelligibility Ratings
Use CS sample for MLUm and Structural Analysis if formal language testing is not possible
Look for silent posturing/groping
Is the prosodic contour of utterances/sentences intact on imitation?
Contrastive stress (I **WANT** one/I want **ONE**/I want one)
Rule a dysarthria component out or in if possible (Skinder-Meredith, A43)
Rule a phonological component out or in if possible

---

10. Speech characteristics rating (Table A43.1)

---

[a]'Parents will often say that their child 'understands everything' or is 'very bright' and many can give excellent examples of why they see their child this way, but it is essential to test receptive skills. Parent report may be positive but testing tells you about co-operation and attention too, possibly revealing subtle deficits in comprehension. This can come as a shock to parents and requires sensitive handling – don't assume they 'know'.

[b]Consider offering one piece of advice in the initial visit. At this point parents are usually not ready to absorb a lot of new information, but they will usually remember one important suggestion. Recommending a regular 5–7 minute 'story time' or 'communication time' or 'talking time' when a parent engages quietly with the child with books, pictures or 'literacy-like' activities, sends a message about the importance of both literacy and 1:1 child–adult communication opportunities, and once established can become the basis for a speech homework routine. Suggest concrete ways that this might be accomplished even with children who don't like books, keeping the demands on the parent reasonable and practical as they adjust to the diagnosis or suspected diagnosis.

Table 6.3 Motor Speech Examination Worksheet

This worksheet was designed by Edythe Strand, and is used by permission (Bowen, 2009, pp. 212–213). The stimuli used as examples in this version are from the DEMSS (Strand, A45).

(A) Observations during connected speech Example for a young child or one with very Severe impairment

	Vowels	Consonants	Typical maximum word length	Syllable shapes C, CV, VC	MLU
Conversation					
Picture description					
Narrative					

(B) Observations of elicited utterances Example for a young child or one with very Severe impairment Examine, dynamically, the child's ability to sequence movement for phonetic sequences in various contexts: (1) Vowels (2) CV VC CVC (3) Monosyllabic, bisyllabic, polysyllabic words (4) Phrases (5) Sentences of increasing length looking at the child's: **Movement accuracy; Vowel production; Consistency;** and **Prosody**, and the level of support required. You don't have to use the DEMSS stimuli (below); use stimuli that 'suit' the child.

	Immediate repetition	Repetition after delay – no cues	Simultaneous production needed	Gestural/tactile cues needed
Isolated vowels				
CV me hi				
VC up eat				
Reduplicated syllables mama booboo				
CVC1 mom peep pop				
CVC2 mad bed hop				
Vowel errors Note the different coarticulatory contexts				
Utterances of increasing length (Note the use of *simple* words)				
Bi-syllabic 1 baby puppy				
Bi-syllabic 2 bunny happy today canoe				
Multi-syllabic banana video				
Phrases Make up stimuli to suit the child being tested Me too; Big boy				
Sentences Make up stimuli of increasing length to suit the child. Dad. Hi dad. Hi daddy.				

regarding his or her probable performance. The worksheet is intended to help the investigator confirm or reject CAS as a diagnosis, bearing in mind that any determination of oral apraxia would have been made during the structural–functional examination (Skinder-Meredith, A43).

As with the assessment prompt (Table 6.2), the procedures in Table 6.3 overlap, and not all will be done with every client. There is no particular order of presentation of these tasks, other than the logical hierarchy that the clinician deems appropriate for the particular individual.

Multi-Syllabic words

James (A50) identified the following 10 words as being the most 'clinically useful' or most revealing diagnostically: *ambulance, hippopotamus, computer, spaghetti, vegetables, helicopter, animals, caravan, caterpillar* and *butterfly*, in her study of polysyllabic words and words containing consonant clusters. These words are displayed in Figure 6.1.

Reading and reviewing the literature

In order to adequately inform and support families, and to fulfil the requirements of evidence-based and ethical practice (Powell, A39), we must be *au fait* with the relevant literature, whether by reading it diligently as a component of a personal learning plan or within a professional learning network (PLN), or by absorbing it in 'distilled' form at CPD/CEU events, where it is often presented by individuals pursuing, or holding, doctoral degrees and who have truly immersed themselves in a topic.

Among the first steps in the PhD process (Mewburn, 2013; Petre & Rugg, 2010) are choosing both a topic area and a research question or questions. This requires the identification of a 'do-able' (by one person) piece of *original* research, and then the development of a proposal: which is probably when the real work of the dissertation begins. Completing a focused literature review around the

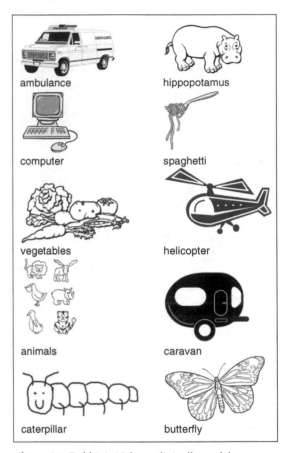

Figure 6.1 Debbie's 10 long clinically useful words

research topic and questions is an important aspect of this endeavour, with the review itself eventually becoming the essence of the introduction to the doctoral dissertation. In response to what is found in the literature, and in response to what emerges from discussion with advisors or supervisors (Deem & Brehony, 2000) and mentors, the potential doctoral candidate may reach a point of wanting to reformulate the topic and/or questions, abandoning some questions and honing and sharpening others. The aim of the review is to frame and shape the research, demonstrate that it can fill a crucial gap, and link it to the larger body of knowledge (Mullins & Kiley, 2002). Ultimately, according to Sternberg (1981), the literature review tells readers that the candidate has grasped the subject, has connected the topic to larger historic and current themes, can demonstrate that the proposed contribution is unique, and that the candidate can produce and critically evaluate an astutely refined and focused bibliography.

Dr. Chantelle Highman is an Australian SLP working as a clinician and researcher in Perth, Western Australia. She completed her doctoral degree in School of Psychology and Speech Pathology at Curtin University, investigating potential early speech motor and language precursors in infants at risk of CAS, and looking for evidence for a motor-specific core deficit for the disorder (Maassen, 2002). Her methodology across three studies has involved a combination of retrospective reports by parents of children with CAS, case study analyses of retrospective CAS data and a prospective longitudinal study of siblings of children with CAS, providing an insight into the potential earliest features of disordered speech motor control (Highman, Hennessey, Leitão & Piek, 2013; Highman, Hennessey, Sherwood & Leitão, 2008; Highman, Leitão, Hennessy & Piek, 2012). One driver of this research is a question often asked by parents of children with CAS regarding the 'early warning features' they should be watchful for in their younger children, an obvious one that most families probably think we would be able to answer quite easily.

By some quirky synchronicity, Dr. Highman completed her literature review just as the final draft of the ASHA Draft Technical Report on CAS was circulated for comment. In her response to Q41, she discusses the role and process of reading the literature as it relates to practice, and the therapy and research implications of the ratified report (ASHA, 2007a) and position statement (ASHA, 2007b).

Q41.   Chantelle Highman: Staying current with published research

The ASHA (2007a) Technical Report on CAS is wide ranging and comprehensive, prompting more questions than it answers, and some of those questions will likely be answered by SLPs/SLTs undertaking higher degrees. The report also makes for absorbing reading for those with the interest and inclination. A recurring theme in discussion with clinical SLPs/SLTs is that, although they would like to, they rarely read the literature for a range of reasons that include lack of time and limited access to journals and other publications (like professional association reports and position statements). On the other hand, for SLPs/SLTs with a theoretical or research bent, reading the literature is routine, time is set aside, and new articles are eagerly awaited and consumed. Can you suggest strategies that clinicians might employ to make the task of keeping abreast with the published evidence base less challenging and more enjoyable; suggest what readers of the Technical Report might gain from it in a practical, clinical sense; and indicate the key areas for further CAS and other child speech research that it points to?

A41.   Chantelle Highman: Keeping up to date with the literature

The literature corroborates the many practical issues faced by clinicians when they attempt to implement Evidence-based practice (EBP). These include lack of time, lack of ready access to published literature and lack of skill in evaluating the evidence (e.g., Bernstein Ratner, 2006; Gosling & Westbrook, 2004; Jansen, Rasekaba, Presnell & Holland, 2012; Johnson, 2006; Roddam & Skeat, 2010; Rose & Baldac, 2004; Vallino-Napoli & Reilly, 2004). Daunting though these barriers may appear to be, clinicians know from their professional associations' Codes of Ethics that keeping up to date with relevant literature is integral to SLPs'/SLTs' responsibilities. Indeed, when surveyed, most clinicians report placing a high value on the importance of research, and desire to keep up to date with the evidence-base underpinning practice (Stephens & Upton, 2012; Vallino-Napoli & Reilly, 2004). These are worthy aspirations, because in combining our clinical knowledge with new evidence and theories, we may be better positioned to provide more effective, efficient and appropriate services (Reilly, Douglas & Oates, 2004).

Keeping up with the literature

Drawing on the suggestions provided by Johnson (2006) and Reilly et al. (2004), and from my own experience as a clinician and researcher, practical strategies to make keeping up with the literature less challenging and more enjoyable for the clinician include:

- Identifying a particular area of interest or a current focus, such as diagnosis of CAS, or treatment approaches for phonological disorders. Allowing your focus to be directed by clinical cases and questions can be particularly motivating.
- Linking up with other clinicians and researchers. Tackling one focussed area as a 'team' will ensure practical implications can be maximised. This may include joining, or forming a relevant interest group or journal club, or extend to partnering with students and universities for joint benefits.
    Making use of the information available on reputable websites (e.g., Bowen, 1998; Childhood Apraxia of Speech Association of North America, CASANA site (www.apraxia-kids.org), see Gretz, A7). Joining the associated discussion groups to receive posts, which often include relevant abstracts, is a time-efficient way of staying connected with clinical and research issues. Making use of the archives and files areas allows clinicians to search for clinically relevant topics, articles and associated discussions with ease.
- The advent of online social networking, in particular Twitter and selected blogs,

can make 'following' a line of research (or researcher) easier.
- Investigating your access to online journals and setting up automatic alerts for particular topics and journals' table of contents will allow you to stay informed without having to repeatedly search for new information.
- Checking association websites (e.g., the Mutual Recognition of Professional Association Credentials signatories: ASHA, IASLT, NZSTA, RCSLT, SAC-AOC and Speech Pathology Australia) for information regarding EBP and continuing professional development, as well as for access to technical reports, position statements and clinical guidelines. For example, the ASHA (2007a) CAS Technical Report and the Royal College of Speech and Language Therapists' policy statement on Developmental Verbal Dyspraxia (DVD) (RCSLT, 2011) provide syntheses of the relevant literature relating to CAS/DVD. SLPs/SLTs who reside outside of the United States can join ASHA as international affiliates and access many resources including all editions of the ASHA journals, and enquiries should go to joinasha@asha.org.
- Utilising available published conference proceedings on topics of interest (e.g., Shriberg & Campbell, 2002). Some of these contain not only the presentations, but also transcripts of frank discussions between the top researchers in the field, affording a more in-depth understanding of topic areas. Videos of topic and panel presentations from the 2013 CAS Research Symposium (www.apraxia-kids.org/symposium-videos) are readily available; ensuring that keeping up to date is only a mouse-click away.
- Making use of sources that have already synthesised information for you, such as review articles, book chapters, meta-analyses and databases of interventions (e.g., speechBITE, www.speechBITE.com). Johnson (2006) provided a list of speech

and language-relevant sources, as well as practical examples of how to apply such information to clinical problems.

- Attending relevant CPD/CEU events, especially those that present a synthesis of the available literature on a given topic.

Practical, clinical applications of the technical report and position statement

The ASHA CAS Technical Report (2007a) and position statement (2007b), as well as the RCSLT (2011) policy statement on DVD are examples of readily available resources that synthesise the literature. The documents provide clinicians with a review of CAS-related literature, referring often to typical development and other speech sound disorders. As such, they provide the busy clinician with a current perspective on this controversial area. As indicated earlier, many questions remain unanswered. However, a number of directly relevant and clinically applicable recommendations were presented in the reports. These are summarised below in terms of the four questions referred to previously:

Is it (CAS) a recognised clinical disorder?

The ASHA Technical Report and accompanying Position Statement clearly support the existence of CAS as a recognised paediatric speech sound disorder. The literature suggests that CAS is a complex disorder, characterised by particular speech production and prosodic features, warranting clinical services and further research. However, the report also acknowledges the overlap of features with other speech sound disorders, and the present lack of a set of validated, differentially diagnostic criteria for CAS. The committee suggested that the term CAS be applied to the idiopathic form as well as

those occurring in the context of neurological and neurobehavioural disorders, and suggests using the qualifier *suspected* (i.e., *suspected* Childhood Apraxia of Speech, sCAS) in cases where the diagnosis is provisional. The RCSLT policy statement on DVD (2011) also supported the existence of the symptom complex of CAS (using the terminology DVD; see the policy statement for a discussion). In contrast to the ASHA CAS Technical Report, the RCSLT policy statement recommended the term DVD *should only* apply to idiopathic cases, where there is not an associated known neurological or neurobehavioural disorder.

What are its core characteristics?

In the committee's proposed definition of CAS, 'a core impairment in planning and/or programming [the] spatiotemporal parameters of movement sequences' is described (ASHA, 2007b, p. 1), highlighting the importance of skilled motor movements underlying speech production. Such impairment results in speech production and prosodic errors. Despite recognising the lack of a validated set of differentially diagnostic criteria that reliably distinguish CAS from other speech sound disorders, the committee did report on features likely to be diagnostic. Based on the reviewed research and consensus opinion, the following three segmental and suprasegmental core characteristics were proposed (ASHA, 2007b, p. 2) and also included in the 2011 RCSLT position statement

1. inconsistent errors on consonants and vowels in repeated productions of syllables or words,
2. lengthened and disrupted coarticulatory transitions between sounds and syllables and
3. inappropriate prosody, especially in the realisation of lexical or phrasal stress.

The ad-hoc CAS committee acknowledged that an affected child's speech characteristics may change over time, and that the three features 'are not proposed to be the necessary and sufficient signs of CAS' (ASHA, 2007b, p. 2). That is as there is no set of validated criteria, one cannot diagnose (or rule out) CAS on the presence (or absence) of these features alone. A number of additional features often observed in CAS are discussed in detail within the report. These include those features that often comprise clinical diagnostic checklists for CAS (e.g., vowel errors, increased errors as syllable and word complexity increase) and those also observed in children with other speech sound disorders (Forrest, 2003; McCabe, Rosenthal & McLeod, 1998).

How should it be assessed?

The CAS Technical Report does not incorporate definitive assessment guidelines or a single diagnostic test for CAS, due to the lack of evidence supporting such specific recommendations (Caspari, 2007). However, guidance for assessment, based on theoretical and research findings, was presented. A key recommendation from the report was that SLPs/SLTs (and not other professionals) are responsible for diagnosing CAS. Assessment should involve sampling speech and language skills across a range of task difficulties, and considering detailed case history information.

Of the available research reviewed, maximal performance tasks of multi-syllable production (e.g., diadochokinetic tasks, nonword repetition, and multi-syllabic word production) and observation of prosody (especially lexical stress) were reported to be the most informative. However, until validated protocols are identified, assessing CAS remains a cautious exercise, where the clinician must assess broadly and in detail, and usually over time. This is particularly the case for younger or less verbal children who are not yet able to take part in detailed speech assessments that sample speech production abilities across contexts (Davis & Velleman, 2000, but see Strand, McCauley, Weigand, Stoeckel & Baas, 2013). All areas of speech and language, including receptive language, expressive language, speech sequencing, phonological development (including inventory, independent and relational analyses), oral-motor skills, communicative intent, compensatory strategies, facilitative techniques and pre-literacy skills need to be considered in identifying the strengths and weaknesses of the individual child.

The report documented assessment considerations from researchers with substantial clinical experience (ASHA, 2007a, p. 54), which included the importance of differentiating performance on

- functional/automatic versus volitional actions,
- single [speech] postures versus sequences of postures,
- simple contexts versus more complex or novel contexts,
- repetitions of the same stimuli versus repetitions of varying stimuli (e.g., sequential motion rates vs. alternating motion rates), and
- tasks for which auditory versus visual versus tactile versus a combination of cues are provided.

As is often the case clinically, a 'working' diagnosis may need to be considered, with diagnostic therapy (Davis & Velleman, 2000) further informing us of the nature of the deficit and relative contribution of speech motor planning and phonological abilities to the child's communication impairment. A recently developed assessment tool, the dynamic evaluation of motor speech skill (DEMSS, Strand et al., 2013; Strand, A45) addresses the challenge of assessing younger or less verbal children by using dynamic assessment at varying utterance levels. The DEMSS profiles overall accuracy, vowel accuracy, prosodic accuracy and consistency across utterance types from simple consonant–vowel to multi-syllabic words and longer utterances and has been shown to have sound psychometric properties (Strand, A45).

How should it be treated?

There were few treatment efficacy studies relating to CAS available to the ASHA CAS committee (reflecting the state of the literature at the time), and none that met the highest levels of scientific rigour (Reilly et al., 2004). However, the report provided guidance on treatment approaches and supporting efficacy data, where available, including discussions on intensity of intervention and funding issues. Descriptive and single subject experimental designs provided preliminary support for the use of augmentative and alternative communication (AAC) devices to improve overall communicative competence in children with severely compromised speech production abilities (e.g., Bornman, Alant & Meiring, 2001, cited in ASHA, 2007a). In addition, research describing intervention approaches that specifically target speech production has provided preliminary efficacy information and direction for practice. In particular, the integral stimulation (Strand & Debertine, 2000), and Dynamic Temporal and Tactile Cueing (DTTC, Strand, Stoeckel & Baas, 2006) approaches that incorporate principles of motor learning (McCabe & Ballard, A47; Strand, A45).

Since 2007, exciting treatment research has begun to emerge, exploring intervention approaches for CAS (McCabe & Ballard, A47; Strand, A45; Williams & Stephens, A46). The RCSLT policy statement on DVD (2011) summarised and grouped some of these approaches, with emerging support for interventions that target

- expansion of phonetic inventory
- tactile cueing to facilitate sound, syllable and word production

- consistency of word production
- frequent and repetitive practice
- incorporation of phonological awareness (PA)
- prosodic aspects of speech production

Subsequently, specific treatment approaches have been investigated using progressively stronger levels of rigour. For example, Rapid Syllable Transition Treatment (ReST), which directly targets dysprosody in CAS by using intensive practice of accurate stress patterns in multi-syllable non-words, has shown positive effects in small treatment studies (Ballard, Robin, McCabe & McDonald, 2010; McCabe, Macdonald-DaSilva, van Rees, Arciuli & Ballard, 2010) and is now being investigated via a randomised control study (e.g., Murray, McCabe & Ballard, 2012a,b; and see McCabe & Ballard, A47).

Key areas for further CAS and child speech research

Research on CAS is still in its infancy, with the lack of consensus about core diagnostic features presenting a significant barrier to progress (ASHA, 2007a, 2007b). Despite this, there has been a flurry of research addressing some important questions about CAS (e.g., the core features of CAS via longitudinal case studies, Highman, Hennessey, Leitão & Piek (2013), perceptual aspects of CAS, Froud and Khamis-Dakwar (2012; A42), and treatment protocols, Murray, McCabe and Ballard, (2012; A42)). As with speech sound disorders in general, there is still much scope (and an urgent need) for research addressing areas such as:

- Diagnostic criteria
- Cross-cultural features and presentations
- Genetic and neurological factors
- Epidemiological factors (e.g., prevalence)
- Treatment efficacy
- Long-term outcomes
- Potential early markers

Perhaps after implementing strategies to keep up to date with the literature, *you* will be motivated to make a positive contribution to addressing some of these areas, and in doing so, improve the outlook for our clients.

Neurophysiological investigations

The reader has been introduced to Dr. Karen Froud in the preamble to her essay on non-linearity in the previous chapter (Froud, A38). Her co-author in A42 is Dr. Reem Khamis-Dakwar.

Dr. Khamis-Dakwar holds a PhD in speech-language pathology from Teachers College, Columbia University, and is currently working as assistant professor in the Department of Communication Sciences and Disorders at Adelphi University in Long Island, New York. She is the director of the Neurophysiology in Speech Language Pathology Lab, where she conducts research into the neural correlates of linguistic processing and representation in specific sociolinguistic situations, such as Arabic diglossia, and functional changes related to SLP treatment and language learning. She is an expert in speech-language service provision for culturally and linguistically diverse populations, especially Arabic-speaking communities.

Q42.   Karen Froud and Reem Khamis-Dakwar: Neural underpinnings of CAS

It is commonly stated that children diagnosed with primary CAS often present with speech output difficulties that have a phonological basis *as well as* their speech difficulties that have a motoric basis. Your work on neural correlates of speech sound perception does not support a view of CAS as a pure motor planning deficit that is often associated with 'additional' cognitive-linguistic difficulties. Rather, it suggests a motor planning component and a phonolog-

ical component are integral to CAS. How did you use neurophysiological methodologies to examine the neural underpinnings of CAS, and how can your findings help us understand the neural underpinnings of CAS and other speech sound disorders in children?

A42.   Karen Froud and Reem Khamis-Dakwar: Neural correlates of speech sound perception in childhood apraxia of speech

Our attempt to examine the neural underpinnings of CAS using neurophysiological methods was undertaken against a backdrop of conflicting research showing lack of agreement with regards to the aetiology, symptoms, and most effective treatment of CAS (e.g., Davis et al., 1998; Forrest, 2003; Shriberg, Aram & Kwiatkowski, 1997b). The prevailing view in the United States is that CAS is primarily a motor planning impairment affecting voluntary movement sequences for speech (ASHA, 2007a). This is despite extensive research (documented in detail elsewhere in this volume) providing evidence of CAS as involving impairment or delay of aspects of language-specific phonological representation (PR), from a number of different domains: auditory speech sound perception (Bridgeman & Snowling, 1998; Maassen, Groenen & Crul, 2003); language and literacy development in CAS (Adel Aziz, Shohdi, Osman & Habib, 2010; Crary, 1984; Davis & Velleman, 2000; Lewis, Freebairn, Hansen, Iyengar & Taylor, 2004; Marion, Sussman & Marquardt, 1993; Marquardt, Sussman, Snow & Jacks, 2002); phonetic and perceptual analysis of speech of individuals with CAS (Munson, Bjorum & Windsor, 2003).

Against this background, we found it difficult to ignore the notion that CAS might in fact involve a representational component. The major advantage of working on communication impairments from a neurophysiological perspective is that we can often examine complex processes that underpin surface behaviours, capitalising on the millisecond timing precision of electroencephalography (EEG) to gain information about brain responses as they unfold over time. In considering whether CAS might in fact involve a representational component, we had recourse to literature from several distinct (though related) disciplines: foundational understanding of typical phonological development and representation; the neuroscientific literature on phonological processing, specifically the mismatch negativity (MMN) component; and previous studies that had examined acoustic parameters in acquired apraxia of speech (AOS) in adults. By bringing together insights from these various fields, we were able to develop and test a hypothesis concerning a specific neural signature of phonological processing in CAS. This process, our preliminary findings (Froud & Khamis-Dakwar, 2012), and some implications for our understanding of CAS and other speech sound disorders, are described here.

Speech sound representations in typical language development and in CAS

Typically developing infants are able to respond to native and non-native speech sounds, words and grammatical structures (Kuhl, Conboy, Padden, Nelson & Pruitt, 2005). Through the course of language acquisition, there is a gradual process of 'tuning' to the native language that results in an eventual insensitivity to non-native speech sounds, indicating a 'neural commitment to the acoustic and statistical properties of native language phonetic units' (Kuhl et al., 2005, p. 238). One perspective on this tuning

process is that, as native phonology develops, fine-tuning of the native-language sound system results in *under-specification* of particular features in the phonological system of the language (Bauman-Waengler, 2004; Bernhardt & Stoel-Gammon, 1994). For example, an articulatory feature that is non-contrastive in a specific language (e.g., aspiration in English stops), gradually ceases to be specified, whereas the same feature value is retained in a linguistic system that treats it as contrastive (e.g., aspiration in Hindi stops). These changes to the available feature values of speech-sound representations are necessary for rapid, automatic and efficient processing (Dinnsen, 1996).

Some studies of acquired apraxia of speech in adults showed that acoustic parameters changed following brain damage. Specifically, coarticulation effects were shown to be disturbed in the speech production of adults with a diagnosis of AOS (Mayer, 1995; Dogil & Mayer, 1998), with the typical ratio of speech transitions (i.e., the time spent transitioning from one speech sound to another) being greatly reduced. Dogil and Mayer suggested that these changes could be related to 'over-specification' at the phonological level, leading to difficulties in transferring phonological representations to phonetic (articulatory) gestures. Specifically, coarticulation and feature spreading – which are interactions at phonetic boundaries – become compromised or impossible if individual segments are fully specified at the level of phonological representation.

Using this theoretically motivated approach as a basis, we hypothesised that atypical speech behaviours in CAS could stem from phonemic representations that have not been subjected to the typical developmental process of under-specification. This would result in a representational deficit involving the availability of *too many* options for articulation and processing. One way to evaluate this hypothesis is to examine the neural mechanisms associated with speech sound perception and processing in CAS.

EEG, ERPs and CAS

Recent years have seen the incorporation of neurophysiological methods into investigations of underlying functional impairments in speech and language disorders. In particular, EEG studies that examine fluctuations in the electrical fields generated by brain activity have proved useful in advancing understanding of the very rapid processes involved in speech and language. EEG is a non-invasive method for measuring electrical potentials generated in the brain, by measuring voltage fluctuations at the scalp via electrodes that are connected to highly sensitive amplification and digital recording equipment. Event-related potentials (ERPs) are derived from continuous recordings of EEG by repeatedly presenting stimuli and averaging together sections of the recorded EEG that are concurrent with stimulus presentation. ERPs therefore represent the electrical potentials that are time-locked to particular cognitive processes. Neurophysiological methods with high temporal precision, such as EEG, can capitalise on the very fine temporal distinctions between different domains of language processing (Osterhout, 2000), and the ERP method has been successfully used to isolate specific neural responses implicated in distinct linguistic processes, including syntax, semantics and phonology (Rugg & Coles, 1995; see Friederici, 2000 for an overview).

There is only one study so far that reports EEG data recorded from children with CAS (Rosenbek & Wertz, 1972), which the authors, using the terminology of the day, called developmental apraxia of speech (DAS). This was a retrospective study that examined continuous EEG recordings, finding focal or diffuse abnormalities in 15 out of 26 children with DAS. The examina-

tion of specific neurological features associated with CAS is different from ERP approaches, and cannot answer questions related to specific levels of linguistic processing and representation. However, other ERP studies have revealed the existence of a specific signature of phonological memory, referred to as the MMN component (Näätänen, Kujala & Winkler, 2011). The MMN is a fronto-central ERP component that can be elicited by the presence of a 'deviant' sound in a sequence of repetitive auditory stimuli (referred to as an 'oddball paradigm'– see Dehaene-Lambertz & Gliga, 2004, for a review). Several studies revealed that MMN responses to speech sounds that constitute language-specific phonological contrasts are greater in native speakers of that language than in control participants who do not speak that particular language (Cheour et al., 1998; Dehaene-Lambertz, 1997; Dehaene-Lambertz, Dupoux & Gout, 2000; Näätänen et al., 1997; Pulvermüller et al. 2001). Such evidence suggests that MMN can be used as an index of the activation of language-specific phonological memory traces. The advantage of this method is that children (with or without speech sound disorders) do not need to produce any speech, and indeed do not even need to pay attention to the speech sounds as they are being processed; the MMN happens very fast (around 150 milliseconds post stimulus presentation) and is considered an automatic, pre-attentional brain response that indexes unconscious mapping between an incoming stimulus and a pre-existing phonological representation.

For our experiment, we selected pairs of speech sounds that are phonemically and allophonically distinct in English phonology (/pa/ vs. /ba/, and /pa/ vs. /pʰa/). We recorded continuous EEG from children with and without CAS while they listened to sequences of these speech sounds, and interrogated the recordings offline for evidence of MMN responses. Our prediction was that children without CAS would show MMN responses to the phonemically distinct pairs of speech sounds, but not to the allophonic contrast; whereas children with CAS, in the event that CAS is associated with a representational deficit like that proposed by Dogil and Mayer (1998), should show abnormalities in MMN. Our participants were groups of right-handed children who were monolingual English speakers, five each in two groups: typically developing (TD) children, and children with a CAS diagnosis. There were three males in the comparison group, four males in the CAS group; and the children were between 5;1 and 8;9 years of age, with normal hearing.

Our findings revealed the expected dissociation between allophonic and phonemic contrasts in the TD group, with the phonemic speech sound contrasts being associated with a significant MMN response, and no MMN observed in response to the allophonic contrast – as predicted for a typically underspecified phonological system. However, the children with CAS responded quite differently, showing a typical MMN in response to the allophonic contrast only. In response to the phonemic condition, children with CAS showed a positive ERP response, rather than the negative-going electrical potential that was expected. Interestingly, a positive-going MisMatch component has been reported previously in infants, and has been taken to indicate an immature or underdeveloped response to phonemic speech sound contrasts (Dehaene-Lambertz & Dehaene, 1994; Friederici, 2002; Leppänen, Pihko, Eklund & Lyytinen, 1999; Pihko et al., 1999;Rivera-Gaxiola, Silva-Pereyra & Kuhl, 2005; Weber, Hahne, Friedrich & Friederici, 2004).

Neural underpinnings of speech sound disorders

Although inconclusive about the nature of the underlying impairment at this stage, our preliminary investigation of CAS using neurophysiological methods strongly suggests that there is some representational involvement that is impacting the speech sound production disorder. The direction of causality remains opaque and it may not be possible to fully determine the causal relationships between the different components of a symptom complex like CAS. Nevertheless, we have provided preliminary evidence that both a motor planning component and a phonological component appear to be crucially involved in speech apraxia, and this in turn suggests research directions for the elucidation of causal mechanisms underpinning observable changes in speech sound production in CAS, as well as in other speech sound disorders.

One possible approach to the interpretation of the very limited available evidence on the neural underpinnings of speech sound disorders could be that CAS constitutes part of a spectrum. We propose, pending further investigation, that speech sound disorders as a broad category involve differential degrees of impairment to a complex network that regulates interactions between phonological representations, their phonetic instantiations, and the motor realisations of speech sounds. Research in the next decade will capitalise on the greater accessibility of neuroimaging methodologies and the increasing application of such approaches to speech and language disorders. It is our hope that rigorous, theoretically motivated investigations that exploit the precise temporal and spatial capabilities of brain-imaging techniques will shed light on the underlying mechanisms that characterize and distinguish the disorders from one another. Such work should be considered a prerequisite to the development of finely tuned and efficacious therapeutic protocols that can be used to attenuate the impact of speech sound disorders on social participation and educational attainment in affected children.

Characteristics and general observations of CAS

Adopting the suggestions of Shriberg, Campbell, Karlsson, McSweeney and Nadler (2003), the segmental and suprasegmental characteristics the clinician will look for with CAS as a suspected, provisional or working diagnosis are listed below. Then follows a guide to the general observations an SLP/SLT might make during differential diagnosis. These are arranged under the overlapping section headings of: general characteristics, phonetic characteristics/phonetic error-types, sound sequencing difficulties, timing disturbances, disturbed temporal–spatial relationships of the articulators, contextual changes in articulatory proficiency, phonological awareness, receptive language and expressive language.

Segmental characteristics of CAS

1. Articulatory struggle and silent posturing
2. Transpositional substitution errors
3. Marked inconsistency (especially token-to-token variability)
4. Sound and syllable deletions
5. Vowel and/or diphthong errors

Suprasegmental (prosodic) characteristics of CAS

6. Inconsistent realisation of stress
7. Inconsistent realisation of temporal constraints on both speech and pause events
8. Inconsistent oral–nasal gestures underlying the percept of nasopharyngeal resonance

General observations of CAS

1. Inability to imitate sounds and segments in the absence of structural or functional abnormalities of the speech mechanism.
2. Refusal or definite reluctance to imitate sounds and segments. Such refusal is often obvious and remarkable in otherwise biddable children

and may be an indication of a child knowing his or her limitations, and it may sometimes signal that a child has been 'pushed' to imitate beyond realistic expectations (for him or her).

3. Decreased proprioceptive awareness of where the articulators are and what they are doing.
4. Difficulty achieving and maintaining articulatory postures and configurations.
5. Silent posturing, groping for articulatory placement, mouthing utterances, or other trial-and-error articulatory behaviour. Although such behaviour may be a characteristic of CAS, it is probable for some children that it appears as an artefact of therapy or being instructed by therapist and parents 'how to' articulate.
6. Distinctive resonance, particularly hypernasality and nasality applied unexpectedly.
7. Prosodic disturbances, notably excessive or equal stress, or excessive and equal stress.

Phonetic characteristics/phonetic error types in CAS

1. Multiple speech sound errors that include: omissions (which is the most common error type), substitutions, distortions, additions, voicing and aspiration errors, vowel errors and errors related to complexity of articulatory adjustment (Grigos & Kolenda, 2010).
2. Independent phonetic inventory (what the child can produce) is larger than relational phonetic inventory (what the child actually says).

Sound sequencing difficulties in CAS

1. Metathesis; for example, Brian (26), an academically gifted comparative theology student and seminarian who was diagnosed at 4;1 and treated for CAS over a 7-year period, pronounced relevant as [ɹɛvələnt], evolution as [ɛləvuʃn], cavalry as [kæləvɹi], sepulchre as [sɛpləkə], employee as [impɔli], Cathedral as [kɹəθɹidɹl], and Sydney as [sɪndi], while making typical, atypical and variable errors when saying commonly mispronounced words, such

as *ask*, *diphthong*, *espresso*, *et cetera*, *height*, *mischievous*, *nuclear*, and *percolate*. For example, the common errors for *ask*, *diphthong*, and *mischievous* are [aks], [dipθɒŋ], and [mistʃiviəs]; but Brian typically pronounced them as [atsk], [diθfɒŋ] (a good example of 'complexification'), and [misvətʃəs]. His sister Bethany (11), also diagnosed with CAS, and whom Brian called [bɛnəθi] unless he really concentrated, pronounced *tomato* as [mətatou] and *wattle tree* as [tɹɒtlwi], as did Daniel at age 6.7 (see point 5 below).

2. Difficulty with a particular phonotactic combination of sounds produced correctly in isolation or in CV or CVC combinations; for example, William (7;8) could say *tip*, *rip*, *tipped*, *ripped*, but not *trip*, which he pronounced homophonously with *ripped* ([ɹɪpt]).

3. Sounds correct in some sequences are erred in other sound sequences, as in the case of Madison (7;0), who pronounced her name correctly as [mædisn] but called the *Radisson* Hotel near her home the [wætisn], replacing /d/ with /t/.

4. Producing clusters is more difficult than producing than singletons.

5. Transposition of sounds and syllables. Daniel (6;7) said [lʌndəwænd] for Wonderland.

Timing disturbances in CAS

1. Word and sentence durations may be longer due to lengthening of both speech events and pause events.

2. The slope of the second formant may be shallower if the tongue is taking longer to get into position.

3. Longer duration of voice onset times may be present, and this can explain voicing errors.

Disturbed temporal–spatial relationships of the articulators in CAS

1. There may be imprecise, non-specific, 'wandering' speech gestures.

2. Palatometry data indicate that children with CAS do not develop the fine-tuned speech movements with the same specificity and precision that typically developing children (and possibly children with other SSDs) exhibit.

Contextual changes in articulatory proficiency in CAS

Note that points 1, 6 and 7 below suggest intervention strategies.

1. Errors increase with increasing length of the word or utterance.

2. Imitation results in better articulatory performance than in spontaneous production, *except* in highly rehearsed spontaneous utterances.

3. Target sounds are easier to produce in single words than in conversational speech.

4. Errors vary according to the phonetic complexity of the utterance.

5. Errors are inconsistently produced (high token-to-token variability).

6. Articulatory accuracy increases if rate is decreased (e.g., if vowels are lengthened).

7. Articulatory accuracy increases with simultaneous visual and auditory models.

Phonological awareness and CAS

As Hesketh (A28) explains, children with SSD have been shown to have difficulties with literacy (Lewis et al. 2011; Wellman et al. 2011), Phonological Awareness in general (Anthony et al. 2011; Carroll & Snowling, 2004) and Phonological Representations in particular (Anthony et. al. 2011; James, A50; Sutherland & Gillon, 2007). PA is an essential skill in literacy acquisition and a necessary aspect of making sense of an alphabetic script, and output phonology plays an important role in learning to read (Snowling, Goulandris & Stackhouse, 1994). Larrivee and Catts (1999) warned that SSDs *alone* are not strongly related to problems with early reading skills, but that when phonological disorders are accompanied by *another* speech or language impairment, such as CAS, reading and writing disabilities may emerge. Children with impaired phonological output are at increased risk for impaired phonological awareness skills. Many children diagnosed with CAS also exhibit Phonemic Awareness difficulties; that is, difficulty reflecting on and manipulating the structure of an utterance as distinct from its meaning (Stackhouse, 1997, p. 157).

Receptive language and CAS

A receptive–expressive (receptive higher than expressive) gap is often cited as a diagnostic characteristic of CAS. This gap is not necessarily across the board but may vary according to the particular language test task. Single-word (SW)-receptive vocabulary on the PPVT-3 (Dunn & Dunn, 1997) may be age-typical, whereas, at the same time, sentence comprehension may be impaired. Similarly, receptive skills for simple sentences may be age-appropriate, whereas comprehension of complex sentences is impaired. With these variations in performance in mind, Crary (1993) advocates testing, at a minimum, three areas: SW-receptive vocabulary, semantic comprehension and syntactic comprehension. Air, Wood and Neils (1989) investigated 'older' children, finding that those who had apparently adequate language comprehension earlier on tended to have difficulty in language processing fundamentals involving categories, organisation and abstract concepts in years (grades) 3 and 4 at school.

Expressive language and CAS

Pronoun errors are common in children with CAS. Morphemic and syntactic errors may be due to phonological simplifications (e.g., omitting /s/, /t/, /d/ word finally in tense and plural markers). Word omissions are a frequent finding (Ekelman & Aram, 1983), and speech may be telegrammatic. Speculatively, this may be an adaptive strategy to reduce linguistic load.

Rating speech characteristics

Having conducted the case history interview (Table 6.2), worked through the motor speech examination worksheet (Table 6.3) and made pertinent observations, the clinician may wish to rate the child's speech characteristics systematically. This can be done by using a procedure devised by Dr. Amy Skinder-Meredith, a Clinical Associate Professor in Speech and Hearing Sciences at Washington State University, Spokane. Dr. Meredith's research interests are in CAS and teaching pedagogy. She has studied prosodic differences, voice onset time, vowel errors, and early literacy skills in children with CAS. She is currently interested in treatment efficacy of implementing both principles of motor learning and phonologic awareness in the treatment of CAS. She is also passionate about service learning locally and globally and works regularly with Hearts in Motion to provide Speech Language Pathology services in Zacapa, Guatemala.

Q43.   Amy E. Skinder-Meredith: Speech characteristics ratings in differential diagnosis

In implementing your speech characteristics rating (Skinder-Meredith, 2000) in the course of differential diagnosis of children with sCAS, the clinician records, on a series of 5-point scales displayed in Table A43.1, quick but detailed observations of speech prosody, fluency and rate; and, voice quality, loudness, pitch and resonance. Can you lead the reader through this process, discussing these and other suprasegmental aspects of speech output, and the segmental aspects that you would include in your descriptive analysis? The nature of assessment for sCAS varies with the age, cognitive capacity, attention span and compliance of the child. In general terms with a child who can cooperate well with testing, in an initial diagnostic workup at say, 3;0, 5;0 and 9;0 years of age, what procedures do you regard as essential components of a test battery? With children whose ability to cope with formal testing is compromised, what advice would you offer the clinician in terms of the observations he or she can make in the assessment process?

A43.   Amy E. Skinder-Meredith: Speech characteristics rating form

Standardised tests are integral to core test-batteries, and necessary when qualifying children for services, but they are limited in usually only addressing segmental (phonetic) performance and phonemic organisation. The errors of children with CAS are not exclusively segmental or phonological (ASHA, 2007a; Highman, A41), posing an assessment challenge. The speech characteristics rating form (SCRF), displayed in Table A43.1 was created in response to this challenge, to allow a thorough, more encompassing, *suprasegmental* view of a child's output. As clinicians, we know that some children diagnosed with CAS progress well with phonetic production accuracy while remaining poorly intelligible due to some combination of atypical prosody, resonance, voice quality and fluency. Moreover, disordered prosody in CAS is a prominent research finding (Shriberg, Aram & Kwiatkowski, 1997a,b,c; Velleman & Shriberg, 1999).

Key elements of CAS assessment

The purpose of the assessment process is to understand the nature of the suspected motor planning deficit relative to any other deficits, such as cognitive, linguistic and motor execution ones, so as to determine the relative contribution of the disorder to the child's overall communicative performance (Strand & McCauley, 1999). Taking into account the age, compliance and developmental status of the child, I typically obtain information in the following order, which can be varied: available test results (e.g., audiology, psychology); developmental and family history; speech, language, PA and literacy assessment data; observations of any groping or silent posturing; oral musculature/structural–functional examination; physiological functioning; inconsistency assessment (Stoel-Gammon, A9; Betz & Stoel-Gammon, 2005; Dodd, Zhu, Crosbie, Holm & Ozanne, 2002; Strand et al., 2013); and, the motor speech examination (displayed in Table 6.2) and diadochokinesis (DDK). It is highly desirable, if possible, for the clinician to video tape the assessment to facilitate the observations required for differential diagnosis. For all children with suspected CAS my *highest* priority is the motor speech evaluation, pinpointing best speech performance and where it breaks down. Applying the principles of dynamic assessment (Strand, A45, Strand et al., 2013), I also want to know whether varying the tactile and temporal cues provided to the child enhances output.

The SCRF is administered *after* the case history interview and an initial core test-battery comprising the *key elements of CAS assessment*. The core battery will have included a structural–functional examination, identifying structural constraints (as in cleft palate), or physiological constraints (as in dysarthria) to speech production. Mixed resonance or inconsistent nasal resonance may indicate CAS, with the child struggling with timing velopharyngeal contraction, versus constant hypernasality suggesting structural anomalies (e.g., cleft palate) or cranial nerve (CN) damage (e.g., spastic or flaccid dysarthria). Once dysarthria is ruled out (see Table A43.2 for a comparison of dysarthria and CAS), close inspection of prosody may help differentiate children with phonological issues only, from those with CAS (or CAS plus phonological issues).

Table A43.1 Speech Characteristics Rating Form (SCRF)

Speech characteristics rating					
Circle the number that, in your judgement best correlates with the corresponding speech characteristic: 1, never present; 2, rarely present; 3, sometimes present; 4, frequently present; 5, always present					
Speech characteristics		Rating scale			
		never	rarely	sometimes	frequently	always
Prosody						
1	Monotone	1	2	3	4	5
2	Hyperprosodic, e.g., sing-song, EES	1	2	3	4	5
3	Dysprosodic, e.g., word stress errors	1	2	3	4	5
4	Appropriate prosody	1	2	3	4	5
Comment						
Voice quality/Resonance						
1	Hoarse voice quality	1	2	3	4	5
2	Breathy voice quality	1	2	3	4	5
3	Glottal fry	1	2	3	4	5
4	Appropriate voice quality	1	2	3	4	5
5	Hypernasal	1	2	3	4	5
6	Hyponasal	1	2	3	4	5
7	Appropriate resonance	1	2	3	4	5
Comment						
Pitch/Loudness						
1	High pitch	1	2	3	4	5
2	Low pitch	1	2	3	4	5
3	Appropriate pitch	1	2	3	4	5
4	Loud voice	1	2	3	4	5
5	Soft voice	1	2	3	4	5
6	Appropriate loudness	1	2	3	4	5
Comment						
Rate/Fluency						
1	Slow rate	1	2	3	4	5
2	Fast rate	1	2	3	4	5
3	Appropriate rate	1	2	3	4	5
4	Dysfluent	1	2	3	4	5
5	Appropriate fluency	1	2	3	4	5
Comment						

Adapted from Skinder-Meredith (2000).

Working with the SCRF

Administration

Rapport with child and parent(s) is established and a high-quality recording of a connected speech sample is obtained for independent and relational analysis (Stoel-Gammon, A9). Narrating a wordless picture book may quickly yield a dense corpus and reading ability is not a factor. With

Table A43.2 Comparison between dysarthria and Childhood Apraxia of Speech (Strand & McCauley, 1999).

Characteristics	Dysarthria	Childhood Apraxia of Speech
Neurological	Decreased strength, coordination and range of motion of the jaw, tongue, lips and/or soft palate.	No weakness of the articulators.
Feeding	Potential long-term difficulty with tongue and jaw control for feeding.	Involuntary motor control for chewing and swallowing is typically normal, unless there is an oral apraxia.
Physiological	Possibility of poor respiratory and phonatory control as noted by decreased subglottal pressure, weak cough, and poor ability to sustain phonation, breathy or strained voice quality.	Respiratory function and phonatory control are within normal limits.
Resonance	Hypernasality with nasal emission if there is flaccid dysarthria of the soft palate or hypernasality without emission for spastic dysarthria.	Disordered resonance is sometimes noted, but when it is observed it is typically mild or inconsistent.
Language	Receptive language scores/performance may or may not be higher than expressive language scores/performance (i.e., a RLS/ELS gap is not typical of dysarthria).	Receptive language scores are typically higher than expressive language scores (RLS–ELS gap).
Prosody	Rate, rhythm and stress are typically disordered depending on the type of dysarthria. (e.g., ataxic dysarthria is characterised by scanning speech; flaccid and spastic dysarthria are characterised by monotonous speech).	Speech is characterised by equal and excessive stress, sounding robotic, with reduced prosodic contours.
Speech	Consistently slurred and distorted in general regardless of the utterance length and complexity. No qualitative difference between automatic speech and novel utterances. Vowels may be distorted.	Errors are inconsistent and increase with utterance length and complexity. Automatic speech (counting, saying the alphabet) is better than novel speech. Vowel errors are a frequent finding.

reticent children, I model the narrative and then have them try. Failing this, a CS sample is obtained through play. Preferably, listen to the sample once per speech characteristic being rated, including separate ratings for hyper- and hyponasality. Additional observations are recorded in the comments sections.

Comments sections

The comments section might include observations of groping (silent posturing); articulatory struggle; word retrieval difficulties; error consistency (suggesting phonological disorder) or inconsistency (suggesting inconsistent speech disorder) or inconsistency and consistency (suggesting CAS); dysfluency; receptive language issues; and, vowel neutralisation errors. In terms of comprehension, children with CAS may perform well on SW-receptive vocabulary, but have difficulties with comprehending sentences, particularly as sentence-length increases. With vowels, the child may be stimulable for isolated vowels, but unable to produce them in syllables or words.

Prosody

Speech may be hypoprosodic (monotone) *and* hyperprosodic (excessively inflected), making it essential to hear entire samples before rating in order to perceive any variation. Excessive stress (choppy, 'robotic sounding speech'), if present may be due to the inherent nature of CAS (Shriberg, Aram & Kwiatkowski, 1997a,b,c) and/or the effects of speech therapy. For example, children focusing on the correct sequencing of syllables in multi-syllabic utterances may be trained to compensate by speaking one syllable at a time, creating staccato, monotonous delivery (Meredith, 2002).

Voice quality/resonance/glottal fry

The intelligibility of children with CAS may reduce when they use less than optimal voice quality. Some (not all) develop hoarseness secondary to vocal nodules, consequent to poor vocal hygiene. Interestingly, in a study by Skinder-Meredith, Lommers and Yoder (2007) 60% of parents reported that their child with CAS often exhibited frustration. Those who express communicative frustration strongly and overtly are prone to hyperfunctional voice disorders. Glottal fry ('creaky voice' or 'pulse register'), a common physiological occurrence at the ends of sentences, manifests when a speaker is running out of air and attempting to vocalise at too low a fundamental frequency. Constant glottal fry greatly reduces intelligibility. *Some* children may be *more* at risk of going into glottal fry due to poor timing between respiration and phonation.

Boone and McFarlane (2000) determined that SLPs/SLTs easily spot resonance disorders, but have difficulty in distinguishing hyper- from hyponasal quality, so listening once for hypernasality, once for hyponasality, and once for mixed nasality is advisable. Children with CAS may have difficulty planning movements of the velum, as they do with other articulators (Hall, Hardy & La Velle, 1990; Weiss, Gordon & Lillywhite, 1987). Consistent with this assumption, researchers have found 50% or more of the children with CAS in their studies to have disordered resonance (Ball, Beukelman & Bernthal, 1999; Hall et al., 1990; Skinder-Meredith, 2000; Skinder-Meredith, Carkowski & Graff, 2004; Weiss et al., 1987).

Pitch/loudness

Many parents observe that their children with CAS have difficulty modulating loudness, and I have noted that they have similar problems with pitch. Speculatively, this might be due to either poor speech monitoring, or to difficulty in coordinating respiration and phonation sufficiently to allow appropriate pitch and loudness variation, or both.

Rate/fluency

When observing rate, note the speed–accuracy trade-off. Children speaking at fast or normal rates may omit syllables and segments. Children using slow speech-rates may be doing so deliberately to maintain segmental or structural accuracy. Skinder-Meredith (2000) found that children with better segmental accuracy tended towards slower speech while children with poor segmental accuracy spoke at either a normal or fast rate.

Fluency is of considerable interest. Many parents report dysfluent periods as the phonetic repertoire of their child with CAS increases, and it is interesting to speculate about causes. Caruso (Caruso & Strand, 1999) considers stuttering to be related to motor planning and thus dysfluency and apraxia of speech could be viewed as being related. But the dysfluency of children with CAS may differ from that of children who stutter. For example, a client of mine only repeated word-final syllables (e.g., fish-ing-ing-ing) a perseverative pattern rarely attested in conventional stuttering.

Procedures to employ in structural–functional evaluation

Respiratory function

Use a static blowing task to evaluate adequacy of respiratory support. The child blows bubbles in a cup of water with a straw placed 10 cm below the surface. If bubbles are produced, the child can generate enough subglottal pressure for speech (Hixon, Hawley & Wilson, 1982). For children with VPI, occlude the nares, preventing nasal air escape (Golding-Kushner, A17).

Sustained phonation

Determine the child's ability to imitate steady phonation for at least 5 seconds with adequate loudness and normal voice quality.

Velopharyngeal function and resonance

Employing a 'listening tube' (e.g., aquarium tubing) or a straw about 45 cm long, position one end close to the child's nares and the other to your ear. Have the child repeat words and phrases (e.g., 'sixty-six', 'Buy Bobby a puppy') with high-pressure oral sounds, and utterances with nasal consonants ('ninety-nine'; 'My mama makes lemonade') (Kummer, 2014). If nasal emission is present, the examiner will feel the air and if there is hypernasality oral sounds will be amplified similarly to nasal sounds.

Comparison of resonance with nares occluded and open

Pinch and release the nares while the child says /pa/. Resonance should be the same in both conditions. If hypernasality occurs, structurally or neurologically based VPI warrants investigation.

Soft palate movement

Check that when producing 'a-a-a' quickly and loudly velar movements are forceful and quick.

Laryngeal function

Having the child cough provides an opportunity to listen for adequate vocal fold adduction. Eliciting *even, sustained phonation* allows observations of voice quality. Breathiness may indicate flaccid dysarthria while strained, strangled quality may signal a spastic dysarthria.

Diadochokinesis

Compare production rates of /pa/, /ta/, /ka/, and /pataka/ to developmental norms. Normative data are provided by Fletcher (1972) for ages 6–13; Yaruss and Logan (2002) for boys 3–7; and Williams and Stackhouse (1998) for ages 3–5. During DDK testing note syllable sequencing, rhythm, voicing errors, and coordination of respiration, phonation, and articulation, and above all, any performance change between duplicated syllables (/papapa/) and sequencing a variety syllables (/pataka/).

Cranial Nerve Examination

The functions of CNs V (jaw), VII (face and lips) and IX and X (pharynx and larynx) are addressed by default during DDK, phonatory and resonance tasks. In addition, observing symmetry of movement, strength, range of motion and coordination while doing the following allows quick assessment of the cranial nerves for speech:

- **CN V** Observe jaw opening, closing and side-to-side movements. Palpate the masseter and have the child bite down, feeling for (appropriate) bulging as the muscle contracts.
- **CN VII** Observe the child smiling, eating, laughing and puckering-and-smiling. Test resistance of the four quadrants of the lips, with either your finger or a tongue depressor, while the child keeps his or her lips closed tightly
- **CN XII** Check tongue protrusion, retraction, lateral movement, and elevation. Check strength by pushing against the tongue with a tongue depressor.

It is important to note that these tasks are only for evaluative purposes to assess if there is a dysarthric component. They are not suggestions for treatment.

Diagnosis and reporting

In reporting the diagnosis, the key symptoms that explain *why* a clinician believes a child has CAS should be clearly specified. Bearing in mind that these features may overlap with other child SSDs, these might include: token-to-token inconsistency, vowel errors, disordered prosody, increased errors on increased length of utterance, groping and difficulty sequencing sounds and syllables. The speech characteristics that argue against alternative diagnoses should also be stated, for example that: structures have adequate range of motion, speed, strength and coordination; age-appropriate receptive language or a receptive–expressive gap; error types consistent with the CAS picture. From my observations, it is a rare child who presents with pure CAS.

Other speech issues or symptoms in a child with CAS should be specified. These symptoms might include those that suggest a dysarthric or a phonological component, or that signal intellectual delay and disability, or hypo- or hypertonicity (as in cerebral palsy and some syndromes). Finally, the clinician must communicate clearly with caregivers about *all* of the factors contributing to the child's communication disorder (Stoeckel, A40).

Education of caregivers cannot be emphasised enough. The diagnosis of CAS can be overwhelming for parents (Hennessy & Hennessy, 2013; Miron, 2012). It can be difficult enough to understand the concept of CAS (motor planning/programming), never mind adding to the list of other issues that may be occurring (Bitter, A15). Parents may wonder why their child is having such difficulty with speech acquisition and some may be told that their child will 'grow out of it' by well-meaning friends and family. To assist the layperson in understanding how difficult speech is, I ask them to say a simple CVC, such as 'can'. I then ask them what it took movement-wise to be able to say that word. Most answer with how the tongue has to move. When we add to the equation that the person also has to time speech with exhalation, have the vocal folds open, the back of the tongue up and the velum raised for /k/, followed by vocal fold vibration and lowering of the tongue and jaw for /æ/ while the velum is starting to lower, and then raising the tongue tip with continued voicing and a lowered velum for /n/, we realise that speech is a lot of work, and that is only the motor planning and execution part for a single syllable word! We also need to educate about the other skills that are required to make a competent communicator (e.g., communicative intent, sentence formulation, pragmatics). When the SLP/SLT takes the time to educate the caregivers, as well as listen to concerns and questions, the family will better understand their child's communication strengths and needs. This knowledge can then empower the family, which encourages them to be collaborators in the treatment of their child (Miron, 2012).

Overlapping symptoms and treatments

Because phonological disorder and CAS symptoms overlap, at times assessment methods, treatment goals, therapy approaches, procedures and activities will obviously be similar for both populations. As clinicians, our own individual theories of development, disorders and intervention determine our assessment methods and conclusions, and our goals, goal attack strategies and the therapy approaches we select (Fey, 1992b; and see Table 1.3). With regard to the outcomes of assessment, differential diagnosis between phonological disorder and CAS is often lengthy and may be inconclusive. Box 6.3 displays the characteristics and signs of both, to guide the clinician's thinking in this sometimes-challenging process, and Boxes 6.4 and 6.5 provide a comparison between the treatment principles for phonological disorder and CAS, respectively.

Box 6.3 A clinician's prompt for differential diagnosis

Phonological disorder characteristics
1. Static speech sound system
2. Variable production without gradual improvement
3. Persistence of phonological processes
4. Chronological mismatch
5. Idiosyncratic rules/processes
6. Restricted use of contrast

CAS characteristics
(Davis et al., 1998) In an individual child, speech *may* reveal:

- Limited consonant repertoire
- Limited vowel repertoire
- Frequent omissions
- High incidence of vowel errors
- Inconsistent articulation errors
- Altered suprasegmentals (prosody)
- Increased errors with output length/complexity
- Difficulty in imitation (groping/refusal)
- Use of simple syllable shapes

and non-speech characteristics *may* include:

- Impaired voluntary oral movements
- RLS–ELS gap (receptive language better)
- Lower diadochokinetic rates

Six clinical characteristics that CAS and phonological disorder may have in common:

1. Consonant, vowel and phonotactic inventory constraints;
2. Omissions of segments and structures;
3. Segmental errors;
4. Altered suprasegmentals (prosody);
5. Increased errors with utterance length and/or complexity; and
6. Use of simple (but not complex) syllable and word shapes.

CAS: a 'symptom complex' rather than a unitary disorder of:

- Volitional (voluntary) movement
- Spatial–temporal coordination
- Motor sequencing
- Performing or learning complex movements
- Central sensorimotor processes
- Accommodation to context (coarticulatory, phonotactic, voice onset time, etc.)

Phonological disorder signs

1. Puzzle phenomenon
2. Unusual errors
3. Marking
4. Stimulability

Consider the possibility of phonological disorder and a phonological intervention approach if:

- Puzzle phenomenon is evident
- There are unusual errors
- The child is marking contrasts 'oddly'
- Error sounds are readily stimulable

CAS signs

- Speech motor sequencing difficulties
- Prosodic/suprasegmental differences
- Receptive language exceeds expressive language: 'the gap'
- Examples are provided in Chapter 8

Ask: Is it phonological disorder? Is it CAS? Is it a dysarthria? Is it VPI? Or some combination of these? Or SLI plus?

Box 6.4 Treatment principles: Phonological disorder

Phonological therapy

1. is based on the systematic nature of phonology;
2. is characterised by conceptual, rather than motor ('artic drill') activities; and,
3. has generalisation as its ultimate goal.

Phonological therapy approaches are designed to nurture the child's system rather than simply to teach new sounds (Fey, 1992a, p. 277).

Treatment principles for phonological disorder (based on the available literature)

- Work at *word* level.
- Work towards functional generalisation.
- Treat a pattern or patterns of errors.
- If using a three-position SODA test, transcribe entire words to see error pattern(s).
- Teach appropriate contrasts.
- Direct the child's attention to the way that different sounds make different meanings. Make this apparent to parents, e.g., give examples of their child's homonymy.
- Use naturalistic contexts that have *meaning* (hold interest) for the child, because this helps demonstrate to the child that the function of phonology is to make meaning.
- Stack the environment with several exemplars of each individual target word so the child can self-select activities, e.g., for work on eliminating Velar Fronting, for the target words: car, key, core, cow, have available several different cars, keys, etc.
- Select targets with an eye to their potential impact on the child's system.
- Carefully select exemplars of an error pattern/phonological rule. With clever exemplar choices, the rule is learned, and carries over to the other targets.
- In explicitly targeted therapy, it should be unnecessary to work on all possible targets.

- Train sound combinations (CV VC CVC ...) rather than isolated phones.
- Keep the focus in therapy (and at home) on movement performance drill.
- Use repetitive production trials/systematic drill as intensively as possible.
- Carefully construct hierarchies of stimuli, using small steps.
- Use reduced production rate with proprioceptive monitoring (child's self-monitoring).
- Use *simple* carrier phrases and *simple* cloze tasks.
- Pair movement sequences with suprasegmental facilitators: including stress, intonation, and rhythm.
- Use singing, whispering and loudness judiciously.
- Establish a core vocabulary or a small number 'power words' (that make things happen) early in therapy, especially for non-verbal or minimally verbal children.
- Use sign/AAC to facilitate communication, intelligibility and language development, and to reduce frustration. Reassure families that AAC will not deter the child from speaking.
- Be flexible. Treatment changes over time.
- Present regular, consistent, effective homework as a 'given', within reason.
- Expect 'good days and bad days' in terms of the child's performance.

Table 6.1 displayed the typical errors found in phonological disorder *and* CAS relative to each of the error types in common, as well as the typical therapy goals for both. Table 6.4 shows the error types and goals once again, but this time with their corresponding approaches and techniques, or 'how to' address the goals. In the following section, these 18 approaches and techniques are either described briefly or the reader is directed to relevant sections in other chapters. Note that stimulability training, prepractice, phonemic placement techniques, shaping, phonotactic therapy, progressive approximations and techniques to encourage self-monitoring are all mentioned in relation to more than one goal, and each is discussed under one heading below.

Box 6.5 Treatment principles: CAS

Treatment principles for CAS (based on the available literature)

- Use paired auditory and visual stimuli in intensive practice trials.

Table 6.4 Phonological disorder and CAS goals, approaches and techniques in common

Six characteristics that phonological disorder and CAS may have in common	Phonological disorder and CAS 14 typical goals	Phonological disorder and childhood apraxia of speech 20 techniques
1. Consonant inventory constraints; vowel inventory constraints; and phonotactic inventory constraints	1. Consonant inventory expansion 2. Vowel inventory expansion 3. Phonotactic inventory expansion	1. Stimulability training 2. Pre-practice 3. Phonemic placement techniques 4. Shaping
2. Omissions of consonants, vowels and syllable shapes that are already in the inventory	4. Syllable shape inventory expansion 5. Word shape inventory expansion 6. Increased accuracy of production of target structures	5. CV syllable and word drills 6. Phonotactic therapy 7. Metalinguistic approaches 8. Reading
3. Vowel errors	7. More complete vowel repertoire 8. More accurate vowel production	o Stimulability training o Pre-practice o Phonemic placement techniques o Shaping 9. Auditory input therapy/Naturalistic intervention 10. Minimal contrasts therapy
4. Altered suprasegmentals	9. Production of strong and weak syllables. 10. Differentiation of strong and weak syllables	o Phonotactic therapy 11. Melodic Intonation therapy 12. Singing
5. More errors with longer and/or more complex utterances, including the so-called 'SODA' errors of substitution, omission, distortion and addition.	11. Generalisation of new consonants, vowels, syllable structures and word structures, to more challenging contexts	13. Prolongation of vowels 14. Slowed rate of production 15. Progressive approximations 16. SW-production drill 17. Techniques to encourage self-monitoring
6. Use of simple, but not complex, syllable shapes and word shapes.	12. More complete phonotactic repertoire. 13. More varied use of phonotactic range within syllables and words 14. Improved accuracy	1. Phonotactic therapy o Progressive approximations 18. SW and CS production drill 19. Backward build-ups 20. Backward chaining o Techniques to encourage self-monitoring

Symptomatic treatment techniques

1. Pre-practice

Pre-practice is an early step in motor learning that occurs prior to the practice phase. Pre-practice – stimulability training, phonetic placement techniques and shaping – has an important role in consonant and vowel inventory expansion (increasing the child's phonetic inventory). This extends beyond learning new phones in isolation into pre-practice for new syllable shapes, words, and longer utterances. In essence, the client is taught how to reliably produce the tar-

get, or an acceptable (in terms a clinical judgement of what the child is capable of producing) approximation, before entering the practice phase. The child is given frequent models and feedback about his or her movement performance ('knowledge of performance' or KP feedback) during pre-practice. Once the child to the practice phase, KP feedback is only given if necessary (i.e., if production accuracy drops off), and feedback is around 'knowledge of results' (KR feedback) and the child adjusts production independently with minimal, or no, modelling by the clinician (Maas, Butalla & Farinella, 2012; Shriberg & Kwiatkowski, 1990).

2. Stimulability training

Miccio (A23) describes a rationale and a program for stimulability training. Miccio's treatment (Miccio, 2005; Miccio & Elbert 1996; Miccio & Williams, 2010) was evaluated as a stand-alone treatment with children with phonological disorder and not CAS, but it has immediate relevance to all children with depleted phonetic and phonemic inventories. Furthermore, Iuzzini and Forrest (2010) reported successful treatment outcomes for four children diagnosed with CAS who received intervention that combined stimulability training, Core Vocabulary Therapy (citing Crosbie, Holm & Dodd, 2005; Dodd & Bradford, 2000) and complex phonological targets (Baker, A13).

3. Phonetic placement techniques

There are several helpful published sources of techniques for phonetic placement, particularly Bleile (2004, 2013), Hanson (1983), Hegde and Peña-Brooks (2007), Ruscello (2008), Secord, Boyce, Donohue, Fox and Shine (2007) and Winitz (1984). Phonetic placement is precisely what it sounds like—the physical positioning of the client's articulators into the correct place of articulation and associating it with the correct manner of articulation (and of course voicing). Phonetic placement techniques may incorporate a variety of models provided by the clinician or other helper for immediate or delayed or simultaneous imitation. Imagery names, simple verbal cues and reminders and iconic gesture cues, as displayed in Table 6.5, are also employed.

4. Shaping

Shaping involves altering a sound already in the child's repertoire to facilitate acquisition of a new sound. For example, a prolonged, 'fricated' [t] might be shaped into /s/; [t] closely followed by [ʃ] might be shaped into /tʃ/; saying *to-you-to-you-to-you* briskly many times might also be used to elicit /tʃ/; or the voiceless velar fricative /x/ (the final consonant in *Bach* /bax/) can be prolonged and then 'stopped' to elicit /k/.

Phonemic placement, shaping, cues and evidence

The Butterfly Procedure, described in detail at www.speech-language-therapy.com, is a stimulability technique that involves phonemic placement, shaping and imagery to remediate lateral /s/ and /z/ and fricatives and affricates produced with tongue-palate contact. Before the therapist can proceed with the technique, the child must be able to produce the alveolar stop /t/ and/or /d/ and the vowel /i/. Then the SLP/SLT can help him or her assume the 'butterfly position' (the place of articulation for /s/ and /z/) and understand the associated imagery in which the tongue is imagined as a butterfly with a central groove and its wings 'braced' against the teeth. The technique is tried and clinically tested, dating back to at least the 1940s, and it has been on my website since 1998 because in my own clinical experience it has 'worked' more often than not. At a pinch, it could be said to be associated with modest Level IV Evidence, *viz.* 'Expert committee report, consensus conference and clinical experience of respected authorities' (ASHA, 2004, adapted from the Scottish Intercollegiate Guidelines Network (SIGN), and displayed below).

Level	Description
Ia	Well-designed meta-analysis of >1 randomized controlled trial
Ib	Well-designed randomized controlled study
IIa	Well-designed controlled study without randomization
IIb	Well-designed quasi-experimental study
III	Well-designed non-experimental studies, i.e., correlational and case studies
IV	Expert committee report, consensus conference, clinical experience of respected authorities

Levels of Evidence Scottish Intercollegiate Guidelines Network www.sign.ac.uk (ASHA, 2004)

Table 6.5 Information for families: Imagery names and verbal and gesture cues and reminders

Target Modelled in isolation or CV or VC by parent or clinician	Imagery name Provided by parent or clinician and possibly modified by the child	Verbal cue Provided by parent or clinician and possibly modified by the child	Gesture cue Provided by an ADULT (clinician, parent/teacher /'helper')
Stops and nasals			
p b	Popping sounds Poppers Pop sounds	'Where's your pop?' 'You forgot your pop.' 'Let's hear your pop'	Adult puffs cheeks up with air, and 'plodes' /p/ or /b/ onto the child's hand so they feel the 'pop'.
t d	Tippies Tongue ready!	'Use your tippy.' 'Was your tongue ready?'	Adult touches his or her philtrum with a straight finger.
k g	Throaty sounds Throaties Glug-glug sounds	'Where's your throaty?'	Adult makes a 'U' with thumb and index finger, so that they touch the angles of the mandible.
m	Humming sound Yum-yum sound	'Close your mouth and humm ... ' or 'mmm mmm'	Adult hums 'mmm' with lips shut, touching the larynx to feel vibration.
n	'N ... ' sound	'Tongue ready and buzz.'	Adult hums 'nnn' touching the larynx to feel vibration.
Adjuncts and clusters			
Adjuncts st sp sk **2-Element clusters**	Friendly sounds Friends Twins Two-step sounds Two-steps	'You forgot your friend' 'Where's your friend?' 'You forgot his or her twin' 'Let's hear your two steps' 'Where's your other step?' 'And your next step?'	Adult slides an index finger from left to right on a surface while saying /s/, and ends by tapping the finger (silently) when the 'friendly sound' is added. Adult 'walks' with fingers on a surface or up an imaginary ladder saying the first element on the first step and the second on the second step.
Fricatives and affricates			
h	Puppy panting sound Hot puppy sound Open mouth windy	'Where's your puppy? 'Where's your wind?' 'I didn't feel your wind.'	Adult places a flattened hand just in front of his or her or the child's mouth to feel the air.
f v	Bunny rabbit sound Biting lip windy Lip-up sound	'You forgot to bite' 'You forgot your wind' 'Where's your bunny?'	Adult brings his or her lower lip up to touch the teeth and blows, or makes a face like a rabbit.
s z SIWI	Smiley windy; Snake sound Big snake teeth Buzzy bee sound	'Show me your teeth' 'Make it buzzy!'	Adult makes a toothy smile and blows, indicating frontal air-flow with the fingers.
ʃ	Pouty windy 'Be quiet' noise	'Push those lips out'	Adult pouts his or her lips and blows, indicating 'be quiet' and then frontal air-flow with the fingers.
tʃ dʒ	Chomping sound Choo-choo train sound Elephant trunk sound	'Make those lips move!' 'Where's the choo-choo?' 'Where's your trunk'	Adult protrudes his or her lips (like an imaginary trunk) while making a chomping or choo-choo sound.

(continued)

Table 6.5 (*Continued*)

Liquids and glides			
l	Tower sound Up-down sound Tongue ready la-la	'Open up - tongue up.' 'Tongue ready, and down' 'Touch the top!'	Adult assumes a mouth open posture with the tongue up behind upper teeth, then lowers it to behind the bottom teeth, using a mirror to rehearse silently first.
ɹ	'Rrr' sound Growly bear sound	'Push up on the sides and move back with your tongue.'	Adult demonstrates pushing up on sides of tongue in the butterfly position.
w	Pouty face Puffy lips	'OOO-EEE sliding' 'OOO-WEE sliding'	Adult starts out in the 'oo' position with pouting lips then moves to 'ee'.
j	Sliding sound Smiley-pouty sound	'EEE-OR sliding.' 'EEE-YOR sliding'	Adult starts with 'ee' with a wide smile then moves to pouty face (or).
Final consonants			
All final consonants	Sticky sounds	'Where's your sticky?'	Adult moves his or her arm from left to right starting with an open hand and finishing with a closed hand.

Table 6.5 is available at www.speech-language-therapy.com/pdf/metalinguisticcues.pdf
Refer to 'your' pop, 'your' windy, etc. so that the child 'owns' the target.

The Butterfly Procedure stirs questions from SLPs/SLTs and students, such as this: 'I am currently a student with my very first client who has a lateral lisp. I came across the "butterfly procedure" on your website, which I think may be helpful for my client to be successful. I was trying to find empirical evidence for this technique and was not successful in my search. I am curious to know if you are aware of such evidence.' This is a reasonable, frequently asked question, and the answer is that there is no empirical evidence in support of the Butterfly Procedure *per se*. Rather, we know from collective clinical experience that using phonemic placement techniques, shaping techniques and facilitative contexts *such as* the Butterfly Procedure, and employing imagery *in general* with children with SSD may help their stimulability. What works with one child may not be effective with the next and as clinicians we may have to, or even usually have to, try a range of alternatives before settling on the most helpful strategy for a particular client, or the one that is most comfortable for us to employ. That is where clinical reasoning comes in.

5. CV syllable and word drills

CV-syllable drill and CV-word drill involve repetitive practice of spoken, chanted, or sung syllables, such as 'many repeats' of *bye-bye-bye*, or *bay-bee-bay-bee-bay-bee*, or rehearsal of a list of CV syllables with a common phonetic or structural characteristic, such as *fee-fie-foe-fum* or *ha-ha-hee-hee-ho-ho-hoo-hoo-hi-hi* or *up-up-up-up* or *off-off-off-off-off* or *go-go-go-go-go*. Returning to the idea of a clinician being 'comfortable' with a technique, for some SLPs/SLTs singing in therapy sessions is an awkward, embarrassing undertaking that we don't have to experience if we do not wish to.

The term 'drill play' implies that syllable and word drills are performed in the context of play activities. These can be presented via conventional toys and games, electronically on CD-ROM, as Apps (Toynton, A33), or as computer slide shows. Drill and drill play can be accomplished with card games such as *Go Fish* and *Snap*, board games like *Snakes and Ladders*, and toys such as posting boxes, *Pop Up Pirate*, *Coco Crazy* and

Monkeying Around, flip-over easel books such as *Word Flips* (Granger, 2005), card chutes (e.g., *Smart Chute*: www.smartkids.com.au), and dedicated speech therapy programs, notably the Williams and Stephens (2004) Nuffield worksheets, and games invented by child, parent and clinician like variations of *I Spy*, *Simon Says*, and *hide-and-seek* and pen and paper games.

6. Phonotactic therapy

Velleman (2002) described a non-linear intervention framework that she dubbed 'Phonotactic Therapy'. She noted that immature phonotactic patterns require intervention that focuses on the syllable level, and that therapy that addresses syllable shapes has the potential to evoke generalisation well beyond the specific sound or sounds targeted in the particular syllable position.

'Phonotactic patterns' or syllable structure processes (see Table 2.4) that may be problematic for children with phonological disorder, CAS, or a combination of the two are: initial consonant deletion, final consonant deletion, replacement of a VC with a diphthong, reduplication, weak syllable deletion, reduction of multi-syllabic words and cluster reduction. These clients may also only ever produce monosyllables, and they may produce erroneous word stress patterns. Strategies to address these difficulties are suggested below.

6a. Initial consonant deletion

In children with initial consonant deletion (ICD), reinforce any initial consonants in CV syllables irrespective of accuracy, starting with consonants already in the child's inventory. VC combinations, repeated in strings, can be used to facilitate CV syllable shapes. For example, *oak-oak-oak-oak-oak* might be repeated and gradually shaped into *coke-coke-coke-coke*, or *um-um-um-um* might be used to gradually elicit *mum-mum-mum-mum*, and ultimately *mum*.

6b. Final consonant deletion

Final consonant deletion (FCD) past about the age of 2;10 is cause for concern in most languages (see Box 2.2), including English. The majority of consonants in English are mastered first SIWI with the exceptions being velars and fricatives, which are mastered first SFWF. English is a language with many final consonants and many CVC words and syllables. The most prevalent final consonants are velars, fricatives, and voiceless stops. To facilitate the development of final consonants, the clinician can reward *any* final consonant, irrespective of accuracy at first, focusing on sounds already in the child's inventory, and favouring the prominent final consonants in the language—that is, fricatives, velars, and voiceless stops.

It is helpful also to know that, in typical development, children produce their first instances of final consonants (codas) after short (lax) vowels, so success may be optimised by target-word choices such as *buck*, *dove* (the bird) and *foot*, where the vowel is short, rather than *beak*, *bike*, *bake*, *Dave*, *feet* and *fête*, where the consonants are the same but the word contains a long vowel (as in *beak* and *feet*), or a diphthong (as in *bike*, *bake*, *Dave* and *fête*). Three picture and word worksheets (#1–3 below), and a word list (#4 below) with word-final fricatives in CVCs with short vowels are available to download from my website:

1. **Final fricatives with short vowels** www. speech-language-therapy.com/pdf/short vowels_fricatives.pdf
   miss kiss Liz fizz whiff biff live give wish dish mess guess says eff rev chef mesh gas mass jazz Rav cash bus cuff buzz dove rush wash cough mash posh of moss boss Oz glove
2. **Final velars with short vowels** www.speech-language-therapy.com/pdf/shortvowels_velars.pdf
   pick wick fig twig wing lick sing peck neck peg beg pack back pack wag bag bang fang tuck luck bug mug bung rung lock knock fog log song pig book buck wok gong king long
3. **Final voiceless stops with short vowels** www. speech-language-therapy.com/pdf/short vowels_voicelessstops.pdf
   zip dip mitt hit wick sick yep Shep net pet neck deck nap lap bat pat yak pack cup pup nut hut luck buck hot dot wok sock

4. 'Favoured' final consonants and short vowels www.speech-language-therapy.com/pdf/shortvowels.pdf

	ɪ	e	æ	ʌ	ɒ	ʊ
Fricatives	miss	mess	mass	bus	moss	bus
SFWF	kiss	guess	gas	fuss	boss	fuss
Mastered	Liz	says	jazz	buzz	Oz	buzz
first word	fizz	Des	has	fuzz	was	fuzz
finally	whiff	eff	gaffe	cuff	cough	cuff
	biff	chef	graph	tough	off	tough
	live	rev	have	dove	of	dove
	give	Bev	Rav	glove	Dov	glove
	wish	mesh	cash	rush	posh	rush
	dish	flesh	mash	hush	wash	hush
Velars	pick	peck	pack	tuck	lock	tuck
SFWF	wick	neck	back	luck	knock	luck
Mastered	fig	peg	wag	bug	fog	bug
first word	twig	beg	bag	mug	log	mug
finally	wing		bang	bung	song	bung
	sing		fang	rung	long	rung
Voiceless	zip	yep	nap	cup	top	cup
Stops	dip	Shep	lap	pup	pop	pup
SFWF	mitt	net	bat	nut	hot	nut
	hit	pet	pat	hut	dot	hut
	wick	neck	yak	luck	wok	luck
	sick	deck	pack	buck	sock	buck

6c. Replacement of a VC with a diphthong

Due to a syllable weight unit constraint, some children with phonological disorder or CAS will produce CVC words such as *bush* as [buə], *keep* as [kɪə] and *walk* as [wɔə], evidently 'knowing' that something is needed after first vowel but making a mistake about its consonantal nature. This can be attacked by using repeated sequences of CVCVCV (which the child *can* produce) building up to the removal of the second consonant, for example [pʌpʌ-pʌpʌ-pʌpʌ-pʌpʌ-pʌpʌ-pʌp]. Ideal early targets for this are 'harmony words' or 'palindrome words' with short vowels and the same initial and final consonants, such as *Bob, bub, cook, dad, kick, mum, nan, none, pip, pop, pup*, and *sis*. Words and pictures are here: www.speech-language-therapy.com/pdf/palindromes.pdf.

6d. Reduplication

In reduplication, typical early language learners and older children with SSD repeat the first syllable of a two-syllable word or utterance so that *daddy* becomes [ˈdʌˈdʌ], *water* is pronounced [ˈwɔˈwɔ] and *me too* becomes [ˈmiˈmi]. In remediating this in children with SSD, it is useful to know that one of the natural phonological tendencies is for toddlers to produce the high front vowel /i/ as the second vowel of CVCV babble, or CVCV words (e.g., diminutisation such as *blankie*, *horsie* and *cuppy*). We can take advantage of this enjoyable tendency by choosing two-syllable words with alveolar consonants, and /i/ in the second syllable, because high front vowels and alveolars tend to co-occur in English, making these contexts facilitative. Early targets could include *buddy, busy, body* and *messy* (see #5 below), and baby expressions and words like *nighty-night, silly-billy, funny-bunny* and *meanie-beanie* that a given family actually uses in child-directed speech (or 'parentese').

5. Alveolars with high front vowels (Pictures: www.speech-language-therapy.com/pdf/high_front_vowels.pdf

/t/	/t/	/d/	/d/	/s/	/s/
pretty	itty-bitty	daddy	Noddy	pussy	horsie
party	tutti-frutti	tidy	lady	messy	wussy
auntie	empty	body	baddy	bossy	teensy-weensy
dirty	footy	buddy	teddy	fussy	kissy-kissy
/z/	/z/	/n/	/n/	/l/	/l/
busy	buzzy	meanie-beanie	pony	silly	silly-billy
easy	lazy	tiny	funny	billy	telly
cosy	mozzie	shiny	bunny	dolly	lolly
noisy	daisy	Winnie-the-Pooh	money	jelly	chilly

6e. Children who only produce of monosyllables

To increase the number of syllables a child can produce in a word or longer utterance, known vocabulary can be employed in a reduplication strategy. For example, suppose the child can already say *bye*. This might be repeated (modelled and imitated) many times in the context of a fun, silly song, perhaps to the tune of 'There is a tavern in the town' or the 'Colonel Bogey March', both readily 'searchable' and available free as MP3s on the Internet. For parents and clinicians who do not fancy singing, it could be chanted or spoken instead. When the child can say sequences *bye-bye-bye-bye-bye-bye* ('evenly' and deliberately at first) the clinician changes the timing (*bye-bye | bye-bye | bye-bye*), gradually building up to the child being able to say *bye-bye* once.

Not every family (or clinician) will be able to endure words like *poo, pee, foo-foo, kaka* and *wee* said many times, but where they are tolerable, they can be useful as early targets for increasing the number of syllables a child can say, not least because the children themselves are often fascinated by 'rude' words, and their siblings in the younger age group may be delighted to reinforce them! Advantageous early targets are *boo-boo, ho-ho-ho, dah-dah, no-no, Noo-noo* and similar reduplicated combinations. Once a child is producing a range of these easily, a consonant or a vowel in one syllable can be changed to produce a new (real) word or onomatopoeic effect. For example, *wee-wee* might change to *peewee* or *pee-pee* might be changed to *peepaw* for a fire-engine sound effect, and then *pawpaw*.

SLPs/SLTs have a history of adapting card, board and other games such as lotto, go-fish, snap, snakes and ladders, dominoes, I spy, tiddlywinks, and matching, sorting, posting and stacking games, to target speech goals. The card game Spotty Snap (www.speech-language-therapy.com/pdf/spottysnap.pdf), for example, is an adaptation of Snap in which you say 'Spotty!' instead of 'snap' when two spotty things pictured on cards match. Once the child can say 'spotty' (perhaps with cluster reduction) the clinician can introduce a different activity with new vocabulary in the form of more 2-syllable adjectives with an alveolar followed by /i/ (*dirty, naughty, pretty, funny, silly, fussy, messy, easy*).

In addition, spondees (words with two syllables, both strong) can be targeted to encourage the addition of a second syllable. *Choo-choo, tutu, pawpaw, bye-bye, Coco, dodo, Toto, Noo-noo, cha-cha, yoyo, mumu, La-La, wee-wee, tomtom, bonbon, Tintin, Bambam* and others are pictured here: www.speech-language-therapy.com/pdf/metre/spondees.pdf

6f. Weak syllable deletion and reduction of multi-syllabic words

Some children only delete weak syllables if the word or word combination is iambic; that is, if the stress pattern is weak–strong (WS) as in '*around*' or weak-strong-weak-strong (WSWS) as in '*a roundabout*'. So, for example, they can say the trochaic words *monkey, hoping, single* and *fussy* (SW) but not *giraffe, delay, amount* and *command* (WS). This tendency is exacerbated if a weak syllable precedes the iambic word or phrase, as it the following examples where the stress pattern is WSWWS: 'I saw a guitar'; 'we found a balloon'. In these examples, the weak-strong-weak-weak-strong stress pattern (metre) feeds the tendency for the child to pronounce *guitar* as [ta] and *balloon* as [bun].

For carrier phrases in drill or drill play, and for preference, in functional, meaningful contexts for the child these WS words can be made easier for the child to say if the therapist makes the whole utterance iambic, with the insertion of a stressed word. The resultant weak-STRONG-weak-STRONG-weak-STRONG metre 'carries' the utterance, rhythmically facilitating the child's production of it: 'I *saw* a *big* guitar'; 'I *saw* a *nice* guitar'; 'I *saw* a *red* guitar'; 'I *saw* a *great* guitar'; 'I *saw* a *strange* guitar'; and 'We *got* a *long* balloon'; 'We *got* a *round* balloon'; 'We *got* a *square* balloon'; 'We *got* a *weird* balloon'; 'We *got* a *good* balloon'. Functional utterances might include: 'I *want* to *read* a book'; 'We *went* down *to* the lake'; 'He *put* it *back* in there'; Dad *thought* it *was* so good'; 'I *like* it *very* much'; 'The *keys* are *in* the car'; 'Is *yours* as *big* as mine' and 'We *flew* across to Perth'.

6g. Increasing the number syllables a child can produce

Pursuing the goal of increasing the number of syllables a child can produce, we can capitalise on the natural tendency in development for trochees (SW) to be easier for children to say. To this end, we can target trochaic words and sequences first, gradually adding a few of the harder (WS) sequences (*giraffe*) and WSW (*volcano*) sequences when the child is ready. Fun trochaic sequences that lend themselves to word play and promote repetition might include: *silly billy* (SWSW), *polly wolly, dilly dally* and *teeter totter*; and *water pistol, Peter Parker, Wonder Woman, Reader Rabbit, Buster Keaton, Mister Fixit, Henny Penny, Foxy Loxy* and *Lego Island*. An example of pictures and words for trochaic sequences is displayed in Figure 6.2 and

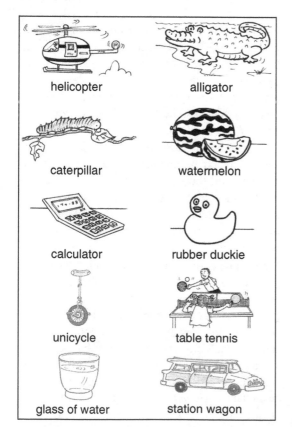

Figure 6.2 Trochaic sequences. Pictures by Helen Rippon.

four worksheets are available on my website, as follows.

Trochees 1: www.speech-language-therapy.com/pdf/metre/trochees1.pdf
Helicopter, locomotive, caterpillar, watermelon, kookaburra, motorcycle, grand piano, alligator, mashed potato, Easter Bunny, creepy crawly, cheeky monkey, clever puppy, birthday present, picking apples, big banana, camel rider, ballerina, taxi driver, soccer player, under water, hula dancer, television, Humpty Dumpty, finger painting, escalator

Trochees 2: www.speech-language-therapy.com/pdf/metre/trochees2.pdf
Letterboxes, tiger lily, very windy, scary monster, service station, stripy tiger, hungry kitty, cosy jacket, clever lady, aviator, tractor driver, unicycle, shopping basket, stacking boxes, supermarket, calculator, shopping trolley, nice tomatoes, laundry basket, rubber duckie, pillowcases, dictionary, competition, excavator, chocolate crackles, agapanthus, Persian carpet, Cookie Monster, grand piano, tiny pencil

Trochees 3: www.speech-language-therapy.com/pdf/metre/trochees3.pdf
Pencil sharpener, birthday candles, tape recorder, suit of armour, asthma puffer, graduation, Viking helmet, Hello Kitty, pressure cooker, motor scooter, airline pilot, ballroom dancing, table tennis, ten pin bowling, table tennis, exercising, scuba diving, entertainer, ballerina, hula dancer, opera singer, film director, portrait painter, carpet layer, fortune teller, respirator, coffee maker, vacuum cleaner, concertina

Trochees 4: www.speech-language-therapy.com/pdf/metre/trochees4.pdf
Ukulele, movie camera, tennis player, toilet paper, salad sandwich, bunch of roses, fortune cookie, apple blossom, window cleaner, paper hanger, teeter totter, vaccination, milk and cookies, bunch of daisies, station wagon, music teacher, salad dressing, taxi driver, glass of water, education, swimming lesson, synthesizer, stormy weather, consultation, swimming teacher, exclamation,

animation, plastic bottle, four-leaf clover, end of freeway

It is relatively easy to think of trochaic and non-trochaic sequences related to a child's interests. For example, for a child who likes the American media franchise character Ben 10, trochees such as *Alan Albright, Armodrillo, Charm of Bezel, Code of Conduct, Colonel Rozum, Cooper Daniels, Doctor Viktor, Kevin Levin, Mr. Smoothy, Spider-monkey, Water Hazard* and *Yamamoto* could be targeted first, before moving on to non-trochaic sequences such as *Omnitrix, Alien Swarm, Amp-Fibian, Rust Bucket III* and *XLR8*.

6h. Cluster reduction

Remarkably, English-learning 2-year olds typically produce some combination of clusters SIWI, SFWF, or both, and by the age of 3;5, full clusters are produced at least 75% of the time! The general trend in acquiring clusters is from complete deletion (which, like initial consonant deletion, is rare in English), such as [ɪm] for *swim*, then deletion of one element, for example, [wim] for *swim*, substitution of one element, for example, [fwim] for *swim*, to correct production, that is, [swɪm] for *swim*. When an element of a two-element cluster is deleted, it is typically, but not always, the most marked one, that is, the one that is most *uncommon* in the languages of the world. For example, /s/ is deleted from *snail, small, swing* and *squash*, and liquids are deleted from *blue, play, tree, cry, drop, flower* and *slug*. Similarly, /s/ is deleted from the adjuncts /sp/, /st/, and /sk/. Note that for some linguists, /sm/ and /sn/ sit somewhere between 'true clusters' (complex onsets) and adjuncts. Baker (A13) provides guidance on cluster target selection and a rationale for prioritising more marked clusters to evoke generalisation to less marked ones, inviting us to put three-element clusters (e.g., /spl, stɹ/) or those with small sonority difference scores, such as /fl, sl, ʃɹ/, first (Bowen & Rippon, 2013).

Morrisette, Farris and Gierut (2006) postulate that initial /s/+ stop 'clusters' are adjuncts and not 'true clusters', demonstrating that they are not subject to the implicational relationships amongst clusters with respect to sonority (and generalisation). Although Gierut (2007) advised against targeting adjuncts because they did not lend themselves to promoting system-wide change, in clinical contexts, it may be tempting, and defensible, to 'break the rules'. This is because /sp/ and /st/ are 'visible' or easily modelled for children. A clinician may make a reasoned decision to target them early on in therapy for a child with no or few clusters, not with a view to system-wide generalisation, but with the intention of giving the child 'the idea' of a 'two-step sound' (see Table 6.5).

7. Metalinguistic approaches

In child speech intervention, metalinguistic approaches involve the child talking about and reflecting upon: (a) the properties of phonemes (e.g., the features of place, voice, and manner displayed in Table 2.5, expressed in age-appropriate language), (b) the structures of syllables and (c) communicative effectiveness. They reflect on the functions of phonemes and syllable shapes in making meaning through a system of contrasts, actively revising and repairing their own error productions (Baker & McCabe, 2010).

If the child is able (this usually means 'old enough'), reading and/or Phoneme Awareness Therapy are incorporated (Hesketh, A28). Auditory Discrimination Training as a component of Traditional Articulation Therapy, Stimulability Therapy (Miccio, A23), Auditory Input Therapy (Lancaster, A24), Perceptually based Interventions (Rvachew, A25), Metaphon (Chapter 4), the four Minimal Pair approaches and Grunwell Therapy (Chapter 4), Core Vocabulary Therapy (Chapter 4), Imagery Therapy (Chapter 4), the Psycholinguistic Framework (Gardner, A27), Vowel Therapy using a contrastive approach (Gibbon, A29), and Parents and Children Together (PACT) (Chapter 9) all rest to a greater or lesser extent on working actively at a metalinguistic level. Relevant activities and procedures include those described in Table 6.5, and those under the heading *Multiple Exemplar Training* in Chapter 9.

8. Reading

When working on syllable shape inventory expansion, word shape inventory expansion, and increased accuracy of production of target structures, as sophisticated metalinguistic tasks, reading and spelling can contribute to speech progress whether the child is being read to or whether the child is doing the reading. Story reading, and spelling and reading games, can help young readers with speech impairment to increase their awareness of the structures of syllables, and the sequences in which sounds occur, while alphabet letters (graphemes) and printed words provide needed cues and prompts. Games that involve letter manipulation, word assembly and word building with concrete media such as letter-tiles, and similar activities are straightforward to incorporate into therapy sessions (Carson, Gillon & Boustead, 2013; Zaretsky et al., 2010).

9. Auditory input therapy/thematic play

In auditory input therapy, also called 'naturalistic speech intelligibility intervention' (Camarata, 2010) incorporates thematic play. Multiple exemplars of targets and contrasts are provided in input, while the child *listens*, or better still *watches* and listens, during enjoyable activities with little or no requirement for the child to imitate adult models or name objects associated with the activity. Described by Lancaster (A24), and an important ingredient of PACT, it is based on the notion that repeated exposure to a word target enhances saliency, thereby increasing learnability.

Figure 6.3 provides an example of a story a child might be told with word-final /f/ as the target. Once the story has been read, it is easy to pursue the goal of 'immersing' the child in final-f by developing games related to the story. For example, the child might make *scarf* after *scarf* for his or her soft toys, or play a game involving zoo animals crowding onto a *roof* one by one to be *safe* from a marauding *wolf*.

Other activities for final-f unrelated to the story might include having the child *stuff* a stocking or long sock to make a caterpillar, carefully cutting lengths of plastic string exactly in half, or feeding a giraffe leaf by leaf.

Another favourite final-f game is to have one *Surf Smurf* after another *surf off* a *roof* (or a *cliff*, or a *wharf*) and into a *trough* of water. It can be a little messy but it's fun! Phonemic contrasts can be introduced in input by saying things like, 'I like this *Smurp* – oops I like this *Smurf*' and then reflecting about it aloud, 'You can't say *Smurp* when you mean *Smurf*'.

A game very young children will often enjoy is to 'refuse' to place a picture or object in a certain spot for an adult unless the adult says its name properly ('Give me the *Smurf*' vs. 'Give me the *Smurp*'), or to put the words said correctly into a container marked with an indication of 'right' (e.g., ✔ or ☺), and the ones said incorrectly into one indicating 'wrong' (e.g., ✖ or ☹).

10. Minimal contrast therapy

The attributes of the four minimal pair approaches, or minimal contrast therapies (Conventional Minimal Pairs, Maximal Oppositions, Multiple Oppositions and Empty Set), are summarised and contrasted in Table 6.6 and described in Chapter 4.

11. Melodic intonation therapy

Melodic intonation therapy (MIT) might be termed a 'prosodic approach' and is based, according to Helfrich-Miller (1983, 1984, 1994) who developed it for children with CAS, on three elements of prosody: melody, rhythm and stress. Although validated as a short-term intervention demonstrating qualitative improvement in the speech of adults with Broca's aphasia (Benson, Dobkin & Gonzalez 1994), its efficacy with children with CAS is currently inconclusive. However, Martikainen and Korpilahti (2011) provide evidence, in a single case study, of an effective treatment for CAS that combined MIT with a

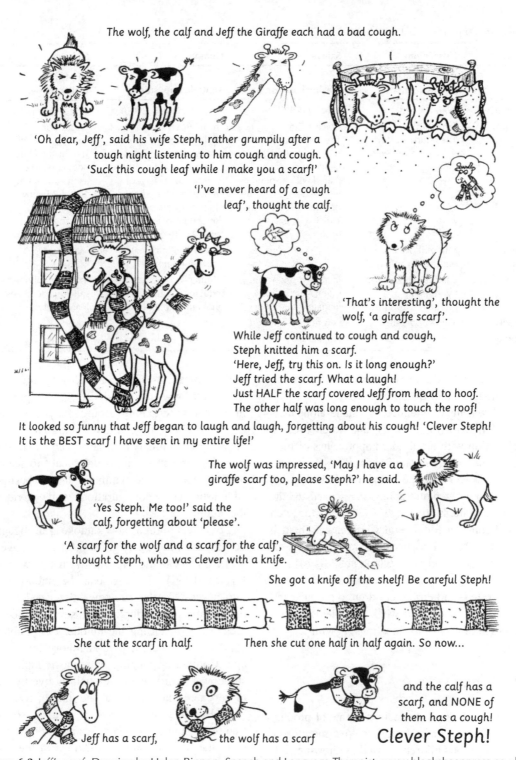

The wolf, the calf and Jeff the Giraffe each had a bad cough.

'Oh dear, Jeff', said his wife Steph, rather grumpily after a tough night listening to him cough and cough. 'Suck this cough leaf while I make you a scarf!'

'I've never heard of a cough leaf', thought the calf.

'That's interesting', thought the wolf, 'a giraffe scarf'.

While Jeff continued to cough and cough, Steph knitted him a scarf. 'Here, Jeff, try this on. Is it long enough?' Jeff tried the scarf. What a laugh! Just HALF the scarf covered Jeff from head to hoof. The other half was long enough to touch the roof!

It looked so funny that Jeff began to laugh and laugh, forgetting about his cough! 'Clever Steph! It is the BEST scarf I have seen in my entire life!'

The wolf was impressed, 'May I have a a giraffe scarf too, please Steph?' he said.

'Yes Steph. Me too!' said the calf, forgetting about 'please'.

'A scarf for the wolf and a scarf for the calf', thought Steph, who was clever with a knife.

She got a knife off the shelf! Be careful Steph!

She cut the scarf in half.   Then she cut one half in half again. So now...

Jeff has a scarf,   the wolf has a scarf   and the calf has a scarf, and NONE of them has a cough! **Clever Steph!**

Figure 6.3 Jeff's scarf. Drawing by Helen Rippon, Speech and Language Therapist, www.blacksheeppress.co.uk

Table 6.6 Comparison of Four Minimal Pair Approaches (described in Chapter 4)

Principle	Homonymy	Saliency	Homonymy	Saliency
	Conventional minimal pairs	Maximal oppositions	Multiple oppositions	Empty set Unknown set
References	Weiner (1981)	Gierut (1989)	Williams (2003, 2006)	Gierut (1989)
Contrasts	Error-Target The child's customary error is paired with the target.	Correct-Target The child's target sound (one that the child cannot say) is paired with a sound the child 'knows' (one that the child can say). The two sounds are maximally distinct.	Error-Targets Up to 4 of the child's targets (sounds they cannot say) are contrasted with an error. Target choices are based on phoneme collapses where the child replaces several sounds with one.	Error-Error Two errors (two sounds the child does not know) are paired as treatment targets. The child knows neither sound, and the two sounds are maximally distinct.
Feature difference	Minimal or maximal, but usually minimal	Maximal	Minimal to maximal across a treatment set	Maximal
Rationale	Eliminate homonymy by inducing a phonemic contrast.	Increased phonemic saliency facilitates learnability.	Eliminate homonymy by inducing multiple phonemic contrasts.	Increased phonemic saliency facilitates learnability.
Severity	Mild–moderate	Severe	Severe	Severe
Approach	Linguistic	Linguistic	Linguistic	Linguistic

touch-cue method that was described by Bashir, Graham-Jones and Bostwick (1984).

MIT was never intended as a stand-alone therapy (Helfrich-Miller, 1994), and when used in conjunction with the kindred approaches of Integral Stimulation (Chapter 7), singing, and prolongation of vowels, it appears to have clinical utility. In MIT, an intoned utterance is lengthened and the rhythm and stress are exaggerated, while the pitch is held constant for several whole notes. In such intoned or chanted 'stylised' utterances, pitch typically varies by only one whole note. Its focus is not on the segmental level, but rather on prosody, and its role is in helping children to produce and differentiate strong and weak syllables and vary the length of notes (vocalisations) at will.

12. Singing

Singing lends itself to decreased rate of production, so it may make proprioceptive monitoring easier for some children, as well as allowing children who have difficulty 'keeping up' with the words of songs to cope better. 'Slowed down' versions of children's songs and nursery rhymes, such

as those on a CD-ROM called *Time to Sing*, available from www.apraxia-kids.org, comprise an invaluable, entertaining resource for younger children, especially those who are minimally verbal. As well as potentially facilitating self-monitoring, the clinician can run a 'visual check' to see that the child has optimal symmetry and the best possible articulatory configurations while producing the 'sung' words.

For older children, slow karaoke is an engaging vehicle for practice (e.g., http://perso.orange.fr/prof.danglais/animations/music/what_a_wonderful_world.swf). Singing can be incorporated into several of the strategies described above, particularly the reduplication strategy (see 6d above) for increasing the number of syllables a child can produce, and for auditory input therapy. Combining singing with the reduplication strategy, a word sequence such as bye-bye can be repeated many times to the tune of a lullaby (e.g., Bye-bye baby, bye-bye-bye to *Doeler* the traditional tune for *Loving shepherd of thy sheep*; or to the tune of *There is a tavern in the town*. The latter lends itself to *Bye-bye bye baby, bye bye-bye, Mum Mum Mumma, Mumma Mum, Dad Dad Dadda Dadda Dad, Pop Pop Poppa Poppa*

Pop, Nan Nan Nanna Nanna Nan, and similar sequences) with a few tiddly-poms thrown in for laughs.

13. Prolongation of vowels

Clinicians can encourage new consonants and vowels, and new syllable structures and word structures to generalise to more challenging contexts by slowing children's utterance rate. It is more effective to prolong the vowels as in *Temporal and Tactile Cueing (DTTC)* (Chapter 7) (e.g., [sæːːːt] for *sat*) rather than consonants (e.g., [sːːːæt] for *sat*). Vowel prolongation is a helpful strategy to apply when a novel word that is difficult for the child to produce is introduced, such as a significant name, like the surname of a new teacher that the child badly wants to say properly. Again, singing or chanting, as in MIT, can be incorporated into this technique, and into #14–16 below.

14. Slowed rate of production

Within *Temporal and Tactile Cueing (DTTC)* (Chapter 7), and in intervention generally, when the aim of an activity is generalisation of newly acquired segments and structures to more difficult contexts for the child (Shriberg & Kwiatkowski, 1990), it can be helpful to instate a 'slow talking time' as part of daily practice. The clinician can model 'slow talking' explaining its purpose to parents and other helpers, and providing models and instruction as well as opportunities for rehearsal *with* the child. It is important not to contrast 'slow talking' with 'fast talking'. It is rarely desirable to have a child with moderate or severe SSD to speak *rapidly*, and it is preferable to suggest to parents that they contrast slow rate with 'normal rate' or even 'ordinary rate' (or 'normal talking' and 'ordinary talking). This may prevent the child from getting the idea of talking quickly, a risky one for many of these children because their intelligibility may deteriorate as they gather speed (Klopfenstein, 2009).

15. Progressive approximations

The technique of progressive approximations, sometimes called successive approximations (Kaufman, 2005), is used with shaping, cuing, and other feedback to 'convert' an utterance that the child can already produce into a new utterance (Shriberg, 1975). Usually the new utterance is not 'perfect' but rather a reasonable approximation to the intended target, intelligible to a familiar or motivated listener.

This technique was used with my client Simon, 19;0 who had Down syndrome. He was learning to travel independently by train and needed to be able to ask for a ticket to Lindfield where his sheltered workplace was. *Lindfield* was beyond his capabilities, but he knew *Lynn* who helped at his school for many years, and associated *peel* with her name because one of her jobs was to assist students to peel and cut up fruit for morning tea. He was trained to say *Lynn-peel* for *Lindfield*, and in the context of the railway station, this was fully intelligible to the ticket seller.

In another example, Max, 6;0, was a late school starter who had delayed speech and language development and cognitive difficulties. He needed to learn how to say the name of his school, *Leura Public* /ˈluˌɹə ˈpʌbˌlɪk/ which he was calling [ˈpʌbˌwiˈluˌwə]. Producing /ɹ/ was beyond Max's capabilities, so we compromised and aimed for /ˈluˌwə ˈpʌbˌlɪk/ (which in any case was the customary pronunciation for many of his age peers). He learned to say it, holding the correct sequence, with picture cues in a slide show representing *loo* (lavatory) *wah* (a crying baby) *pub* (a hotel) and *lick* (a person licking an ice-cream) for the syllable sequence *loo-wah-pub-lick* (see www.speech-language-therapy.com/pdf/max.ppsx). It should be noted that his parents were asked for, and after a little thought gave, permission to use the words *loo* and *pub*.

16. Single word production drill

It is manifest in working with children with moderate and severe SSD, particularly children with

/f/SFWF

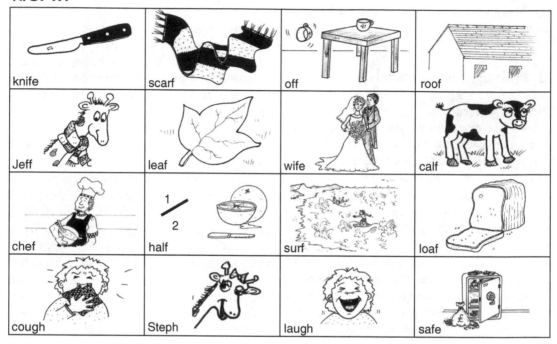

Figure 6.4 /f/ SFWF – knife, Steph, off, roof, etc. Drawing by Helen Rippon, Speech and Language Therapist, www.blacksheeppress.co.uk

CAS that 'practice makes perfect' or at least 'practice makes good enough'. Production practice of single words containing target sounds and/or syllable shapes, or practice of 'difficult' or polysyllabic words, facilitates generalisation of newly learned speech skills. The child might practice a few pictured words with a common phonetic feature, such as the final-f words (*knife, scarf, off, roof,* etc.) displayed in Figure 6.4.

17. Techniques to encourage self-monitoring

Techniques to encourage children to self-monitor their speech production are covered in Chapter 8 (Ruscello, A48; Lowe, A49), and in Chapter 9.

18. Single word and conversational speech production drill

Production drill of single words, combined with production of the same words in phrases and

sentences, and ultimately in controlled conversational contexts can facilitate a more complete phonotactic repertoire, more varied use of phonotactic range within syllables and words, and improved articulatory accuracy and prosody. For example, the words in the Jeff's Scarf story displayed above in Figure 6.3 might be used as the basis for a game in which the child has to use the words in short phrases. Similarly, the child might be asked to formulate short sentences with the words in Figure 6.5 to highlight meaning differences. This could be something simple, such as the child saying, 'You can't say *eight* if you mean *fête*; You can't say *aisle* if you mean *file*; You can't say *ox* if you mean *fox*' etc., or the child instructing an adult to 'Point to *la*; Point to *laugh*'; etc.

19. Backward build-ups

Backward build-ups have long been used in foreign language teaching, and Velleman (2003)

No initial consonant vs. /f/ SIWI

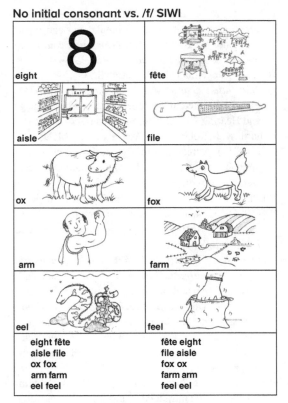

eight fête	fête eight
aisle file	file aisle
ox fox	fox ox
arm farm	farm arm
eel feel	feel eel

Figure 6.5 No initial consonant versus /f/ SIWI – eight fête, aisle file, etc. Drawing by Helen Rippon, Speech and Language Therapist, www.blacksheeppress.co.uk

advocates them as a useful technique for teaching multi-syllabic words, especially with children with CAS. They are also handy for the shorter but 'tricky words', like *yellow*, which may exist as erred fossilised forms. The clinician starts with as much of the *end* of the word a child can say. This might even be all of the word except the first syllable. For example, to teach *dictionary*, the clinician might start by having the child rehearse and strengthen production of *arry*, then *shun-arry*, and finally *dick-shun-arry*, after which the stress and timing are adjusted until the child is saying *dictionary*, naturally with appropriate prosody. *California* might go like this: *yuh*, then *forn-yuh*, then *lee-forn-yuh*, then *callie-forn-yuh*, and ultimately *California*.

20. Backward chaining

Backward chaining is a technique that can be used to facilitate the production of two-syllable words in children who only produce monosyllables. The child produces the second syllable many times (e.g., the *king* in *making* or the *key* in *donkey*) until he or she can say it easily. Then, the highly rehearsed, habituated syllable is alternated with several potential 'first syllables'. For example, the child might practice *king may king way king tay king*, etc. At first, the child is actually saying *king-may, king-way, king-tay*, etc., but then the stress is gradually shifted so that he or she is saying, *making, waking, taking, looking, poking*, etc. It may be necessary to provide simultaneous models at first, and then 'fade' the model, Integral Stimulation style, using DTTC if required. DTTC is described in detail in Chapter 7. There are downloadable 'King Words' and 'Key Words' picture worksheets for backward chaining at www.speech-language-therapy.com, as well as the slideshow used when Jessica, 5;4 learned to say *yellow* (*low* then *yellow*) at the web link www.speech-language-therapy.com/jessica.pps.

It is quite common to find children with SSD who can produce stops (plosives) word finally (SFWF) and syllable finally within words (SFWW) but not word initially (SIWI) and at the beginnings of syllables within words (SIWW). This is particularly the case for /k/ and /g/, where a child can say the velars in *bag*, *back*, *zig-zag* and *tic-tac*, but not in *key* and *go*. A variation of backward chaining can be used to address this difficulty by using final velars that the child *can* already produce, to facilitate initial velars. For example, using the 'King Words' and 'Key Words' worksheets mentioned above to elicit *king* and *key*, the child rehearses *mong*-key, *dong*-key, *bling*-key and so on, emphasising the first syllable. The stress on the first syllable is gradually reduced and shifted to the second syllable, making it more prominent: mong-*key*, dong-*key*, bling-*key*, etc., and then a little 'gap' is inserted between the syllables.

Moving at the child's pace, the clinician works towards just mouthing or cueing the first syllable of *monkey, Blinky, donkey*, etc. (silently), so that the child is saying *key* on his or her own with a strong onset, but not distorted /k/. Once *key* is well established, the child can be encouraged to practice strings of: *key-keep, key-keys, key-keen, key-keel, key-quiche,* etc., before introducing initial /k/ in combination with other vowels. There are pictures and therapy activity sheets for this at www.speechlanguage-therapy.com.

Additional techniques

The available repertoire of approaches and techniques to apply in the symptomatic treatment of SSD does not stop here. There is more to come in Chapter 7, where the focus is on intervention specifically for CAS; in Chapter 8, which covers a range of 'tips' for target selection and intervention for phonological disorder; and in Chapter 9, which contains a detailed account of PACT in action.

References

ASHA. (2004). *Evidence-based practice in communication disorders: an introduction* [Technical Report]. Available from www.asha.org/policy.

ASHA (2007a). *Childhood Apraxia of Speech [Technical Report].* Retrieved 15 Jan, 2014 from www.asha.org/docs/html/TR2007-00278.html

ASHA (2007b). *Childhood apraxia of speech* [Position Statement]. Retrieved 15 January 2014 from www.asha.org/policy

Adel Aziz, A., Shohdi, S., Osman, D. M., & Habib, E. I. (2010). Childhood apraxia of speech and multiple phonological disorders in Cairo-Egyptian Arabic speaking children: language, speech, and oromotor differences. *International Journal of Pediatric Otorhinolaryngology, 74*, 578–585.

Air, D. H., Wood, A. S., & Neils, J. R. (1989). Considerations for organic disorders. In: N. A. Creaghead, P. W. Newman, & W. A. Secord (Eds.), *Assessment and remediation of articulatory and phonological disorders* (2nd ed., pp. 265–301). Columbus: Merrill Publishing Company.

Anthony, J. L., Aghara, R. G., Dunkelberger, M. J., Anthony, T. I., Williams, J. M., & Zhang, Z. (2011). What factors place children with speech sound disorders at risk for reading problems? *American Journal of Speech-Language Pathology, 20*(2), 146–160.

Baker, E., & McCabe, P. (2010). The potential contribution of communication breakdown and repair in phonological intervention. *Canadian Journal of Speech-Language Pathology, 34*(3), 193–204.

Ball, L., Beukelman, D., & Bernthal, J. (1999). *Communication characteristics of children with DAS.* Poster presented to the American Speech-Language and Hearing Association, San Francisco, CA.

Ballard, K. J., Robin, D. A., McCabe, P., & McDonald, J. (2010). A treatment for dysprosody in childhood apraxia of speech. *Journal of Speech, Language, and Hearing Research, 53*(5), 1227–1245.

Bashir, A. S., Graham-Jones, F., & Bostwick, R. Y. (1984). A touch-cue method of therapy for developmental verbal apraxia. *Seminars in Speech and Language, 5*, 127–137.

Bauman-Waengler, J. (2004). *Articulatory and phonological impairments: A clinical focus* (2nd ed.). Boston: Allyn and Bacon.

Benson, D. F., Dobkin, B. H., & Gonzalez, L. J. (1994). Assessment: Melodic intonation therapy. Report of the therapeutics and technology assessment subcommittee of the American Academy of Neurology. *Neurology, 44*, 566–568.

Bernhardt, B., & Stoel-Gammon, C. (1994). Nonlinear phonology: Introduction and clinical application, *Journal of Speech and Hearing Research, 37*, 123–143.

Bernstein Ratner, N. (2006). Evidence-based practice: An examination of its ramifications for the practice of speech-language pathology. *Language, Speech, and Hearing Services in Schools, 37*, 257–267.

Betz, S. K., & Stoel-Gammon, C. (2005). Measuring articulatory inconsistency in children with developmental apraxia, *Clinical Linguistics & Phonetics, 19*, 53–66.

Bleile, K. M. (2004). *Manual of articulation and phonological disorders: Infancy through adulthood* (2nd ed.). Clifton Park, NY: Thomson Delmar Learning.

Bleile, K. M. (2013). *The late eight* (2nd ed.). San Diego: Plural Publishing.

Bornman, J., Alant, E., & Meiring, E. (2001). The use of a digital voice output device to facilitate language development in a child with developmental apraxia of speech: A case study. *Disability and Rehabilitation, 23*, 623–634.

Boone, D. R., & McFarlane, S. C. (2000). *The voice and voice therapy.* Needham Heights, MA: Allyn & Bacon.

Bowen, C. (1996). The quick screener. Retrieved 15 January 2014 from www.speech-language-therapy.com

Bowen, C. (1998). *Speech-language-therapy dot com.* Retrieved 15 January 2014 from www.speech-language-therapy.com

Bowen, C. (2009). *Children's speech sound disorders.* Oxford: Wiley-Blackwell.

Bowen, C. (2010). Child speech assessment resources. Retrieved 15 January 2014 from www.speech-language-therapy.com/index.php?Itemid=117

Bowen, C., & Rippon, H. (2013). Consonant clusters: Alliterative stories and activities for phonological intervention. Cowling, Keighley: Black Sheep Press.

Bridgeman, E., & Snowling, M. (1998). The perception of phoneme sequence: A comparison of dyspraxic and normal children, *British Journal of Disorders of Communication, 23*, 245–252.

Camarata, S. M. (2010). Naturalistic intervention for speech intelligibility and speech accuracy. In: A. L. Williams, S. McLeod, & R. J. McCauley (Eds.), *Interventions for speech sound disorders in children* (pp. 381–405). Baltimore, MD: Paul H. Brookes Publishing Co.

Carroll, J. M., & Snowling, M. J. (2004). Language and phonological skills in children at high risk of reading difficulties, *Journal of Child Psychology and Psychiatry, 45*(3), 631–640.

Carson, K., Gillon, G., & Boustead, T. (2013). 'Classroom phonological awareness instruction and literacy outcomes in the first year of school', *Language Speech, and Hearing Services in Schools, 44*(2),147–160.

Caruso, A., & Strand, E. (1999). Motor speech disorders in children: Definitions, background and a theoretical framework. In: A. Caruso, A., & E. A. Strand(Eds.), *Clinical Management of Motor Speech Disorders in Children.* New York, NY: Thieme.

Caspari, S. (2007). Working guidelines for the assessment and treatment of childhood apraxia of speech: A review of ASHA's 2007 position statement and technical report. Retrieved 30 October 2013 from www.speechpathology.com/articles

Cheour, M., Ceponiene, R., Lehtokoski, A., Luuk, A., Allik, J., Alho, K., & Näätänen, R. (1998). Development of language-specific phoneme representations in the infant brain. *Nature Neuroscience, 1*, 351–353.

Crary, M. A. (1984). A neurolinguistic perspective on developmental dyspraxia. *Journal of Communicative Disorders, 9*, 33–49.

Crary, M. A. (1993). *Developmental motor speech disorders.* San Diego, CA: Singular Publishing Group.

Crosbie, S., Holm, A., & Dodd, B. (2005). Intervention for children with severe speech disorder: A comparison of two approaches. *International Journal of Language and Communication Disorders, 40*, 467–491.

Davis, B., Jakielski, K., & Marquardt, T. (1998). Developmental apraxia of speech: Determiners of differential diagnosis. *Clinical Linguistics and Phonetics, 12*(1), 25–45.

Davis, B. L., & Velleman, S. L. (2000). Differential diagnosis and treatment of developmental apraxia of speech in infants and toddlers. *Infant-Toddler Intervention, 10*(3), 177–192.

Deem, R., & Brehony, K. J. (2000). Doctoral students' access to research cultures – are some more equal than others?. *Studies in Higher Education, 25*, 149–165.

Dehaene-Lambertz, G. (1997). Electrophysiological correlates of categorical phoneme perception in adults. *NeuroReport, 8*, 919–924.

Dehaene-Lambertz, G., & Gliga, T. (2004). Common neural basis for phoneme processing in infants and adults. *Journal of Cognitive Neuroscience, 16*, 1375–1387.

Dehaene-Lambertz, D., & Dehaene, S. (1994). Speed and cerebral correlates of syllable discrimination in infants. *Nature, 370*, 292–295.

Dehaene-Lambertz, G., Dupoux, E., & Gout, A. (2000). Electrophysiological correlates of phonological processing: A cross-linguistic study. *Journal of Cognitive Neuroscience, 12*, 635–647.

Dinnsen, D. A. (1996). Context-sensitive underspecification and the acquisition of phonemic contrasts. *Journal of Child Language, 23*, 57–79.

Dodd, B. J., & Bradford, A. (2000). A comparison of three therapy methods for children with different types of developmental phonological disorder. *International Journal of Language and Communication Disorders, 35*, 189–209.

Dodd, B., Crosbie, S., Zhu, H., Holm, A., & Ozanne, A. (2002). *Diagnostic evaluation of articulation and phonology (DEAP).* London: Psychological Corporation.

Dogil, G. & Mayer, J. (1998). Selective phonological impairment: a case of apraxia of speech. *Phonology, 15*, 143–188.

Dunn, L. M., & Dunn, L. M. (1997). *Peabody picture vocabulary test III.* Circle Pines, MN: American Guidance Service.

Ekelman, B. L., & Aram, D. M. (1983). Syntactic findings in developmental verbal apraxia. *Journal of Communication Disorders, 16*(4), 237–250.

Fey, M. E. (1992a). Phonological assessment and treatment. Articulation and phonology: An introduction. *Language Speech and Hearing Services in Schools, 23*, 224.

Fey, M. E. (1992b). Phonological assessment and treatment. Articulation and phonology: An addendum. *Language Speech and Hearing Services in Schools, 23*, 277–282.

Fletcher, S. G. (1972). Time-by-count measurement of diadochokinetic syllable rate. *Journal of Speech and Hearing Research 15*:757–762.

Flipsen, P., Jr. (2006). Measuring the intelligibility of conversational speech in children. *Clinical Linguistics and Phonetics, 20*(4), 303–312.

Forrest, K. (2003). Diagnostic criteria of developmental apraxia of speech used by clinical speech-language pathologists. *American Journal of Speech – Language Pathology, 12*(3), 376–380.

Friederici, A. D. (2000). The developmental cognitive neuroscience of language: A new research domain. *Brain and Language, 71*, 65–68.

Friederici, A. D. (2002). Towards a neural basis of auditory sentence processing. *Trends in Cognitive Sciences, 6*, 78–84.

Froud, K., & Khamis-Dakwar, R. (2012). MisMatch negativity responses in children with a diagnosis of Childhood Apraxia of Speech (CAS). *American Journal of Speech-Language Pathology, 21*(4), 302–312.

Gierut, J. (1989). Maximal opposition approach to phonological treatment. *Journal of Speech and Hearing Disorders, 54*, 9–19.

Gierut, J. A. (1998). Treatment efficacy: Functional phonological disorders in children. *Journal of Speech, Language and Hearing Research, 41*, S85–S100.

Gierut, J. (2007). Phonological complexity and language learnability. *American Journal of Speech-Language Pathology, 16*(1), 6–17.

Gosling, A. S., & Westbrook, J. I. (2004). Allied health professionals' use of online evidence: a survey of 790 staff working in the Australian public hospital system. *International Journal of Medical Informatics, 73*(4), 391–401.

Granger, R. (2005). *Word flips*. Greenville, SC: Super Duper Publications.

Grigos, M. I., & Kolenda, N. (2010). The relationship between articulatory control and improved phonemic accuracy in childhood apraxia of speech: A longitudinal case study. *Clinical Linguistics & Phonetics, 24*(1), 17–40.

Hall, P. K., Hardy, J. C., & La Velle, W. E. (1990). A child with signs of developmental apraxia of speech with whom a palatal lift prosthesis was used to manage palatal dysfunction. *Journal of Speech and Hearing Disorders, 55*(3), 454–460.

Hanson, M. L. (1983). *Articulation*. Philadelphia, PA: W. B. Saunders Co.

Hegde, M. N., & Peña-Brooks, A. (2007). *Treatment protocols for articulation disorders*. San Diego, CA; Plural Publishing.

Helfrich-Miller, K. R. (1983). The use of melodic intonation therapy with developmentally apractic children: A clinical perspective. *Journal of the Pennsylvania Speech-Language-Hearing Association*. 11–15.

Helfrich-Miller, K. R. (1984). Melodic intonation therapy with developmentally apraxic children. *Seminars in Speech and Language, 5*, 119–125.

Helfrich-Miller, K. R. (1994). Clinical Perspective: Melodic Intonation Therapy for Developmental Apraxia. *Clinics in Communication Disorders, 4*(3), 175–182.

Hennessy, K., & Hennessy, K. (2013). *Anything but silent: Our family's journey through childhood apraxia of speech*. Tarentum, PA: Word Association Publishers.

Highman, C. D., Hennessey, N. W., Leitão, S., & Piek, S. (2013). Early development in infants at risk of childhood apraxia of speech: A longitudinal investigation. *Developmental Neuropsychology, 38*(3), 197–210.

Highman, C., Hennessey, N., Sherwood, M., & Leitão, S. (2008). Retrospective parent report of early vocal behaviours in children with suspected childhood apraxia of speech. *Child Language Teaching and Therapy, 24*, 285–306.

Highman, C., Leitão, S., Hennessy, N., & Piek, J. (2012). Prelinguistic communication development in children with childhood apraxia of speech: A retrospective analysis, *International Journal of Speech-Language Pathology, 14*(1), 35–47.

Hixon, T., Hawley, J., & Wilson, K. (1982). The around-the-house device for the clinical determination of respiratory driving pressure: A note on making the simple even simpler. *Journal of Speech and Hearing Disorders, 47*, 413.

Hodson, B. (2004). *Hodson assessment of phonological patterns* (3rd ed.). Austin, TX: Pro-Ed.

Iuzzini, J., & Forrest, K. (2010). Evaluation of a combined treatment approach for childhood apraxia of speech. *Clinical Linguistics & Phonetics*, *24*(4–5), 335–345.

Jansen, L., Rasekaba, T., Presnell, S., & Holland, A. E. (2012). Finding evidence to support practice in allied health: Peers, experience and the internet. *Journal of Allied Health*, *41*(4), 154–161.

Johnson, C. J. (2006). Getting started in evidence-based practice for childhood speech-language disorders. *American Journal of Speech-Language Pathology*, *15*(1), 20–35.

Kaufman, N. (2005). *Kaufman speech praxis workout book*. Gaylord, MI: Northern Speech Services.

Klopfenstein, M. (2009). Interaction between prosody and intelligibility. *International Journal of Speech-Language Pathology*, *11*, 326–331.

Kuhl, P. K., Conboy, B. T., Padden, D., Nelson, T., & Pruitt, J. (2005). Early speech perception and later language development: implications for the critical period. *Language Learning and Development*, *1*, 237–264.

Kummer, A. W. (2014). Speech and resonance assessment. *Cleft palate and craniofacial anomalies* (3rd ed.). Clifton Park, NY: Delmar Cengage Learning.

Larrivee, L. S., & Catts, H. W. (1999). Early reading achievement in children with expressive phonological disorders, *American Journal of Speech-Language Pathology*, *8*, 118–128.

Leppänen, P. H. T., Pihko, E., Eklund, K. M., & Lyytinen, H. (1999). Cortical responses of infants with and without a genetic risk for dyslexia: II. Group effects. *NeuroReport*, *10*, 969–973.

Lewis, B. A., Avrich, A. A., Freebairn, L. A., Hansen, A. J., Sucheston, L. E., Kuo, I., Taylor, H. G., Iyengar, S. J., & Stein, C. M. (2011). Literacy outcomes of children with early childhood speech sound disorders: Impact of endophenotypes. *Journal of Speech, Language, and Hearing Research*, *54*(6), 1628–1643.

Lewis, B., Freebairn, L., Hansen, A., Iyengar, S., & Taylor, H. (2004). School-age follow-up of children with childhood apraxia of speech. *Language, Speech, and Hearing Services in Schools*, *35*, 122–140.

Maas, E., Butalla, C. E., & Farinella, K. A. (2012). Feedback frequency in treatment for childhood apraxia of speech. *Journal of Speech, Language, and Hearing Research*, *55*(2), 561–578.

Maassen, B. (2002). Issues contrasting adult acquired versus developmental apraxia of speech. *Seminars in Speech and Language*, *23*(4), 257–266.

Maassen, B., Groenen, P., & Crul, T. (2003). Auditory and phonetic perception of vowels in children with apraxic speech disorders. *Clinical Linguistics and Phonetics*, *17*, 447–467.

Martikainen, A., & Korpilahti, P. (2011). Intervention for childhood apraxia of speech: A single-case study. *Child Language Teaching and Therapy*, *27*(2), 9–20.

Marion, M. J., Sussman, H. M., & Marquardt, T. P. (1993). The perception and production of rhyme in normal and developmentally apraxic children. *Journal of Communication Disorders*, *26*, 129–160.

Marquardt, T. P., Sussman, H., Snow, T., & Jacks, A. (2002). The integrity of the syllable in developmental apraxia of speech. *Journal of Communication Disorders*, *35*, 31–49.

Mayer, J. (1995). A representational account for apraxia of speech. *Proceedings of the 13th International Congress of Phonetic Sciences*, 82–85.

McCabe, P., Macdonald-DaSilva, A., van Rees, L., Arciuli, J., & Ballard, K. (2010). *Using orthographic cues to improve speech production in children with & without childhood apraxia of speech*. Paper presented at the Motor Speech Conference, Savannah, Georgia, USA.

McCabe, P., Rosenthal, J. B., & McLeod, S. (1998). Features of developmental dyspraxia in the general speech-impaired population? *Clinical Linguistics & Phonetics*, *12*(2), 105–126.

Meredith, A. (2002). Disordered prosody and articulation in children with childhood apraxia of speech: What's the relationship? Retrieved 30 September 2013 from https://www.kintera.org/site/apps/nlnet/content2.aspx?c=chKMI0PIIsE&b=701773&ct=464245

Mewburn, I. (2013). How to tame your PhD. Raleigh, NC: Lulu.

Miccio, A. W. (2005). A treatment program for enhancing stimulability. In: Kamhi, A. G., & Pollock, K.E. (Eds.), *Phonological disorders in children: Clinical decision making in assessment and intervention* (pp. 163–173). Baltimore, MD: Paul H. Brookes Publishing Co.

Miccio, A. W., & Elbert, M. (1996). Enhancing stimulability: a treatment program. *Journal of Communication Disorders*, *29*, 335–352.

Miccio, A. W., & Williams, A. L. (2010). Stimulability intervention. In: A. L. Williams, S. McLeod, & R. J. McCauley (Eds.), *Interventions for speech sound disorders in children* (pp. 179–202). Baltimore, MD: Paul H. Brookes Publishing Co.

Miron, C. (2012). The parent experience: When a child is diagnosed with childhood apraxia of speech. *Communication Disorders Quarterly, 33*(2), 96–110.

Morrisette, M. L., Farris, A. W., & Gierut, J. A. (2006). Applications of learnability theory to clinical phonology. *International Journal of Speech-Language Pathology, 8*(3), 207–219.

Mullins, G., & Kiley, M. (2002). It's a PhD, not a Nobel Prize: how experienced examiners assess research theses, *Studies in Higher Education, 27*(4), 369–386.

Munson, B., Bjorum, E., & Windsor, J. (2003). Acoustic and perceptual correlates of stress in nonwords produced by children with suspected developmental apraxia of speech and children with phonological disorder. *Journal of Speech, Language, and Hearing Research, 46*, 189–202.

Murray, E., McCabe, P., & Ballard, K. (2012a). A comparison of two treatments for childhood apraxia of speech: methods and treatment protocol for a parallel group randomised control trial. *BMC Pediatrics, 12*(3), 1–9.

Murray, E., McCabe, P., & Ballard, K. J. (2012b). The first randomised control trial for treatment of Childhood Apraxia of Speech (ReST vs Nuffield Dyspraxia Program-3). *Communicate: Our natural state. Speech Pathology Australia National Conference.* Hobart, TAS, Australia.

Näätänen, R., Lethokoski, A., Lennes, M., Cheor, M., Houtilainen, M., Iivonen, A., et al. (1997). Language specific phoneme representations revealed by electric and magnetic brain responses. *Nature, 385*, 432–434.

Näätänen, R., Kujala, T., & Winkler, I. (2011). Auditory processing that leads to conscious perception: a unique window to central auditory processing opened by the mismatch negativity and related responses. *Psychophysiology, 48*, 4–22.

Neilson, R. (2003). *Sutherland phonological awareness test – Revised.* Wollongong: Author.

Osterhout, L. (2000). On space, time, and language: for the next century, timing is (almost) everything. *Brain and Language, 71*, 175–177.

Petrie, M, & Rugg, G. (2010). *The Unwritten Rules of PhD Research* (2nd ed.). Maidenhead, UK: Open University Press.

Pihko, E., Leppänen, P. H. T., Eklund, K. M., Cheour, M., Guttorm, T. K., & Lyytinen, H. (1999). Cortical responses of infants with and without a genetic risk for dyslexia: I. Age effects. *NeuroReport, 10*, 901–905.

Pulvermüller, F., Kujala, T., Shtyrov, Y., Simola, J., Tiitinen, H., Alku, P., Alho, K., Martinkauppi, S., Ilmoniemi, R.J., & Näätänen, R. (2001). Memory traces for words as revealed by the mismatch negativity. *NeuroImage, 14*, 607–616.

RCSLT (2011). *Royal College of Speech and Language Therapists: Developmental verbal dyspraxia [Policy Statement],* Author. Available from www.rcslt.org

Reilly, S., Douglas, J., & Oates, J. (2004). *Evidence-based practice in speech pathology.* London: Whurr Publishers.

Rivera-Gaxiola, M., Silva-Pereyra, J., & Kuhl, P. K. (2005). Brain potentials to native- and non-native speech contrasts in 7- and 11-month-old American infants. *Developmental Science, 8*, 162–172.

Roddam, H., & Skeat, J. (2010). *Embedding evidence-based practice in speech and language therapy: International examples.* London: Wiley-Blackwell.

Rose, M., & Baldac, S. (2004). Translating evidence into practice. In: S.Reilly, J.Douglas, & J.Oates (Eds.), *Evidence-based practice in speech pathology* (pp. 317–329). London: Whurr Publishers.

Rosenbek, J. C., & Wertz, R. T. (1972). A review of 50 cases of developmental apraxia of speech. *Language, Speech, and Hearing Services in Schools, 3*, 23–33.

Rugg, M. D., & Coles, M. G. (1995). The ERP and cognitive psychology: Conceptual issues. In: M.D.Rugg, & M.G.Coles (Eds.), *Electrophysiology of mind: Event-related brain potentials and cognition* (pp. 27–39). Oxford, UK: Oxford University Press.

Ruscello, D. R. (2008). *Treating articulation and phonological disorders in children.* St. Louis: Elsevier.

Secord, W., Boyce, S. Donohue, J., Fox, R., & Shine R. (2007). *Eliciting Sounds: Techniques and Strategies for Clinicians* (2nd ed.). Clifton Park, NY: Thompson Delmar Learning.

Shriberg, L. D. (1975). A response evocation program for /ɚ/. *Journal of Speechand Hearing Disorders, 40*, 92–105. Reprinted in *Contemporary readings in articulation disorders.* C. Bennett, N. Bountress, & G. Bull. Dubuque, IA: Kendall-Hunt.

Shriberg, L. D., Aram, D. M., & Kwiatkowski, J. (1997a). Developmental apraxia of speech: I. Descriptive perspectives. *Journal of Speech, Language, and Hearing Research*, *40*, 273–285.

Shriberg, L. D., Aram, D. M., & Kwiatkowski, J. (1997b). Developmental apraxia of speech: II. Toward a diagnostic marker. *Journal of Speech, Language, and Hearing Research*, *40*, 286–312.

Shriberg, L. D., Aram, D. M., & Kwiatkowski, J. (1997c). Developmental apraxia of speech: III. A subtype marked by inappropriate stress. *Journal of Speech, Language, and Hearing Research*, *40*, 313–337.

Shriberg, L. D., & Campbell, T. F. (2002). *Proceedings of the 2002 childhood apraxia of speech research symposium.* Carlsbad: The Hendrix Foundation.

Shriberg, L. D., Campbell, T. F., Karlsson, H. B., McSweeney, J. L., & Nadler, C. J. (2003). A diagnostic marker for childhood apraxia of speech: The lexical stress ratio. *Clinical Linguistics and Phonetics*, *17*(7), 549–574.

Shriberg, L. D., Fourakis, M., Hall, S., Karlsson, H. K., Lohmeier, H. L, McSweeny, J., et al. (2010). Extensions to the speech disorders classification system (SDCS). *Clinical Linguistics & Phonetics*, *24*, 795–824.

Shriberg, L. D., & Kwiatkowski, J. (1990). Self-monitoring and generalization in preschool speech-delayed children. *Language Speech and Hearing Services in Schools*, *21*, 157–170.

Shriberg, L. D., Lohmeier, H. L., Strand, E. A., & Jakielski, K. J. (2012). Encoding, memory, and transcoding deficits in childhood apraxia of speech. *Clinical Linguistics & Phonetics*, *26*(5), 445–482.

Skinder-Meredith, A. (2000). *The Relationship of prosodic and articulatory errors produced by children with developmental apraxia.* Unpublished Doctoral Dissertation, University of Washington, Seattle.

Skinder-Meredith, A., Carkowski, S., & Graff, N. (2004). Comparison of nasalance measures in children with childhood apraxia of speech and repaired cleft palate, to their typically developing peers. *SpeechPathogy.com.* Retrieved March 21 2008 from http://www.speechpathology.com/articles/index.asp

Skinder-Meredith, A., Lommers, K., & Yoder, J. (2007). Trends in the case histories of 15 children with childhood apraxia of speech. Poster presented at the *American Speech Language and Hearing Convention*, Boston, MA.

Snowling, M., Goulandris, N., & Stackhouse, J. (1994). Phonological constraints on learning to read: Evidence from single case studies of reading difficulty. In: C. Hulme, & M. Snowling (Eds.), *Reading development and dyslexia* (pp. 86–104). London: Whurr Publishers.

Stackhouse, J. (1997). Phonological awareness: Connecting speech and literacy problems. In: B. W.Hodson, & M. L.Edwards (Eds.), *Perspectives in applied phonology* (pp. 157–196). Gaithersburg, MD: Aspen.

Stephens, D., & Upton, D. (2012). Speech and language therapists' understanding and adoption of evidence-based practice. *International Journal of Therapy and Rehabilitation*, *19*(6), 328–334.

Sternberg, D. (1981). *How to complete and survive a doctoral dissertation.* New York, NY: St. Martin's Press.

Strand, E. A., & Debertine, P. (2000). The efficacy of integral stimulation with developmental apraxia of speech. *Journal of Medical Speech-Language Pathology*, *8*(4), 295–300.

Strand, E., & McCauley, R. J. (1999). Assessment procedures for treatment planning in children with phonologic and motor speech disorders. In: A. Caruso, & E. Strand (Eds.), *Clinical management of motor speech disorders in children.* (pp. 73–107). New York, NY: Thieme-Stratton.

Strand, E. A., McCauley, R. J., Weigand, S., Stoeckel, R., & Baas, B. (2013). A motor speech assessment for children with severe speech disorders: Reliability and validity evidence. *Journal of Speech, Language, and Hearing Research*, *56*(2), 505–520.

Strand, E., Stoeckel, R., & Baas, B. (2006). Treatment of severe childhood apraxia of speech: A treatment efficacy study. *Journal of Medical Speech Pathology*, *14*, 297–307.

Sutherland, D., & Gillon, G. T. (2007). The development of phonological representations and phonological awareness in children with speech impairment. *International Journal of Language and Communication Disorders*, *42*(2), 229–250.

Teverovsky, E. G., Bickel, J. O., & Feldman, H. M. (2009). Functional characteristics of children diagnosed with childhood apraxia of speech. *Disability and Rehabilitation*, *31*(2), 94–102.

Vallino-Napoli, L. D., & Reilly, S. (2004). Evidence-based health care: A survey of speech pathology practice. *Advances in Speech-Language Pathology*, *6*(2), 107–112.

Velleman, S. (2002). Phonotactic therapy. *Seminars in Speech and Language, 23*, 43–57.

Velleman, S. L. (2003). *Resource guide for childhood apraxia of speech*. Clifton Park, NY: Delmar/Thomson Learning.

Velleman, S. (2005). Perspectives on assessment. In: A. Kamhi, & K. Pollock (Eds.), *Phonological disorders in children* (pp. 23–34). Baltimore, MD: Brookes.

Velleman, S., & Shriberg, L. (1999). Metrical analysis of the speech of children with suspected developmental apraxia of speech. *Journal of Speech, Language, and Hearing Research, 42*, 1444–1460.

Velleman, S. L., & Strand, K. (1994). Developmental verbal dyspraxia. In: J. E. Bernthal, & N. W. Bankson (Eds.), *Child phonology: Characteristics, assessment, and intervention with special populations* (pp. 110–139). New York, NY: Thieme Medical Publishing, Inc.

Weber, C., Hahne, A., Friedrich, M., & Friederici, A. D. (2004). Discrimination of word stress in early infant perception: Electrophysiological evidence. *Cognitive Brain Research, 18*, 149–161.

Weiner, F. (1981). Treatment of phonological disability using the method of meaningful contrast: Two case studies. *Journal of Speech and Hearing Disorders, 46*, 97–103.

Weiss, C. E., Gordon, M. E., & Lillywhite, H. S. (1987). *Clinical management of articulatory and phonological disorders, treatment of special populations* (pp. 259–260). Baltimore, MD: Williams and Wilkins.

Wellman, R. L., Lewis, B. A., Freebairn, L. A., Avrich, A. A., Hansen, A. J., & Stein, C. M. (2011). Narrative ability of children with speech sound disorders and the prediction of later literacy skills. *Language, Speech, and Hearing Services in Schools, 42*(4), 561–579.

Williams, A. L. (2003). *Speech disorders: Resource guide for preschool children*. Clifton Park, NY: Thomson Delmar Learning.

Williams, A. L. (2006). A systemic perspective for assessment and intervention: A case study. *Advances in Speech-Language Pathology, 8*(3), 245–256.

Williams, P., & Stackhouse, J. (1998). Diadochokinetic skills: Normal and atypical performance in children aged 3–5 Years. *International Journal of Language and Communication Disorders, 33* (Suppl): 481–486.

Williams, P., & Stephens, H. (2004). *Nuffield centre dyspraxia programme* (3rd ed.). Windsor, UK: The Miracle Factory.

Winitz, H. (1984). *Treating articulation disorders: For clinicians by clinicians*. Baltimore, MD: University Park.

Yaruss, J. S., & Logan, K. (2002). Evaluating rate, accuracy, and fluency of young children's diadochokinetic productions: A preliminary investigation. *Journal of Fluency Disorders, 27*, 65–86.

Zaretsky, E., Velleman, S. L., & Curro, K. (2010). Through the magnifying glass: Underlying literacy deficits and remediation potential in childhood apraxia of speech. *International Journal of Speech-Language Pathology, 12*, 58–68.

Chapter 7
Childhood apraxia of speech

This chapter begins with a summary of the principles of motor learning defined as 'a set of processes associated with practice or experience leading to relatively permanent changes in the capability for movement' (Schmidt & Lee, 2011). These principles are central to the dynamic assessment (DA) and treatment of childhood apraxia of speech (CAS). Next, in A44, is Judith Stone-Goldman's schema that allows the clinician to choose an appropriate level of intervention for a client relative to a specified intervention target. Although this chapter is essentially about CAS, it should be noted that Dr. Stone-Goldman's chart is applicable to articulation disorders and phonological impairment as well. We go on to explore more approaches to CAS intervention, and Edythe Strand from the Mayo Clinic, Pam Williams and Hilary Stephens from the Nuffield Centre, and Patricia McCabe and Kirrie Ballard who are based at The University of Sydney talk about 'their' practices and research around CAS in A45, A46 and A47, respectively. The reader is reminded that Gretz (A7) in Chapter 1, and Highman (A41) and Froud and Khamis-Dakwar (A42) in Chapter 6, and a good part of the rest of Chapter 6 also cover CAS topics.

Principles of motor learning

The precursors to motor learning, including speech motor learning are

a. motivation;
b. focused attention; and
c. pre-practice before entering the practice phase.

The clinician and parents may need to consider a behaviour management plan, implemented by a suitably qualified professional, for children who cannot focus or co-operate easily or who have motivation, attention, or compliance difficulties (Bitter, A15). It is important for parents (and us) to know that simply attending intervention sessions will have little or no impact on the speech of children with CAS unless they engage adequately in the motor learning and other aspects of treatment. It is also important that we recognise the limits of our professional expertise and not attempt to address issues, such as behaviour of concern (Chan et al., 2012) that are best managed by a professional counsellor or other professional, or indeed, by the child's own family.

Children's Speech Sound Disorders, Second Edition. Caroline Bowen.
© 2015 John Wiley & Sons, Ltd. Published 2015 by John Wiley & Sons, Ltd.
Companion website: www.wiley.com/go/bowen/speechlanguagetherapy

The conditions of practice for motor learning, including speech motor learning are

a. motivation;
b. goal and target setting (what will be practiced, and how many times);
c. instructions (how directions will be delivered);
d. modelling (e.g., simultaneous production/immediate imitation/delayed imitation); and
e. the setting and with whom (e.g., where the practice take place and who will help).

Other factors may arise specific to a client. For example, the reinforcement (praise) used should not take up too much time, make too much noise, 'interrupt' or distract. It is usually necessary to guide parents in how to deliver reinforcement, providing explicit modelling and practice in sessions (with feedback to them). It is also necessary to choose and develop appealing activities for the child (and to an extent for the parents, too) that will facilitate and invite repeated opportunities for production of target behaviours or utterances.

Repetitive practice (motor drill)

The type of practice we aim for is repetitive practice, sometimes called motor drill. There *must* be sufficient trials (or 'repeats') of the target behaviour within a practice session for any motor learning to take place and for it to become habituated. Habituation is a step towards more automatic speech output processing.

A comparison of practice schedules

There are four types of practice schedule, each with advantages and disadvantages. In the 'real world', we may not *have* much choice regarding practice distribution. We *must* decide, however, which targets to select and how many will be addressed concurrently or sequentially, and communicate this clearly to those concerned: the parents and any other helpers implementing practice away from the treatment room, and where indicated, the child him or herself. The options are:

massed practice versus distributed practice; and random practice versus blocked practice.

Massed practice versus distributed practice

Massed practice involves fewer practice sessions, but the sessions themselves are longer. This promotes quick development of skills, but poor generalisation. Distributed practice, on the other hand, has the same duration (in aggregate) distributed across more sessions. Distributed practice takes longer, and can become tedious, but it has the advantage of promoting better motor learning and is potentially more motivating over time.

Blocked practice versus random practice

In blocked practice, all practice trials ('repeats' of the behaviours) of a stimulus (target) are done in one time block before moving to the next target. This arrangement tends to lead to better performance. By contrast, in random practice, the order of presentation of all stimuli is randomised through the session, and this fosters better retention, better motor learning, and, in many instances, higher levels of motivation.

KP and KR feedback to the child

It is essential during motor drill to give a child frequent information about his or her movement performance, building his or her 'knowledge' of what the speech motor apparatus is capable of, what it is doing 'right now', and what it did a moment before (just then). Interestingly, there are reports in the cognitive motor literature that adults derive most benefit from finely specified feedback. Conversely, if feedback to children is too specific, their performance can decrease. Skilled observations by the SLP/SLT allow the frequency of feedback to be tailored to suit, bearing in mind that it can distract some children and that, for some, saving any 'reward' until the end of a session is the most effective way to proceed.

During pre-practice the clinician models the utterance and provides detailed feedback on 'movement performance' to shape correct responses, and to prepare the child for the practice phase. This is called knowledge of performance (KP) feedback. In the practice phase the child should be able to adjust productions independently in the absence of both models and KP feedback. In the practice phase the clinician minimises the volume of modelling, really aiming to provide no models. Instead, knowledge of results (KR) feedback that diminishes over the course of treatment is provided. This KR feedback is delivered in response to about 80% of the child's responses to start with either in a session or over several sessions, falling off to 10% as his or her capacity for self-monitoring, instating revisions and repairs and engaging in self-reinforcement builds. If the child is not doing well in a practice session with KR feedback only, then some KP feedback may be introduced to get him or her back on track.

Rate of production trials

There is usually a trade-off between rate and accuracy. A slower rate of production will, up to a point, increase accuracy. *Varying the expected rate of production* can be an effective technique to incorporate into motor drill, using speech, chanting (Melodic Intonation Therapy) and singing, because it encourages habituation of articulatory movement accuracy while working towards automaticity, a natural rate and natural prosody.

Finding the right level of intervention

Dr. Judith Stone-Goldman is an Emeritus Senior Lecturer with the Department of Speech and Hearing Sciences at the University of Washington. She has had a long career teaching in the areas of child speech-language disorders, treatment methodology and counselling, as well as working clinically with children and families in early intervention centres, clinics and schools. At present she continues to teach through workshops and individual coaching (see www.judystonegoldman.com), helping SLPs improve communication, relationships and professional satisfaction. In A44, she details a teaching tool she created and found useful for both guiding students and communicating with parents.

Q44. Judith Stone-Goldman: Finding the right level of difficulty in therapy

The grid in Table A44.1 is one of those deceptively simple-looking clinical nuggets! It allows a clinician to choose an appropriate level of intervention for a client relative to the status of a particular therapy target. What prompted its development, and can you walk the reader through the process of using it, with real life examples? How would you suggest presenting the grid to carers and teachers, especially if more than one target and more than one level were involved simultaneously for a client?

A44. Judith Stone-Goldman: Choosing where to start

- A 6-year-old touches his tongue tip with a tongue depressor and then says 'la'.
- A 9-year-old plays a game with hidden clues, using the words 'near' and 'far' to guide the clinician.
- A 4-year-old takes turns with the clinician, rolling cars along a pretend road and saying phrases, such as 'car go!' and 'come on car!'
- A 7-year-old makes up a story from words containing /s/.

Table A44.1 Choosing a level of intervention relative to the status of the therapy target

Status of the therapy target →	Absent →	→	→	Mastered →
Clinical Decisions	Level 1	Level 2	Level 3	Level 4
Assessment: Current level of the target behaviour ↓	a) Absent OR b) Beginning to emerge	Present but limited to certain activities and contexts. Inconsistent at different linguistic levels and/or in different activities	Present across linguistic levels in familiar, rehearsed tasks, but not produced naturally in a variety of situations	Present in all linguistic contexts and environments, with a variety of child and adult communicative partners
Goal: Desired treatment outcome ↓	Establish the new behaviour or increase (reinforce) the emerging behaviour	Make the behaviour more consistent, and establish it in varied linguistic levels, varied activities	Generalise the behaviour to conversational speech, new communicative partners and new situations	Not applicable Treatment not needed Move on, but monitor the new behaviour
Therapy contexts: Situations in which the client will produce the targeted behaviour ↓	Under optimal, often contrived conditions (drill; drill-play), in, simple linguistic forms, in a small range of activities	In new linguistic forms and levels, in a variety of activities, with clear focus maintained on target	In varied, natural interactions and activities, with different communicative partners, in different settings	Not applicable; target is used in naturally occurring events and situations in the child's life
Stimuli: Range of stimuli and materials ↓ **Cues:** Degree of clinician cues **Reinforcement:** Frequency, type **Responses:** Expected responses	A small set of familiar stimuli and predetermined target responses. Responses are tightly linked to treatment. Maximal cues, reinforcement.	An expanding set of practiced stimuli to evoke responses in varied linguistic contexts (naming, question/answer) and levels (phrase, sentence); frequent cues, reinforcement	Less constrained stimuli and materials to allow practice of target responses in natural communicative contexts; overt cues are faded, reinforcement becomes natural, intermittent	Not applicable; real events create opportunities for use of target
Measurement: Treatment: Nature of the stimuli and expected responses as specified in behavioural objective ↓	Practiced stimuli and responses; cues as needed	Practiced stimuli and responses; limited cues	Not practiced:Novel stimuli and unrehearsed responses (these may be sampled within familiar treatment activities); no cues	Not applicable
Measurement: Generalisation: Probable generalisation measures ↓	Probe/explore the next teaching level or new set of responses to see if the child is ready to move on	Probe new, unpractised (unrehearsed) words containing the target or probe new linguistic levels	Objectively probe generalisation beyond therapy activities (Does the child use the target spontaneously?). Probe novel events and contexts (relay a message, tell a story)	Family and teachers may continue to monitor the target behaviour in everyday interactions outside the clinic

Introduction

Activities like these are familiar to SLPs/SLTs who work with children with speech sound disorder (SSD). Although age-appropriate activities are important, they do not by themselves make up good therapy. What is important about the above activities for effective therapy? How might we evaluate their usefulness for a particular child?

A key factor that will affect an activity's usefulness is its *level of difficulty*. Activities that are too easy will not challenge the child sufficiently, but activities that are too difficult are frustrating and limit progress. Through my years of teaching and supervising, I have come to believe that zeroing in on the right level of difficulty, relative to the child's skill level, is critical for developing treatments that yield good outcomes. Finding the right level of difficulty is particularly important for choosing where to *start* intervention.

Determining the level of difficulty raises many questions. Do you practise words or sentences? Should therapy stimuli be familiar and limited in number, or should they be novel and extensive? Is it better to keep an activity focused, or should activities be similar to natural communication? How do we know when it's time to make the work harder? We must ask and answer these questions repeatedly over the course of a client's treatment if we are to work at the right level and support the client's progress.

In my efforts to guide students in coming up with answers to these questions, I sketched out the ideas that are reflected in the chart displayed in Table A44.1. Creating the chart helped me organise clinical concepts that were second nature to me, and using it as a teaching tool brought these concepts to light for students. In our group case conferences, the chart helped us appreciate differences among clients' treatments. It gave students a way to be comfortable with clients who were 'just starting out' in therapy, as well as a way to imagine the future directions a client's treatment might take. Thanks to the initiative of one student, the chart subsequently became a tool for communicating with parents.

Orientation: Reading the chart

First, consider the top row, labelled *'Status of the therapy target'.* This describes how regularly a speech sound target (e.g., word initial /ʃ/) or syllable structure target (e.g., initial consonants) is produced correctly and the variety of contexts in which it is produced. A Level 1 target may be *absent* or just *barely emerging*, in which case it is never produced correctly or under rare conditions only. In contrast, a Level 4 target that is *mastered* is produced reliably in varying linguistic conditions, in different environments, with different communication partners. Levels 2 and 3 refer to targets that are produced with varying consistency, in varying contexts, on a progression towards mastery. The description of each level can be found in the row below the level numbers, labelled *'Assessment: Current level of the target behaviour'*.

Now examine the left-hand column, labelled *'Clinical Decisions'.* Each box in this column refers to an aspect of treatment that the clinician specifies to make treatment at the right level of difficulty. The first four boxes in the *Clinical Decisions* column are important for *planning treatment*: determining the current level; stating the treatment goal; planning therapy contexts; and specifying therapy stimuli, cues, reinforcement, and responses. Roth and Worthington (2005) are helpful on the topic of therapy conditions, such as contexts and stimuli, cues and reinforcement. The remaining two boxes in this column are important for *planning measurement*: measuring treatment progress and measuring generalisation, both of which are typically done using non-standardised probes (see Mowrer, 1985 for a review of basic data collection and measurement issues). Note that, by reading down the column under any of the levels (1–4), you can see the clinical decisions for that level. By reading across a row, you can see how a particular clinical decision changes as the level changes.

Case examples

Two case examples serve to clarify the chart's sections and demonstrate its clinical application. The children described received individual treatment at the *University of Washington Speech and Hearing Clinic* from a graduate student in speech-language pathology, under my supervision. Both children were developing normally in receptive and expressive language, cognition and social skills, and had normal hearing thresholds, with speech being the only area of concern. For the purpose of clear illustration, I chose to discuss children with a small set of speech errors. This chart can lend guidance when working with children with more errors or with additional language problems, or when using other models of treatment, such as those that incorporate phonological analysis.

Case 1

Joanna was a 5-year-old monolingual child whose parents were concerned about intelligibility and age-appropriate speech. Phonological assessment revealed errors on all velars (/k, g, ŋ/) in single words and connected speech. Joanna was not immediately stimulable for velars when given models and simple instructions for making these sounds. All her substitutions and imitated attempts were [t, d, n] for /k, g, ŋ/, respectively.

Joanna is a good example of a child who needed to begin at Level 1. With the potential therapy targets all absent, treatment was, by necessity, narrow in scope. The goals were to establish the new targets /k/ and /g/ in simple phonetic forms, and the therapy contexts were restricted to highly structured practice (e.g., table drill or finding stimulus items hidden around the room). The clinician provided maximal cues: tactile cues with a tongue depressor, descriptive names for sounds (e.g., calling /k/ a 'back sound' and referring to it as 'kay'), gestures towards the back of the mouth, verbal instructions and models were used freely to help Joanna learn about and produce the new velar sounds. The same stimuli were repeated many times, and the only expected responses were /k/ and /g/, first in isolation and then in a few syllables. Concerning /k/ and /g/ 'in isolation', it should be noted that stops cannot exist in isolation, so realisations at this level were actually produced with a whispered or minimally articulated schwa ([kə], [gə]). Reinforcement was frequent and enthusiastic.

Measuring treatment progress at this level was limited to the practice attempts, supported by the clinician cues. Given that Joanna had never produced /k/ or /g/, *any* correct productions were a big step. In the same spirit, our expectations for generalisation were modest, limited to explorations of Joanna's readiness to move ahead to different vowels or new syllable/word positions (i.e., dynamic assessment or stimulability; Hasson and Joffe, 2007). It was too soon to worry about generalisation to novel words or connected speech. We knew that more functional gains would come later in treatment. We also did not treat /ŋ/, even though it was absent, but held it as a control behaviour. Had this target remained absent or inconsistent after /k/ and /g/ developed, treatment would have been introduced. Hegde (2002) provides a discussion of measuring control behaviours for treatment efficacy.

Once Joanna produced /k/ and /g/ in a variety of syllables and in some carefully selected CVC words, she met the definition of Level 2: the targets were present but limited to certain activities and contexts. Now the goal was for Joanna to produce targets in varied linguistic forms (new word positions and phonological forms), linguistic levels (phrases and sentences) and activities. Level 2 treatment involved a larger set of practice words and game-like activities that incorporated different types of responses (naming, answering questions). The treatment still remained sufficiently structured to maintain focus on the target and to permit the clinician to provide cues and reinforcement. Note that the structure of therapy, for example, drill versus free play, is an important variable in choosing the right level of treatment, and related discussion by Roth and Paul (2002) may be helpful.

We anticipated staying at Level 2 for a while longer. We expected to work on the targets in sentences and to fade cues before moving to Level 3, at which point we would help Joanna generalise her productions to conversational speech and natural activities. To our surprise, Joanna suddenly moved to Level 3 independently, using the targets spontaneously throughout the entire session. Parent report supported that changes were occurring at home as well. We therefore used measurements associated with Levels 2 and 3 to document these changes and make further decisions about treatment. Probes of the targets in unpractised words and sentences revealed 100% accuracy; even in conversation and narratives, correct production had risen to slightly above 50%. A probe of /ŋ/ (never treated or practiced) showed 90% correct in words.

Given the speed of these changes, which far outstripped the direct therapy, we concluded that Joanna would likely continue her development independently, especially because her family reinforced her gains and provided a language rich home. Together with her family, we made the decision to discontinue treatment and follow-up as needed at a later time. Subsequently, the family confirmed that Joanna had mastered her sounds and needed no further treatment.

Joanna moved from Level 1 to Level 3 within a 10-week period, which is unusually fast progress, even for a young child. Joanna's strengths were many: she was able to focus and cooperate; she had age-appropriate phonemic awareness and curiosity about what she was learning (e.g., 'Why does that word have a 'kay' sound?'); and, despite her initial lack of stimulability, she had a normal motor speech system. These strengths, coupled with a positive therapeutic environment and supportive parents, added up to rapid, well-maintained changes.

Case 2

Let us briefly consider a child who stands in contrast to Joanna. At age 9, Robert was brought to therapy for remediation of /ɹ/. Robert's family had lived in the Middle East for a number of years, and Robert was exposed to several languages. He produced /ɹ/ correctly some of the time in conversational speech. What level of treatment was the correct level for him?

Despite some spontaneous productions in conversational speech (making him appear to be at Level 3), Robert needed treatment at Level 2. He produced some but not all forms of /ɹ/ in words, and he needed to become consistent in phrases and structured sentences. Robert showed excellent progress in sessions as well as generalisation to unpractised words and sentences. However, he still did not produce the targets consistently in conversation; treatment thus moved to Level 3.

The goal for Level 3 was to extend correct productions to more natural communication. The clinician introduced tasks to evoke connected speech (picture description, structured conversations), create practice with new partners, move treatment out of the familiar room to other parts of the clinic, and replace overt cues with subtle, natural reinforcers. By systematically varying the treatment contexts, stimuli, cues, reinforcement and expected responses, the clinician helped Robert meet Level 3 goals of generalisation. Follow-up after a 3-month break showed that Robert was maintaining his progress and doing well in his daily environment.

Why did Robert begin treatment at Level 2 if he was already producing some correct targets in conversational speech? Robert needed better consistency of his productions, even in simpler tasks. Treatment at Level 3 did not allow sufficient control of therapy conditions to build up that consistency. We did not know if his early multilingual experiences had influenced his articulation development, but the more obvious explanation lay in his speech musculature. Robert had mild low tone in his face and lips, and his speech was sometimes imprecise or weak sounding. He needed to work at a level where he could refine and stabilise his /ɹ/ productions before reinserting them into increasingly complex speech. Though he developed /ɹ/ on his own, he needed treatment to shape his best productions and maintain them under the high processing demands of complex, natural speech.

Conclusion

Working at the right level brings confidence to children and patience to both clinicians and families. By discussing with parents the basics about a child's current level, we can promote realistic expectations and suggest appropriate participation. A simplified chart of levels and corresponding treatment conditions aids the discussion. If more than one target is involved, parents can easily see each target's level on the chart. Even a smart, motivated child can grasp the levels: one 9-year-old girl volunteered that, while she was thrilled to be saying a correct /ɹ/, practising words in the session simply was not the same as the way she spoke at home! This led to a discussion of how her treatment would progress in time, and the clinician introduced some functional phrases to support the girl's interest in meaningful communication.

I hope the reader will see that this chart is not meant to impose rules or restrict creativity but to foster logical, careful planning. The concepts it covers are essential to therapy, but the chart is not exhaustive, and a clinician should individualise the activities (even Level 1 activities can be made enjoyable). Although the chart emphasises production practice, other types of learning, such as discrimination exercises or phonemic awareness, can be added. In addition, creative homework assignments can be used at every level, from word awareness or key word assignments at Level 1 to at-home word diaries and creative writing at Levels 3 and 4.

Further, children will vary in how slowly or quickly they progress through the levels. Children may work on different targets at different levels, and some children will need treatment at every level before completing therapy. The guiding principles are to begin at a level that allows a child to be successful, build steadily and systematically towards natural communication, and collect data that support treatment decisions.

Integral stimulation

In the mid-1950s, Robert L. Milisen published an article about a multi-layered program for articulation therapy incorporating imitation and auditory and visual models (Milisen, 1954). Milisen's method, called integral stimulation, has shaped the treatment of functional articulation disorders, the dysarthrias, and acquired apraxia of speech. It utilises hierarchical cueing procedures that begin with high levels of support via simultaneous production of slowly spoken simple utterances with visual and tactile cues. The cues are subtly, and expertly faded and amplified as required until, at the lowest level of support, they disappear completely and the client produces delayed repetition of increasingly complex stimulus items. Research by Rosenbeck, Lemme, Ahern, Harris and Wertz (1973) and Strand and Debertine (2000) shows that integral stimulation intervention in treatment of individuals with apraxia of speech is efficacious.

Although they may be unaware of its precise origins, the children's version of integral stimulation is widely used by SLPs/SLTs who treat children's speech and language difficulties. It involves a familiar procedure in which the clinician models an utterance and the child *imitates* it, while the clinician ensures that the child's attention is as focused as possible on *listening to* the model while *looking at* the clinician's face (watching the model, if you like).

Integral stimulation proceeds from bottom up, starting with simple phonetic segments and sequences and then short utterances; building in a hierarchy of difficulty to longer and more phonetically complex stimuli. Integral stimulation can be used alone when working with children with CAS, but it is thought to be more effectively applied in combination with tactile and gesture cues that shape the accuracy of articulatory gestures and prosodic cues (Strand, 1995; Strand, Stoeckel & Baas 2006), involving melodic intonation therapy techniques (Helfrich-Miller, 1983, 1984, 1994) or contrastive stress (Velleman, 2002). A prominent feature of the application of the integral-stimulation-combined-with-prosodic-cues approach with children with CAS is that syllable, word and sentence stress are emphasised early in therapy, that is, from the outset, and with young children *if possible*.

Dynamic temporal and tactile cueing

For non-verbal children with severe CAS, for whom the method described above is too difficult, Strand has developed and tested (Strand et al., 2006; see also Jakielski, Kostner & Webb, 2006)

a variation of integral stimulation called *Dynamic Temporal and Tactile Cueing (DTTC) for Speech Motor Learning*. Incorporating the principles of motor learning (see above), it can be used with the non-verbal children who struggle unsuccessfully with the task of articulatory imitation and who seem unable to achieve even the remotest approximation for consonants or vowels. DTTC is an explicitly principled, modified version of the *Eight-Step Continuum for Treatment of Acquired Apraxia of Speech* (Rosenbeck et al., 1973), originally designed for adult clients with AOS. It allows for what Strand calls 'a continuous shaping of the movement gesture', to (1) improve motor planning and (2) program speech processing as speech and language acquisition progresses. The tiny steps and essential adjustments of the therapy dance within DTTC will have a familiar ring to many clinicians, and are as follows.

1. *Imitation*
   In its implementation, DTTC begins with direct, immediate imitation of natural speech.
2. *Simultaneous production with prolonged vowels (most clinician support)*
   If the child cannot imitate, the task is changed to the simplified, more 'supported' one of *simultaneous production*. At this easier level, the SLP/SLT says the utterance at normal volume *with* the child first, very slowly with the addition of touch cues and/or gesture cues as required. Slowing the utterance by sustaining the *vowel* ([si::::] rather than [ssssi], as explained in Chapter 6) helps the child, and at the same time lets the SLP/SLT run a visual check to see that the jaw and lip postures are correct (e.g., ensuring that there is no jaw slide and that there is acceptable facial symmetry).
3. *Reduction of vowel length*
   As the simultaneous production phase of therapy advances the rate of stimuli production is increased (i.e., vowel length is reduced) allowing the child's speech output to sound more natural.
4. *Gradual increase of rate to normal*
   Practice continues at this level to the point where the child synchronises effortlessly

with the therapist at normal rate, with normal movement gestures, and without silent posturing.

5. *Reduction of therapist's vocal loudness, eventually miming*

Using delicate timing, the SLP/SLT is then in a position to reduce his or her vocal volume, eventually reaching a point where the clinician is producing a mime (mouthing the utterance) as the child says it aloud. Because of the intellectual closeness within the dyad, this can be a tricky point in therapy, and some children will dutifully follow *exactly* what the adult is doing so that the two are miming at each other! 'Like a pair of goldfish' as one parent commented. This is obviously not the goal, and children may need explicit instruction to keep their voice or voice box 'turned on' even though the adult's is 'off'. The gesture and touch cues may still be needed at this point and will almost certainly be necessary in the next step: the integral stimulation method proper.

6. *Direct imitation*

Ensuring that the child is secure and comfortable with moving to this harder level, the SLP/SLT instructs the child to watch the adult's face (Look at me for help) while an auditory model is delivered. The child attempts to repeat the model and, if successful, does so many times. If unsuccessful, the therapist may backtrack to the simultaneous model or silent mouthing/miming level described above. Eventually all miming is faded, and the child directly imitates and 'repeats' targets numerous times before the final step – step 7 – is introduced.

The key to successful implementation of integral stimulation is the clinician's empathic, informed observations of and sensitivity to what the child is 'giving' by way of responses. The professional skill and flexibility involved in continually fine-tuning the hierarchy of stimuli *and* fine-tuning the amount of support provided to enable the child to imitate spontaneously, is critical. Auditory (including prosodic), visual, and tactile cues and the level of demand on the child are continually aug-

mented and faded in each practice trial according to the child's responses.

The clinician's alertness to the child's responses is especially important with the CAS population, who have good and bad days with their speech-processing capacities. The SLP/SLT must be always be prepared to take the therapy 'down a notch' if required, and to explain to parents why this is happening.

7. *Introduction of a one-or two-second S-R delay (least support)*

Once the child is directly imitating the therapist's model with normal rate, with prosody he or she can vary, and with appropriate articulatory gestures, the therapist inserts a new requirement. This is in the form of a one- to two-second delay before the child imitates, so that the child produces a *slightly* delayed response. To facilitate this for the children who find the delay difficult and want to 'jump in', miming while the child produces the delayed response can prove helpful.

8. *Spontaneous production*

Finally, the SLP/SLT elicits short and long spontaneous utterances, for example, by asking the child, 'What is this called?' using cloze tasks such as '*Twinkle, twinkle ___ ___*', sentence completion such as '*Mother elephant is very big, her baby is ___ ___*', 'Three things I like about the beach are ___', engaging in story telling (e.g., with wordless picture books), picture and object description, narrative and role play, and the like.

Dr. Edythe Strand, who developed DTTC, is a consultant in the Department of Neurology, Division of Speech Pathology, at the Mayo Clinic in Rochester, Minnesota, and a Professor in the Mayo Medical School. Professor Strand's primary research and clinical interests have been in neurologically mediated communication disorders, especially developmental and acquired AOS, dysarthria and neurogenic voice disorders. She has published articles and chapters regarding the clinical management of motor speech disorders in children, including treatment efficacy. Responding to Q45, she talks about DA, the *Dynamic*

Evaluation of Motor Speech Skill (DEMSS) and DTTC.

Q45. Edythe A. Strand: Dynamic assessment, DEMSS and DTTC

Child-centred DAs (Feuerstein, Rand, Jensen, Kaniel & Tzuriel, 1987; Vygotsky, 1978) such as DEMSS are comfortable partners with DTTC and integral stimulation, especially early in the suspected CAS (sCAS) therapeutic encounter, when it is impossible to divorce evaluation from treatment. Hasson and Joffe (2007) write that a DA approach sees the positive relationship between therapist and child potentially enhancing the child's performance, feelings of competence, and levels of motivation both in assessment and in therapy, cautioning that these benefits must be balanced against the need to obtain reliable and replicable test results. What is the potential contribution of DA, including DEMSS, to differential diagnosis of SSD; to short-term and longer-term goal setting, or 'choosing where to start' (Stone-Goldman, A44) for children with severe CAS; and how does it interface with DTTC and integral stimulation?

A45. Edythe A. Strand: Dynamic assessment of motor speech disorders in children

Dynamic Assessment (DA) offers several contributions to simplifying the sometimes-difficult task of differential diagnosis of SSDs, especially when CAS is suspected. First, DA facilitates eliciting behaviours that the clinician can then compare to accepted phenotypes for different types of SSD. Second, DA allows the clinician to make more accurate judgements of severity and prognosis. Finally, DA is very helpful to the clinician in choosing initial stimuli and determining those types of cues that are likely to best assist the child's motor speech performance.

Dynamic assessment

DA utilises interaction and support to maximise the child's potential performance. In DA multiple attempts may be elicited, with the clinician using different types of cues, with scoring reflecting the child's change in performance (Glaspey & Stoel-Gammon, 2007; Lidz & Peña, 1996). Researchers have studied the role of dynamic assessment in language disorders (e.g., Bain & Olswang, 1995; Hasson & Joffe, 2007; Olswang & Bain, 1996), and phonological disorders (e.g., Glaspey & Stoel-Gammon, 2005), but its role in childhood motor speech disorders has had little discussion.

The role of DA in differential diagnosis

When CAS is suspected, differential diagnosis is complicated because children with SSD present with co-morbidities such as global developmental delay, hearing loss, language disorders (including pragmatic difficulties), phonological disorders and/or dysarthria (McCauley, A14; Stoeckel, A40). In order to plan appropriate treatment, the clinician must determine the relative contribution of different types of cognitive, linguistic and motor influences. One of the biggest challenges for the SLP/SLT is determining whether or not *motor* speech impairment is contributing to the child's SSD. Identification of CAS in particular, is not at all easy because in many cases segmental errors due to difficulty with producing the movement gestures for the sound targets are especially hard to differentiate from phonologically based segmental errors.

The ASHA position statement concerning CAS (ASHA, 2007) provided a welcome definition of the disorder with a list of behavioural characteristics that should be associated with the label (Highman, A41). Because DA examines the child's responses in varying contexts, the clinician may elicit more observations of these characteristics. In contrast, observations of spontaneous speech only afford a view of the child's customary production. In standardised test formats, we make observations of a child attempting an utterance they may be unable to say correctly, with the child frequently producing a habituated response, or making a minimal attempt at correct production. Binary scoring tells us they cannot say the utterance, without suggesting *why* they cannot say it. But what we see and hear produced spontaneously and in static testing is different from what we perceive when they actively *try* to correctly produce a new word or one that they typically mispronounce. The cueing involved in DA enables observations of what the child does while really attempting specific movement gestures (i.e., when they are 'trying hard'. In the case of children with sCAS, we have the opportunity to evaluate discrete characteristics associated with that label. For example, we may see groping that is not evident in spontaneous speech, but evident in when cues are used to encourage accurate imitation of an articulatory gesture. Inconsistency is likely more evident across repeated trials as cueing occurs, as is segmentation of syllables which may occur only when the child really concentrates on producing correct articulatory movement gestures.

The role of DA in short- and long-term goal setting

DA is an important resource for determining the severity of the child's motor speech disorder and the prognosis, both of which are important when it comes to setting appropriate and realistic goals. DA is sensitive to changes that result from the child's *responses* to cueing; in other words, his or her *learning*. This is very different from standardised tests that must show stability over time (Lidz & Peña, 1996). Traditional standardised tests allow comparison of a child's performance on a task (e.g., articulation performance) with the performance of a normative group, at one point in time. While this may allow some idea of severity, it is quite conceivable that two children may exhibit the same standard score on a measure, but have very different levels of severity and different prognoses for change. This is because most standardised tests do not provide the clinician with the opportunity to observe the child's responses to different types of cueing, or their potential to learn via such cueing. DA can greatly facilitate judgements regarding severity and prognosis because the therapist is engaging the child across contexts, providing different levels of support such as tactile cueing, visual attention to the clinician's face, having the child produce the response more slowly, and/or having the child produce the utterance simultaneously with the examiner. Judgements can then be made regarding the child's response to these types and levels of cueing. Such observations facilitate the clinician's judgements of how much cueing will be *needed* in early therapy, to induce improvement in performance, and how long it may take to achieve initial progress.

Prognostic decisions lead the clinician to short- and long-term goal setting. Parents of non-verbal children often come with the question, 'Will my child ever talk?' If the child's responses to cueing and facilitation during DA indicate potential as a verbal communicator, then the long-term goal is to establish functional verbal communication. DA also facilitates short-term goals, and they are closely tied to decisions about where to start. Rather than examining at what level (V vs. CV and VC vs. CVC, etc.) the child is successful, using binary scoring, DA allows observations of practice as well as the level of cueing needed to improve production at varying levels of phonetic complexity. Consider a non-verbal child who exhibits numerous vowel distortions in isolation, syllables and words, but improves production in all contexts when the clinician helps him or her achieve the initial articulatory position and stay in the steady state of (sustaining) the vowel for longer. Logically, this would lead to the decision to work at *and beyond* the CV, VC and CVC levels. On the other hand, if a child cannot improve vowel production even with maximum cueing and slowed rate, the clinician would begin with a smaller stimulus set, fewer vowel targets and CV and VC syllable shapes.

Dynamic evaluation of motor speech skill

Because DA has much to contribute to differential diagnosis and treatment planning, I have been working to develop a DA tool, the DEMSS, designed specifically for younger children and/or those who have more severe SSD. The purpose of the DEMSS is to facilitate differential diagnosis of speech sound disorders that are due to difficulty with speech praxis, distinguishing them from speech sound errors with other bases. It utilises systematic, progressive cueing to facilitate imitative production of utterances that vary in length and phonetic complexity. Construct validity and reliability of the DEMSS (Strand, McCauley, Weigand, Stoeckel & Baas, 2013) have been demonstrated, and we are in the process of completing the manual and training tape.

The interface between DTTC and integral stimulation

Integral stimulation (Milisen, 1954) denotes a therapy approach focused on imitation of auditory and visual models. DTTC (Strand et al., 2006) is just one type of integral stimulation, which uses auditory, visual and tactile cueing. DTTC, however, emphasises varying the temporal relationship between the stimulus and the response, maximising cueing at first, then fading cues over continued practice. This variation in levels of cueing characterises the similarity between DTTC and DA. In DA, however, cues are progressively *added* to determine how *much* help the child needs to improve accuracy of movement gestures. In DTTC, cues are maximised at first for utterances the child cannot produce, and *then gradually faded* as improvement occurs. This strategy helps the child to take increasing responsibility for the planning/programming and execution of the movement gestures for the target utterance; so in a sense, the child takes responsibility for his or her motor learning.

Case example

Peter aged 4:2 came for speech and language evaluation due to his continued delayed speech acquisition. Since 2:6 he had received individual speech therapy: once weekly at first, building to thrice weekly for the previous 14 months. Traditional articulation therapy approaches had evoked little speech progress. His parents' chief concern was whether or not he would ever talk. They were considering abandoning work on his speech to focus only on augmentative communication.

Peter's receptive language was in the normal range with standard scores between 94 and 101. He initiated communication readily, using sign and gestures, a few intelligible words, and many word approximations understood only by his mother. His Goldman–Fristoe (Goldman & Fristoe, 2000) standard score was <40. A DA of motor speech skill (DEMSS) was administered, revealing numerous CAS characteristics including difficulty achieving initial articulatory configurations, with instances of groping and trial and error behaviour; frequent vowel distortions which varied with co-articulatory context; prosodic errors; and token-to-token inconsistency across trials. He was able to produce only 6 of the 68 items correctly in direct imitation without any cues (*do*; *up*; *mama*; *papa*; *booboo*; and *mom*). These results were consistent with the Goldman Fristoe scores. His DEMSS scores, however, also reflected *improvement* with visual attention to the clinician's face, tactile cueing, slowing-down and simultaneously producing the movement gesture *with* the clinician. His performance improved with progressive cueing on over 65% of utterances, and correct production after cues on 28% of incorrect items, although it usually took the maximum cues to achieve correct production. Because of his ability to benefit from cues focused on movement accuracy, a favourable prognosis for functional communication was determined. Because of the severity of his apraxia of speech, and therapy progress to date, intensive therapy was recommended.

Peter was seen for two daily 30-minute therapy sessions over 6 weeks. DTTC was used to help Peter take increasing responsibility for planning/programming and executing movement gestures for the selected stimuli. Initial goals focused on producing correct movement gestures for speech; improving his ability to produce the syllable shapes of CVC, VC and CV CVC (as in *hi Mom*); and improving accuracy for (/i/, /æ/ and the diphthong /aɪ/. Seven functional words and short phrases were chosen for the initial stimulus set to allow enough massed practice for attaining movement accuracy, yet some distributed practice to facilitate motor learning: *me, bye, dad, eat, home, himom* and *mine*. By the end of the 6 weeks, he had mastered 6/7 of his original training items and had generalised them to spontaneous speech. He had improved his ability to produce five

new items (added in one at a time as he mastered an original item) as well several other phrases that were not in the stimulus set but that had been modelled for him at other times throughout the day and through play, such as, *I win, I won, me too, I'm home* and *I want*.

This fairly rapid improvement likely occurred as a result of more frequent therapy, an approach that focused on facilitating accurate movement for segmental and syllabic sequences, *and* therapy that was based on the principles of motor learning. We maximised the number of practice trials within sessions by using reinforcers that were quick, and given only after several responses. Early in treatment feedback was frequent, immediate and contained specific information regarding movement performance (KP feedback) to maximize movement accuracy. As therapy progressed, feedback was provided less frequently, with slightly longer delays, and with less specificity to maximise motor learning (KR feedback). We varied rate of movement, starting with slow movement and prolonged vowels to achieve accuracy, gradually increasing rate to normal by reducing vowel length. We worked to vary prosody to avoid habituation of rote prosodic contours. As therapy continued, progress towards correct production of words and phrases became faster. He now has many functional words and phrases, and continues in therapy.

NDP3

Well known and widely used in Australia, Ireland, New Zealand, Singapore and the United Kingdom, the *Nuffield Centre Dyspraxia Programme, Third Edition: NDP3* (Williams & Stephens, 2004) is continually amended and updated to reflect current research findings (Williams & Stephens, 2010). A progressive step in 2013 was the removal of informational pages about, and 35 worksheets devoted to NS-OME (Hodge, A31; Lof, A35;

Powell A39), or 'oro-motor work', to give its usual UK handle. The most exciting recent development, however came with the publication of Murray, McCabe and Ballard (2012b) reporting initial comparative outcomes for children aged 4;0 to 12;0 treated with rapid syllable transition training (*ReST*) and children treated with Nuffield Centre Dyspraxia Programme, in the first randomised controlled trial (RCT) to test treatment for CAS (McCabe & Ballard, A47).

NDP3 intervention is described as a bottom-up, motor skills learning approach, focusing on motor programming skills, and in its implementation requires from the client frequent, repetitive practice to learn and establish new speech production skills. The approach is described in A46 by the *NDP3* co-authors, Pam Williams and Hilary Stephens.

Mrs. Pam Williams is a consultant SLT and team manager (developmental disorders) at the Nuffield Hearing and Speech Centre (NHSC). Pam has conducted research into the rate, accuracy and consistency of the diadochokinetic (DDK) performance of young children with typical speech development (Williams & Stackhouse, 1998, 2000) and is currently pursuing doctoral studies on DDK performance of children with speech difficulties. In 2013 she was awarded a Fellowship of Royal College of Speech and Language Therapists in the category of clinical expertise. She is widely known in the United Kingdom and Ireland for her workshop presentations on the Nuffield Program.

Ms. Hilary Stephens works as a principal Speech and Language Therapist in the developmental disorders team at the NHSC. For many years she worked at the Nuffield Speech and Language Unit, providing assessment services and intensive treatment to children, aged 4–7 years, with very severe speech and language disorders, including CAS. Hilary is an officer of the Royal College of Speech and Language Therapists London Speech Disorders Special Interest Group (SIG). In addition to her current clinical duties, Hilary is involved in developing new resources for *NDP3*.

Q46. Pam Williams and Hilary Stephens: The Nuffield Dyspraxia Programme

The skills that children with CAS need to acquire are conceptualised metaphorically in the *NDP3* as a 'brick wall', with speech motor skills and single C and V sounds seen as the foundations, and word level skills built up in layers of bricks on top of the foundations. Simple CV and VC syllables comprise the first layer, moving up in layers through CVCV, CVC, CVCVC and multi-syllabic words, clusters, word combinations of phrases and sentences, finally reaching the top layer of connected speech. Since its publication in 2004, the NDP3 has been continually modified and has seen various changes in content and form. As well, it has been included in an RCT comparing it with ReST (Murray et al., 2012b; McCabe & Ballard, A47). Can you describe for clinicians interested in using the approach the steps used in this 'multi-layered, multi-target treatment', highlighting the suggested dosage and recent developments?

A46. Pam Williams and Hilary Stephens: The Nuffield approach to CAS and other motor speech disorders

The *NDP3* (Williams & Stephens, 2004) is a comprehensive, flexible treatment package that provides a set of therapy procedures, techniques and pictorial materials, designed primarily for children aged 3–7 years. *NDP3* aims to support children with CAS and other motor speech disorders in building accurate motor programs (Stackhouse & Wells, 1997) for individual speech sounds, syllables and words of varying phonotactic complexity, through a fine-tuned therapy hierarchy and frequent repetitive practice.

Dosage

Typically, we recommend the *NDP3* approach be delivered directly by an SLP/SLT on a regular, on-going basis. By this we mean the child should receive a direct therapy session once a week or once fortnightly, continuously, without breaks, for as long as needed. For many children, this will amount to 2 years or more of *NDP3* intervention. Between therapy sessions, the child should do homework provided by the SLP/SLT, based on targets worked on in the direct therapy sessions. These targets should be practised daily for a minimum of 15–20 minutes per day (*NDP3* manual, p. 80). For some children, teaching assistants in school may also be involved in delivering the practice to provide the child with maximum practice opportunities.

For children with very severe speech difficulties, it may be appropriate for *NDP3* to be delivered more intensively, up to once or twice daily during school term time. In such a scenario, homework is not needed, except during holiday periods. Children with co-occurring speech and learning difficulties may require less frequent direct therapy, since such children are likely to require longer periods of practice between the therapy sessions, to establish and consolidate target single sounds, syllables and words.

At the NHSC, our therapy sessions last for 1 hour and are usually observed by the child's parent/carer. Each session includes around four to six different activities, to address the child's current goals on the multi-level treatment hierarchy. For each single sound, syllable or word targeted in a task, we aim for the child to do(say) a minimum of four to eight productions. The same target can be included in several activities, and therefore the SLP/SLT will often elicit 50–100 productions of a particular target within a session.

Preliminary results from an RCT (Murray et al., 2012b; and see McCabe & Ballard, A47 for this and subsequent work), showed NDP3, administered intensively as described above, to be an effective treatment approach for children with CAS.

New developments

Since 2009, we have modified the early stages of our treatment approach, to reflect the current evidence base, and expanded our range of supporting pictorial resources that can be purchased online via www.ndp3.org. In particular, we have published *NDP3® Speech Builder*, a software package, which offers the SLP/SLT the flexibility of creating tailor-made pictures and worksheets, specific to the needs of individual clients, in a simple, time efficient manner. Recent developments are highlighted in the following description. The reader should note that when V is used to describe a constituent of a phonotactic structure, such as CVCV or CVC, 'V' represents either a pure vowel or a diphthong.

Treatment planning

Treatment planning using the *NDP3*, is based on the *NDP3* assessment procedure. Data derived from the *NDP3* assessment enable the SLP/SLT to establish a baseline for a child's speech production capabilities. In practice, most children, start therapy at a single-sound and CV level, with the following two aims. First, to extend the child's phonetic repertoire to include: /p, b, t, d, k, g, m, n, h, f, s, w, j/ and possibly /ʃ/ and /l/, long vowels and if possible, some short vowels and diphthongs. Second, to increase the number of CV syllables and words the child can produce. In pursuing these aims, the syllables and words that are targeted for production practice are carefully selected so as to include as many sounds as possible already present in the child's phonetic repertoire.

In the *NDP3* approach, therapy proceeds in a hierarchy, with the ability to produce words with complex phonotactics, or word combinations, being dependent on mastery of single phones and simple phonotactic structures. As the child's speech production abilities develop, treatment generally involves a multi-level, multi-target approach, whereby the SLP/SLT works concurrently on several targets at a particular level and also targets at different levels (Stone-Goldman, A44). For example, a child might be working on producing /l/, /f/, /ɔ/ and /ɜ/ at single-sound level, voicing contrasts for plosives (stops) at CV level, and CVCV words with /b, d, m, n/ in a variety of contexts.

Sound-cue pictures

The *NDP3* uses sound-cue pictures representing consonants, vowels and diphthongs (e.g., /b/ is represented by a picture of a ball; /aɪ/ is represented by a picture of an eye), and it is therefore necessary, early in therapy, to teach the child to associate the sound-cue pictures with the sounds they represent. These sound–picture associations are used to help the child create or modify motor programs (Stackhouse & Wells, 1997), for sounds that they cannot say or that they say incorrectly. Typically, the use of the sound-cue pictures is augmented by a range of other facilitators such as: verbal cues, for example, 'open your mouth wide for this one'; manual cues such as *Cued Articulation* (Passy, 1993); informal tactile cues, for example, the therapist gently pushing the child's lips together for bilabial placement; orthographic prompts (graphemes) and/or diagrammatic cues, for example, articulograms (Stephens & Elton, 1986) as shown in Figure A46.1, to represent a particular sound's features. Coloured A5 (210 × 297 mm) sound-cue cards for each consonant and vowel have now been published, and these incorporate articulograms.

Oro-motor activities (NS-OME)

In light of increasing concerns around the use of NS-OME when treating speech disorders (McCauley, Strand, Lof, Schooling & Frymark, 2009), we have modified our approach and replaced the oro-motor advice worksheets with Early Sound Making sheets. If the SLP/SLT considers it necessary to elicit a component movement, such as tongue or lip placement, it is recommended that this should be closely linked to production of the target (Royal College of Speech and Language Therapists, 2011).

Single sounds and CV words

To begin, the clinician introduces four to six sound-cue pictures of consonants and vowels that the child can already produce spontaneously, or imitate. Preferably, these should include sounds from different sound classes, to facilitate the retrieval of separate motor programs. The tasks, games and activities that are provided in the *NDP3* reinforce auditory and visual discrimination, and production, thereby consolidating the ability to associate the sounds with the related pictures, and produce the sounds. Additional sound–picture associations are gradually introduced for sounds the

b /b/

Say the sounds Say each syllable three times

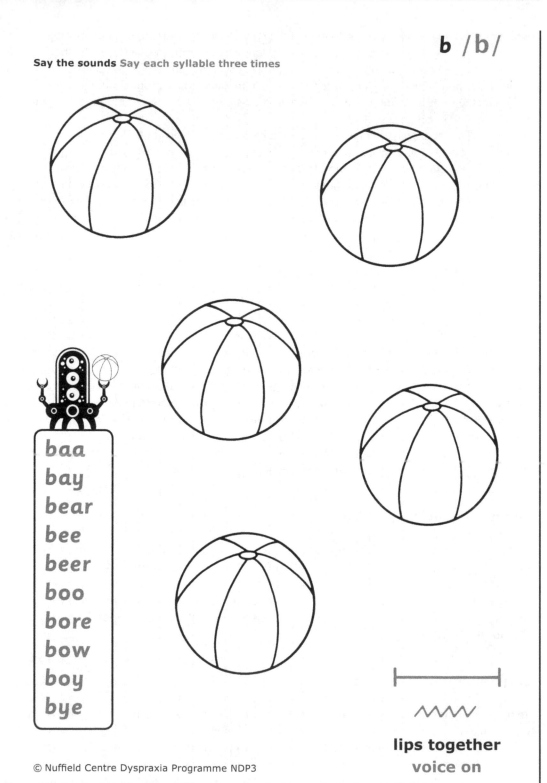

baa
bay
bear
bee
beer
boo
bore
bow
boy
bye

lips together
voice on

© Nuffield Centre Dyspraxia Programme NDP3

Figure A46.1 Articulograms: CV syllables. Reproduced with permission from Nuffield Dyspraxia Programme 3rd Edition.

child can already say, while continuing to reinforce those introduced at the beginning, so that the sounds are not 'lost'. Cues and feedback are provided, as required, to ensure articulatory accuracy and consistency of best production. The child also practices vocal control and prosody: for example by imitating intonation patterns (rising and falling pitch). As well as working on isolated phones, the child's CV repertoire is expanded through repetitive babble and sound play for any consonants or vowels within their current phonetic inventory. Pictures of CV words are also introduced, again building on the child's strengths by starting with words the child can already say.

Teaching new sounds

Once the child has some familiarity with a number of consonant and vowel sound-cue pictures and is able to produce the corresponding sounds accurately and consistently, the clinician teaches one or more sounds that the child cannot currently produce spontaneously or imitate. It is not possible or desirable to be prescriptive about the choice of target. The SLP/SLT should consider such factors as: stimulability (Miccio, 2005; Miccio, Elbert & Forrest, 1999) and whether to work in typical developmental acquisition order, or take a complexity approach (Baker, A13). When imitation is not possible various strategies are utilised, including phonetic placement techniques (Bleile, 2013; Secord, Boyce, Donahue, Fox & Shine, 2007), visual, verbal, tactile and kinaesthetic cues, and facilitative contexts, described in Appendix 4 of the NDP3 manual. While teaching new sounds, interim 'approximations' or 'best productions', such as interdental or dental placements for alveolars, may be accepted at first and later refined.

Introducing sequencing

Once new motor programs (Stackhouse & Wells, 1997) have been established and the child has practised producing sequences involving at least eight repetitions of the same sound (e.g., /b b b b b b b b/), contrastive sequencing (e.g., /b s b s b s b s/ can be introduced, using the *NDP3* worksheets. This challenges the child to retrieve two different motor programs and to utilise motor planning skills to maintain accurate production of the individual sounds throughout the sequence. At the outset, the SLP/SLT aims for a slow production rate (Strand, A45) and contrasts involving two or more distinctive features, to facilitate retrieval and avoid perseveration. Closer feature contrasts should be controlled carefully by the SLP/SLT and introduced gradually, with each step challenging the child only slightly. For example, for a child with a /t/ for /k/ replacement: contrastive sequencing might start with /m-k/, then /b-k/, /p-k/ and finally /t-k/. Speed of production can gradually be increased, and rhythmic and stress patterning incorporated.

Teaching new CV words

If a child is unable to imitate the clinician's spoken model, the SLP/SLT may facilitate the development of new CV words by combining two already established motor programs (C + V = CV). This presents a major challenge for many children, since the process of motor programming is one of the core deficits in CAS (ASHA, 2007). The child needs to learn how to modify the two existing motor programs so that they join smoothly, without the 'gap' in production left earlier in sequencing tasks. Transition worksheets, specifically designed for this purpose, present the sequence of a consonant and a vowel, followed by the CV word created as they join, for example,

/m/ +/u/ = 'moo'; /p/+/aɪ/= 'pie'. The process of 'sound joining' (co-articulation) is supported by careful modelling and by making explicit, using KP feedback (McCabe & Ballard, A47), the articulatory changes the child needs to achieve, for example, the inclusion of /h/ or a 'puff of air' between the consonant and vowel, to produce a CV word with a voiceless plosive (stop).

Recognising that this approach is not appropriate for all children in the 3–7 age-range, we have produced additional CV babble cards and worksheets, to support the imitation of CV syllables, for example, for consonant /b/, the SLP/SLT could model some or all of: *baa, boo, bee, bye, boy, bay, bow, beer, bear*. First, the child is asked to copy the model once, and then to repeat it 5–10 times in a babble string.

Incorporating new CV words into the child's repertoire

As at single-sound level, each newly created CV word has to be practised and consolidated by frequent repetitive practice to establish the new motor program, utilising the *NDP3* pictorial materials. Once established, newly created CV words need to be incorporated into the set of CV words the child can already produce, thereby allowing the development of a system of contrasts at the CV level. This aim may be achieved through minimal pair activities (Bowen & Cupples, 2006, pp. 287–288), incorporating discrimination and production, and using the therapy cards and the many prepared minimal pair worksheets in *NDP3*.

The SLP/SLT needs to select suitable worksheets carefully to ensure the child achieves success but is increasingly challenged, in small graded steps, by the phonetic demands of the individual words in the sequence. For example, for a child who has recently learned to produce *key* accurately, having previously produced it as *tea*: sequencing might move from a vowel change, for example, *key, coo*, to an easy phonetic placement change, for example, *key, bee* to a harder placement change, for example, *tea, key* (see Figure A46.2). Verbal cues (e.g., 'remember this one starts with a /k/') and visual cues using the picture symbols (e.g., a small picture of a camera to represent /k/ placed next to the car picture) make the phonetic composition of words explicit, helping to clarify phonological representations, as well as establishing the motor program.

Moving beyond CV words

CVCV words with the same phone duplicated (e.g., *mummy, daddy, baby, nanny*) and simple CV + CV 'phrases' (e.g., two-word combinations like *no bee, bye boy*) can be introduced, using the *NDP3* pictures and worksheets, as soon as the child has established CV syllables involving /b d m n/. Such activities enable children with restricted phonetic repertoires to experience accurate production of two-word utterances and this can be highly motivating for both the child and parents.

Once able to produce a range of consonants, vowels and CV syllables and words, the child has the building blocks to create words of increasing phonotactic complexity such as CVCV, CVC, CCV, CVCVC and multisyllabic words. Once again the child is required to modify two or more existing motor programs, so that they join together smoothly. Strategies for supporting each level of difficulty, in terms of maintaining accuracy, avoiding sound additions, such as schwa insertion or addition, syllable or glottal insertion or addition, and ensuring appropriate placement of word or syllable stress, are provided in the manual.

The *NDP3* provides transition, blending worksheets for CV + CV = CVCV (e.g., *toe + bee = Toby* as shown in Figure A46.3), CV + C = CVC (e.g., *boo + t = boot* as shown in Figure A46.4)

CV–CV Sequencing: tea–key

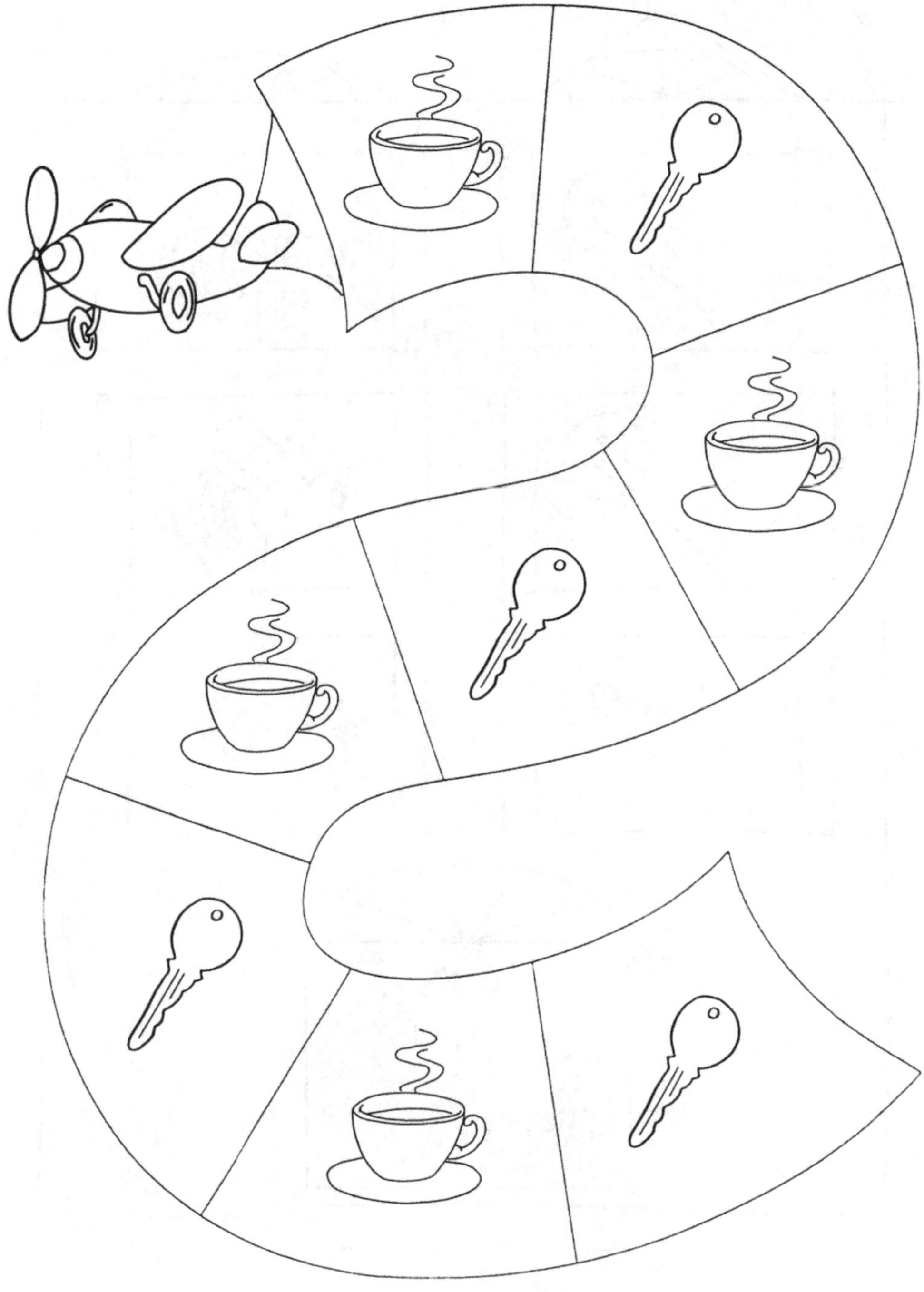

Figure A46.2 CV–CV sequencing. Reproduced with permission from Nuffield Dyspraxia Programme 3rd Edition.

Transition (CV + CV = CVCV): toe + bee = Toby

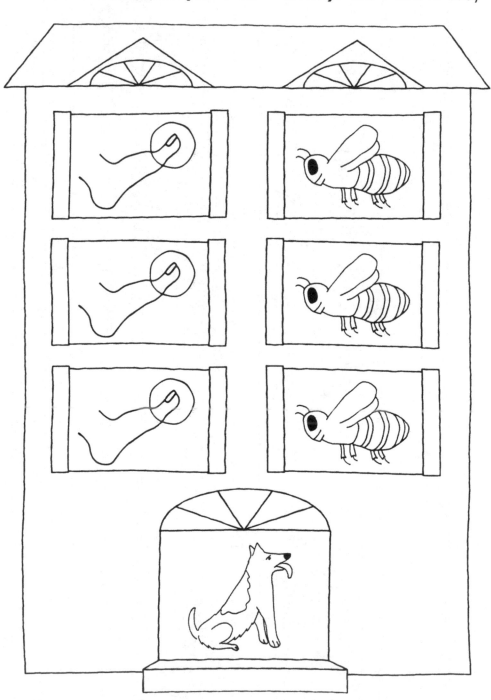

Figure A46.3 CV + CV = CVCV toe + bee = Toby. Reproduced with permission from Nuffield Dyspraxia Programme 3rd Edition.

Transition (CV + C = CVC): boo + t = boot **and** bow + t = boat

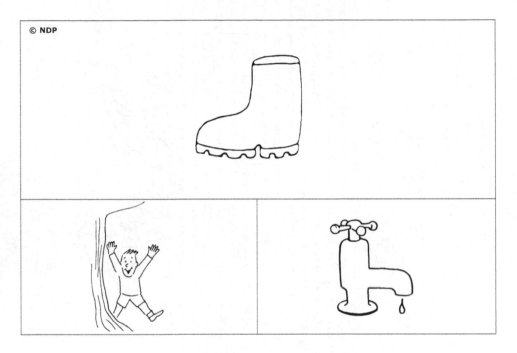

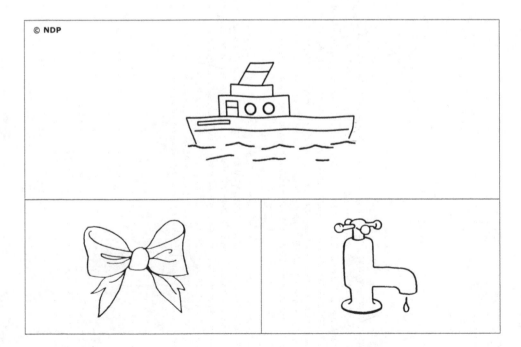

Figure A46.4 CV + C = CVC boo + t = boot, bow + t = boat. Reproduced with permission from Nuffield Dyspraxia Programme 3rd Edition.

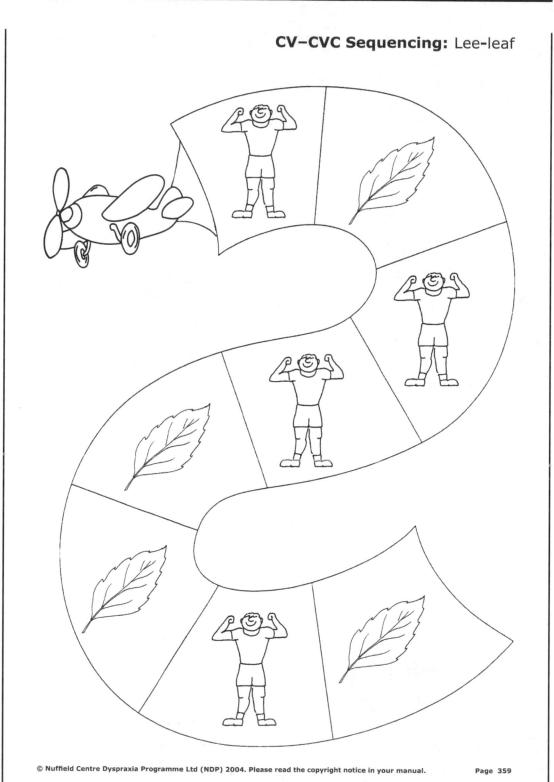

CV–CVC Sequencing: Lee-leaf

Page 359

Figure A46.5 CV–CVC sequencing. Reproduced with permission from Nuffield Dyspraxia Programme 3rd Edition.

and C + CV(C) = CCV(C) (e.g., *s* + *tar* = *star*) levels; contrastive sequencing worksheets for CVC and CCV(C) levels (e.g., the minimal and near-minimal pairs: *Lee-leaf* (as shown in Figure A46.5), *Kate-cake*, *bed-bread*, *tar-star*) and sets of pictures and cards for all levels.

As at single-sound and CV levels, the aim when working at each phonotactic level is to develop accurate motor programs for as wide a range of words as possible and to develop a contrastive system. At the same time, other psycholinguistic processes should be facilitated including accuracy of phonological representations and phonological awareness skills, as described above for the CV level.

Word combinations

Once speech production skills have been established in single words, more word combinations can be introduced, starting with simple and then more complex phrases and clauses, moving on to sentences, and ultimately to connected speech. At each of these levels, the child is challenged to maintain accurate and consistent production as utterances increase in length and complexity, but also to incorporate prosodic features (stress, intonation, rate, rhythm) and word joining strategies.

Conclusion

In conclusion, the *NDP3* provides both a set of therapy procedures and techniques, and a flexible resource of pictorial materials, from which the SLT/SLP can select appropriate components to plan and deliver treatment for individual children. The SLP/SLT should deliver therapy directly typically on a once weekly or once fortnightly basis continuously for a period of around 2 years. Parents/carers and school staff play an important role in treatment success, by carrying out daily practice of target sounds, syllables and words between therapy sessions, using the *NDP3* worksheets and materials.

The key aim of *NDP3* is to support children with CAS and other motor speech disorders in building accurate motor programs (Stackhouse & Wells, 1997) for individual speech sounds, syllables and words of varying phonotactic complexity, through a fine-tuned therapy hierarchy and frequent repetition. The goal of functional speech requires that children are able to use motor programs within a contrastive phonological system. This is also fundamental to the *NDP3* approach, as seen in the use of many contrastive worksheets and activities at each level. The materials can also be used to support the development of a range of phonological processing skills, such as auditory discrimination, segmentation and blending (Stackhouse & Wells, 1997).

An intervention for CAS with a prosodic emphasis

The changes in duration, loudness and pitch across words and longer utterances that express linguistic and affective information are referred to collectively as prosody, and lexical stress is one aspect of prosody. Cutler and Carter (1987) determined that over 90% of English words have more than one syllable. So, children with typical speech and language capabilities learning English acquire the ability to apply lexical stress to most of the words they speak. It appears that prosodic difficulties are a core deficit in CAS, and this includes difficulty with lexical stress. There is a tendency for affected children to apply excessive and/or equal stress, impacting their speech acquisition, naturalness and intelligibility. Coupled with this, their well-recognised difficulties with phonetic production also impact intelligibility. ReST, an intervention for CAS, developed by Kirrie Ballard, Tricia McCabe and their collaborators, has a prosodic as well as a segmental focus and is intended for school-aged children.

Dr. Tricia McCabe's research, teaching and clinical practice all focus on improving treatment outcomes for children and adults with severe or difficult to treat speech disorders, particularly those with CAS. Associate Professor McCabe is the leader of the CAS Research Group at The University of Sydney and has driven the research program that developed ReST.

Dr. Kirrie Ballard is an Associate Professor and Australian Research Council Future Fellow at The University of Sydney, Australia. Her research has focused on understanding the nature and treatment of speech motor disorder in children and adults, and an area of particular interest is the application of principles of motor learning to interventions for speech production.

Q47.   Patricia McCabe and Kirrie Ballard: Rapid syllable transition training

Embracing the Principles of Motor Learning (Maas, 2010), ReST is a new approach to the treatment of school-aged children with CAS in which complex, varied, multi-syllable non-word strings are practised intensively, providing children with repeated opportunities to transition between segments and syllables with unpredictable stress patterns, at the same time increasing segmental accuracy. Within a treatment session the child encounters a low frequency of feedback on response accuracy. Can you walk the reader through the theoretical rationale for ReST, its development, testing, implementation, effects and probable future in day-to-day clinical practice? Is there place for homework with caregivers in a ReST regimen and if so how might non-SLPs/SLTs be trained to provide appropriate feedback, is there scope for children to practice independently without close supervision, and might treatment and homework sessions include stimuli delivered electronically?

A47.   Patricia McCabe and Kirrie Ballard: The ReST program

ReST is a treatment designed for children with CAS and other motor speech disorders that include motor-based errors of linguistic prosody, such as lexical stress errors, with or without articulation errors. Don Robin initially devised the approach (see Maas, Barlow, Robin and Shapiro (2002), for an example using single-syllable words). The primary goal of ReST is to simultaneously address difficulties transitioning from sound to sound or syllable to syllable, difficulties with lexical stress production, and impaired articulatory accuracy. It uses pseudo-word stimuli to practice rapid and natural sounding multisyllabic sequences without interference from the linguistic/semantic system or ingrained error patterns on familiar words.

So far we have completed six studies of ReST treatment for children with CAS (Ballard, Robin, McCabe & McDonald, 2010; McCabe & Ballard, 2008; McCabe, Macdonald-DaSilva, van Rees, Arciuli & Ballard, 2010; Murray, McCabe & Ballard, 2012a), one for children with typically developing speech (van Rees, Ballard, McCabe, Macdonald-D'Silva & Arciuli, 2012) and one single case study for a child with acquired ataxia following removal of a cerebellar tumour (Murray, McCabe & Ballard, 2011).

We have completed an RCT (Murray.et al., 2012a) comparing ReST with the Nuffield Dyspraxia Programme (3rd ed.) (Williams & Stephens, 2010; A46) that is commonly used in both Australia and the United Kingdom among a number of countries. This RCT has shown that ReST is effective (Murray et al., 2012b) with children aged 4–12 years, when used according to the manual. Although children made better initial progress using the NDP3 than in ReST, the children who received ReST had better maintenance and generalisation than those in the NDP3 group. So, all things being equal, a clinician focused on immediate change in younger or more disabled (in terms of their speech or concomitant disorders) children might choose NDP3 but an SLP/SLT focused on long term or sustainable change in older or less disabled children would choose ReST.

ReST uses pseudo-words as the practice targets. These are chosen for each child using a set of principles that includes a hierarchy of difficulty. The default starting-place for therapy is three syllable CVCVCV nonsense words where each consonant and vowel differs from the other. Children who will not cope with this level can start with simpler structures such as two-syllable CVCV words with differing consonants and vowels or two-syllable CVCV nonsense words which differ in consonants or vowels only while the other remains static. Children who are not suitable for this level should not complete a ReST treatment. Once children are able to say the three-syllable target pseudo-words to 80% correct over three sessions the difficulty and complexity of the stimuli should increase. For example, words can be placed in carrier phrases and/or additional consonants and vowels as well as consonant blends can be added to the stimulus set.

Pseudo-word structures should comply with the rules of the child's language and dialect. To date ReST for CAS has only been trialled in Australian English where the pseudo-words have one strong syllable and one to two weak syllables. Each pseudo-word is provided as a written stimulus, with the spelling of the pseudo-word orthographically biased, which means there should only be one primary way to say the syllable from the written language (Arciuli & Cupples, 2006). Sounds included in the words should be minimally present in the child's phonemic inventory. So a child who once in the initial assessment produces an accurate /s/ could have this sound in his or her pseudo-words.

We use pseudo-words because we want to target speech motor learning with as little reference as possible to the underlying linguistic system. Using complex real words, which are unlikely to be in the child's vocabulary, poses the risk that existing morphemes within the real word will have a stored motor form which the child will use automatically. In addition, pseudo-words allow the clinician to re-sort the syllables randomly so that the child's task is to compile new motor plans/programmes for each stimulus presented. In this way we hope we are treating the underlying motor planning/programming problem in CAS.

A correct production is one with correct articulation, lexical stress and syllable transition and is identical to the clinician's model if one was provided. These three concepts are directly taught to the child and are what any feedback is based upon. For younger children these are called sounds, beats and smoothness. Older children can read the stimuli, if their reading accuracy permits, but the same standard of correctness applies. Lexical stress accuracy relies not only on marking only one strong syllable but using schwa correctly in weak syllables. Lexical stress accuracy can be achieved through increasing the pitch, loudness or duration of stressed syllables relative to unstressed ones. Syllable transition accuracy is determined by a smooth, normal rate production of the target word so hesitations, restarts or staccato speech are clearly incorrect.

In trialling ReST treatment with typically developing children, we found that they were able to learn how to say the pseudo-words very quickly and most reached the ceiling of 80% correct across three sessions in the minimum three sessions (van Rees et al., 2012).

Treatment sessions for ReST apply PML, which although widely used in sport and physical skills development, are currently individually less tested in speech treatment, particularly with children (Bislick, Weir, Spencer, Kendall & Yorkston, 2012; Maas et al., 2008). To structure a treatment based on the PML a couple of concepts must be incorporated. First, we need to think about learning as being a relatively permanent change in behaviour, which means change within any session is less important than maintenance of change over time. Second, we need to recognise that expertise in any skill required many hours of practice. It is said in folklore that it takes 10,000 hours of practice to become a concert pianist or a top-100 tennis player. Although we cannot say speech equates to piano playing or tennis, it is important to consider how much practice may be required to correct a motor speech disorder.

When we set out to manualise and test ReST intervention we used many of the PML with strongest evidence for facilitating long-term skill maintenance and generalisation of treatment gains. This included attending to practice conditions including intensity and frequency of practice and random presentation of both stimuli and feedback. We were also keen to ensure feedback during practice told the child whether they had said the word correctly or not but did not say how to fix it. This type of feedback is called KR. KR feedback in ReST is provided on a reducing scale with the child receiving feedback on 80% of attempts in the first set of stimuli and 10% on the final set in any session. Finally, if the child will tolerate it, we delay giving feedback for 3–5 seconds after the child has made an attempt. This delayed, randomised, reducing frequency KR feedback has been shown to facilitate real learning and naturally encourages the child to self-correct and self-evaluate. 'Real learning' is a change in behaviour that remains when a stimulus or practice condition is not present.

Treatment sessions last 50–60 minutes and have two components, consistent with the PML framework. The first component is pre-practice. This may be up to 20 minutes in the first few sessions and becomes shorter with subsequent sessions. The goal of pre-practice is to provide the child with both an understanding of the task and success at producing target behaviours. To help the child to produce the target words correctly the clinician uses all of the tricks in his or her tool bag. These may include articulatory cueing, metaphor, modelling, instruction, feedback, visual aids such as pictures and blocks, drumming or clapping the rhythm and any other idea that may facilitate the child's success. In pre-practice the clinician provides both KR feedback on correctness and, if required, knowledge of performance feedback that tells the child what he or she did correctly or incorrectly. Once the child has produced any five targets correctly then pre-practice is complete and the session moves on to the practice phase.

The practice phase should include at least 100 trials of randomly selected stimuli, broken into sets of 20–25 with a 2-minute break between sets. In the break the child chooses an activity that is engaging and rewarding to them.

In most of the research to date, ReST has been provided 4 days per week for 3 weeks by a clinician with no homework. This is a model of service delivery that we recognise is not commonly provided internationally and we are exploring alternate service delivery models to see if we can obtain the same treatment effect as in the intensive model however our preliminary work suggests a reduced frequency of treatment is less efficacious. In Thomas, McCabe and Ballard (2013) we showed that for four children treated with ReST at the same total dose but reduced dose frequency (i.e., 2 days per week for 6 weeks), with no other changes to the protocol, all children showed a similar treatment effect as reported in the RCT.

However, there was less maintenance of skill and less generalisation to real words. In fact, the two children with lower starting accuracy did not generalise their treatment gains to untreated pseudo-words although they did generalise to real words of similar complexity as the treated pseudo-words. In addition all four children showed stable maintenance of treatment effects for up to 4 months after treatment, which differed to the RCT where children continued to improve following completion of treatment. Together, these findings suggest that while change might be observed in treatment provided at the lesser schedule of two times per week, the follow-on effects may be different and perhaps demonstrate less efficiency overall.

We have completed a pilot study of parent training of ReST intervention (Thomas, McCabe & Ballard, 2014). In this study we maintained intensity and frequency of treatment but transitioned from clinician provided treatment to parent provided treatment in the following schedule: Week 1, three clinician sessions: one parent session; Week 2, 2:2 clinician: parent provided sessions and Week 3, 1:3 clinician: parent provided sessions. An additional change in this treatment was that clinicians provided pre-practice and practice and trained parents within the 60-minute clinic session where parents provided only practice in their home-based sessions.

Three out of four parents were able to provide the practice component at home with while one was not. All parents were quite anxious about the accuracy of their feedback but when we measured it their accuracy ranged between 69% and 87% agreement with the clinician (Thomas et al., 2014). Surprisingly none of the parents reported difficulties getting their children to complete the homework despite the drill nature of ReST practice.

The training provided in this pilot mimicked the parent training provided in the Lidcombe programme (Australian Stuttering Research Centre, 2012; Jones et al., 2005) and was supported by written materials. We intend to continue this research and improve the training so that parents and therapy aides can effectively deliver the practice component of ReST.

At this stage we have also conducted a small feasibility study of ReST delivered via Skype and it appears that assuming a quiet space can be found at home and parents have sufficient technology skills to use a lapel microphone then treatment may be delivered via the Internet.

Ideally a computer program or smart phone app could be developed which could judge correct and incorrect productions. If this were possible then electronic gaming could be used to provide treatment, independent of direct parent or clinician input. However the program would need to contain algorithms to analyse pauses between syllables, relative syllable stress between strong and weak syllables and phonemic accuracy. While each of these tasks is technologically feasible, we do not have normative information for them and so the design of such an app is still embryonic. We have shown through good reliability scores that the trained human brain makes these judgements quickly and without much error so any app would need to be able to mimic that capacity. We are exploring these options concurrently with improving the delivery of ReST on a number of other fronts.

Early days

In the initial stages of assessment and intervention for children with CAS or suspected CAS (sCAS), parents embark on a huge learning trajectory and may feel overwhelmed with information. It is also a time for hard work for parents as they adjust to their changed situation (Hennessy & Hennessy, 2013), keeping the child occupied with fun, relevant activities stemming from the child's needs and strengths (Hammer & Stoeckel, 2001). According to Hammer and Stoeckel, at this early stage it is important to help parents to:

- work *with* the therapist or team, particularly in terms of encouraging the child's motivation, participation and cooperation in therapy sessions and homework;
- learn about CAS and relevant techniques to employ at home;
- question anything not understood, or anything worrying, straight away;
- be available at key times for participation in sessions, observations or video viewing;
- report openly about home practice frequency and the child's responses;
- work within realistic parameters;
- understand treatment limitations and prognostic indicators; and
- have high and reasonable expectations of the child.

Parents, according to Hammer and Stoeckel, will do best if they are shown how to

- organise the environment to facilitate communication;
- make some homework 'invisible' or 'indirect';
- provide input without always insisting on a response;
- make some of the homework visible and direct;
- identify nursery rhymes, songs and stories that can be used relative to particular targets;
- use communicative temptations/'desired objects' that are visible but not accessible;
- employ modelling and recasting techniques optimally;
- choose targets that will be functional and powerful to motivate the child to *try*; and
- use fun games and drill-play with frequent 'communication temptations'.

Potential pitfalls parents may be alerted to include

- over cueing; for example, providing exaggerated, distorted models;

- introducing many new targets quickly: new content is best balanced with older content;
- tackling targets that are too difficult for the child;
- avoiding practising things the child is 'good at': this is not a waste of time!
- burnout of child, parents and other helpers. This is an issue that needs to be considered in relation to homework. Sometimes parents are so eager to do as much as they can that they quickly kill off any good will on the part of the child, exhaust themselves, and face thorny cooperation issues. In the early months, it may be helpful to limit the duration of speech focus at home, and then to expand it gradually if need be so parents are not overwhelmed, and the child is not put off.

Within intervention, the clinician's overriding goal is for the child to become as fully functional a communicator as possible by teaching needed skills based on individual and on-going assessment. Parents need to know that the clinician sees them as the most important members of the treatment team, and integral to any progress, and that he or she will

- educate them about CAS and its management;
- provide information about networking opportunities and available support;
- teach them specific strategies relative to their child's intervention needs;
- be flexible with targets and strategies and programme implementation;
- maximise production practice;
- maximise functional communication goals;
- maintain high and reasonable expectations of the child within his or her capabilities; and
- maintain high and reasonable expectations of *them*, within *their* capabilities.

To accomplish these objectives, the therapist must be able to

- explain goals in clear language and explain changes in treatment strategies, particularly as changes may be misinterpreted as a sign of failure on the part of child, parent or clinician;
- genuinely welcome parents' 'why' questions;

- ensure opportunities for participation, observation and discussion; and
- work with parents to motivate and reinforce child's learning.

The child has responsibilities, too. He or she must accept help from the parents and SLP/SLT in the process of learning to communicate more effectively; and ultimately, as an older child or adult, with on-going professional or non-professional support if wanted, they need to start taking responsibility for maintaining skills, using adaptive strategies and accepting that there will be communicative consequences when they do not.

Taking responsibility

At the same time, we must be aware that children and youth can tire of 'trying all the time' and many hit a point where they have effectively 'grown out of therapy'. Andy (Hennessy & Hennessy, 2013, p. 148) writes:

I was in and out of therapy from the earliest time that I can remember and continued until just about the end of my eighth grade year of school. By that point in my life I was sick of speech therapy. Skipping class had changed from being cool to being annoying... I just wanted to be like the other kids. I actually wanted to go to all of my classes... So, I told my mother I was done with speech therapy.

My client James, with CAS was referred at the age of 4;0 and came happily to once weekly, and at times twice-weekly 50-minute sessions with one or other parent and me until he was 6;0, making good progress with his speech and language. At that time his diplomat father was posted overseas to a country in which SLP/SLT services were generally unavailable and they were fortunate enough to find a retired British expatriate SLT who was able to help on a voluntary basis. Sadly, when he was 7;1 his father died suddenly, and James and his mother returned to Australia to live with her mother and sister. James, finding his life dominated by women – his mother, aunt, a series of teachers and me – continued to see me for help

with his speech, and an SLP colleague for literacy intervention until he was 11;6, when he was fed up with it. It all came to a head for him one day in a treatment session when, to his mother's horror, he told me to f-off. His mother had to agree that it was time to take a break. James greeted my assurance that my door would be open if he wanted to come back when he was older with disdain. But when he was 14, and wanting to ask a girl to a school social, he asked his mother if he could come back to see me. She agreed, but said he had to take responsibility for making and keeping appointments, and complying with any programme set up, mentioning to him that I might not want to see him, as he had been rude to me the last time we all met!

He telephoned me to make an appointment and then attended weekly, working on a few late developing sounds with a strong focus on prosody and fluency, for about a year, primarily motivated by wanting to 'talk to girls'. He returned for brief intervention – 8 sessions – at 19, as a university student needing help with acute performance anxiety experienced when speaking to a tutorial group. James assumed that his 'stage fright' was due to having CAS, and was relieved and reassured when it was normalized as something may people, even actors and seasoned public speakers, experience, and heartened by Mark Twain's 'How I conquered stage fright' speech (Twain, 1910).

Still initiating contact, he returned at 22 wanting to role-play job interviews. The last I saw of him was when he was 25 when the request was for help rehearsing his wedding speech. The speech was sounding good at the end of the second session, and James sat back in his seat and said, 'Do you think I'll always need to come and see you?' One thing led to another, and I asked him whether his fiancée ever remarked on his speech. He said that Hannah did, and that he appreciated it when she corrected his pronunciation, or helped him say new or difficult words such as the names of people and places. The following week he came with Hannah who turned out to be someone he had known for many years. She greeted me with, 'I've always wanted to meet *you*!'

I tell the story because we do not often see the positive effect of what we do as SLPs/SLTs quite so clearly from the perspective of someone close to an adult with CAS. James had told Hannah the whole story. How he had been a 4-year-old that none of the children or the teachers at his pre-school could understand. How, as he saw it, his parents and I had taught him to speak intelligibly, but not perfectly. How they, as a family, had a thrilling overseas adventure that stopped abruptly with his father's death when James was 7. How my colleague and I had helped him, and been important to him, in pre-adolescence, and how he had been 'horribly rude' to me nonetheless; and how we had 'been there for him' intermittently ever since. The way she told it, often quoting James, it was a moving and inspiring story, and a wonderful example of an adult maturely taking responsibility for his own communication needs. For complete-ness I should add that Hannah and I had three ses-sions alone to explore simple strategies she could employ to help James with particular utterances and speaking situations, and a final session with the three of us working together.

Homework and the homework habit

No matter how 'in tune', creative, flexible, encour-aging and motivating we, as clinicians, are in ther-apy sessions, the necessary carryover is unlikely without solid family support. So, homework has to be understood and implemented properly, one-to-one in good listening and learning conditions, and often. It is essential to impress upon parents that we see this is a collaborative process, that they are not expected to do all the work or to perform miracles, and that their suggestions and feedback are welcome. As the people who know their child best, it is often the parents who can tell us how to get things done without a battle: which rewards will be effective, which activities will be appeal-ing, and the signs we should look for that tell us that the child wants or needs us to 'back off' a little.

If parents can be encouraged to regard 'speech homework' as part of the family's normal rou-tine, it can help enormously. If brief, regular 5- to 7-minute bursts of homework are as usual as

mealtimes and bathing, and as non-negotiable as wearing a car seatbelt or looking both ways before crossing the road (and hopefully not just a job for *one* parent to do with the child), explicitly princi-pled homework is not so difficult for most families to accomplish despite other family commitments, work and other responsibilities and life-events. Distributed, random bursts of practice with appro-priate reinforcement, taken cumulatively, can contribute to significant change. Rehearsal of homework tasks during therapy sessions, and 'coaching' of parents by the clinician, is valu-able as it helps parents build confidence in their skills, and it lets their child know that *their* par-ents really are part of *their* treatment team. Parents can be engaged early as 'the homework experts' for their own child, compiling power word and phrase lists (words and phrases that are impor-tant to the child), collecting speech samples and making a 'brag book'.

Brag book

A brag book is a small, durable album or picture book, owned by the child and devoted to what the child *can* do, even if it only contains a couple of signs and a few sound effects. It is not a collec-tion of words the adults in the child's life would *like* him or her to say! There is no 'right way' to compile one of these books, but it is quite popu-lar (with children) to start with a few pictures of the child, so that when asked 'Who's this?' they can point to indicate 'me' even if they cannot say it yet; or simply nod when asked 'Is this you?' if they are not yet able to respond with 'Mmm', 'Uh-huh' or 'Yes'. If the child has a few signed or spoken verbs (e.g., *go, stop, eat*) or verbal approx-imations, these could follow, with photographs of the child engaged in the actions. Favourite toys or foods and drinks that they have a sign, sound or word for might come next, followed by impor-tant people (parents, siblings and grandparents, perhaps), pets, places (e.g., *home, my room, my bed*) and possessions. Next come all the words and approximations the child can say (including *poo, wee, bum*, etc. if they are in the repertoire) and the child's sound effects for vehicles, machines, animals and appliances. For all of the images in the brag book, it is important to print, in lower case, the intended word or sound effect (e.g., *ee-ee* or *ee ee* for mouse and not *EE-EE* or *EE EE*, and instructions for executing any signs or gestures, so that *anyone* who picks up the book knows how to enjoy it with the child. If touch cues, prompts and imagery are being used, include appropriate graphics and instructions. 'Favourite words' (e.g., *Bob*) or 'good words' (words or phrases that the child says well or is proud of) can go in several times, making sure that there are some easy, fun words at the beginning of the book and again at the end. Songs, rhymes, rebus and cloze where the child *can* provide the punch line can be included. As the book grows, the pictures can be rearranged so that they are loosely organised by theme and initial sound, encouraging everyone to think in terms of patterns and prosody from early on.

The brag book can include a note or letter from the therapist in accessible, jargon-free language to let the family and significant others know that

- the emphasis should be on *meaningful* word production and syllable production (e.g., *bee, boo, moo, neigh, go, me too, no way, bye-bye, up*) and that isolated sounds are really only a goal if they carry meaning (e.g., *sh* for be-quiet, *ss* as a snake sound, *ee-ee* for a mouse sound-effect, *mm* for yes and yum), and as a means to an end in stimulability therapy (Miccio, A23; Williams & Stephens, A46).
- isolated sound production *may* be used briefly as a means to an end, but that *ba-baba, bee-bee-bee, ta-ta-ta*, etc. are more desirable than practice drills comprising sequences such as [b-b-b-b-b-], [t-t-t-t-], [p-t-p-t-p-t-p-t-p-t-p-t-], etc.
- suprasegmentals (rhythm, melody, stress, loudness, pitch, rate, resonance including nasal resonance, and intonation) should be emphasised from the start. This may promote more natural-sounding speech earlier, as opposed to the 'programmed' sound with odd prosody, and the excessive and equal stress (EES) characteristic of many children who have been treated for CAS.

- the desired goal is *many* 'repeats' of therapy targets whether they are syllables, syllable sequences, single words or word sequences. The 'repeats' or 'practice trials' are needed to facilitate optimal, 'automatic' speech production.
- parents' ingenuity and input, particularly in the initial stages, are necessary to get therapy off to a good start, and we rely on them to help find activities and rewards that are beneficial and also motivating and fun for toddlers and pre-schoolers.
- they can be reassured that, with appropriate support, most children will start to 'bring the homework to parents', understand what the therapy is for, and take some responsibility for their own practice needs.

Ten tips for intervention for young children with severe CAS

With children who are non-verbal or who have few word approximations, early goals are to:

1. establish a 'core vocabulary' (a selection of 'power words' or words to 'sign and say' like *no, more, go* and *me too*);
2. select phonetic stimuli, favouring ones that are already spontaneously produced;
3. start with CV and VC and CVC combinations, *definitely* including isolated vowels, but avoiding isolated consonants unless they carry meaning;
4. establish the most beneficial facilitators for the child (ask the parents, or *tell* them!);
5. establish an appropriate stimulus/response relationship (How many models and how many repeats?);
6. set criteria for subsequent changes in stimuli (How many correct trials?);
7. choose reinforcers carefully, knowing that achieving the necessary intensity of drill is difficult and that it is often hard to maintain the child's attention and cooperation. The aim here is to ensure a sufficient number of responses within a practice session.

8. watch linguistic load. Keep it simple. Do not use complex carrier phrases or cloze, or awkward prosody.

9. use alternative and augmentative communication (AAC), including sign and picture exchange to augment verbal attempts, to enhance language development and to reduce the child's frustration. Reassure parents that AAC will not stifle verbal communication.

10. keep therapy fresh—sameness and boredom kill *everyone's* motivation.

Controversial interventions for CAS

In Chapter 2, under the heading: 'The questions families ask: Which method do you use?' are some thoughts about, and examples of, popular but nonevidence-based interventions for SSD generally, some of which are widely promoted to SLP/SLT professionals and families on the Internet, and to SLPs/SLTs by a few continuing professional development providers. Some of the SSD products are directly marketed to the parents and other family members of children with CAS, and to the clinicians working with them.

People explore these intervention options with the best of motives, and some are advised in good faith to pursue treatments that are supported by neither theory nor evidence, but which may appeal to them because they sound more exotic, interesting and exciting, and even more 'scientific' than mainstream speech and language therapy. Even some clinicians seem to believe that a therapy that comes in a box has more appeal than one that comes in the form of a journal article.

It may be beneficial to counsel some parents and colleagues that not all treatments suit every child and that all treatments must be individually, carefully and expertly tailored in response to the child's needs, strengths, challenges, co-morbidities, assessment and re-assessment outcomes, and response to intervention. In that sense, there is no 'preferred method'. A 'good method' is one that is evidence based or theoretically sound, *adaptable* to short-term changes in the child (in terms of attention, interest, motivation, and well-

being 'on the day'); *flexible* over time (as the child develops); *adjustable* for different settings (e.g., clinic, home, pre-school and 'out') and *modifiable* to suit different service delivery conditions (e.g., in a dyad, and in a group). The same applies to the target selection approaches and therapy techniques we adopt, and some of these are presented in Chapter 8.

References

ASHA (2007). *Childhood Apraxia of Speech [Technical Report]*. Retrieved 4 September 2013 from www.asha.org/docs/html/TR2007-00278.html

Arciuli, J., & Cupples, L. (2006). The processing of lexical stress during visual word recognition: Typicality effects and orthographic correlates. *Quarterly Journal of Experimental Psychology, 59*(5), 920–948.

Australian Stuttering Research Centre. (2012). Lidcombe Program. Retrieved September 7 2013 from http://sydney.edu.au/health-sciences/asrc/clinic/parents/lidcombe.shtml

Bain, B. A., & Olswang, L. B. (1995). Examining readiness for learning two-word utterances by children with specific expressive language impairment: Dynamic assessment validation. *American Journal of Speech Language Pathology, 4*(1), 81–91.

Ballard, K. J., Robin, D. A., McCabe, P., & McDonald, J. (2010). A treatment for dysprosody in childhood apraxia of speech. *Journal of Speech, Language, and Hearing Research, 53*(5), 1227–1245.

Bislick, L. P., Weir, P. C., Spencer, K., Kendall, D., & Yorkston, K. M. (2012). Do principles of motor learning enhance retention and transfer of speech skills? A systematic review. *Aphasiology, 26*(5), 709–728.

Bleile, K. M. (2013). *The Late Eight* (2nd ed.). San Diego, CA: Plural Publishing.

Bowen, C., & Cupples, L. (2006). PACT: Parents and children together in phonological therapy. *Advances in Speech Language Pathology, 8*(3), 282–292.

Chan, J., Arnold, S., Webber, L., Riches, V., Parmenter, T., Stancliffe, R. (2012). Is it time to drop the term 'challenging behaviour'? *Learning Disability Practice, 15*(5), 36–38.

Cutler, A., & Carter, D. M. (1987). The predominance of strong initial syllables in the English vocabulary. *Computer Speech and Language, 2*, 133–142.

Feuerstein, R., Rand, Y., Jensen, M. R., Kaniel, S., & Tzuriel, D. (1987). Prerequisites for assessment of learning potential: the LPAD model, In: C. S. Lidz (Ed.): *Dynamic assessment: an interactional approach to evaluating learning potential.* New York, NY: The Guilford Press.

Glaspey, A. M., & Stoel-Gammon, C. (2005). Dynamic assessment in phonological disorders: The scaffolding scale of stimulability. *Topics in Language Disorders: Clinical Perspectives on Speech Sound Disorders, 25*(3), 220–230.

Glaspey, A. M. & Stoel-Gammon, C. (2007). A dynamic approach to phonological assessment. *International Journal of Speech-Language Pathology, 9*, 286–296.

Goldman, R., & Fristoe, M. (2000). *Goldman-Fristoe Test of Articulation* (2nd ed.). Circle Pines, MN: American Guidance Service.

Hammer, D., & Stoeckel, R. (2001). Teaching and talking together: Building a treatment team. Presentation at the annual convention of the American Speech-Language Hearing Association, New Orleans, Louisiana.

Hasson, N., & Joffe, V. (2007). The case for dynamic assessment in speech and language therapy. *Child Language Teaching and Therapy, 23*(1), 9–25.

Hegde, M. N. (2002). *Treatment procedures in speech-language pathology* (3rd ed.). Austin, TX: Pro-Ed.

Helfrich-Miller, K. R. (1983). The use of melodic intonation therapy with developmentally apractic children: A clinical perspective. *Journal of the Pennsylvania Speech-Language-Hearing Association.* 11–15.

Helfrich-Miller, K. R. (1984). Melodic intonation therapy with developmentally apraxic children. *Seminars in Speech and Language, 5*, 119–125.

Helfrich-Miller, K. R. (1994). Clinical perspective: Melodic intonation therapy for developmental apraxia. *Clinics in Communication Disorders, 4*(3), 175–182.

Hennessy, K., & Hennessy, K. (2013). *Anything but silent: Our family's journey through childhood apraxia of speech.* Tarentum, PA: Word Association Publishers.

Jakielski, K. J., Kostner, T. L., & Webb, C. E. (2006). Results of integral stimulation intervention in three children. Paper presented at the *5th International Conference on Speech Motor Control.* Nijmegen: the Netherlands.

Jones, M., Onslow, M., Packman, A., Williams, S., Ormond, T., Schwarz, I., & Gebski, V. (2005). Randomised controlled trial of the Lidcombe programme of early stuttering intervention. *BMJ, 331*(7518), 659.

Lidz, C. S., & Peña, E. D. (1996). Dynamic assessment: The model, its relevance as a nonbiased approach, and its application to Latino American preschool children. *Language, Speech and Hearing Services in Schools, 27*, 367–372.

Maas, E. (2010). Conditions of practice and feedback in treatment for apraxia of speech. *Perspectives on Neurophysiology and Neurogenic Speech and Language Disorders, 20*(3), 81–87.

Maas, E., Barlow, J., Robin, D., & Shapiro, L. (2002). Treatment of sound errors in aphasia and apraxia of speech: Effects of phonological complexity. *Aphasiology, 16*(4/5/6), 609–622.

Maas, E., Robin, D. A., Austermann Hula, S. N., Freedman, S. E., Wulf, G., Ballard, K. J., & Schmidt, R. A. (2008). Principles of motor learning in treatment of motor speech disorders. *American Journal of Speech-Language Pathology, 17*(3), 277–298.

McCabe, P., & Ballard, K. J. (2008). *An Innovative Syllable Transition Treatment Trial for Childhood Apraxia of Speech.* Paper presented at the Motor Speech Conference, March 2008, Monterey, CA, USA.

McCabe, P., Macdonald-DaSilva, A., van Rees, L., Arciuli, J., & Ballard, K. (2010). *Using orthographic cues to improve speech production in children with & without childhood apraxia of speech.* Paper presented at the Motor Speech Conference, Savannah, Georgia, USA.

McCauley, R. J., Strand, E., Lof, G. L., Schooling, T., & Frymark, T. (2009). Evidence-based systematic review: Effects of nonspeech oral motor exercises on speech, *American Journal of Speech-Language Pathology, 18*, 343–360.

Miccio, A. W. (2005). A treatment program for enhancing stimulability. In: A. G. Kamhi, & K. E. Pollock (Eds.), *Phonological disorders in children: Clinical decision making in assessment and intervention* (pp. 163–173). Baltimore, MD: Paul H. Brookes Publishing Co.

Miccio, A. W., Elbert, M., & Forrest, K. (1999). The relationship between stimulability and phonological acquisition in children with normally developing and disordered phonologies. *American Journal of Speech-Language Pathology, 8*, 347–363.

Milisen R. (1954). A rationale for articulation disorders. *Journal of Speech and Hearing Disorders.* (Monograph supplement), *4*, 6–17.

Mowrer, D. E. (1985). The behavioral approach to treatment. In: N. A. Creaghead, P. W. Newman, & W. A. Secord (Eds.), *Assessment and remediation of articulatory and phonological disorders* (pp. 159–192). Columbus, OH: Merrill.

Murray, E., McCabe, P., Ballard, K. (2011). Using ReST intervention for paediatric cerebellar ataxia: A pilot study. *Stem-, Spraal-en Taalpathologie*, (*17*), S55.

Murray, E., McCabe, P., Ballard, K. (2012a). A comparison of two treatments for childhood apraxia of speech: methods and treatment protocol for a parallel group randomised control trial. *BMC Pediatrics*, *12*(3), 1–9.

Murray, E., McCabe, P., & Ballard, K. J. (2012b). The first randomised control trial for treatment of Childhood Apraxia of Speech (ReST vs Nuffield Dyspraxia Program-3). *Communicate: Our natural state. Speech Pathology Australia National Conference.* Hobart, TAS, Australia.

Olswang, L. B., & Bain, B. A. (1996). Assessment information for predicting upcoming change in language production. *Journal of Speech and Hearing Research*, *39*, 414–423.

Passy, J. (1993). *Cued Articulation.* Ponteland, Northumberland: STASS Publications.

RCSLT (2011). *Royal College of Speech and Language Therapists: Developmental verbal dyspraxia [Policy Statement]*, Author. Available at www.rcslt.org.

Rosenbek, J. C., Lemme, M. L., Ahern, M. B., Harris, E. H., & Wertz, R. T. (1973). A treatment for apraxia of speech in adults. *Journal of Speech and Hearing Disorders*, *38*, 462–472.

Roth, F. P., & Paul. R. (2002). Principles of intervention. In R. Paul (Ed.), *Introduction to clinical methods in communication disorders* (pp. 160–181). Baltimore, MD: Paul H. Brookes Publishing Co.

Roth, F. P., & Worthington, C. K. (2005). *Treatment resource manual for speech-language pathology.* San Diego, CA: Singular.

Schmidt, R. A., & Lee, T. D. (2011). *Motor control and learning: A behavioural emphasis* (5th ed.). Champaign, IL: Human Kinetics.

Secord, W., Boyce, S. Donohue, J., Fox, R., & Shine R. (2007). *Eliciting Sounds: Techniques and Strategies for Clinicians* (2nd ed.). Clifton Park, NY: Thompson Delmar Learning.

Stackhouse, J., & Wells, B. (1997). *Children's speech and literacy difficulties I: A psycholinguistic framework.* London: Whurr Publishers.

Stephens, H., & Elton, M. (1986). Description of systematic use of articulograms. *College of Speech and Language Therapists Bulletin*: December.

Strand, E. (1995). Treatment of motor speech disorders in children, *Seminars in Speech and Language*, *16*(2), 126–139.

Strand, E. A., & Debertine, P. (2000). The efficacy of integral stimulation with developmental apraxia of speech. *Journal of Medical Speech-Language Pathology*, *8*(4), 295–300.

Strand, E. A., McCauley, R. J., Weigand, S., Stoeckel, R., & Baas, B. (2013). A motor speech assessment for children with severe speech disorders: Reliability and validity evidence. *Journal of Speech, Language, and Hearing Research*, *56*(2), 505–520.

Strand, E., Stoeckel, R., & Baas, B. (2006). Treatment of Severe Childhood Apraxia of Speech: A Treatment Efficacy Study. *Journal of Medical Speech Pathology*, *14*, 297–307.

Thomas, D., McCabe, P., & Ballard, K. J. (2013). *Treatment for Childhood Apraxia of Speech: Does Rapid Syllable Transition (ReST) treatment work when it's done twice rather than four times per week?* Paper presented at the Speech Pathology Australia Annual National Conference, Gold Coast, QLD, Australia.

Thomas, D., McCabe, P., & Ballard, K. (2014). *Parent Training for Rapid Syllable Transitions Treatment for Childhood Apraxia of Speech: Fidelity of parent conducted treatment.* Paper presented at the Motor Speech Symposium, Sarasota, Fl, USA, March 2014.

Twain, M. (1910). How I conquered stage fright. Published as "Mark Twain's First Appearance" in *Mark Twain's Speeches*, New York, NY: Harper & Brothers.

Van Rees, L. J., Ballard, K. J., McCabe, P., Macdonald-D'Silva, A. G., & Arciuli, J. (2012). training production of lexical stress in typically developing children using orthographically biased stimuli and principles of motor learning. *American Journal of Speech-Language Pathology*, *21*(3), 197–205.

Velleman, S. (2002). Phonotactic therapy. *Seminars in Speech and Language*, *23*, 43–57.

Vygotsky, L. S. (1978). Mind in society, In: M. Cole, V. John-Steiner, S. Scribner, & E. Souberman (Eds.), *The development of higher psychological processes.* London: Harvard University Press.

Williams, P., & Stackhouse, J. (1998). Diadochokinetic skills: Normal and atypical performance in children aged 3–5 years. *International Journal of Language and Communication Disorders*, *33* (Suppl): 481–486.

Williams, P., & Stackhouse, J. (2000). Rate, accuracy and consistency: diadochokinetic performance of young normally developing children. *Clinical Linguistics and Phonetics*, *14*(4), 267–293.

Williams, P. & Stephens, H. (2004). *Nuffield Centre Dyspraxia Programme* (3rd ed.). Windsor, UK: The Miracle Factory.

Williams, P., & Stephens, H. (2010). The Nuffield Centre Dyspraxia Programme. In: A. L. Williams, S. McLeod, & R. J. McCauley (Eds.), *Interventions for Speech Sound Disorders in Children* (pp. 159–177). Baltimore, MD: Paul H. Brookes Publishing Co.

Chapter 8

Treatment targets and strategies for speech sound disorders

Hollywood cameraman John Alton wrote the first book on cinematography in 1949, calling it *Painting with Light*. This title may have been the inspiration for *The Publicity Photograph* (Galton & Simpson, 1958), a radio sketch for *Hancock's Half Hour*. Persuaded by Miss Pugh (Hattie Jacques), Bill (Bill Kerr) and Sid (Sid James) that he needs to update his image, Hancock (Tony Hancock) and Sid consult flamboyant theatrical photographer Hilary St. Clair (Kenneth Williams, he of the soaring triphthongs). When Sid tells St. Clair, 'I want you to take some snaps', he is outraged! '*Snaps*, Sidney? I don't take *snaps*; I *paint* with *light!*'

The topic of 'therapy tips' often arises in social media discussions and at professional development events. When it does, there can be an urge to mount one's high horse and emulate St. Clair's retort. '*Tips? Tips?* I don't do *tips!* I put solid theory and evidence into practice!' or whatever the SLP/SLT equivalent of painting with light might be. But as seasoned interventionists know, therapy breakthroughs often come when, without abandoning evidence-based practice, we play educated clinical hunches, have a good idea, apply inspired

brainwaves shared by mentors and colleagues, simply try something different, or implement a tip or trick from our repertoire that has worked for us before in making our jobs as scientific clinicians easier, especially with more complex clients. This chapter holds a compilation of such tips, tricks and insights, and pointers for where to find more.

Phonological disorder signs

As shown in Boxes 6.1 and 6.4, points 7, 8, 9 and 10, there are four signs that may help us determine whether a child's speech difficulties, or at least *some* of them, are phonological in nature. We should consider the possibility of phonological disorder and a phonological intervention approach if the puzzle phenomenon is evident, if there is a pattern of unusual errors, if the child is marking contrasts 'oddly', and if error sounds are readily stimulable. Two of these giveaway signs, the puzzle phenomenon and marking, can be difficult to 'pick' unless the clinician is actively looking for them, so examples are provided below.

Puzzle phenomenon

The puzzle phenomenon occurs when a child consistently mispronounces sounds where they should occur, but uses them as substitutes where they should not! A 'demonstration' by Dane, father of Quentin, 6;1, exemplifies this.

Dane: Show her how you say *thumb*.

Quentin: *Fum*.

Dane: Now say *sum*.

Quentin: *Thum*.

Dane: If he can say *thumb* when he means *sum*, how come he says *fum* when he means *thumb*? I think he's just lazy.

A second example of the puzzle phenomenon comes from Andrew, 4;6.

yellow	/lɛloʊ/	brother	/bwʌzə/
then	/dɛn/	globe	/bloʊb/
those	/doʊz/	rabbit	/bɹæbɪt/
glove	/gwʌb/	some	/θʌm/
breathe	/bwiv/	thumb	/sʌm/
snooze	/ðuð/	zoo	/ðu/

Marking

Some of the errors children make deceive our trained ears; but when we listen closely, we may find that the errors provide hints that a child knows more than he or she is able to produce, and that their difficulties are phonological and not phonetic. They do so by 'marking' the presence of the correct sound, with nasality and/or with vowel length.

Marking with nasality

Uzzia, 5;1, with extensive final consonant deletion, talked about going to [bɛ](*bed*) and referred to her brother as [bɛ̃]. Although it was easy to hear these as homonyms, it was apparent that Uzzia was *marking* the presence of the /n/ in *Ben* by nasalising the preceding vowel. This hint of a nasal final consonant was consistent with what happens normally, in that vowels preceding nasal consonants are usually nasalised.

Marking with vowel length

Like Uzzia, Owen, 4;3, also exhibited final consonant deletion, producing bus as [bʌ] and Buzz Lightyear's name as [bʌː], and again these two productions, [bʌ] and [bʌː], were readily mistaken for homonyms. But when we recall that vowels are typically longer before voiced consonants, we would be on safe ground to assume that Owen's lengthening of the short vowel /ʌ/ to [ʌː] meant that he 'knew' the difference between /s/ and /z/ but was not yet able to produce them SFWF.

Individualised education programs: IEPs

Individualised Education Programs (IEPs) or Individualised Education Plans (IEPs) for articulation therapy tend to be along the lines of the following ones for Alison 7;1 who had /s/ as a phonetic target. These goals are based on those in the IEP Goal Bank provided at www.speakingofspeech.com/IEP_Goal_Bank.html#artic.

Long-Term Goal: Alison will produce the /s/ speech sound with 90% mastery.

Short-Term Objectives:

1. Alison will produce /s/ in isolation with 90% accuracy.
2. Alison will produce /s/ in syllables with 90% accuracy.
3. Alison will produce /s/ in all positions of words with 90% accuracy.
4. Alison will produce /s/ in sentences with 90% accuracy.
5. Alison will produce /s/ in oral reading tasks with 90% accuracy.
6. Alison will produce /s/ in structured conversation with 90% accuracy.
7. Alison will produce /s/ in spontaneous speech with 90% accuracy.

8. Alison will improve self-monitoring skills for /s/ with 90% accuracy.

9. Alison will improve carry-over of /s/ outside of the therapy setting with 90%.

Chapter 6 contains an exploration of the six-shared characteristics of phonological disorders and childhood apraxia of speech (CAS) (see Tables 6.1 and 6.4 and associated discussion) and 14 goals in common. The six character-istics are: (1) Consonant inventory constraints; vowel inventory constraints; phonotactic inven-tory constraints. (2) Omissions of consonants, vowels and syllable shapes that are already in the child's inventory. (3) Vowel errors. (4) Altered suprasegmentals. (5) More errors with longer and/or more complex utterances, including the so-called 'SODA' errors of substitution, omission, distortion and addition. (6) Use of simple, but not complex, syllable shapes and word shapes.

The 14-shared goals are: (1) Consonant inven-tory expansion. (2) Vowel inventory expansion. (3) Phonotactic inventory expansion. (4) Syllable shape inventory expansion. (5) Word shape inven-tory expansion. (6) Increased accuracy of produc-tion of target structures. (7) More complete vowel repertoire. (8) More accurate vowel production. (9) Production of strong and weak syllables. (10) Differentiation of strong and weak syllables. (11) Generalisation of new consonants and vowels, syl-lable structures, and word structures, to more chal-lenging contexts. (12) More complete phonotac-tic repertoire. (13) More varied use of phonotactic range within syllables and words. (14) Improved accuracy.

Clearly, when goal setting and writing IEPs for children with phonological disorder and/or CAS these 14 goals cannot be expressed in the same way articulation goals usually are, using 'mas-tery' criteria and percentages. So, what follows is a suggested guide for wording IEP goals, based on the six characteristics common to both diagnoses, and the 14 treatment goals in common. Then fol-low examples of IEPs that were used for Tad who had CAS in combination with significant phono-logical issues. Tad's IEP goals encompassed 1, 2, 4 and 8 in the guide.

Guide to expressing IEP goals phonological disorder and CAS

1. Expanding the consonant inventory; promoting more accurate consonant production.
2. Expanding the vowel inventory; promoting more accurate vowel production.
3. Expanding the syllable shape inventory; pro-moting accurate syllable shapes.
4. Expanding the word shape inventory; promot-ing more accurate word structures.
5. Expanding the capacity to produce/differen-tiate accurate strong and weak syllables.
6. Promoting more varied and accurate use of phonotactic range in syllables and words.
7. Promoting more effective accurate supraseg-mental use prosody.
8. Promoting generalisation of accurate new: segments, syllable structures, word structures and prosodic features – to more challenging contexts.

Tad's IEP goals

1. **Expanding the consonant inventory; pro-moting more accurate consonant produc-tion.**

   Long-Term Goal: Tad will produce the stops /p b t d k g/ and the fricatives /f s ʃ/ or close approximations in CV and VC syllable and word contexts.

   Short-Term Objectives
   1. Tad will perceive and produce /p b t d/ in CV and VC words.
   2. Tad will perceive and produce /k g/ in iso-lation and CV and VC syllables.
   3. Tad will perceive and produce /k g/ in CV and VC words.
   4. Tad will perceive and produce / f s ʃ / in CV and VC words

2. **Expanding the vowel inventory; promoting more accurate vowel production.**

   Long-Term Goal: Tad will produce all vow-els and diphthongs in CV and VC syllable and word contexts.

   Short-Term Objectives

1. Tad will discriminate /ɜ/ from /ɔ/ in single word contexts.
2. Tad will discriminate /ɜ/ from /ɔ/ in short sentences.
3. Tad will produce /ɜ/ from /ɔ/ in isolation.
4. Tad will produce /ɜ/ in CV and VC non-words and words.

3. **Expanding the word shape inventory; promoting more accurate word structures.**

   Long-Term Goal: Tad will produce the clusters /pl bl kl and gl/ or close approximations in CCV and CCVC word contexts.

   Short-Term Objectives
   1. Tad will produce /pl bl kl and gl/, or close approximations, in CCV words.
   2. Tad will produce /pl bl kl and gl/, or close approximations, in CCVC words.
   3. Tad will produce /pl bl kl and gl/, or close approximations, in CCV and CCVC words, in short utterances.

4. **Promoting generalisation of accurate new: segments, syllable structures, word structures and prosodic features – to more challenging contexts.**

   Long-Term Goal: Tad will produce segmentally correct trochaic sequences, with appropriate prosody (stress and intonation), in word and sentence contexts.

   Short-Term Objectives
   1. Tad will produce two-syllable trochaic words with Strong-Weak stress (e.g., *many*)
   2. Tad will produce four-syllable trochaic sequences with Strong-Weak-Strong-Weak stress (e.g., *many people*)

Target selection

A tradition is a ritual, belief or object passed down within a society, maintained in the present, with origins in the past. A scientist embarking on a research trend inherits the tradition of preceding scientists, along with their conclusions and critical discussion. A sense of such a crucial inheritance of tradition is what sets apart the best scientists; those who change their fields through their embrasure [widening] of tradition.

(Kuhn, 1977)

In the left column of Table 8.1 is a list of eight familiar, traditional target selection criteria that are not strongly based, if at all, in evidence or solid theory. In the right column are eight newer criteria with stronger linguistic underpinnings and empirical support. The implication here is *not* 'out with the old criteria, and in with the new(ish)'! We can combine all of these criteria to bring the evidence, theory and critical discussion of science, and the wisdom of tradition, to the same table while respecting the characteristics and preferences of the child, the family and the clinician, and the individual child's intervention needs.

Traditional target selection criteria

1. Work in developmental sequence

Working on sound targets in the typical sequence of acquisition is done on the logical assumption that earlier developing sounds are easier for a child to learn first, less frustrating for them to attempt,

Table 8.1 Traditional and newer criteria for treatment target selection

Traditional selection criteria Associated with: little or no evidence, logic, intuition, experience, hunches	Newer selection criteria These tend to be evidence-based, linguistically driven, theoretically sound
1. Work in developmental sequence	9. Work on later developing sounds/structures first
2. Choose socially important targets	10. Work on marked consonants first
3. Work on phonemes that are stimulable	11. Work on non-stimulable phonemes first
4. Use minimal feature contrasts in treatment	12. Use maximal feature contrasts in treatment
5. Choose unfamiliar words as targets	13. Use a systemic approach to analyse the child's rules
6. Work on inconsistently erred sounds	14. Apply the sonority sequencing principle
7. Target sounds most destructive of intelligibility	15. Prioritise least knowledge sounds in treatment
8. Target non-developmental errors	16. Consider lexical properties of 'therapy words'

or easier for the clinician to teach (Hodson, 2007, 2010; Van Riper & Irwin, 1958). A clinician using this strategy might prioritise intervention targets following Shriberg's (1993) early, middle, and late eight acquired sounds, displayed in Table 1.2, proceeding from the early eight: /m n j b w d p h/ to the middle eight: /t ŋ k g f v tʃ dʒ/ to the late eight: /ʃ ʒ l ɹ s z θ ð/, or they might refer to any number of 'age of acquisition tables' (McLeod, 2013) or 'phonetic mastery tables' (Kilminster & Laird, 1978, also displayed in Table 1.2), or Hodson's (2007, 2010) target selection guidelines.

2. Choose socially important targets

The notion of 'social importance' usually implies a significant target for the child or parents in terms of how the child is perceived, and may relate to avoiding embarrassment, as in the following examples. Stoel-Gammon (A9) describes Brett, 4;9, who was teased for saying *Bwett*. Tired of the hilarity it generated, the Ayres family were anxious for Gerri, 5;3, to stop calling herself /dɛɹieːz/ (example used by permission); and Shaun, 4;9, was eager to work on /ʃ/ because he was taunted for saying his name /dɔn/. Many SLPs/SLTs have been asked by parents if the word *truck* might be considered as a target in children who pronounce /tɹ/ as in *tree* as /f/.

3. Work on phonemes that are stimulable

Prioritising for intervention the child's stimulable, most knowledge phonemes (see Table 8.4) is based on the interwoven ideas of developmental readiness, ease of learning, and early success as a motivator (Hodson, 2007, 2010) for the child, and ease of teaching (for the clinician). Traditionally, 'stimulable' has meant that a consonant or vowel can be produced in isolation by the child, in direct imitation of an auditory and visual model with or without instructions, cues, imagery, feedback, and encouragement. For example, a clinician might elicit /f/ simply by providing placement cues and modelling it.

4. Use minimal feature contrasts in treatment

Meaningful minimal word-pairs, or real words contrasted with each other, can be maximally opposed, like *sick-wick*, which differs in place, voice, manner and major class (and markedness); 'nearly maximally opposed', like *big-jig*, which cuts across many featural dimensions but shares the voicing feature; or minimally opposed, like *pat-bat* differing in voice only, *tip-sip* differing in manner only, and *cap-tap* differing in place of articulation only. Targeting error phonemes, or error patterns, using *minimally* opposed words is done on the understanding that it is the most direct way of demonstrating (his or her own) homophony to a child (Dean, Howell, Waters & Reid, 1995; Grunwell, 1989). So, in choosing treatment words for a child exhibiting voiced velar fronting SFWF, word contrasts such as *bug-bud, cog-cod, beg-bed* and *mug-mud* would be selected, with just one feature difference (in place) between error and target. In the process of constructing minimal pair sets, the clinician would attempt to find phonetically appropriate picturable words representing age-appropriate vocabulary that lend themselves to activities for pre-readers, and in most instances would include printed captions, in lower case, on picture cards and worksheets. For example, *peel* would be printed 'peel', not 'PEEL' or 'Peel' and *Paul* would be printed 'Paul' not 'PAUL' or 'paul', to be consistent with the way early literacy instruction is commonly delivered.

Note that a near minimal pair is formed with the addition or removal of a sound, or in other words, a change in syllable structure, as in *lap-clap*, *blimp-limp, moat-most*, and *mild-mile*. Bound morphemes used to mark inflection generate morphosyntactic minimal pairs (e.g., *jumps-jumped, drags-dragged*) and morphosyntactic near minimal pairs (e.g., *book-books, run-runs*).

5. Choose unfamiliar words as targets

Choosing unfamiliar words or low-frequency words (in terms of their usage) for treatment stimuli is based on the premise that a child's error production of seldom-spoken or novel words (like *yowie*, *yeti*, and *yen*) will not be as habituated as familiar words (such as *yes*, *yell*, *you* and *yet*), or well-established, frozen (fossilised) forms like /lɛloʊ/ for *yellow*.

6. Work on inconsistently erred sounds

The principle governing the selection of sounds that are sometimes pronounced correctly is that, because the child demonstrates some knowledge of an inconsistently erred target, it will be easier to learn and teach than a sound for which a child has less (or no) knowledge. For example, following the developmental trend, a child receiving intervention might have acquired velar stops word finally in words like *shake* and *big*, but not in other syllable contexts, encouraging the clinician to target /k/ and /g/ pre-vocalically, inter-vocalically, and in clusters, perhaps using facilitative contexts containing final velars (see Backward Chaining in Chapter 6). Similarly, a child might be producing the /k/ and /g/ in /kl/ and /gl/ clusters but not in other positions, as can happen in typical acquisition, prompting the construction of near minimal pairs, such as *clap-cap*, *clean-keen*; *glow-go*, *glad-lad*, to facilitate velar stops SIWI. Again, a child may be able to produce the voiceless affricate only in words ending with /ntʃ/, suggesting that practising words such as those found here: www.speech-language-therapy.com/pdf/clustersNCHsfwf.pdf, might be facilitative.

7. Target sounds most destructive of intelligibility

Sometimes an error has such a pervasive, negative impact on intelligibility that it compels consideration as a high treatment priority (Grunwell, 1989). My client Yoshi, 4;2, with English as his first language had a PCC below 30% in both Japanese and English. His mother's second language was Japanese, English was his monolingual father's only language, and his Japanese au pair communicated with him in Japanese and German. In English, Yoshi had widespread glottal insertion before and after utterances and pre- and post-vocalically (as in Japanese). This, coupled with a complete absence of voiced stops had a devastating effect on his intelligibility. Early treatment goals included achieving stimulability of /b d g/ to two-syllable positions and elimination of glottal insertion. Yoshi's phonology was unusual in there being no glottal *replacement* evident, only glottal insertion.

Another client Sam, 4;1, had the unusual pattern of replacing stops with /f/ or /v/ which I saw only twice over 40 years of clinical practice, and had no clusters (e.g., *boo* → /vu/ *blue* → /vu/ *Pooh* → /fu/ *do* → /vu/ *coo* → /fu/ *goo* → /vu/). Note that Sam marked the voiced-voiceless cognate correspondences. The effect of these idiosyncratic errors meant that stops and clusters virtually *had* to be early targets for him.

8. Target non-developmental errors

Flipsen Jr. and Parker (2008) drew upon Dodd and Iacono (1989), Edwards and Shriberg (1983) and Khan and Lewis (1983) to make lists of non-developmental and developmental patterns, based on the 1983 and 1989 authors' interpretation of what was 'developmental' and what was not. Flipsen Jr. and Parker reported that the non-developmental patterns include: initial consonant deletion; within word consonant deletion (SIWW and SFWW); deletion of unmarked elements of clusters; within word consonant replacement (SIWW and SFWW); errors of insertion and addition (e.g., schwa insertion or addition; vowel addition word finally) and intrusive consonants; backing of stops, fricatives, and affricates; denasalisation; devoicing of stops; idiosyncratic systematic sound preferences; and glottal replacement, unless it is dialectal. Developmental patterns include final consonant deletion; reduplication; weak syllable deletion; cluster reduction; context-sensitive voicing; depalatalisation; fronting of fricatives, affricates, and velars; alveolarisation of stops and fricatives; labialisation of stops; stopping of fricatives and affricates; gliding of fricatives and liquids; deaffrication; epenthesis; metathesis; migration; and vocalisation.

Grunwell (1989) recommended that patterns that 'deviated most from normal development' (i.e., non-developmental phonological patterns) should be given priority as treatment targets, particularly initial consonant deletion, which is not attested in normal development in English, and glottal replacement where it is not dialectal. These non-developmental patterns often beg to be eliminated because they can sound 'odd' even to the untrained ear, and they can disrupt prosody and affect intelligibility. Non-developmental phonetic errors are also often given priority. These include lateral fricatives and affricates, ingressive fricatives, phoneme specific nasality and vowel errors.

Prevalent or inconsistent vowel errors are a diagnostic marker for CAS. Children with CAS and those with moderate/severe phonological disorder frequently experience difficulties producing vowels (Gibbon, A29). Vowel errors may occur in as many as 50% of children with these diagnoses (Eisenson & Ogilvie, 1963; Pollock & Berni, 2003). Depending which study is consulted, 24%–65% typically developing children below 35 months have a high incidence of vowel errors. This is a wide range that it is difficult to interpret. A more meaningful, useful piece of information for clinicians' guidance is that by 35 months errors are far less prevalent, ranging from zero to 4% (Pollock & Berni, 2003).

Newer target selection criteria

9. Work on later developing sounds and structures first

Some research suggests selecting later developing sounds (e.g., the late eight acquired consonants: /ʃ ʒ l ɹ s z θ ð/ in Table 1.2), complex targets (e.g., the marked consonants from a choice of /p t k f v θ ð s z ʃ ʒ tʃ dʒ/ that are missing from the child's inventory), and the more marked of the clusters: /spɹ/, /stɹ/, /skɹ/, /spl/ and /skw/, and /sm/, /sn/, /fl/, /fɹ/, /θɹ/, /sl/, /ʃɹ/, /bl/, /bɹ/, /dɹ/, /gl/, /gɹ/ and /sw/ (see points 10 and 14 below) as early treat-

ment targets because training them will result in greater system-wide change (Gierut, Morrisette, Hughes & Rowland, 1996). Gierut and colleagues furnish persuasive arguments in favour of devising complex targets that are marked, non-stimulable, late acquired, consistently erred, and presented to the child in high-frequency words representing maximally distinct feature oppositions (Baker, A13).

10. Work on marked consonants first

A distinctive feature, or 'feature', is an acoustic or articulatory parameter whose presence of absence defines a phonetic category, distinguishing it from another phonetic category (Chomsky & Halle, 1968). Targeting the marked properties (features) of phonemes is prioritised on the understanding that it may well facilitate acquisition of unmarked aspects of the system. Markedness is a concept from the study of the sound systems of all natural languages. A marked feature in a language *implies* the necessary presence of another feature, hence the term '*implicational* relationship'. There are languages, like English, that have stops *and* fricatives. There are languages that have stops, but *no* fricatives. But no language has fricatives and no stops. This means that fricatives are a marked class of sounds because the presence of fricatives necessarily implies the presence of stops in a particular language. Thus, it is said that there is an implicational relationship between the fricatives /f v θ ð s z ʃ ʒ/ and stops (Elbert, Dinnsen & Powell, 1984).

Another way of putting this is to say that the fricatives, /f v θ ð s z ʃ ʒ/, are marked because they imply stops. Similarly, the voiceless stops that occur in /s/ clusters (/p t k/) are marked because they imply voiced stops: /b d g/. Furthermore, according to this interesting but somewhat controversial body of research, consonants imply vowels (Robb, Bleile & Yee, 1999); affricates /tʃ and dʒ/ imply fricatives (Schmidt & Meyers, 1995); clusters (except for /sp, st, sk/) imply affricates (Gierut & O'Connor, 2002); and true clusters with small sonority differences imply true clusters with larger sonority differences (Gierut, 1999).

David Ingram (personal correspondence, May 2011) notes that Jakobson discussed the voiceless stops /p/, /t/ and /k/ as unmarked, and that this is common in the linguistic literature. This general claim, however, is based on languages where the voiceless stops are unaspirated and have roughly a zero voice onset time (VOT). English speaking children start out with stops that are characterised by 0 VOT, but English speaking parents (including researchers) hear and often transcribe these as voiced because they are within the VOT boundaries for English voiced stops. So, the unmarked stop for English children is neither the English voiced nor voiceless aspirated stop, but those stops that occur after 's' in clusters (i.e., /st/, /sp/ and /sk/). Based on judgements of accuracy, the voiced stops in English actually are acquired before the voiceless ones, and can be interpreted as the unmarked ones.

Interestingly, the opposite occurs in Spanish where the voiceless stops are 0 VOT and the voiced stops are prevoiced. Spanish children start out doing well with voiceless stops, which are perceived by Spanish speakers as voiceless, and have errors with the voiced ones, sometimes making them fricatives, something rarely if ever seen in children with English as their first language (L1). So the markedness of stops has to be viewed in relation to whether a language has one, two or even three series of stops, and in relation to their VOT values.

In summary then, some research suggests we should target the *marked* consonants and clusters, particularly those with small sonority differences (see point 14 below), to facilitate the acquisition of unmarked ones. Clinicians interested in applying these ideas in intervention can be guided as follows:

FRICATIVES imply **STOPS**
Target fricatives to promote functional generalisation to (other) fricatives and stops.
VOICELESS STOPS that occur in /s/ clusters (adjuncts) imply **VOICED STOPS**
Target voiceless stops to promote functional generalisation to voiced and voiceless stops.
AFFRICATES imply **FRICATIVES**

Target affricates to promote functional generalisation to affricates and fricatives.
CLUSTERS imply **SINGLETONS**
Target clusters to promote functional generalisation clusters and singletons.

11. Work on non-stimulable phonemes first

Since the mid-1990s, sections of the research world have encouraged clinicians to target non-stimulable sounds because if a sound *is* stimulable, or if it *becomes* stimulable, it is likely to be added to a child's inventory without direct treatment (Miccio, A23; Miccio, Elbert & Forrest, 1999). As sounds that are *not* stimulable have poorer short-term prognosis than those that are, treatment outcomes are likely to be enhanced when SLPs/SLTs use their unique skills to address the production of those non-stimulable sounds – to *make* them stimulable. Once the sounds are stimulable, in two-syllable positions (e.g., /f/ SIWI and SFWF in *fie* and *off*, respectively; or alternatively /f/ SIWI and SIWW in *far* and *Sophie*, respectively), they are likely to progress and become established in the child's productive repertoire even if not targeted directly for treatment beyond that level.

This has strong implications for clinicians who, for whatever reason, can only see a child with significant inventory constraints infrequently. The available time to provide intervention in such circumstances may be best spent doing stimulability therapy, something we are exclusively qualified to do, rather than expect an unskilled non-SLP/SLT, perhaps armed with a 'home program', to teach sounds absent from the child's repertoire.

Targeting stimulable sounds yields short-term but limited gains, in terms of generalisation (Powell & Miccio, 1996), whereas targeting *non-stimulable* sounds via stimulability therapy (Miccio, A23), exploratory sound play, and phonetic placement techniques increases the probability of generalisation, once stimulability has been achieved (Rvachew, Rafaat & Martin, 1999). Rvachew & Nowack (2001) determined that clinicians can be reasonably confident that provided the child has relatively greater productive phonological knowledge for them, that is, the child is stimulable for them, developmentally earlier targets will be easier for pre-schoolers to acquire than target phonemes that are *both* unstimulable *and* late developing.

12. Use maximal feature contrasts in treatment

The rationale for using maximally opposed, non-proportional contrasts (Gierut, 1992) is that the heightened perceptual saliency of the contrasts so formed increases learnability, facilitating phonemic change. This is discussed under *Maximal Oppositions and Empty Set* in Chapter 4 with examples of treatment targets for Xing-Fu, 4;5, and Vaughan, 5;8, and elaborated by Baker (A13). A maximal opposition cuts across many featural dimensions. For example, by referring to the Table 2.5 and Table 8.2 we see that the contrast between /b/ and /s/ in the word pair *bun-sun* is in place (labial is distinct from coronal), manner (stop is distinct from fricative) and voice (/b/ is voiced and /s/ is voiceless). The contrast between /f/ and /n/ in *fat-gnat* is in place, manner, voice and major class (/f/ is an obstruent; /n/ is a sonorant).

13. Use a systemic approach to analyse the child's rules

Williams (A26; 2010) describes a non-traditional approach to target selection, based on analysis of the function of the sound in the child's own system, as having maximal impact on phonological restructuring. This is explained with examples in Chapter 4 under the heading *Minimal Pair Approaches: Multiple Oppositions*, and by Williams herself in A26.

14. Apply the sonority sequencing principle

Sonority is the amount of 'sound' or 'stricture' in a consonant or vowel, represented numerically in a 'sonority hierarchy' devised by Steriade (1990). Steriade's proposed hierarchy was from most to least sonorous: vowels (=0) were most sonorous, followed by glides (=1), liquids (=2), nasals (=3), voiced fricatives (=4), voiceless fricatives (=5), voiced stops (=6) and finally voiceless stops (=7), the least sonorous.

Markedness data tell us that consonant clusters are more marked than singletons (see point 10 above). Sonority theory adds to the picture by ranking two-element consonant clusters (note: just the two-element ones) in terms of markedness according to their sonority difference scores (Ohala, 1999), as displayed in Table 8.3.

For example, /kl/ (7 minus 1 in Steriade's hierarchy) has a sonority difference score of 6, whereas /fɹ/ (5 minus 2) scores 3. As Baker (A13) discusses, *small* sonority differences of 3 (like /sl/ and /ʃɹ/) or 4 (like /gl/), and the three-element clusters may promote generalised change

Table 8.2 'Place-Voice-Manner Chart' for PVM Analysis, after Kleinschmidt, in Hanson 1983, pp. 132–133. Reproduced with permission from Elsevier

		English Phonemes							
				Place					
Manner		Labial		Coronal				Dorsal	
NOTE cognate pairs: voiceless on the left		Bilabial	Labiodental	Interdental	Alveolar	Palato-alveolar	Palatal	Velar	Glottal
Obstruents	Stop	p b			t d			k g	ʔ
	Fricative		f v	θ ð	s z	ʃ ʒ			h
	Affricate					ʧ ʤ			
Sonorants	Nasal	m			n			ŋ	
	Liquid				l		ɹ		
	Glide	w					j	w	

Table 8.3 Sonority Difference Scores

Most Complex			Sonority Difference
⬆	Voiceless fricative + nasal	sm sn	2
	Voiceless fricative + liquid	fl fɹ θɹ sl ʃɹ	3
	Voiced stop + liquid or voiceless fricative + glide	bl bɹ dɹ gl gɹ sw	4
⬇	Voiceless stop + liquid	pl pɹ tɹ kl kɹ	5
	Voiceless stop + glide	tw kw	6
Least Complex			

Consider targeting three-element clusters, and two-element clusters with smaller sonority differences 2 or 3 or 4.

to singletons *and* clusters (Gierut, 1999; Gierut & Champion, 2001; Morrisette, Farris & Gierut, 2006) than other two-element clusters. It should be noted again here that Morrisette et al. (2006) count initial /s/ + stop 'clusters' as adjuncts and not 'true clusters'.

15. Prioritise least knowledge sounds in treatment

Some research suggests selecting sounds for which the child has 'least knowledge' in terms of the 'knowledge types' described in Table 8.4, because they will be easier to learn (Barlow & Gierut, 2002; Gierut, 2001; Williams, 1991). Applying learnability theory, Gierut (2007) provides support for the position that, in order for efficient learning to occur, we should teach phonologically impaired children complex aspects of the target system, outside of what they have learned already.

16. Consider the lexical properties of 'therapy words'

We can consider word properties when we choose words to use in intervention. In this respect we have the choice of selecting words that are either of '*high frequency*' in the language, or words with '*low neighbourhood density*'.

High-frequency words are those words that occur often in the language. They are recognised (comprehended) faster *by children* than low-frequency words.

High neighbourhood density words are phonetically similar to many other words. Children recognise and repeat high-density words slower and with less accuracy than low-density words. As well, children name high-density words more accurately than low-density words, suggesting that lexical processing in children entails a high-density disadvantage in recognition and a high-density advantage in production (Storkel, Armbruster & Hogan, 2006).

In view of this, in choosing stimulus words, or 'treatment words', the clinician might consider those that are either high frequency or have low neighbourhood density (Storkel & Morrisette, 2002).

High-frequency words

By way of example, Table 8.5 contains high-frequency words with /s/ SIWI and SFWF, and /s/ words and pictures are available at www.speech-language-therapy.com/pdf/SwordsHF.pdf.

Low neighbourhood density words

High-density words are phonetically similar to many other words and have 11 or more neighbours. The words in a neighbourhood are based on one sound substitution, for example, *sat* to *pat*, one sound deletion, for example, *sat* to *at* or one sound addition, for example, *sat* to *scat*. The word *bat* is in a dense neighbourhood of 40, according to the Washington University Neighborhood

Table 8.4 Knowledge Types. Reproduced with permission from the American Speech-Language-Hearing Association

Description	Examples	
Type-1 knowledge – Most knowledge A child displaying type-1 knowledge of target [s] would produce this sound correctly in all word positions and for all morphemes; [s] would never be produced incorrectly.	sun /sʌn/ soup /sup/ messy /mesi/ missing /mɪsɪŋ/ miss /mɪs/	
Type-2 knowledge A child displaying type-2 knowledge of target [s] would produce this sound correctly for all morphemes and positions. However, a phonological rule would apply to account for observed alternations between, for example, [s] and [t] in morpheme final position.	sun /sʌn/ soup /sup/ messy /mesi/ ice /aɪs/	BUT miss /mɪt/ kiss /kɪt/
Type-3 knowledge A child displaying type-3 knowledge of target [s] would produce this sound would produce this sound correctly in all positions. However, certain morphemes that were presumably acquired early and acquired incorrectly 'fossilised' would always be produced in error.	sun /sʌn/ messy /mesi/ miss /mɪs/	BUT Santa /næntə/ juice /wu/
Type-4 knowledge A child displaying type-4 knowledge of target [s] would produce this sound for all morphemes, in, for example, initial position. However, production of [s] would be incorrect in within-word and word final positions.	sun /sʌn/ soup /sup/	BUT messy /meti/ missing /mɪtɪŋ/ miss /mɪt/ kiss /kɪt/
Type-5 knowledge A child displaying type-5 knowledge of target [s] would produce this sound correctly in, for example, initial position. However, only some morphemes in this position would be produced correctly. All [s] morphemes in post-vocalic positions would be produced incorrectly.	sun /sʌn/ soup /sup/	BUT soap /təup/ sock /sɔk/ messy /meti/ kiss /kɪt/
Type-6 knowledge – Least knowledge A child displaying type-6 knowledge of target [s] would produce this sound incorrectly in all word positions and for all morphemes; [s] would never be produced correctly.	sun /tʌn/ soup /tup/ missing /mɪtɪŋ/ miss /mɪt/ kiss /kɪt/	

Database: www.psych.wustl.edu/sommers. Its 39 neighbours are: *back bad badge bag baht bait ban bang bash bass bast batch bath batteau batten batter battle beat bet bight bit boat boot bought bout brat but cat chat fat gnat hat mat pat rat sat tat that* and *vat*.

It is interesting to consider words with /dʒ/ word initially in terms of neighbourhood density. The words *gym, jack, jam, jet, jig, jog, juice, joke* and *jug* are often chosen as stimulus items (word targets to use in therapy sessions). If we want to let neighbourhood density inform our choices,

Table 8.5 Selected, picturable, 'child friendly' high-frequency words for /s/

	/s/SIWI				/s/SFWF			
cell	sat	summer	seam	audience	face	miss	police	space
city	saw	seven	sun	case	force	office	press	us
say	scene	six	sent	class	house	peace	price	voice
same	season	small	science	close	less	place	race	yes

however, we would avoid these particular words because *gym* has 14 neighbours, *jack* 17, *jam* 16, *jet* 20, *jig* 17, *jog* 11, *juice* 13, *joke* 11 and *jug* 16. Instead we would opt for words with fewer than 11 neighbours such as *germ* with 7, and *giant* 0, *jaguar* 0, *jalopy* 0, *jester* 1, *jazz* 7, *jeans* 4, *jelly* 5, *jetty* 4, *jewel* 6, *joey* 0, *joust* 5, *judo* 1, *jump* 8 and *junk* with 9. It is not necessary or advantageous to give preference to words with the lowest possible numbers, aiming for zeros, ones and twos, just so long as the word resides in a sparse neighbourhood of 10 or fewer other words. Low-density /ʤ/ words and pictures can be downloaded at www.speech-language-therapy.com/pdf/dg-siwi.pdf.

Picturable, child friendly low neighbourhood density verbs

blink block blow bounce bring broke brush bump camp carve change chirp clean climb clip cough count crawl crush cry dance dream dress drill drink drip drive drop dry faint film flap flip frown fry gasp give grab grow growl help honk hunt iron jive join judge jump love march pinch plant point push quack scan scold scream shrug ski skid skip smash smell smile snap sneeze snooze snore snort speak speed spell spend spill spit splash splat spray spread spy squash squawk squeak squeal stand start stay steal step stir stitch stomp stop surf sweat sweep swish swoop thank throw trim trot waltz want wash watch whoosh woof zoom

Picturable, child friendly low neighbourhood density nouns

ant arch ark arm axe bench blade blind block blood blouse branch breath bridge brooch broom brush bulb bump bunch bush champ child chimp church clamp clasp claw clay cliff clog cloth clove clown club couch crab craft cream crop crow crowd crown crumb crust crutch cube desk dial disc disk dog drain drawer dress drill drum farm fence five flag flake flame flash flask fleece flex flock flood floor flower fluff flute fog foot frame fridge friend fringe frog front frost froth fruit fudge geese germ gift glass glove glue golf gown grouch knife ground group grub harp hinge hoist ink jazz jewel junk lion lounge lump lunch lamp mask milk month moth mouth mulch mumps noise nurse palm plan plane plant plough plug

plum plus pond porch pouch pram prawn price prince print pulse queen quiche quilt choir ramp ranch scab scar scarf school scone scoop score screen screw shark shelf shield shrub chef silk skin skirt skull skunk sky sleeve slice slime slug smock smog smoke snack snail snake snow salt spa space spark speech spice spire sport spring sprout spud square squid staff stag stage stalk stamp star steam steel stem stilt store stork storm stove straw stream street string stripe stump stunt swag swamp swan swarm swatch thatch thief thong thread three throat throne thud thump torch towel track tram trap trash treat tree troll trout trowel truck trunk sty tube tusk twig twin view voice wasp watch web whale wharf wheat wheel whip wolf world worm yolk zinc

Picturable, child friendly low neighbourhood density adjectives

black brave brown clean crisp cross cute damp dark flash fresh glad good grey huge large old proud quick real sharp short smart small soft strong sweet white

Targeting speech perception

There is ample evidence to show that a large component of the SSD population has more difficulty with speech perception than their peers with age-typical speech (Munson, Baylis, Krause & Yim, 2006; Munson, Edwards & Beckman 2005; Rvachew, 2007; Rvachew & Brosseau-Lapré, 2012; Sutherland & Gillon, 2007). In an individual client, it is possible that one or more errors are due to the child's inability to hear the difference between his or her customary production and the target correctly produced, but this difficulty may not be readily apparent.

Locke's (1980) procedure takes the guesswork out of trying to decide whether a child actually can hear the difference between error and target, at word level, when an adult says them. The form displayed in Table 8.6a allows testing for two different discrimination errors (or to test and re-test one), and instructions for the task are in Table 8.6b. For a discussion of perceptually based interventions, see Rvachew (A25).

Table 8.6a Locke's Speech Perception Task

Date: Task 1 / / →/ / Target / / Error / / Control / /		Date: Task 2 / / →/ / Target / / Error / / Control / /	
Stimulus –Class	**Response**	**Stimulus –Class**	**Response**
1. / / -Control	yes -NO	1. / / -Target	YES -no
2. / /-Error	yes -NO	2. / /-Control	yes -NO
3. / / -Target	YES -no	3. / / -Target	YES -no
4. / / -Target	YES -no	4. / / -Control	yes -NO
5. / / -Error	yes -NO	5. / / -Error	yes -NO
6. / /-Control	yes -NO	6. / /-Error	yes -NO
7. / / -Control	yes -NO	7. / / -Target	YES -no
8. / / -Target	YES -no	8. / / -Error	yes -NO
9. / /-Error	yes -NO	9. / /-Target	YES-no
10. / / -Target	YES -no	10. / / -Control	yes -NO
11. / / -Error	yes -NO	11. / / -Control	yes -NO
12. / / -Control	yes -NO	12. / / -Error	yes -NO
13. / / -Error	yes -NO	13. / / -Target	YES -no
14. / / -Target	YES -no	14. / / -Control	yes -NO
15. / / -Control	yes -NO	15. / / -Error	yes -NO
16. / / -Error	yes -NO	16. / / -Target	YES -no
17. / / -Target	YES -no	17. / / -Error	yes -NO
18. / / -Control	yes -NO	18. / / -Control	yes -NO
Mistakes: Error Control Target		Mistakes: Error Control Target	

Table 8.6b Instructions for Locke's Speech Perception Task

1. Under 'Task', enter the target word and the substitution. For example, if the child said /fʌm/ for *thumb*, enter thumb→/fʌm/, or /θʌm/→/fʌm/

2. Indicate the target sound in the space marked Target /θ/ in the above example, the substituted sound in the space marked Error /f/ in the above example, and a related sound as a control in the space marked Control. /s/ might be chosen for this example with the word *sum*. So the three contrasting words will be thumb (the target), Fum (the error, represented by an imaginary character) and sum (the control item).

3. In each of the 18 spots under 'Stimulus – Class' fill in the appropriate sounds from #2 above depending on which item is listed. For example if the item says Target, write /θ/, if it says Error write /f/, and if it says Control write /s/. This creates the stimuli for the test. Now familiarise the child with the three pictures and word before proceeding to step 4.

4. To administer the test, *only* show the child the picture of the target (thumb). Ask the speaker to judge whether or not you said the right word. For example:
   1. Is this *fum*?
   2. Is this *sum*?
   3. Is this *thumb*?
   4. Is this *thumb*?
   5. Is this *fum*? … etc

   If the speaker says 'yes', circle yes next to the item. If the speaker says 'no' circle no. '**YES**' and '**NO**' indicate correct answers; '**yes**' and '**no**' indicate incorrect responses.

5. Count the mistakes 'yes' and 'no' in each category Target, Error, Control.

6. The speaker is said to have a problem with perception if 3 or more mistakes in perception are noted in response to the Error stimuli out of 6 Error stimuli. 3/6 indicates that at least half the child's responses are incorrect indicating that the child may have trouble distinguishing their customary production from the adult target.

7. Repeat the process for each erred sound suspected to have a perceptual basis.

The column headed Task 2 can be used to re-test, or to test another error sound.

Targeting compensatory errors in the cleft palate population

Velopharyngeal dysfunction (VPD) is most commonly associated with bilateral or unilateral cleft palate or submucous cleft, but there are other causes, including a short soft palate, adenoidectomy, any neuromotor disorder that causes velopharyngeal insufficiency, craniofacial anomalies, enlarged tonsils, or irregular adenoids. Karen Golding-Kushner discusses issues in speech development, assessment, and intervention for children with craniofacial disorders, cleft palate, and VPD in A17; and in this chapter, Dennis Ruscello describes intervention techniques to use (and *not* to use) with this population.

Dr. Dennis Ruscello is a practitioner with an interest in the assessment and treatment of children with SSD, particularly those with structurally based deficits. His research and teaching have focused primarily on this population. Dennis is a member of the West Virginia University Cleft Palate Team and West Virginia University Center for Excellence in Disabilities Pediatric Feeding Team. He holds the Certificate of Clinical Competence in Speech-Language Pathology and is an ASHA Fellow. Dr. Ruscello is the author of a comprehensive book on therapy for child speech impairment (Ruscello, 2008a) that includes step-by-step treatment strategies for SSDs with functional, structural, sensory or neurological bases. What better person to ask in Q48 about the tricks-of-the-trade in the evaluation and treatment of resonance disorders and nasal emission, including context specific nasality, using low tech and 'no tech' procedures?

Q48. Dennis M. Ruscello: Compensatory errors and cleft lip and palate

Many generalist paediatric SLPs/SLTs rarely encounter children with speech and resonance disorders secondary to cleft palate, craniofacial anomalies and VPD. Terms like pressure-sensitive consonants, nasal rustle (turbulence), compensatory

articulations, prosthetic management, phoneme- specific hypernasality, glottal substitutions and the like may be only dimly understood. Karen Golding-Kushner addresses some of the 'big picture' issues in assessment and treatment in A17. Can you share with the non-specialist reader the practical strategies and techniques they should know about when approaching this population, and the therapy tools they should have to hand, and dispel some of the myths surrounding VPD and its management?

A48. Dennis M. Ruscello: Treating compensatory errors in the cleft palate population: some treatment techniques

Before discussing treatment techniques for children with VPD, it is important to emphasise several points. First, these patients have a structurally based problem that can manifest in different resonance and speech disorders. Second, many SLPs/SLTs see such clients infrequently; so have limited relevant content knowledge and clinical skills. Third, these children have heterogeneous speech production characteristics that may include developmental variation, obligatory errors and compensatory errors.

Developmental variation occurs in the speech of children acquiring the sound system(s) of their language(s) (Bernthal, Bankson & Flipsen Jr., 2013). These may be outgrown or persist, requiring treatment and are unrelated to structural problems. Obligatory errors result from structural differences, which influence negatively the physiologic movement(s) requisite to correct sound production (Golding-Kushner, 2001; Peterson-Falzone, Hardin-Jones & Karnell, 2009). Generally, obligatory errors are distortions of the intended sound and they typically resolve spontaneously once structural defects are corrected (Kummer, Strife, Grau, Creaghead & Lee, 1989; Moller, 1994). Finally, compensatory errors involve substitutions of individual sounds or sound classes and are typical in children with VPD (Golding-Kushner, 2001; Kummer, 2001a). They include glottal stops, nasal snorts, velar fricatives, pharyngeal fricatives, pharyngeal stops and mid-dorsum palatal stops.

A study conducted by Hardin-Jones and Jones (2005) gives the reader an impression of the incidence of resonance and speech production errors in children with repaired cleft palate. Of 212 pre-school children, 78 subjects (approximately 37%) had moderate-to-severe hypernasality, whereas 53 (25% of the group) had compensatory errors. The most frequent compensatory errors, in order, were glottal stops, glottal fricative /h/, nasal substitutions, mid-dorsum palatal stops, pharyngeal fricatives and posterior nasal fricatives.

Treatment techniques for compensatory errors

The treatment of hypernasality is generally accomplished through surgery or speech prosthetics; treatment of compensatory errors, however, is the responsibility of the SLP/SLT. Such treatment is important since research demonstrates that elimination of compensatory errors positively influences velopharyngeal movement (Henningsson & Isberg, 1986). Treatment techniques for compensatory errors have been described in several study reports, treatment reviews and texts (Golding-Kushner, 1995, 2001, 2004; Kummer, 2001b; Peterson-Falzone, Trost-Cardamone, Karnell & Harden-Jones, 2006; Peterson-Falzone et al., 2009; Ruscello, 2008a; Trost-Cardamone, 2009). The techniques are based primarily on judicious clinical decision-making and a modicum of treatment efficacy research, as the evidence base (Baker & McLeod, 2004) is limited. Comprehensive reviews by Bessell et al. (2013) and Peterson-Falzone et al. (2009)

support the efficacy of treatment, but the studies do not provide extensive information on the modification of compensatory errors. I use the following treatment techniques differentially with children with cleft palate who have compensatory errors. Each has a specific purpose and rationale, tied to the research literature. They are divided into techniques used during acquisition (while a child is acquiring correct conscious production of a target sound), and during automatisation (when *automatic* spontaneous correct production is becoming established) or techniques that may be used in both phases of phonetic target sound practice when using a motor learning paradigm (Maas et al., 2008; Ruscello, 1993). The acquisition techniques are suitable for pre-schoolers as young as 3;0, with stimuli presented in a picture-reading format. The automatisation tasks are appropriate for school-aged children from 6;0 and beyond. Self-monitoring incorporates acquisition and automatisation activities for children aged 3;0 upwards.

Acquisition

Imitative modelling

Imitative modelling is important in early treatment. Stimuli are spoken with normal loudness, because excessive loudness or overstimulation may cause children to produce practice stimuli similarly, thereby distorting them. More particularly, this is best avoided, since children with cleft palate are at risk for hyperfunctional voice disorders (Peterson-Falzone et al., 2006), and undue loudness may mask the SLP's/SLT's perception and accurate assessment of imitative productions.

Non-speech sound stimulation and nonce words

Eliciting a target 'pressure sound' (obstruent) can be very difficult with some children, because they revert to their customary substitution during sound stimulation trials or, if they are backing, produce another posterior-based articulation (i.e., a non-target glottal or velar production). Accordingly, it is helpful to begin with the sound in *isolation* for target fricatives. Stops and affricates are elicited in CV contexts, since they are produced with obstruction of the vocal tract prior to release to an adjacent vowel. I have also found it useful to incorporate non-speech sounds, to reduce error sound interference (Ruscello, 2008a). For example, I may ask children to whistle with their tongue for /s/, which of course they say they cannot do! I then furnish instructions regarding tongue placement and lip position. I follow this with a whistle sound made with the tongue tip. Sometimes, the child's imitative token is judged to be /s/ in isolation. The child receives positive verbal feedback, continuing to practice until the target is elicited with the verbal cue alone ('Make the whistle sound'). After /s/ production has stabilised through practice, I inform the child that the 'whistle sound' is really /s/.

Another approach to reducing contextual interference is the use of nonce words. A nonce item is a sound combination that is not a free morpheme, with or without a permissible phonological structure. It is generally paired with a picture or line drawing, for example ⊕, to assign meaning to it. 'Billy, this is a sud'. (the clinician proffers ⊕) 'Say sud'. In this way the child rehearses a 'word unit', absent from his or her lexicon to reduce interference from the error response.

Nasal occlusion

During practice trials at the isolation, nonce and word levels, I have children gently pinch their nostrils with their thumb and forefinger (Golding-Kushner, 2001). I emulate this while producing the stimuli, to cue them. Since the children have obligatory VPD, nasal occlusion helps them generate and sustain adequate oral air pressure for plosive, frica-

tive and affricate target production. It also provides auditory and tactile feedback for the child, while practicing in this manner (Kummer, 2001b).

Imagery

For some children, using imagery helps them distinguish between target sound(s) and their substitution error(s). Since many compensatory errors preserve manner of articulation, but change place to a more posterior point of articulation (Trost-Cardamone, 2009), a place distinction can be made. For example, if a child substituted /ʔ/, for /t/ and /d/, a place-based distinction between 'throaties' and 'tippies', respectively can be made (Klein, 1996b; and see Chapter 4 for a discussion of Imagery Therapy, and Table 6.5 for imagery names and verbal and gesture cues and reminders). Introductory identification trials contrast glottal error productions and the alveolar target(s), enabling the child to make the appropriate auditory distinction with the associated image. Once able to make the distinction, children are queried periodically during practice trials. 'Billy, did you make the tippy sound or the throaty sound? Yes, you did make the tippy sound. Good job!'

Automatisation

Speed drills

Speed drills can assist in the automatisation of a target sound (Ruscello, 1993). The child practises the target in context, while the SLP/SLT manipulates speaking rate to transition from conscious to automatic production. The goal is to increase rate of production, while maintaining high levels of response accuracy. Speed drills consist of speech output by the client in practice sets, across training trials, with a gradual reduction in the time necessary to produce it. For instance, the clinician may present 20 phrases, to be read or 'picture-read' citation-naming style. The client has to read (or 'read') aloud the phrases using the target sound correctly. The time needed to produce the phrases and the accuracy rate for the practice set are recorded and shared with the child, providing feedback. The client is then instructed to read the 20 phrases taking less time, while maintaining the accuracy rate. Time and accuracy rate are taken and the results discussed with the client. Additional practice sets can be completed, aiming to reduce time and sustain accuracy. Speed drills may also be performed with words or sentences, at the therapist's discretion. A variation is to have the client practice lists that contain target and non-target items presented in random order. Speed drills can be interspersed throughout treatment as a supplementary activity. If the child's performance deteriorates during speed drills, the SLP/SLT should withdraw them, re-introducing when the child appears ready (applying clinical judgement).

Auditory masking

Manning, Keappock and Stick (1976) originally developed auditory masking for the purpose of *assessing* the automatic use of a target sound. The authors hypothesised that a client relies on auditory information during the automatisation phase of treatment and interfering with auditory information provides an indication of the extent to which an individual is using a target sound automatically. The following is a description of a potentially effective treatment variation I employ. The client reads or picture-reads a list of words, phrases or sentences containing the target, and an accuracy rate is established. The client is then instructed that he or she will read the material again, wearing a headset through which noise will be played. Masking noise from an audiometer is audio recorded or digitised and the signal played through a headset, while the client produces the practice material. Comparative accu-

racy rates between the masking and non-masking conditions are then presented to the client.

Acquisition/Automatisation

Self-monitoring

Self-monitoring tasks are included in a number of treatments (Bernthal et al., 2013; Shriberg & Kwiatkowski, 1987), and the author has found that self-monitoring can be useful for children with cleft palate. Tasks include the client: (1) monitoring correct and incorrect productions of targets in production practice, (2) identifying, discriminating and/or monitoring the production of another speaker such as the clinician or caregiver, and (3) assessing the accuracy of his or her productions in more spontaneous treatment activities, such as conversation (Koegel, Koegel & Ingham, 1986). My preference is to employ self-monitoring in conversation or during other automatisation tasks. Initially, a topic is introduced and the child is instructed that 'one idea at a time' will be discussed and to be sure to make the 'new sound' correctly. The use of limited spontaneous speech reduces any possible frustration for the child without diminishing spontaneity. When the conversation ends, the child is queried regarding a word or words containing the target sound. The child identifies words containing the target sound, indicating the accuracy of those productions. As the child's self-monitoring skills improve, conversations increase in length so that the dialogues approximate actual interchanges.

Caregiver involvement

Ideally, caregivers are involved in their children's treatment but the type of involvement varies as most SLPs/SLTs can attest (Ruscello, 2008a). I meet with the caregiver, discuss the child's speech sound disorder and any coexisting communication disorders, and the proposed treatment, answering their questions. Stressing the importance of careful monitoring of hearing acuity, in light of the high incidence of conductive hearing loss in this population (Peterson-Falzone et al., 2009), I ask caregivers to provide verbal feedback to the child regarding speech progress, and to project a positive attitude to treatment. If a caregiver is willing to take a more active role, I involve the person in the treatment process, encouraging observation of some treatment sessions, and providing home activities that offer additional opportunities for practice. A brief written contract that succinctly describes the parent's (or parents') responsibilities is prepared. Crucially, the actively involved caregiver must first be trained to discriminate between correct and incorrect responses, because the child must receive reliable response information from both caregiver and SLP/SLT. I recommend that the caregiver carry out short practice sessions of approximately 8–10 minutes daily, recording the accuracy of the child's responses. These data are discussed each week with the caregiver and modifications to practice material or sessions are made as needed.

Non-speech oral motor exercises (NS-OME)

One treatment technique that I do not recommend is non-speech oral motor exercises/non-speech oral motor therapy (Bowen, 2005; Golding-Kushner, A19; Hodge, A31; Lof, A35; Powell; A39; Ruscello, 2008b). The overwhelming majority of children with cleft palate do not have muscle weakness or muscle tone problems, and even if they did, NS-OME divorced from speech production activities would not be indicated (Golding-Kushner, 2001). Non-speech oral motor treatment techniques, such as blowing, sucking or specific resistance exercises to 'improve' lip, tongue or palate strength are not indicated and lack an evidence base

(McCauley, Strand, Lof, Schooling & Frymark, 2009). Moreover, studies designed to improve velopharyngeal function for speech through non-speech oral motor treatment have largely been unsuccessful (Ruscello, 2008b; Tomes, Kuehn & Peterson-Falzone, 2004). The clinician (and parent) should avoid non-speech oral motor exercises and treat compensatory speech errors by using task-specific speech therapy.

Summary

The techniques described herein are used by the author in the treatment of children with cleft palate who present with compensatory errors. Most are based on research, but the reader must be mindful that large-scale RCT treatment studies have not been undertaken to validate the treatment efficacy of each. Consequently, it is important for the SLP/SLT to measure the client's performance, so that the efficacy of the techniques can be assessed empirically and necessary changes made.

Competence, focus and motivation

As discussed in Chapter 7, for therapy to work, child, family and therapist all need to share the inherent responsibilities of the therapeutic encounter. There is a mutual obligation for families and clinicians to work with each other to facilitate progress, and for children to be as cooperative in the process as they can be. Simply put, we are unable to work effectively with children who cannot attend – even if only for brief flashes – to the business of therapy. At a minimum, they must possess some level of competence, focus and intrinsic motivation.

Intrinsic motivation

Intrinsic motivation as it relates to children's contributions to progress in therapy has been a strong interest of Dr. Robert J. Lowe. A graduate of Ohio University, Dr. Lowe received his doctorate in speech pathology in 1986. His work experience includes several years as a school clinician in Iowa before beginning university teaching at the University of South Dakota. Now enjoying retirement, from 1985 to 2011 he was a professor at Bloomsburg University of Pennsylvania, where he taught courses in phonetics, diagnostics, fluency and phonology. Dr. Lowe is author of the *ALPHA-R Phonology Test* (Lowe, 2000) available as a free download from www.speech-language-therapy.com, a textbook on phonology (Lowe, 1994), and a workbook on phonological processes (Lowe, 2002).

Q49. Robert J. Lowe: Motivation and generalisation of treatment targets

There is a certain pre-occupation in our work with speech-impaired children with the tasks of choosing the right therapy approach, treatment objectives, reinforcement schedules and initial target words. These are important priorities that tend to focus practitioners on assessment data analysis and matching those data with suitable interventions and therapy materials that will trigger new learning, new patterns of generalisation, new levels of intelligibility and hopefully a new and improved PCC. Amid this busy process, we probably sometimes do not look closely at the characteristics of the child, the family and ourselves, and how these qualities might impinge upon speech progress. Can you explore for us the place in the therapy equation of levels of self-efficacy, valence (the degree of attraction or aversion that an individual feels towards a specific object or event), and attribution of behaviour, on the part of the child?

A49. Robert J. Lowe: The role of intrinsic motivation in learning of new speech behaviours

In 1993, Kwiatkowski and Shriberg proposed a framework for intervention in which the two parameters of capability and focus were viewed as an interactive system impacting the learning and generalisation of speech sounds. They called this two-factor approach the 'capability-focus treatment framework'. Capability included linguistic variables, such as productive phonology and risk factors (e.g., mechanism constraints, cognitive-linguistic constraints). Kwiatkowski and Shriberg (1998) elaborate on capability and ascribe to it both the ability to produce sound targets and the ability to use self-monitoring processes in the learning of new targets. Focus included attention, motivation and effort that basically would reflect the child's interest or disposition towards change. In Shriberg's (1997) review of the model, he points out clinician comments suggesting that lack of focus is associated with minimal treatment progress. Clinicians made comments such as: 'lack of motivation for speech change', 'fear of failure', 'unwilling to risk being incorrect', and 'easily frustrated'. He suggests that, for some children, this lack of focus will interfere with learning and generalisation, even when they have strong capabilities.

Weiss (2004) expanded this view of focus as she explored the research literature outside of the speech-language field. Her paper looked at the role the client plays in the intervention process, and she notes that this role is largely ignored in the treatment of children with speech and language disorders. The exception appears to be the area of stuttering, which has looked at the roles of motivation, temperament, the client's belief in the clinician and belief in the potential success of treatment.

Weiss tells of an unintelligible five-year-old client (Sid) who made remarkable progress over a 4-week period during which he was not seen for therapy. The progress followed a conversation in which Sid asked if Weiss could understand his younger sister's speech better than his own. The answer was 'yes', to which Sid replied, 'But she's a baby'. Four weeks later, they met again for a therapy session and his speech had improved remarkably. Weiss suggests that the dramatic improvement was in part due to a change in the child's motivation or perhaps to a realisation that his speech was something that he must take responsibility for and work to correct. In other words, the child had chosen to change his speech system, believed he could, and did. In terms of the Kwiatkowski and Shriberg model, the child's disposition had changed, and he was now willing to apply his production skills and make use of self-monitoring and regulation to learn the new sound targets.

This choosing to change and believing that it can be done are associated with the constructs of intrinsic motivation, self-efficacy and valence. Speech-language clinicians are familiar with the construct of motivation. We typically motivate our clients by offering rewards for their good work. Sometimes it is verbal praise or a pat on the back, and often we use prizes (e.g., stickers, toys and special privileges). These are *extrinsic* motivators in that they come from outside of the client. Intrinsic motivation comes from within the individual. It is all about doing something because you want to do it and is considered to be more powerful than extrinsic motivation. In the Weiss example, her client displayed intrinsic motivation by showing that he wanted to change his speech.

Intrinsic motivation can be developed by the use of extrinsic reinforcers. Henderlong and Lepper (2002), in their review of the literature on praise, note several studies that have shown verbal praise to increase a child's desire to engage in tasks or spend more time

at a task. However, in some cases, reinforcers have also been shown to actually inhibit the development of intrinsic motivation. This phenomenon is sometimes referred to as the 'over justification effect'. The child may initially engage in an activity because it has some intrinsic value, but as the adult continues to reinforce or reward the behaviour, there is a shift so that the activity is done to gain adult approval or the prize. In other words, the adult's judgement or approval of the performance becomes the child's goal. As a result, when there is not the likelihood of a reward, the child will not voluntarily engage in the behaviour. This effect has been documented in children as young as 4 years of age.

Henderlong and Lepper (2002) and Malone and Lepper (1987) note several factors that can promote intrinsic motivation. Several of the factors are described below.

Praise

Verbal praise is a common component of the speech therapy session. Praise is more effective when it is perceived by the client to be sincere, and if it is associated with a specific aspect of the client's performance rather than just a general 'Good job!' Sincerity is more important for older children than it is for preschoolers, who are not as discerning. Older children have a good sense of how well they should perform, thus praising a child's effort for work on a task that should be easy may not be well received and could actually lead to discouragement. On the other hand, praise for effort on a difficult task would be appreciated and promote intrinsic motivation.

Praise can function to recognise a client's work, and recognition in itself can be a strong motivator. Who doesn't feel some satisfaction when others recognise our efforts and results? One cautionary note: when giving praise, be sure to centre that praise on the client's efforts and successes towards reaching his or her goals. If the child begins working to please the clinician and meet the clinician's goals, then intrinsic motivation suffers.

Cameron, Banko and Pierce (2001) reviewed more than 100 experimental studies on the impact of praise and rewards on intrinsic motivation. They conclude that rewards given for low-interest tasks increase intrinsic motivation. For high-interest tasks, rewards have a negative effect if they are tangible, offered beforehand, and if loosely tied to performance level. If the rewards are clearly linked to performance, the measures of intrinsic motivation increase or are equivalent to non-rewarded controls.

Attributions

What the child attributes success or failure to can also influence the effects of praise. Performance attributions refer to the inferences children make about the causes of their successes or failures. Healthy attributions are those that the child can control. For example, a child believing he was successful because he kept trying shows a healthy attribution because the child has control of how hard he or she tries. But, if the child attributes his success to luck or to the task being easy, then that is not a healthy attribution as the child does not have control of how lucky they are or the difficulty of the task. The clinician can encourage healthy attributions through his or her comments and use of praise. Pointing out that their continued efforts resulted in success reinforces a healthy attribution ('If I keep at it, I can succeed').

Meaningful goals

Setting goals that are meaningful to the client can promote motivation. In the Weiss article, Sid recognised that his younger sister, 'a baby', was a better talker. After that realisation, his goal was to improve speech production. That, of course, was the clinician's goal from day one. The difference was that now it

was also *Sid's* goal. Choosing goals that are meaningful to the client and that are seen as obtainable work to promote intrinsic motivation. Valence is the perceived strength or value of the reward that will result from the performance. In the case of Sid, the value of talking better than his baby sister was very motivating. Whenever the clinician can 'sell' the value of change, motivation will result.

Fantasy

Children love to play games. Placing speech activities within game or fantasy contexts will tap into a natural play mode of young children. It is okay to practice production of the /s/ sound in different word contexts, but it is much more motivating to practice those words if they are the key to finding clues to a hidden treasure. Once children understand the concept that speech is a tool to help them acquire their needs, activities can then be designed to use this tool in fantasy games, which are highly motivating. An example would be a game where the child is searching for clues that would help locate a hidden treasure. The clinician would serve as the 'clue master', and in order to reveal a clue to the child, a secret code would have to be uttered. It might simply be the saying of three target words in a particular order with correct articulation. The clinician would be aware of the order (it could be written down), and the child would try the different sequences until he or she hit on the correct one. The target words could be pictured so that the child could change the order as each attempt is made. This activity points out the value of correct articulation in accomplishing a desired end (finding the treasure), while at the same time being fun!

Self-efficacy

Self-efficacy is an individual's belief in their ability to perform a particular task. More formally, Bandura (1994) described it as a person's beliefs in their capabilities to produce designated levels of performance. Self-efficacy beliefs can determine how you feel, think and behave. They can also influence motivation. Individuals with good self-efficacy for a particular task are more likely to engage in the task, show more perseverance in completing the task, and are more likely to use self-regulation in learning.

It should be emphasised that efficacy appears to be task- or behaviour-specific. For example, you may have good self-efficacy for successfully reading a romance novel, but poor self-efficacy for reading a textbook on organic chemistry. Bandura (1994) notes several influences on the development of self-efficacy. Past experiences, for example, can promote good self-efficacy. In relation to speech and language, a client is much more likely to approach learning a new speech sound if they have already had success in learning other speech sounds. Successful past experiences build a child's confidence, or their belief that they can succeed in the future. On the other hand, a series of past failures would increase the child's belief that they will fail at future attempts. It is here that I would suggest that some of the recent literature on choosing sound targets might be misleading. Some of the work summarised by Gierut (2001) suggests that treatment of more complex properties of the phonological system appears to result in the greatest generalisation. I'd argue that it might depend on the child's temperament. For a child who is a risk taker, this may be the approach to take; but for a shy child who is reluctant to try new sound targets, I would suggest starting with easier, less phonologically complex sound targets. Once the child has a history of success, then I would move to more complex sound targets.

Another factor that promotes self-efficacy is vicarious learning. If a client sees a peer successfully learning a new sound target, it may increase his or her confidence and encourage him or her to keep trying. Again, it would be important for the client to hear praise for efforts so that the idea of perseverance is being promoted. Along with that, the clinician can also express his or her confidence in the client's abilities, which also promotes self-efficacy.

The last influence on the development of strong self-efficacy is the reduction of stress reactions. The client must recognise that it is okay to fail. Failing is part of the process of learning the new skill. Any emotional distress associated with failing will only interfere with learning the new behaviour. In the clinical situation, the client should be experiencing success more than failure. An occasional failure is needed to develop perseverance, but those failures need to be surrounded by successes. The speech-language clinician can be proactive in this area by developing an atmosphere where failure is recognised as part of the learning process but not penalised. We all fail, and often it is by failing that we learn how to succeed.

Summary

Intrinsic motivation represents an intangible that can be tapped by the speech-language clinician and used to promote the learning of new speech targets. It is influenced by a number of factors, including praise, attributions, goals and self-efficacy. Its value is that it can take the speech and language goals of the clinician and make them into what the client wants to accomplish. Once that occurs, our job becomes a whole lot easier!

Words and pictures

Words familiar to children in one linguistic milieu may be unfamiliar in another. For example, the luggage compartment of a car is called a *trunk* in the United States and a *boot* in Australia; a *jersey* or *pullover* in the United Kingdom is called a *sweater* in the United States and a *jumper* in Australia and New Zealand; a *pacifier* in the United States is a *dummy* in the United Kingdom, Australia and New Zealand. Depending on where you are, a *dumpster* is a *skip*, a *lorry* a *truck*, an *elevator* a *lift*, a *queue* is a *line*, a *quay* is a *wharf* and a *courgette* is a *zucchini*. Because of these semantic differences, vowel variation between varieties of English, and other difficulties associated with commercially available picture resources, clinicians often elect to make 'homemade' materials that are linguistically, developmentally and culturally suited to their clients.

At www.speech-language-therapy.com the reader will find, or judging by the millions of hits the site receives each month, may *already* have found, free, homemade worksheets. They include singleton consonant worksheets, vowel and vowel contrast worksheets, minimal pair and near minimal pair resources, worksheets based on facilitative contexts and complexity principles, worksheets to address self-monitoring (the fixed-up-one routine). They can be located by clicking on the RESOURCES tab at the top of every page of the site. Also on the RESOURCES tab are links to Assessment Resources, Forms, Handouts, Slideshows and Word Lists. There is also a drop down menu on the RESOURCES tab containing a Reference list and a Glossary.

Most, but not all of the vocabulary used in these resources represents non-rhotic Australian English pronunciation, and although most of the words and minimal pairs will 'work' in other varieties of English, users may need to discard some.

The resources were made using the insert table feature in Microsoft Word, with royalty-free pictures from Microsoft Images, royalty free Google Images (readers can go to http://www .google.com/advanced_image_search, and select 'free to use or share' [or similar] under *usage rights* to locate these), and original photographs. The Word documents were converted into portable document files (pdf) using Adobe Acrobat software. Colleagues are free to save them to their own computers and customise them to suit individual clients and service delivery models. Copyright

information is on the ABOUT tab which appears on every page of the www.speech-language-therapy.com website. The resource pages that attract the most downloads are the consonants clusters and vowels page, the minimal pairs page and the near minimal pairs page, described and discussed in the next three sections.

Consonants, clusters and vowels

There is a page on the site devoted to consonants, consonant clusters and vowels. The consonant pictures are organised by major class: Obstruents: Stops, Fricative and Affricates; and Sonorants: Nasals, Liquids and Glides. There is a selection of cluster worksheets with consonant clusters SIWI and SFWF, and vowel worksheets. There are also worksheets for working with facilitative contexts such as the aspiration trick for voiceless fricatives and stops, chaining for /k/, /f/, /s/, /n/ and /ɹ/, and additional facilitative contexts for /s/, /tʃ/, /ɹ/ and /l/.

Minimal pairs

The quest for picture pairs with age-appropriate vocabulary can be disappointing. Many of the published cards and worksheets intended for child speech intervention involve words that have been selected because an artist can represent them pictorially. In fact, it often appears that word-choices may have been *decided* by an artist, a publisher, or at least by someone minimally acquainted with child phonology. It is rare to encounter materials that take account of the necessary linguistic and developmental criteria, and consequently, clinicians often need to discard minimal word-pairs because they are too challenging. For example, picturable word-pairs like *kite-tight, coat-tote, cart-tart, can-tan, Ken-ten, corn-torn, code-toad* are usually unsuitable in the early stages of working on voiceless velar fronting because the assimilatory effects of the alveolars /t/, /d/, and /n/ will likely promote productions like [taɪt] for *kite* and [tɛn] for *Ken*.

On the topic of velars, there are few picturable English CVCs for the voiced velar–alveolar opposition SFWF to select from without resorting to proper nouns (e.g., *Doug-Dud*) and fictional words, such as the names of 'aliens', monsters, and creatures (e.g., *Zig-Zid*). The picturable real words are *big-bid, bag-bad, bug-bud, cog-cod, beg-bed, mug-mud, leg-lead, hag-had, rig-rid, dig-did, rogue-road, sag-sad*, available at www.speech-language-therapy.com/pdf/mpDvsGsfwf.pdf, and not many more. Of these, *dig-did* probably needs to be rejected because *did* may feed the tendency for *dig* to be pronounced [dɪd]; *bag-bad, hag-had* and *rogue-road* will not be suitable if clinicians or parents regard *bad, hag* and *rogue* as scary, pejorative or politically incorrect. Some children don't like pictures of *sad* because it makes them feel sad, so *sag-sad* may be unacceptable; and *big-bid, cog-cod, beg-bed, leg-lead, hag-had, rig-rid, dig-did, rogue-road* and *sag-sad* are likely to be problematic because *bid, did* and *rid* are difficult conceptually, and *cod, cog, lead* (/lɛd/), *hag* and *rogue* may be unfamiliar to the child. That leaves three potential pairs, which may actually be enough to work with (Elbert, Powell & Swartzlander, 1991): *bug-bud, beg-bed* and *mug-mud*.

A similar process of elimination may be necessary with minimal pairs for the voiced velar–alveolar contrast SIWI (www.speech-language-therapy.com/pdf/mpDvsGsiwi.pdf). The word-pairs are: *go-dough, gown-down, game-dame, got-dot, gull-dull, guy-dye, gear-deer, ghee-D, guide-died*, and SLPs/SLTs will quickly realise that *gig-dig, gown-down, got-dot, guide-died* may promote unwanted assimilation.

Near minimal pairs

A minimal pair is formed when two words differ by one sound, as in *tap-tip, bed-Ted* and *limb-lip*. A near minimal pair is formed when adding or removing a sound, as in *tap-trap, tip-trip, bed-bread, Ted-tread, limb-limp* and *limb-slim*, changes the structure of the syllable. Near minimal pairs are often used to work on cluster reduction, and by clinicians interested in

complexity approaches (e.g., applying markedness theory and the sonority sequencing principle discussed above) employ them to facilitate widespread generalisation.

Alliterative stories and activities

Frustrated in 2013 by the dearth of therapy materials for 'experimenting with' and developing a feel for complexity approaches to intervention, with the help of my colleague Helen Rippon a UK-based SLT and Illustrator, I wrote a resource pack for Black Sheep Press entitled: Consonant Clusters: Alliterative Stories and Activities for Phonological Intervention (PW12). Sample pages from PW12 are in Figures 8.1, 8.2, 8.3, 8.4 and 8.5. The PW12 pack (Bowen & Rippon, 2013) contains activities for the more marked, or more complex clusters: namely, /spɹ/, /stɹ/, /skɹ/, /spl/ and /skw/, and /sm/, /sn/, /fl/, /fɹ/, /θɹ/, /sl/, /ʃɹ/, /bl/, /bɹ/, /dɹ/, /gl/, /gɹ/ and /sw/ - eighteen in all. There are five pages for each cluster.

1. **Story or Verse**
   First, there is an illustrated alliterative story, for example, Grass Karting displayed in Figure 8.1, which has /sl/ 21 times. It is suggested that when a new target is introduced the clinician starts by reading the story or verse to the child, preferably with a parent present. Following the reading of the story or verse the clinician talks about it, weaving in additional repetitious input, and involving parent and child, fuelling their interest and creativity, triggering language play (Crystal, 1996).

2. **Pictures and words**
   There are six pictures and words for the cluster in question, for example, sleep, sleeve, slope, slip, slime, slow for /sl/, as shown in Figure 8.2. They can be used for input activities such as listening and judgement of correctness, and output activities including production practice.

3. **Talk about**
   Third, there is a Talk About picture, for example, A Slippery Slope for /sl/ (Figure 8.3) with

/sl/

Grass Karting

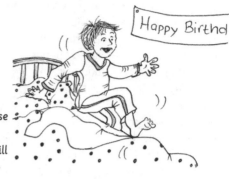

Time seemed to pass very slowly for Ike while he waited for his ninth birthday. Turning nine was important to him because at that age he would be old enough to go grass karting. Grass karts are off-road thrill machines with four-wheel steering, shock-absorbing pump-up tyres, and friction brakes. In bed at night, before he went to sleep, Ike imagined what it would be like to sling on a long-sleeved grass karting jacket, slide into the driver's seat of one of those karts and slowly gather speed as his kart slammed its way downhill through the short grass that covered the long, gradual slope. He imagined himself avoiding slippery moss and slimy mud patches and turning the wheel slightly in order to slosh through a puddle, slicing through piles of white sand and sliding slickly to a standstill at the end of the run. But Ike had to wait.

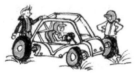

Finally the big day came. On his ninth birthday Ike and two of his friends went grass karting. It was the best fun! They slid and sliced their way down the slippery surface of the sloping run, coming to a slick standstill at the bottom. There they attached their karts to a mechanical lift and were pulled slowly back up to the top in grand style, ready to zoom down the inviting slope again.

Figure 8.1 Alliterative story for /sl/

a suggested 'script' for guidance for clinicians and parents who do not find it easy, or who do not wish to extemporise. Just as an aside, sometimes parents are given tasks to perform that do not come easily to them. For example, a parent might be asked to help their child 'make a poster with sl-words on it, and then talk about the words'. They might make a great job of producing the poster, but then not provide sufficient 'inputs' of the words, resorting to 'point to the slimy things', 'how many people have short sleeves', how many people have long sleeves' and so on, so that the child hears the sl-words just a few times. A script for guidance may help solve this problem. As with the stories and verses the idea here is for the child to hear the target in an alliterative context many times (12 to 18 times within a minute, at least).

Pictures and Words for /sl/

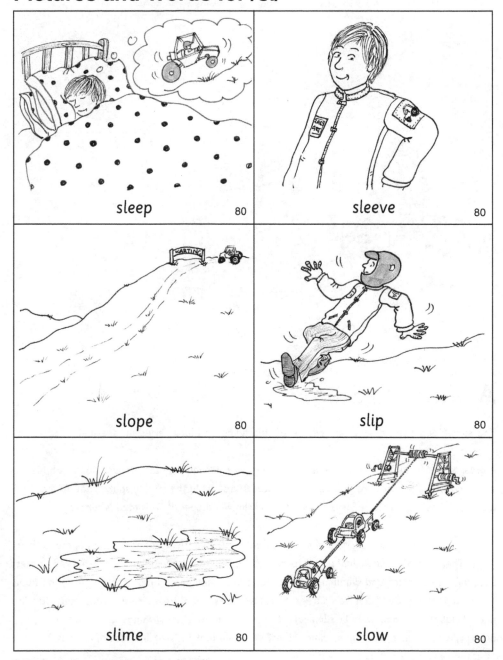

sleep   80

sleeve   80

slope   80

slip   80

slime   80

slow   80

Figure 8.2 Pictures and words for /sl/

/sl/ Talk about the picture using the following text as a guide.
The aim is for the child to hear (but not say) the /sl/ words many times.

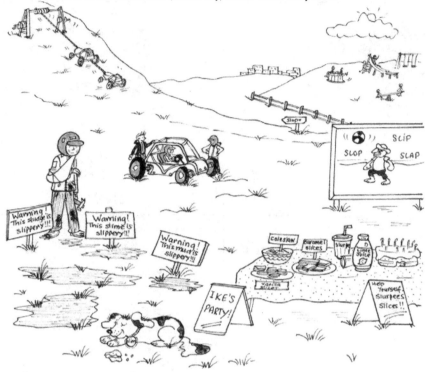

A Slippery Slope

This sleepy dog is called Slim. He looks sleepy, but he doesn't look very slim, does he?

A grass karter has hurt his arm and it is in a sling. He can't manage the slippery slope with his arm in a sling, so he is just looking sadly at the sludge and slime in the muddy spot. What do these warning signs say? 'This sludge is slippery!' 'This slime is slippery!' 'This mud is slippery!'

On the slate it says, 'Ike's party' and here are Ike and his two friends at the bottom of the slippery slope. There is a Slip! Slop! Slap! poster to remind everyone about slipping on long-sleeved clothes, slopping on sunscreen and slapping on hats, and a small sign pointing to the slow lift on the slope. There are lots of sl-things on Ike's party table: slaw, slices and Slurpees™. But what's this? It's lime juice. Maybe it is supposed to be slime juice to go with all the other sl-things. Can you think of a good recipe for slime juice, full of slimy things? We could look in The Slimy Book for ideas.

Figure 8.3 'Talk About' picture for /sl/ with a 'script' for guidance

/sl/

Listening List

slow	slam	sly
slip	slop	slap
sling	slaw	slim
slink	slash	slate
sleep	slice	slide

Near Minimal Pairs

low - slow	seat - sleet
leap - sleep	sew - slow
lime - slime	sip - slip
lap - slap	Sam - slam
late - slate	sink - slink

© 2013 Caroline Bowen, Helen Rippon, Black Sheep Press

Figure 8.4 Listening list and near minimal pairs for /sl/

4. **Listening lists**

   Fourth, there are listening lists with the cluster in the word initial position, for example, slow, slip sling, slink, sleep, slam, slop, slaw, slash, slice, sly, slap, slim, slate and slide and the near minimal pairs: low-slow, leap-sleep, lime-slime, lap-slap, late-slate; and seat-sleet, sew-slow, sip-slip, Sam-slam and sink-slink for /sl/ (Figure 8.4).

5. **Word pairs**

   Finally, there are pictured word-pairs (e.g., low-slow, leap-sleep and lime-slime for /sl/ shown in Figure 8.5). Only a few word-pairs are provided for each cluster, bearing in mind the findings of Elbert et al. (1991) who determined that as few as three to five minimal pairs were all that were necessary for generalisation to occur. It should be noted that in

Word Pairs for /sl/

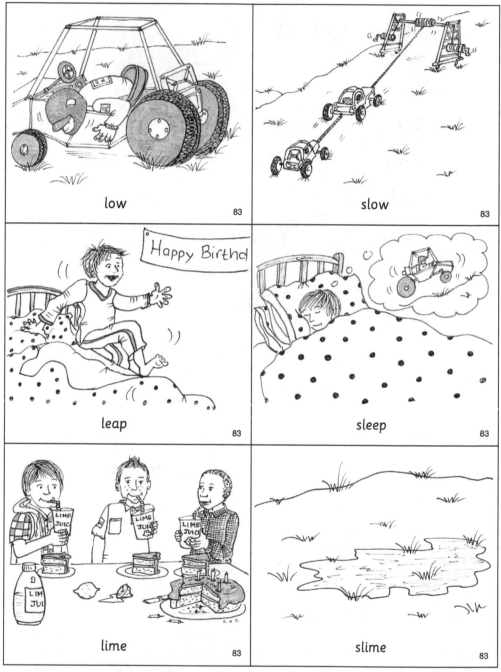

low 83

slow 83

leap 83

sleep 83

lime 83

slime 83

Figure 8.5 Word-pairs for /sl/

order to maintain a child's interest, clinicians might sometimes want to use more than five word-pairs and these are available from various sources including Black Sheep Press and www.speech-language-therapy.com.

In similar vein, Taps Richard (2012) developed a set of 88 modestly priced picture cards and an App (Taps Richard, 2014), to employ in targeting 10 of the more complex clusters: /skɹ/, /spɹ/, /stɹ/, /spl/, /skw/, /fl/, /fɹ/, /θɹ/, /ʃɹ/ and /sl/ in word initial position. She also provides free information about assessment and intervention based on complexity principles and a 4-page handout describing 25 activities that can be used with the cards at www.slpath.com.

Inspiration online

A final source of tips, tricks and insights, not to mention good solid theory and evidence, can be found in the currently sporadic discussion among members of the phonologicaltherapy group (www.groups.yahoo.com/neo/groups/phonologic altherapy, Bowen, 2001), in the extensive message archive, and in the group's outstanding collection of links and resource files. Over the years, people have joined phonologicaltherapy for a variety of reasons. Some enjoy sharing their knowledge, many love a good exchange of ideas, and lots like to ask questions and have them answered – and they usually *are* answered. Others, especially those in academic settings, have been eager to stay in touch with the 'clinical reality' and stay appraised of what clinicians in the field are thinking and doing, whereas people in isolated work settings join for support and contact with peers. Many members appreciate, and constantly access, the extensive collection of child speech-related links and informational files, including important journal articles, available on the group website.

The primary topic for the group is children's speech sound disorders, including phonological disorders, CAS, functional articulation disorders and speech production difficulties associated with craniofacial differences, and syndromes.

Discussions also concern 'older' children whose phonological or other speech sound difficulties persist, and who have phonological awareness, literacy, and language-processing problems. Most members of the group are SLPs/SLTs and Linguists, including clinicians, university teachers and researchers. There are also many undergraduate and graduate students of communication sciences and disorders, and a few consumers.

Alongside the rise of Facebook (www.face book.com), Twitter (https://twitter.com), Pinterest (www.pinterest.com) and other social media (Bowen, 2012, 2013b) for SLP/SLT professional purposes has come a reduction in the use of SLP/SLT-related electronic mailing lists such as LISTSERV®, MAJORDOMO, Yahoo Groups and Google Groups. It is difficult to know what will happen to the established mailing lists over the next few years, but the current plan is to leave phonologicaltherapy in place, even if the discussion dwindles away, so that the profession can access the resources.

References

Baker, E., & McLeod, S. (2004). Evidence-based management of phonological impairment in children. *Child Language Teaching and Therapy, 20*(3), 265–285.

Bandura, A. (1994). Self-efficacy. In: V.S. Ramachaudran (Ed.), *Encyclopedia of human behavior* (Vol. 4, pp. 71–81). New York, NY: Academic Press. (Reprinted in H. Friedman [Ed.], *Encyclopedia of mental health*. San Diego, CA: Academic Press, 1998).

Barlow, J. A., & Gierut, J. A. (2002). Minimal pair approaches to phonological remediation. *Seminars in Speech and Language, 2*(1), 57–67.

Bernthal, J. E., Bankson, N. W., & Flipsen, P., Jr. (2013). *Articulation and phonological disorders* (7th ed.). Boston, MA: Pearson Education.

Bessell, A., Sell, D., Whiting, P., Roulstone, S., Albery, L., & Persson, M. (2013). Speech and language therapy interventions for children with cleft palate: A systematic review. *The Cleft Palate-Craniofacial Journal, 50*, e1–e17.

Bowen, C. (2001). *Children's speech sound disorders (phonologicaltherapy) discussion group. Retrieved*

15 January 2014 from http://groups.yahoo.com/neo/groups/phonologicaltherapy/info

Bowen, C. (2005). What is the evidence for . . . ? Oral motor therapy. *ACQuiring Knowledge in Speech, Language, and Hearing*, 7, 144–147.

Bowen C. (2012). Webwords 44: Life online. *Journal of Clinical Practice in Speech-Language Pathology*, *14*(3), 149–152.

Bowen C. (2013b). Webwords 46: social media in clinical education and continuing professional development. *Journal of Clinical Practice in Speech-Language Pathology*. *15*(2), 104–106.

Bowen, C., & Rippon, H. (2013). *Consonant Clusters: Alliterative Stories and Activities for Phonological Intervention*. Cowling, Keighley: Black Sheep Press.

Cameron, J., Banko, K. M., & Pierce, W. D. (2001). Pervasive negative effects of rewards on intrinsic motivation: The myth continues. *The Behavior Analyst*, *24*, 1–44.

Chomsky, N., & Halle, M. (1968). *The sound pattern of English*. New York, NY: Harper and Row.

Crystal, D. (1996). Language play and linguistic intervention. *Child Language Teaching and Therapy*, *12*, 328–344.

Dean, E.C., Howell, J., Waters, D., & Reid, J. (1995). *Metaphon*: A metalinguistic approach to the treatment of phonological disorder in children. *Clinical Linguistics and Phonetics*, *9*, 1–19.

Dodd, B., & Iacono, T. (1989). A longitudinal study of the speech of children with phonological disorders. *British Journal of Disorders of Communication*, *24*, 333–351.

Edwards, M. L., & Shriberg, L. D. (1983). *Phonology: Applications in communicative disorders*. San Diego, CA: College-Hill Press.

Eisenson, J., & Ogilvie, M. (1963). *Speech correction in the schools*. New York, NY: Macmillan.

Elbert, M., Dinnsen, D., & Powell, T. (1984). On the prediction of phonological generalisation learning pattern. *Journal of Speech and Hearing Disorders*, *49*, 309–317.

Elbert, M., Powell, T. W., & Swartzlander, P. (1991). Toward a technology of generalization: How many exemplars are sufficient? *Journal of Speech and Hearing Research*, *34*, 81–87.

Flipsen, P., Jr., & Parker, R. G. (2008). Phonological patterns in the speech of children with

cochlear implants. *Journal of Communication Disorders*, *41*(4), 337–357.

Galton, R., & Simpson, A. (1958). *The Publicity Photograph*, Hancock's Half Hour, BBC, Retrieved 15 January 2014 from www.youtube.com/watch?v=EHijvPFMdlg

Gierut, J. A. (1986). On the assessment of productive phonological knowledge. *National Student Speech-Language-Hearing Association Journal*, *14*, 83–101.

Gierut, J. A. (1992). The conditions and course of clinically induced phonological change. *Journal of Speech and Hearing Research*, *35*, 1049–1063.

Gierut, J. A. (1999). Syllable onsets: Clusters and adjuncts in acquisition. *Journal of Speech, Language and Hearing Research*, *42*, 708–726.

Gierut, J. (2001). Complexity in phonological treatment: Clinical factors. *Language, Speech, and Hearing in Schools*, *32*, 229–241.

Gierut, J. (2007). Phonological complexity and language learnability. *American Journal of Speech-Language Pathology*, *16*(1), 6–17.

Gierut, J. A., & Champion, A. H. (2001). Syllable onsets II: Three-element clusters in phonological treatment. *Journal of Speech, Language, and Hearing Research*, *44*, 886–904.

Gierut, J. A., Morrisette, M. L., Hughes, M. T., & Rowland, S. (1996). Phonological treatment efficacy and developmental norms. *Language, Speech and Hearing Services in Schools*, *27*, 215–230.

Gierut, J. A., & O'Connor, K. M. (2002). Precursors to onset clusters in acquisition. *Journal of Child Language*, *29*, 495–517.

Golding-Kushner, K. J. (1995). Treatment of articulation and resonance disorders associated with cleft palate and VPI. In: R. J. Shprintzen, & J. Bardach (Eds.), *Cleft palate speech management: A multidisciplinary approach* (pp. 327–351). St. Louis, MO: Mosby.

Golding-Kushner, K. J. (2001). *Therapy techniques for cleft palate speech and related disorders*. San Diego, CA: Singular.

Golding-Kushner, K. J. (2004). Treatment of sound system disorders associated with cleft palate speech. *SID 5 Newsletter*, *14*, 16–19.

Grunwell, P. (1989). Developmental phonological disorders and normal speech development: A review and illustration. *Child Language Teaching and Therapy*, *5*, 304–319.

Hanson, M. L. (1983). *Articulation*. Philadelphia, PA: W. B. Saunders Co.

Hardin-Jones, M. A., & Jones, D. L. (2005). Speech production of preschoolers with cleft palate. *Cleft Palate-Craniofacial Journal*, *42*, 7–13.

Henderlong, J., & Lepper, M. R. (2002). The effects of praise on children's intrinsic motivation: A review and synthesis. *Psychological Bulletin*, *128*(5), 774–795.

Henningsson, G., & Isberg, A. (1986). Velopharyngeal movements in patients alternating between oral and glottal articulation: a clinical and cineradiographical study. *Cleft Palate Journal*, *23*, 1–9.

Hodson, B. (2007, 2010). *Evaluating and enhancing children's phonological systems: Research and theory to practice.* Wichita, KS: PhonoComp Publishers.

Khan, L., & Lewis, N. (1983). *Khan–Lewis phonological analysis.* Circle Pines, MN: AGS.

Kilminster, M. G. E., & Laird, E. M. (1978). Articulation development in children aged three to nine years. *Australian Journal of Human Communication Disorders*, *6*(1), 23–30.

Klein, E. S. (1996b).*Clinical phonology: Assessment and treatment of articulation disorders in children and adults.* San Diego, CA: Singular Publishing Group, Inc.

Koegel, L., Koegel, R., & Ingham, J. (1986). Programming rapid generalization of correct articulation through self-monitoring procedures. *Journal of Speech and Hearing Disorders*, *51*, 24–32.

Kuhn, T. S. (1977). *The essential tension: Selected studies in scientific tradition and change.* Chicago, IL: University of Chicago Press.

Kummer, A. W. (2001a). Perceptual assessment. In: A. W. Kummer (Ed.), *Cleft palate and craniofacial anomalies: The effects of speech and resonance* (pp. 265–292). San Diego, CA: Singular.

Kummer, A. W. (2001b). Speech therapy for effects of velopharyngeal dysfunction. In: A. W. Kummer (Ed.), *Cleft palate and craniofacial anomalies: The effects of speech and resonance* (pp. 459–482). San Diego, CA: Singular.

Kummer, A. W., Strife, J. L., Grau, W. H., Creaghead, N. A., & Lee, L. (1989). The effects of Le Fort I osteotomy with maxillary advancement on articulation, resonance, and velopharyngeal function. *Cleft Palate Journal*, *26*, 193–199.

Kwiatkowski, J., & Shriberg, L. D. (1993). Speech normalization in developmental phonological disorders: A retrospective study of capability-focus theory. *Language, Speech, and Hearing Services in Schools*, *24*, 10–18.

Kwiatkowski, J., & Shriberg, L. D. (1998). The capability-focus treatment framework for child speech disorders. *American Journal of Speech-Language Pathology*, *7*, 27–38.

Locke, J. L. (1980). The inference of speech perception in the phonologically disordered child. Part II: Some clinically novel procedures, their use, some findings. *Journal of Speech and Hearing Disorders*, *45*, 445–468.

Lowe, R. J. (1994). *Phonology: Assessment and intervention application in speech pathology.* Baltimore, MD: Williams & Wilkins.

Lowe, R. J. (2000). *ALPHA-R: Assessment link between phonology and articulation – Revised.* Mifflinville, PA: ALPHA Speech & Language Resources.

Lowe, R. J. (2002). *Workbook for the identification of phonological processes and distinctive features* (3rd ed.). Austin, TX: Pro-Ed.

Maas, E., Robin, D. A., Austermann Hula, S. N., Freedman, S. E., Wulf, G., Ballard, K. J., & Schmidt, R. A. (2008). Principles of motor learning in treatment of motor speech disorders. *American Journal of Speech-Language Pathology*, *17*(3), 277–298.

Malone, T. W., & Lepper, M. R. (1987). Making learning fun: A taxonomy of intrinsic motivations for learning. In: R. E. Snow & M. J. Farr (Eds.), *Aptitude, learning and instruction: III. Conative and affective process analysis* (pp. 223–253). Hillsdale, NJ: Erlbaum.

Manning, W. H., Keappock, N. E., & Stick, S. L. (1976). The use of auditory masking to estimate automatization of correct articulatory production. *Journal of Speech and Hearing Disorders*, *41*, 143–149.

McCauley, R. J., Strand, E., Lof, G. L., Schooling, T., & Frymark, T. (2009). Evidence-based systematic review: Effects of nonspeech oral motor exercises on speech, *American Journal of Speech-Language Pathology*, *18*, 343–360.

McLeod, S. (2013). Speech sound acquisition. In: J. E. Bernthal, N. W. Bankson, & P. Flipsen, Jr. (Eds.), *Articulation and phonological disorders: Speech sound disorders in children* (7th ed., pp. 58–113). Boston, MA: Pearson Education.

Miccio, A. W., Elbert, M., & Forrest, K. (1999). The relationship between stimulability and phonological acquisition in children with normally developing and disordered phonologies. *American Journal of Speech-Language Pathology*, *8*, 347–363.

Moller, K. T. (1994). Dental-occlusal and other oral conditions and speech. In: J. Bernthal, & N. Bankson (Eds.), *Child phonology: Characteristics, assessment, and intervention with special populations* (pp. 3–28). New York, NY: Theime Medical Publishers.

Morrisette, M. L., Farris, A. W., & Gierut, J. A. (2006). Applications of learnability theory to clinical phonology. *International Journal of Speech-Language Pathology, 8*(3), 207–219.

Munson, B., Baylis, A., Krause, M., & Yim, D-S. (2006). *Representation and access in phonological impairment.* Paper presented at the 10th Conference on Laboratory Phonology, Paris, France, June 30–July 2.

Munson, B., Edwards, J., & Beckman, M. E. (2005). Relationships between nonword repetition accuracy and other measures of linguistic development in children with phonological disorders. *Journal of Speech, Language, and Hearing Research, 48,* 61–78.

Ohala, D. K. (1999). The influence of sonority on children's cluster reductions. *Journal of Communication Disorders, 32,* 397–422.

Peterson-Falzone, S., Trost-Cardamone, J., Hardin-Jones, M., & Karnell, M. (2006). *The Clinician's Guide to Treating Cleft Palate Speech.* St. Louis, MO: Mosby.

Peterson-Falzone, S. J., Hardin-Jones, M. A., & Karnell, M. (2009). *Cleft palate speech* (4th ed.). St. Louis, MO: Mosby.

Pollock, K. E., & Berni, M. C. (2003). Incidence of non-rhotic vowel errors in children: Data from the Memphis Vowel Project. *Clinical Linguistics and Phonetics, 17,* 393–401.

Powell, T. W., & Miccio, A. W. (1996). Stimulability: A useful clinical tool. *Journal of Communication Disorders, 29,* 237–253.

Robb, M. P., Bleile, K. M., & Yee, S. S. L. (1999). A phonetic analysis of vowel errors during the course of treatment. *Clinical Linguistics and Phonetics, 13*(4), 309–321.

Ruscello, D. M. (1993). A motor skill learning treatment program for sound system disorders. *Seminars in Speech and Language, 14,* 106–118.

Ruscello, D. R. (2008a). *Treating Articulation and Phonological Disorders in Children.* St. Louis, MO: Elsevier.

Ruscello, D. M. (2008b). Oral motor treatment issues related to children with developmental speech sound disorders. *Language, Speech, and Hearing Services in Schools, 39*(3), 380–391.

Rvachew, S. (2007). Phonological processing and reading in children with speech sound disorders. *American Journal of Speech-Language Pathology, 16,* 260–270.

Rvachew, S., & Brosseau-Lapré, F. (2012). *Developmental Phonological Disorders: Foundations of Clinical Practice.* San Diego, CA: Plural Publishing.

Rvachew, S., & Nowak, M. (2001). The effect of target-selection strategy of phonological learning. *Journal of Speech, Language and Hearing Research, 44,* 610–623.

Rvachew, S., Rafaat, S., & Martin, M. (1999). Stimulability, speech perception and the treatment of phonological disorders. *American Journal of Speech-Language Pathology, 8,* 33–43.

Schmidt, A. M., & Meyers, K. A. (1995). Traditional and phonological treatment for teaching English fricatives and affricates to Koreans. *Journal of Speech and Hearing Research, 38,* 828–838.

Shriberg, L. D. (1993). Four new speech and prosody-voice measures for genetics research and other studies in developmental phonological disorders. *Journal of Speech and Hearing Research, 36,* 105–140.

Shriberg, L. D. (1997). Developmental phonological disorders: One or many? In: B. W. Hodson, & M. L. Edwards (Eds.), *Perspectives in applied phonology* (pp. 105–132). Gaithersburg, MD: Aspen.

Shriberg, L.D., & Kwiatkowski, J. (1987). A retrospective study of spontaneous generalization in speech-delayed children. *Language, Speech, and Hearing Services in Schools, 18,* 144–157.

Steriade, D. (1990). *Greek prosodies and the nature of syllabification (Doctoral dissertation, Massachusetts Instituted of Technology, 1982).* New York, NY: Garland Press.

Storkel, H. L., Armbruster, J., & Hogan, T. P. (2006). Differentiating phonotactic probability and neighborhood density in adult word learning. *Journal of Speech, Language, and Hearing Research, 49,* 1175–1192.

Storkel, H. L., & Morrisette, M. L. (2002). The lexicon and phonology: Interactions in language acquisition. *Language, Speech and Hearing Services in Schools, 33*(1), 24–37.

Sutherland, D., & Gillon, G. T. (2007). The development of phonological representations and phonological awareness in children with speech impairment.

International Journal of Language and Communication Disorders, *42*(2), 229–250.

Taps Richard, J. (2012). *Complex cluster cards*. San Diego, CA: SLPath.

Taps Richard (2014). *Clusters Complex*. Computer Software. *Apple App Store*. Version 1.0.3. SLPath, 2014. Accessed 5 June 2014.

Tomes, L. A., Kuehn, D. P., & Peterson-Falzone, S. J. (2004). Research considerations for behavioral treatments of velopharyngeal impairment. In: K. Bzoch (Ed.), *Communicative disorders related to cleft lip and palate* (5th ed., pp. 797–846). Austin, TX: Pro-Ed.

Trost-Cardamone, J. E. (2009). Articulation and phonologic assessment procedures and treatment decisions. In: K. T. Moller, & Glaze, L. E. Starr (Eds.), *Cleft lip and palate: Interdisciplinary issues and treatment* (2nd ed., pp. 377–414). Austin, TX: Pro-Ed.

Van Riper, C., & Irwin, J. V. (1958). *Voice and articulation*. Englewood Cliffs, NJ: Prentice Hall.

Weiss, A. L. (2004). The child as agent for change in therapy for phonological disorders. *Child Language Teaching and Therapy*. *20* (3), 221–244.

Williams, A. L. (1991). Generalization patterns associated with training least phonological knowledge. *Journal of Speech and Hearing Research*, *34*, 722–733.

Williams, A. L. (2010). Multiple Oppositions Intervention. In: A.L. Williams, S. McLeod, & R. J. McCauley (Eds.), *Interventions for speech sound disorders in children* (pp. 73–94). Baltimore, MD: Paul H. Brookes Publishing Co.

Chapter 9

Parents and children together in phonological intervention

PACT is an acronym for a family-centred phonological assessment and intervention approach to speech sound disorders called *Parents and Children Together* (Bowen, 2010; Bowen & Cupples, 2006). PACT could just as easily stand for 'parents and child, and therapist' and implies an arrangement in which all are actively involved in the intervention process, while the name itself reflects the child and family focus of the approach. Administered in planned blocks and breaks, PACT is termed 'broad-based' because, while concentrating mostly on the phonemic (phonological or cognitive–linguistic) level, it *also* takes account of phonetic and auditory perceptual factors. This is because the difficulties children diagnosed with phonological disorders experience may not be exclusively 'phonological'. PACT directly targets speech perception and production, and hence intelligibility, in children with phonological disorder. It may also indirectly impact morphosyntax and phonological awareness (particularly phonemic awareness) and hence literacy acquisition. In Chapter 9, PACT is described and illustrated with a case study of Josie, augmented by a contribution by Debbie James in A50, relating to issues that arose.

More PACT information can be accessed at www.speech-language-therapy.com. Click on the ARTICLES tab in the header of any page, and go to 'Intervention'. On that page are links to four PACT-related pages: *Implementation*, *Publications*, *Theory and Evidence* and *Therapy for Josie*. On the latter page is a slide show about Josie's intervention and progress, and links to activities and resources used in treating her severe phonological disorder that involved a mix of phonemic, perceptual and phonetic issues.

Primary population

PACT was designed for 3- to 6-year olds and validated as an effective treatment for children in this age range diagnosed with mild, moderate and severe phonological disorders (Bowen, 1996a; Bowen & Cupples, 1999a, b). The children in the efficacy study were typical of children with intelligibility difficulties in that they did not necessarily have 'pure' phonological disorder. Whereas children with language impairment, including SLI, were excluded from the study, and each of the children's major communication difficulty was

Children's Speech Sound Disorders, Second Edition. Caroline Bowen.
© 2015 John Wiley & Sons, Ltd. Published 2015 by John Wiley & Sons, Ltd.
Companion website: www.wiley.com/go/bowen/speechlanguagetherapy

at the phonological level, the major contributing component was often accompanied by phonetic execution and auditory perceptual difficulties. Moreover, some participants were treated for stuttering (Unicomb, Hewat, Spencer & Harrison, 2013) during the intervention process.

Why 3- to 6-year olds?

We had a twofold rationale for developing a therapy for pre-schoolers and younger school children. First, intelligibility difficulties may be obvious in 2- and 3-year olds (Dodd, A10; McIntosh & Dodd, 2011), but diagnosis of SSD is usually elusive until sometime in a child's fourth year. Withholding intervention, however, until diagnosis is 'definite' can prove counterproductive in the longer term. Second, we wanted to develop an intervention that families could access before their children started formal schooling, potentially 'catching' many of the children before they were busy (and often tired) and inaccessible – in the sense of not wanting to miss school – to attend speech therapy, and pre-empting or minimising literacy acquisition difficulties.

Secondary populations

Clinicians have reported acceptable outcomes with PACT with other populations, but such implementation has not been tested experimentally. The 'other' children have included 3;0- to 6;11-year olds with language processing and production issues *and* SSD; and children with speech production issues ≤10 years with SLI; ≤10 years with pragmatic issues; growing up bilingual (and multilingual; Goldstein, A19; McLeod, Verdon & Bowen, 2013; Ray, 2002) and with developmental delay; as well as children with clefts, autism spectrum disorder, Down syndrome, Fragile X syndrome, Williams syndrome and cochlear implants. Although not designed specifically for children with CAS, it has been incorporated, with integral stimulation (Strand, Stoeckel & Baas, 2006), and compatible techniques that follow the principles

of motor learning (Schmidt & Lee, 2011), to help treat children diagnosed with CAS.

Theoretical basis

PACT is based on the assumptions that phonemic change is (1) gradual and motivated by homophony (Grunwell, 1987); (2) enhanced through metalinguistic awareness of phones (the phonetic level) and the phonemic system (the phonological level); and (3) facilitated by heightened perceptual saliency of contrasts because it increases their learnability. PACT embraces the foundations of all minimal pair approaches (Fey, 1992) by systematically modifying groups of sounds produced in error; emphasising the elimination of homophony (i.e., different words pronounced the same way) and the establishment of feature contrasts to mark meaning distinctions, rather than putting the spotlight on accurate sound production; and making it explicit to children that the function of phonology is communication. This is achieved in PACT by working at word level and above, using naturalistic parent–child communicative contexts, increasing the child's (and parents') metaphonological awareness, and targeting, as required, phonological, phonetic, phonotactic and perceptual goals.

Empirical support

In the efficacy study, a longitudinal matched groups design was employed, with assessment, treatment and reassessment (probe) phases. Fourteen children were treated under typical clinical conditions, and treatment was withheld from eight matched children on waiting lists. At probe, the treated children showed accelerated and highly selective improvement in their productive phonology [$F(1,20) = 19.36$, $P < 0.01$], whereas the untreated eight did not. No such selective improvement was observed in the treated children in either receptive vocabulary or Mean Length of Utterance in Morphemes, attesting to the specific effect of the therapy. PACT is practicable (Robey &

Schultz, 1998) under conditions of everyday practice in terms of the in-clinic component (Bowen & Cupples, 1998, 1999a), and it is feasible and often enjoyable for interested families implementing homework and follow-up away from the clinic (Bowen & Cupples, 2004).

Assessment

A 200-utterance conversational speech (CS) sample, or a 200-word CS sample, *and* single words (SWs) elicited using the *Quick Screener* (Bowen, 1996b, after Dean, Howell, Hill & Waters, 1990) usually provide sufficient data to allow independent and relational analyses (Stoel-Gammon, A9) and diagnosis, or provisional diagnosis, of phonological impairment. Additional testing is sometimes necessary, and this might entail administration of the DEAP (Dodd, Crosbie, Zhu, Holm & Ozanne, 2002) or the HAPP-3 (Hodson, 2004), the Locke Speech Perception Task (Locke, 1980; see Tables 8.6a and 8.6b), and an imitative PCC (Johnson, Weston & Bain, 2004). Speech assessment within the PACT approach, whether initial or ongoing, is integral to intervention. As parents play a central role in management, it is highly desirable for them to be aware—through observation, participation and explanation—of the speech-language assessment process. Essential components of data gathering are the case history interview; an audiological evaluation by an Audiologist; screening for language, pragmatics, voice and fluency strengths and difficulties; an oral musculature examination; and, as noted above, a CS sample of 200 utterances, if possible, remembering that, for some children, single word tokens may predominate. Within the case history interview, parents are asked to provide an intelligibility rating using a scale of 1–5: (1) completely intelligible; (2) mostly intelligible; (3) somewhat intelligible; (4) mostly unintelligible; and (5) completely unintelligible. This is recorded at the top of the *Quick Screener* data collection form displayed in Figure 9.1.

If the child's output is so unintelligible that the clinician cannot even guess the content, or if time is short or the child's cooperation difficult to establish, an imitative PCC procedure is used rather than the conversational PCC procedure (Flipsen Jr., A11). Johnson et al. (2004) found that PCCs derived from conversational samples did not differ significantly from PCCs drawn from sentence imitation, using age-appropriate vocabulary, syntax and representative distribution of speech sounds in children aged 4–6. They concluded that 'the sentence imitation procedure offers a valid and efficient alternative to conversational sampling'. In their experiment, an almost wordless picture book, *Carl Goes to Daycare* (Day, 1993), provided visual stimuli for the repetition task, and the 36 short sentences, potentially containing 273 consonants, the children repeated after the examiner included, 'Watch them dance', 'He got cold', and 'Time to go home'.

Quick Screener

Speech assessment begins with the administration of the *Quick Screener*, while parents observe, using the data collection form displayed in Figure 9.1. The SLP/SLT phonetically transcribes in full, with necessary diacritics, the child's production of the first word 'cup' and immediately assigns a score that goes in the 'CC' (consonants correct) column. For example, if the child says [kʌp] the score is 2; if he or she says [kʌ], [ʌp], [tʌp] or [gʌp] the score is 1; and if he or she says [ʌ] or [tʌ] the score is zero. Each word is scored for consonant production in this way. There are approximately 100 consonants in the sample, depending on the dialect of English, so a tentative single-word PCC can be estimated quickly, with parents watching, by adding the figures in the CC columns and calling the sum a percentage. For example, if the child scores 55 consonants correct, his or her tentative PCC, or screening PCC, is 55%. There is also provision on the form to record vowel errors. The vowel and diphthong targets on the data collection form reflect non-rhotic Australian English. Therapists working with children speaking other varieties of English can change the vowel symbols, and 'vowelless' forms are

Quick Screener

SINGLE-WORD SCREENING SAMPLE USING THE METAPHON STIMULUS VOCABULARY

Dean, E., Howell, J., Hill, A., & Waters, D. (1990). Metaphon Resource Pack. Windsor, Berks: NFER Nelson

Date of Birth	Observer(s)
Today's date	Examiner

① completely intelligible ② mostly intelligible ③ somewhat intelligible ④ mostly unintelligible ⑤ completely unintelligible

#	TARGET	TRANSCRIPTION	CC	#	TARGET	TRANSCRIPTION	CC
1	cup	ʌ		23	jam	æ	
2	gone	ɒ		24	house	aʊ	
3	knife	aɪ		25	path	a	
4	sharp	a		26	door	ɔ	
5	fish	ɪ		27	smoke	oʊ	
6	kiss	ɪ		28	bridge	ɪ	
7	sock	ɒ		29	train	eɪ	
8	glass	a		30	chair	ɛə	
9	watch	ɒ		31	red	ɛ	
10	nose	oʊ		32	spoon	u	
11	mouth	aʊ		33	plane	eɪ	
12	yawn	ɔ		34	fly	aɪ	
13	leaf	i		35	sky	aɪ	
14	thumb	ʌ		36	sun	ʌ	
15	foot	ʊ		37	wing	ɪ	
16	toe	oʊ		38	splash	æ	
17	snake	eɪ		39	tent	ɛ	
18	van	æ		40	salt	ɒ	
19	fast	a		41	crab	æ	
20	girl	ɜ		42	sweet	i	
21	stairs	ɛə		43	sleeve	i	
22	big	ɪ		44	zipper	ɪ ə	

Check ɔɪ boy ɪə ear   **SUBTOTAL CC:**   **TOTAL CC:**

TENTATIVE single word phonetic inventory (≈100 consonants in sample) and PVC (47 vowels/diphthongs in sample)

Vowels	i	ɪ	ɛ	æ	a	ʌ	ə	ɜ	ɒ	ɔ	ʊ	u	**Vowels correct (47)** %
Obstruents	p	b	t	d	k	g	f	v					**Consonants correct (≈ 100)** %
Obstruents	θ	ð	s	z	ʃ	ʒ	tʃ	dʒ	**STIMULABILITY**				
Sonorants	m	n	ŋ	l	r	w	j	h					**MARKED** p t k f v θ ð s z ʃ ʒ tʃ dʒ

List phonological processes/record observations

Figure 9.1 The Quick Screener data collection form. From Bowen (1996b), after Dean et al. (1990).

available at www.speech-language-therapy.com. If the child mispronounces the vowel or diphthong in a word, the vowel or diphthong is circled by the therapist and later tallied to calculate a screening, single-word, percentage of vowels correct (PVC) using the formula VOWELS CORRECT ÷ 47 × 100 = PVC (again, while parents observe). It should be remembered that the PCC and the PVC derived from the screener are *screening* (tentative) measures, although it has been observed clinically that there is little variation in PCC and PVC scores between data gathered via the *Quick Screener* and larger data sets.

Using the *Quick Screener* analysis form displayed in Figure 9.2, the clinician summarises the child's phonological processes as percentages of occurrence, if this is considered useful, and records pertinent observations, including the therapist's own intelligibility rating. These outcomes are discussed in the child's hearing. It is explained to parents that the child's continued presence during discussion demonstrates to the child that his or her parents are important partners in the therapy process. It also helps to acknowledge parents, up front, as the homework experts and experts where their own child is concerned.

The word set contained in *Quick Screener* is based on the *Metaphon Resource Pack Screening Test* developed by Dean et al. (1990) with the word 'gun' changed to 'gone'. The stimulus pictures, data collection forms and analysis form are freely available at www.speech-language-therapy.com. Word productions can be elicited using the *Metaphon Resource Pack Screening Test* easel book (now unfortunately out of print), or the *Quick Screener* pictures presented as a slide show, or printed on cards. I prefer the slide show option, not least because children usually find it interesting and fun, *and*, quite remarkably, frequently ask to do it 'again'! The data collection form has space for recording stimulability data and the child's inventory of marked consonants. In stimulability testing, the child is asked to directly imitate vowels in isolation and CVs, usually [ba bi bu] etc. focusing on vowels and diphthongs already circled on the form; and consonants of interest in CV or VC contexts, or both, but not usually in

isolation. Marked consonants in the child's inventory are circled, from a choice of /p t k f v θ ð s z ʃ ʒ tʃ ʤ/. The stimulability and markedness data are later used in the decision-making process for treatment target selection, as outlined in Chapter 8.

Assessing progress

It is usual to reassess, using the *Quick Screener*, with parent observation, at the beginning of each intervention block (immediately after a break from intervention), allowing parents, who are often particularly interested in the inventories and percentages, to observe and discuss any changes. Additional testing may be required; for example, the DEAP, HAPP-3 or the Locke Task might be repeated. Any decision to terminate or continue therapy is made jointly with parents (see Baker, 2010 for thoughtful discussion).

Goals and goal attack

Table 1.3 provides a schema within which to view three levels of intervention goal. The basic goal of PACT is to work at word level or above to encourage phonological reorganisation, thus facilitating the emergence of clear speech. This basic goal is achieved by increasing a child's consonant, vowel, syllable-shape, syllable-stress, phonotactic and suprasegmental repertoires and accuracy; and by promoting generalisation of new segments, structures and prosodic features to increasingly challenging contexts and situations. The intermediate goal is to target groups of sounds related by an organising principle (processes, rules or patterns), addressing phonetic and perceptual levels as required. Specific intervention goals are to target a sound, sounds or syllable structures, using horizontal strategies: targeting several sounds within a sound class or manner of production, or syllable structure category, and/or targeting more than one process or deviation or structure simultaneously.

Velar fronting

#	Target SI	0 / 1	#	Target SF	0 / 1
1	cup		7	sock	
6	kiss		17	snake	
2	gone		22	big	
20	girl		37	wing	
	TOTAL	/4		TOTAL	/4

Palato-alveolar fronting

#	Target SI	0 / 1	#	Target SF	0 / 1
4	sharp		5	fish	
30	chair		9	watch	
23	jam		28	bridge	
	TOTAL	/3		TOTAL	/3

Word-final devoicing

#	Target	0 / 1	#	Target	0 / 1
41	crab		43	sleeve	
31	red		10	nose	
22	big		28	bridge	
				TOTAL	/6

Backing

#	Target SI	0 / 1	#	Target SF	0 / 1
16	toe		15	foot	
39	tent		42	sweet	
26	door		31	red	
	TOTAL	/3		TOTAL	/3

Stopping of fricatives

#	Target SI	0 / 1	#	Target SF	0 / 1
5	fish		13	leaf	
15	foot		11	mouth	
14	thumb		6	kiss	
7	sock		38	splash	
36	sun		43	sleeve	
4	sharp		10	nose	
18	van				
44	zip(per)				
	TOTAL	/8		TOTAL	/6

Stopping of affricates

#	Target SI	0 / 1	#	Target SF	0 / 1
30	chair		9	watch	
23	jam		28	bridge	
	TOTAL	/2		TOTAL	/2

Pre-vocalic voicing

#	Target	0 / 1	#	Target	0 / 1
25	path		5	fish	
16	toe		14	thumb	
6	kiss		36	sun	
			4	sharp	
				TOTAL	/7

Liquid/glide simplification

#	Target	0 / 1	#	Target	0 / 1
9	watch		12	yawn	
13	leaf		31	red	
				TOTAL	/4

Initial consonant deletion

#	Target	0 / 1	#	Target	0 / 1
3	knife		7	sock	
22	big		30	chair	
18	van		12	yawn	
				TOTAL	/6

Final consonant deletion

#	Target SI	0 / 1	#	Target SF	0 / 1
23	jam		10	nose	
44	zip		5	fish	
31	red		28	bridge	
				TOTAL	/6

Initial cluster reduction

#	Target SI	0 / 1	#	Target SI	0 / 1
33	plane		43	sleeve	
8	glass		27	smoke	
28	bridge		17	snake	
29	train		32	spoon	
41	crab		21	stairs	
34	fly		35	sky	
42	sweet		38	splash	
				TOTAL	/14

Final cluster reduction

#	Target	0 / 1	#	Target	0 / 1
19	fast		40	salt	
39	tent				
				TOTAL	/3

Figure 9.2 Quick Screener analysis form

Goal selection and attack strategies are primarily therapist-driven and explained to parents. Multiple goals are addressed in and across treatment sessions and within homework, sequentially and simultaneously, and rarely cyclically. For example, Emeline, 5;1, in Session 4 of her second therapy block, had three concurrent goals. First, a phonetic goal to produce /dʒ/ and /tʃ/ in onset and coda in six practice words; second, a phonological goal to recognise distinctions in input, and to mark distinctions in output in short phrases between the cognate pairs /p b/, /t d/ and /k g/ (e.g., with Emeline instructing and adult to 'Touch the *pea/bee'*, 'Touch the *toe/doe'*, 'Touch the *cap/gap'*; and then switching roles); and a generalisation goal to use the voiceless fricatives /f/, /s/ and /ʃ/ in conversational speech in untrained words in the therapy session and during an agreed daily period at home.

Materials and equipment

The materials and equipment required consist of toys, vowel and consonant pictures on cards and worksheets, a 'speech book' (exercise book, ring binder or scrapbook), drawing and 'making' materials and equipment, rewards such as stamps and stickers, a desktop, laptop or tablet computer for slide shows and the administration of the *Quick Screener* and an audio recorder to record therapy snippets. It is helpful but not essential for the family to have a computer and audio recorder. One option is for them to use a tablet (e.g., iPad or Android and an inexpensive voice recorder App such as *iTalk Recorder Premium* from Griffin Technology (http://store.griffintechnology.com/italk-premium). Pictures in speech books and on cards usually include printed captions to clarify what the target words are meant to be. Captions are printed consistent with the way in which early literacy instruction is commonly delivered, with all words printed in lower case, and capital letters used only for the beginnings of proper nouns. Suitable pictures are available to clinicians and families, at no cost, at www.speech-language-therapy.com.

Intervention

Therapy sessions

The clinician sees the child for 50–60 minutes (usually 50 minutes) once per week in therapy blocks. The minimum parent participation involves the parent joining the therapist and child for 20 minutes at the end of a session, or 10 minutes at the beginning and end; and the maximum parent participation sees parents staying 50–60 minutes. The parent assumes the role of a dynamic collaborator in a treatment triad with child and therapist. Segments of parent participation always require the child's continued involvement, to properly demonstrate what should happen at home. The following is an outline of a 50-minute session for Iain, 5;7, with his father Gordon and a therapist, towards the end of his second treatment block (of three) in which one treatment target was addressed.

Iain had a persistent [n] for /l/ sound replacement SIWI, and over the previous 2 weeks, had *finally* become stimulable for /l/ in CVs by dint of every phonetic placement technique the therapist knew—or at least it felt that way! Gordon left Iain with the therapist for 15 minutes while he dropped his wife Lucinda at a railway station and took 7-year old Bruce to school, returning for the final 35 minutes of the session with Iain's brother Fergus, 18 months, who played happily alone while work proceeded. Iain had already engaged in items 1–3 with the therapist.

1. Rhyming auditory bombardment using five pictured, captioned (in lower case printing), minimal pairs: *snip-slip, snap-slap, snow-slow, snug-slug, sneak-sleek*, was presented. The pairs were spoken to Iain at a comfortable conversational loudness level, and then he played a quick game of 'Point to the one I say', with the therapist saying the words and Iain pointing.

2. Next was auditory input cloze with the same captioned pictures, with Iain saying the sn-words that he was already able to pronounce correctly: Adult: *Slow* rhymes with ... Iain:

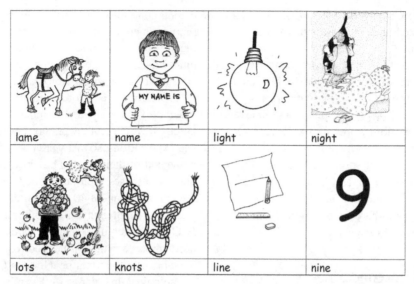

lame	name	light	night
lots	knots	line	nine

Figure 9.3 /l/ versus /n/ minimal word pairs. Drawings by Helen Rippon, Speech and Language Therapist, www.blacksheeppress.co.uk

snow Adult: *Slap* rhymes with . . . Iain: *snap*, etc.

3. A minimal pairs 'silent sorting' task followed. Four cards (*name, night, knots* and *nine*) were placed on the table, and Iain was encouraged to 'think the words' as he placed a rhyming word (from a choice of *lame, light, lots* and *line*) beside each (see Figure 9.3).

4. Gordon began participating in the session at this point. Iain was shown a page of pictures of late, lei, lap, let, light, lock, lick, lame, lead, lit and lice, and told, 'This time, Iain, you be the teacher and tell me if I say these words the right way or the wrong way'. Taking the role of 'student', Gordon made deliberate random errors, emulating Iain's sound replacement (e.g., 'Nate' for 'late', 'neigh' for 'lei', 'nap for 'lap' as single word inputs or in short utterances, e.g., 'He is *late* for school' vs. 'He is *Nate* for school'). All Iain had to do was tell the 'student' whether he was right or wrong without modelling correct pronunciation.

5. The therapist, and then Gordon, presented a 'fixed-up-one routine' for /n/ versus /l/.

6. The clinician presented a homophony confrontation task with *lei-neigh, lap-nap, lame-name* and *low-no*, and this was the one task not included in homework.

7. All three rehearsed a Knock-Knock joke (Knock, knock. Who's there? Lettuce. Lettuce who? Lettuce in!). This was then recorded several times on the same recording, with Iain saying 'Lettuce' and 'Lettuce in' and his father saying 'Who's there' and 'Lettuce who?'

8. The auditory bombardment was delivered again and recorded, so that it followed the 'lettuce' humour. It consisted of *snip-slip, snap-slap, snow-slow, snug-slug, sneak-sleek*, as in item one above, followed by 15 words in sequence: *leaf, lamb, lock, label, lead, lie, lake, lion, lip, letter, lunch, llama, lamp, lettuce.*

9. Homework, comprising activities 2–4 and 6–8, was explained by the clinician, demonstrated by the clinician and Iain, and then rehearsed by Iain and Gordon. Iain tried the Knock-Knock joke out on his father several more times, and the recording with the joke and bombardment sequences, with a running time of 2.5 minutes, was played.

10. In the context of putting 'children' on a toy school bus, Gordon, therapist, and Iain sang 'Lettuce-in, lettuce-in, lettuce-in', 'Lettuce-go, lettuce-go, lettuce-go', and 'Lettuce-out, lettuce-out, lettuce-out' to the tune of 'Here

we go, here we go, here we go' on the recording to take home, increasing the running time to 4 minutes.

11. How to reinforce /l/ using frequent recasting was discussed with Gordon (parent education), and suggestions for thematic play were made around the words 'llama' and 'line' and making up more words for the 'lettuce song' ('Lettuce stop', 'Lettuce start', 'Lettuce see', etc.). They were to do all the activities except number 6 at home, and instructions and pictures were included in Iain's speech book for Lucinda, who shared over half the homework-load with Gordon.

Intervention scheduling

A unique feature of PACT is its administration in planned blocks and breaks (Bowen & Cupples, 2004) that are intended to

- accommodate the gradualness of speech acquisition, mimicking typical development;
- allow for spurts and plateaus in development;
- make 'space' for consolidation of new speech skills;
- make 'space' for phonological generalisation;
- make 'space' for untrained spontaneous gains; and
- provide periodic respite, allowing families to refresh and regroup.

Dosage

The initial block and break are usually about 10 weeks each, and then the number of therapy sessions per block tends to reduce while the period between blocks remains more or less constant at 10 weeks. A typical schedule is 10 weeks on, 10 weeks off, 8 weeks on, 10 weeks off, 4–6 weeks on. It is suggested to parents that, during the breaks, they do no formal practice for up to 8 weeks. In the 2 weeks prior to the next block, they are asked to enjoy looking through the speech book with the child a few times and to do any activities the child wants to do. Although they do not do homework or revision in the breaks, the child's

parents continue to provide modelling corrections, reinforcement of revisions and repairs and pursue metalinguistic activities, incidentally, as opportunities arise, using the strategies learned in 'parent education' in the therapy block(s).

Typically those children with phonological disorder *only* have needed a mean of 21 consultations for their output phonology to fall within age-expectations, so many are ready for discharge at the end of their second block (about 30 weeks after initial assessment) or immediately after their second break (about 40 weeks after initial assessment). A small number of children engaged in PACT have required a third block; fewer have needed four; and there is no record of a child needing more than four treatment blocks. Children with phonological disorder as well as mild language or fluency difficulties have required about the same volume of therapy for speech, but most have continued having intervention for longer to address their other, non-speech goals.

Target selection

Like goal selection and attack, target selection (with exceptions like Shaun's wanting to work on /ʃ/ to pronounce his own name correctly) is therapist-driven, and the reasons certain targets are given preferential treatment are explained to parents. As part of a stopping pattern, Shaun, 4;9, mentioned in Chapter 8, called himself 'Dawn'. An adult neighbour whose name actually was Dawn, apparently oblivious to the misery it evoked and angry requests from Shaun to 'Stop it', teased him endlessly to the point where *all* he and his mother were interested in doing in therapy was to work on /ʃ/ in just one word – *Shaun* (which we did, with a successful outcome). In selecting treatment targets, the clinician uses linguistic criteria, taking into account motivational factors and attributes of the child and parents; is flexible in terms of feature contrasts; and applies evidence and clinical judgement. Traditional and newer criteria (see Table 8.1 and the discussion that follows it) may be applied to isolating optimal targets.

Sometimes it is necessary to fall back on other, more traditional criteria. Take Tessa for example

(Bowen, 2010). Superficially, Tessa 5;10, was a perfect candidate for a least knowledge approach using high-frequency lexical targets because she had a phonetic inventory of only 13 consonants, a PCC of 38%, and extensive homophony. Or *was* she? She was a fretful, diffident child with wary, apprehensive parents, ready to abandon therapy if the clinician attempted anything 'too hard'. These three were unsuited to complex maximal oppositions or empty set feature contrasts, for which Tessa had least knowledge. They needed to ease into intervention via a gentler, albeit less potent, approach using unmarked, stimulable, inconsistently erred, early developing sounds; low-frequency words with low neighbourhood density; and minimal feature contrasts. Once they were all ready to trust the clinician's target choices and confront more difficult tasks, Tessa took more risks, handling the challenges of multiply opposed word sets within the Multiple Exemplar Training component of PACT.

PACT components

PACT has five dynamic and interacting components: Parent Education (Family Education), Metalinguistic Training, Phonetic Production Training, Multiple Exemplar Training (Auditory Input and Minimal Contrasts Therapy), and Homework. The therapy involves the child, primary caregiver(s) and therapist; and sometimes significant others, including older siblings, grandparents and teachers, become involved in homework.

Parent education (Family education)

Rationale

Recognising that PACT will not suit every child or every family, we hypothesised that arming interested parents with techniques (e.g., modelling, recasting, fostering repair strategies and providing alliterative input in thematic play contexts) related to their own child's intervention needs, and by working with them collaboratively, we would tap a unique and powerful 'therapeutic resource'. Unique because a child (usually) only has one set

of parents, and powerful because (usually) parents likely spend the most time with their child and are most motivated to help. Through supportive parent education, they would be guided to use 'speech time' optimally in homework and incidentally in real (not contrived) communicative contexts as natural opportunities arose. This might lead to the need for less consultation and fewer child–clinician contact hours, and ensure that planned breaks from therapy were used more productively.

Methods

Incorporating simple principles of adult learning (Knowles, 1970), parents learn techniques, explained in plain-English (Bowen, 1998a, b), including: delivering modelling and recasting, encouraging self-monitoring and self-correction, using labelled praise and providing focused auditory input. Employing clinical judgement and responding to parent feedback, parent education is delivered according to need (Bowen & Cupples, 2004). It may happen in the form of modelling, counselling, direct instruction, observation, scripted routines, participation and discussion in assessment and therapy sessions, as well as role-playing, 'coaching' and rehearsal. For some families, this involves independent reading of handouts and publications (Bowen, 1998a, b; Flynn & Lancaster, 1996) and viewing informational slide shows that are e-mailed to them or accessed from www.speech-language-therapy.com, viewed on home computers, and later discussed. Some families need more support than this and are 'talked through' informational handouts and view individualised (for them and their child) slide shows in-clinic, explained carefully by the therapist.

Written information is provided in a speech book that often becomes a prized possession of the child's, particularly if it features his or her own artwork. It is used to facilitate communication between therapist, family and others involved (e.g., grandparents or teachers). It includes current targets and goals, a progress record, homework activities, developmental norms and information about intervention for SSD. Parents and teachers are encouraged to contribute to the book: recording progress, commenting on homework content and performance, noting favourite activities or their own innovations and often giving important pointers to the therapist that might otherwise be unavailable. For instance, Bowen & Cupples (2004) reported that Sophie, 4;3, with a moderate-to-severe SSD, talked constantly at home and was animated and chatty in the clinic, but that her teacher surprised (and enlightened) the therapist and her parents when she wrote in the speech book: 'I enjoy working with Sophie and doing the activities in her book. She is very responsive in the one-on-one – loves it – but if I try to involve another child or two she clams up completely. I think you should know that she never speaks to her kindy peers – only to teachers and the aide, and only one-to-one, and in a quiet voice we can hardly hear'. The teacher's insightful note led to providing pre-school personnel with strategies that fostered Sophie's ability to communicate with her peers (see 'Adult Communicative Styles and Encouraging Reticent Children to Converse' at www.speech-language-therapy.com).

Discussion

Parents of the children in the efficacy study were not 'selected' in any sense and were not forewarned prior to initial consultation that they would be asked to participate in the therapy. Nonetheless, all the families rose to the task willingly, becoming actively involved in therapy sessions and in homework which they did in 5- to 7-minute bursts once, twice or three times daily, as recommended. On average, homework was done 24 times per week (4 families), 18 times per week (1 family), 12 times per week (7 families), 8 times per week (1 family) and 6 times per week (1 family) (Bowen, 2010; Bowen & Cupples, 2004).

Parents vary in the amount and style of information they need, some performing well with little explanation, learning best via observation and rehearsal. Others want a lot of 'training' before being comfortable performing activities at home. Although it is encouraged without insisting, some parents are shy when it comes to rehearsing

homework tasks in the clinic with the therapist watching. Educational levels appear to have little bearing on how readily parents comprehend and work with concepts, expressed in plain-English, such as 'sound patterns', 'sound classes', 'reinforcement', 'modelling', 'labelled praise', 'revisions and repairs', 'progressive approximations', 'shaping' and 'gradualness of acquisition'. Subjectively, it seems some parents have an instinct, 'feel', or 'gene' for this sort of thing, and some appear to have missed out! Some are intuitive 'natural teachers', and some are not. Despite this, it is amazing what parents will *learn* to do well with adequate levels of support when they perceive that their child stands to benefit. Parents with personal histories of communication difficulties similar to their child's may be endowed with a special empathy, although some of them may have residual issues affecting their capacity to reflect on language function and to enjoy language play (Crystal, 1996, 1998).

In delivering parent education, it is imperative to

- avoid overwhelming families with information at any point;
- circumvent giving them the impression that they have to become 'mini-therapists';
- provide parents with opportunities to rehearse new skills if appropriate, while being sensitive that some adults find it embarrassing and difficult (or culturally inappropriate) to play (Watts Pappas & Bowen, 2007);
- create an atmosphere in which parents can feel comfortable in questioning anything not understood, share their perspectives, and exercise choice; and
- listen to their ideas respectfully and incorporate them where possible.

Metalinguistic training

Rationale

This component was inspired by a fascinating article by Dean and Howell (1986) that proposed a role for guided discussion and meta-language in helping children reflect on the features or properties of phonemes, and the structure of syllables, with a view to improving their awareness of when and how to apply phonological repair strategies. Dean, Howell and colleagues went on to develop *Metaphon*, described in Chapter 4, an approach that centres on dialogue between therapist and child with only passing references to parents. We wanted to take these ideas in a new direction, actively engaging parents, still with the aim of increasing children's metaphonological awareness, and their capacity to reflect on their own speech performance.

Excited by the practical connections between Ingram's (1976) schema of underlying representation, surface form and mapping rules, and the Dean and Howell (1986) suggestions for developing linguistic awareness, it struck us that, if they were only implemented for a short period in weekly therapy sessions, their effects might not be optimal. Our plan was to provide parents with training, scripts and informational handouts (later to become Bowen, 1998a, and in French, Bowen, 2007). We reasoned that if *child*, and *clinician* and *parents*, and *teachers* where applicable, used a common language around sound and syllable properties, and the reasons for, and the communicative consequences of homophony, it would improve the accuracy of that child's knowledge of the system of phonemic contrasts and increase the likelihood of spontaneous self-corrections. This would be especially the case if *all* the adults involved (not just the SLP/SLT) knew how to reinforce them. Metalinguistic training fosters 'phonological discoveries' by the child. His or her capacity to *perceive, talk about, reflect upon* and *revise and repair* homophonous productions is enhanced via simple routines and systematic feedback delivered by parents.

Methods

Using guided discussion (Dean & Howell, 1986), child, parents and clinician talk and think about the properties of the speech sound system and how it is organised to convey meaning, incorporating simple metaphonological and phonological

awareness (Hesketh, A28) activities. In finding a common language to describe phonemic features and syllable shapes, the clinician can borrow from many sources, including Klein's (1996a, b) 'imagery terms' or 'imagery labels' (e.g., poppy, windy, throatie and tippy, discussed in Chapter 4); the *Metaphon* (Dean et al., 1990) terms such as long, short, front, back, noisy, growly, whisper and quiet; and the imagery names and cues in Table 6.5.

Activities, at home and in therapy, involve sound picture associations (e.g., /ɹ/ is a roaring lion sound; /tʃ/ is a choo-choo train; /f/ is a bunny rabbit sound, because it is made with teeth like a bunny); phoneme segmentation for onset matching (e.g., kangaroo starts with /kə/, or for preference, /k/); awareness of rhymes and sound patterns (e.g., games with minimal pairs like *tie-die*; and near minimal pairs like *tie-tight*); rudimentary knowledge of the concept of 'word'; understanding the idea of words and longer utterances 'making sense'; awareness of the use of revision and repair strategies using 'judgement of correctness' games (e.g., *The boy tore his shirt* vs. *The boy tore his cert*) and the 'fixed-up-one routine'; and playing with morphophonological structures to produce lexical and grammatical innovations (e.g., *pick* vs. *picks*).

The use of spontaneous revisions and repairs is fostered, particularly at home, by use of the fixed-up-one routine. The routine is a metalinguistic technique that allows adults to talk simply to children about revisions and repairs (or self-corrections). Scripts, such as the one displayed in Figure 9.4, are provided to introduce them to the technique, and various versions of it are available, with an instructional slide show at www.speech-language-therapy.com. Also with regard to self-monitoring and making revisions and repairs, the child is encouraged to *notice* phoneme collapses or homonymy (e.g., *boo* and *blue* realised homophonously as /bu/).

Discussion

The 1986 suggestions of Dean and Howell were adopted and extended, allowing metalinguistic

seal

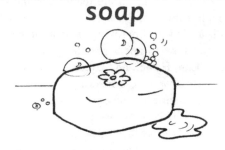

1. Say to your child, "Listen. If I said 'heel', it wouldn't sound right. I would have to fix it up and say 'seal'".

soap

2. Say to your child, "'Hope' isn't right, is it? I need to do a fixed-up-one and say 'soap'".

soup

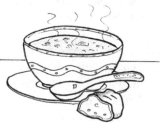

3. "Would I have to do a fixed-up-one if I said 'hoop' for this one?"

sand

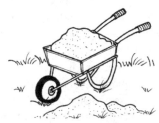

4. "What would I have to do if I accidentally said 'hand' for this one? I would have to do a ..." [fixed-up-one]

sauce

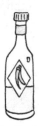

5. "If I said 'horse' instead of 'sauce' I would have to do a fixed-up-one again. I would have to think to myself not 'horse' it's 'sauce'. Did you hear that fixed-up-one?"

sun

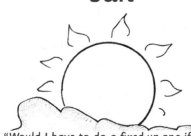

6. "Would I have to do a fixed-up-one if I said 'hun' for this one?"

Self-corrections
Adults continually make little mistakes when they speak. They barely notice these mistakes at a conscious level, and quickly correct themselves, and go on with what they are saying. This process of noticing speech mistakes and correcting them as we go is called making revisions and repairs, or self-corrections. Many children with speech sound difficulties are not very good at self-correcting. They find it difficult to monitor their speech (i.e., listen to it critically) and make corrections.

Fixed-up-ones
At home this week, introduce the idea of a "fixed-up-one", or the process of noticing speech mistakes and then saying the word(s) again more clearly, specifically in relation to the consonants at the beginnings of the six words featured on this page. Go through the following routine two or three times, and talk about fixed-up-ones. Have some fun making up other "mistakes" with words, that need correcting.

Figure 9.4 An example of a fixed-up-one routing. Drawing by Helen Rippon, Speech and Language Therapist: www.blacksheeppress.co.uk.

awareness to be targeted in naturalistic, supportive clinic *and home* settings. Expressions that crop up constantly in the context of PACT being discussed with parents are 'talking task', 'listening task', 'thinking task', 'fixed-up-ones', 'word', 'rhyme', 'making sense', 'make the words sound different from each other', 'two-step word' and 'remember the 50:50 split'. The latter refers to the general recommendation that the 50:50 split between 'talking tasks' versus 'thinking and listening tasks' that is observed in therapy sessions is also observed at home.

Sometimes a family will generate its own appropriate terminology, and memorable offerings have included 'Bob', 'Bobs' and 'fix-its' in relation to 'fixed-up-ones' (Bob the Builder's motto is 'Can we fix it? Yes we can') and 'Einstein Time' in relation to listening and thinking tasks! 'Einstein Time' and 'Nice one, Einstein!' were the brainchild of Sebastian's father, who was intrigued by my framed picture of Einstein, adorned with a thinks bubble that read 'THINKING'. The picture is sometimes put on the table during 'thinking tasks', such as judgement of correctness games, silent sorting of word-pairs, 'point to the one I say' activities, and word classification games, to cue everyone that (quiet) 'thinking' is supposed to be happening! Readers who would like to experiment with this idea can download Einstein pictures from www.speech-language-therapy.com.

Phonetic production training

Rationale

'Phonological disorders arise more in the mind than in the mouth', according to Grunwell (1987), and phonological therapy is, by definition, linguistic, meaning-based, focused on activating a child's underlying system for phoneme use, and 'in the mind'. But, having said that, some children with phonological disorder need help at the phonemic level *and* the perceptual and phonetic levels. In other words, they must be taught to perceive (discriminate) sounds, and make the sounds and structures.

Methods

Phonetic production training is integrated with metalinguistic training and multiple exemplar training. It uses, as required, auditory discrimination activities, stimulability techniques (Bleile, 2004, 2013; Miccio, 2005) and sound elicitation and phonemic placement procedures (Secord, Boyce, Donohue, Fox & Shine, 2007) wherein the therapist teaches a child to perceive and generate absent phones *beyond* isolated sound level, or failing that, to produce approximations of consonants in the same sound class in CV (onset) and VC (coda) combinations. Homework for phonetic targets includes listening and production, observing the 50:50 split.

Discussion

It is rarely necessary to train intervocalic (SIWW or SFWW) stimulability or to train all vowel and diphthong contexts. For instance, having taught /tʃu/ and /utʃ/, one seldom has to teach /tʃu tʃi tʃɔ tʃaɪ tʃoʊ tʃeɪ tʃa/ and /utʃ itʃ ɔtʃ aɪtʃ oʊtʃ eɪtʃ atʃ/, etc. Children usually proceed from syllable to word level, having demonstrated the capacity to produce the phone in CV and/or VC contexts. Introductory stimulability or pre-practice tasks may be at individual sound (segment) and 'nonsense syllable' level, even involving 'syllable drill', but not for long. Once a child is stimulable for a target, or is producing a passable approximation, or a phone in the same sound class, in syllables or words, therapy moves onto the phonemic level and all activities are 'meaning-based' at word level and beyond (Bowen & Cupples, 2006). The child does production practice of a few target words, usually no more than six. It is important to know that 'phonetic production training' does not imply traditional articulation therapy (Van Riper, 1978) or adaptations of it (e.g., Raz, A4).

Multiple exemplar training

Rationale

Focused auditory input and the heightened perceptual saliency of phones, structures and contrasts, provided by the therapy activities, increases the learnability of new sounds, syllable structures and word contrasts.

Methods

Multiple exemplar training has two overlapping aspects: auditory input and minimal contrast (minimal pair) therapy. Auditory input involves listening lists, alliterative input and thematic play; and minimal contrast therapy uses minimal, maximal or multiple oppositions between words. Listening lists comprise word lists of up to 15 words with a common phonetic feature (e.g., *sail, seat, sigh, sew, seed, sum, sack, sun, sand, sea, sock, soup, silly, seal, saw, soap*) or up to seven word pairs (e.g., *sock-shock, sour-shower; sack-shack, sip-ship, sell-shell, Sue-shoe, save-shave*) or triplets (e.g., *seat-sheet-cheat, sigh-shy-chai, sip-ship-chip, sore-shore-chore, Sue-shoe-chew*) or target, error, and 'foil' (e.g., *pie-bye-boo, pig-big-boo, Paul-ball-boo, pin-bin-boo, pug-bug-boo, pat-bat-boo, poi-boy-boo*) to the child. Foils are introduced to make some sequences more rhythmical and fun, and more enticing for the child to dance, jog, march, rap or bop to. Sometimes the words are pictured and sometimes not. Alliterative input can be provided via stories, songs, rhymes, games and worksheets, such as one for /k/ SIWI depicting a *cat*: in a *cupboard*, with a *kite*, in a *coat*, in a *corner*, in a *kennel*, being *carried*, behind a *curtain* and in a *cap*.

Thematic play or auditory input therapy (Lancaster, A24) involves playing games and reading books to the child that give rise to frequent repetitions of targets. Bowen (2010) describes an activity for 'Bruno', 4;2, who was learning /f/ SFWF. In one therapy session, and for a week in homework, he listened to the story of Jeff and Steph and the scarf (shown in Figure 6.3). In related homework, Bruno played minimal contrast games using the work sheet illustrated in Figure 9.5. At intervals, outside of formal homework, Bruno played a game with his father where a superhero jumped off a roof, and he played with Smurf figurines with both parents. In fact, he took the Smurfs almost everywhere, constantly

pretending to be a Smurf; and, for a period, Smurfs became his main conversational topic (briefly supplanting Thomas the Tank Engine)—exactly what was needed to provide intense and interesting (to him) input for final /f/.

In minimal contrast therapy, a child sorts, with as much help as is required, words pictured and captioned on cards according to their sound properties, in sessions and for homework, and engages in homophony confrontation tasks (in sessions but not for homework), such as the ones below. With activities 6, 7 and 8, it is important to explain clearly to parents that the child does not have to 'correct you'. All the child is required to do is to judge the correctness of the adult's production.

1. **'Point to the one I say'.**

   The child points to pictures of the words, spoken by the adult in random order (e.g., *sheet, sip, sell, ship, shell, seat*) or rhyming order (e.g., *seat-sheet, sip-ship, sell-shell*).

2. **'Put the rhyming words with these words'.**

   Three to nine cards are presented (e.g., *pin, pea, pack, pole*), and the child puts rhyming cards beside them (*bin, bee, back, bowl*).

3. **'Say the word that rhymes with the one I say'.**

   The adult says words with the target phoneme; the child says rhyming non-target words (adult: *floor*; child: *four*; adult: *flake*; child: *fake*), with the child saying carefully selected words that he or she can already say.

4. **'Give me the word that rhymes with the one I say'.**

   The adult says the non-target word, and the child selects the rhyming word containing the target sound. For example, in working on velar fronting: Adult says 'tea'; Child selects a picture of 'key'. Adult says 'tool'; Child selects a picture of 'cool'. Adult says 'tape'; Child selects a picture of 'cape'.

5. **'Tell me the one to give you'.**

   This is a homophony confrontation game, and it is the only task that it not included in homework. It needs a skilled, light touch and can easily go wrong, especially if the child

Rhyming Pairs /f/ SFWF

laugh	scarf	off	cough
Jeff	Steph	wife	knife
half	calf	laugh scarf off cough Jeff Steph wife knife calf half	scarf laugh cough off Steph Jeff knife wife half calf

/f/ vs. /p/ SFWF

cough	cop	Steph	step
wife	wipe	cuff	cup
sniff	snip	cough cop Steph step wife wipe cuff cup sniff snip	cop cough step Steph wipe wife cup cuff snip sniff

Final /f/ vs. no final consonant

la	laugh	Y	wife
Lee	leaf	low	loaf
scar	scarf	la laugh Y wife Lee leaf low loaf scar scarf	laugh la wife Y leaf Lee loaf low scarf scar

Figure 9.5 Minimal pair and near minimal pair sets. Drawing by Helen Rippon, Speech and Language Therapist, www.blacksheeppress.co.uk.

is pushed too hard. In a game context, the adult responds to the word actually said (e.g., the child says [tɪn] for 'chin' and is handed 'tin'). The aim is for the child to recognise communicative failure (i.e., recognise his or her own homophony) and attempt a revised production.

6. **'You be the teacher: tell me if I say these words the right way or the wrong way'.**

    The adult says individual words or phrases, and the child judges whether they have been said correctly; for example, *puddy tat* versus 'pussy cat'. The child judges: right/wrong; yes/no; OK/silly. The child does not 'correct' the adult.

7. **'Silly sentences'**

    The child judges whether or not a sentence is a 'silly one'; for example, One-two buckle my doo versus One-two buckle my shoe; Mary had a little lamb versus Mary had a whittle wham. The order of presentation of the correct and incorrect sentence is varied. The child does not 'correct' the adult.

8. **'Silly dinners'**

    The adult says what he or she wants for dinner, and the child judges whether it is a 'silly dinner': I want jelly/deli; I want fish and chips/ships; I want green peas/bees; I want a cup of coffee/toffee. The child does not 'correct' the adult.

9. **'Shake-ups and match-ups'**

    The child is shown four pictures, for example, tie-time, two-toot. The pairs are said to the child rhythmically several times. Cards are 'shaken up' in a container and tipped out. The child then arranges them, with help if necessary, 'the same as they were before' (i.e., in near minimal pairs).

10. **'Find the two-step words'.**

    With adult assistance, the child sorts pictured near minimal pair words with consonant clusters SIWI or SFWF from contrasting words with singleton consonants SIWI or SFWF (e.g., feet-fleet, fat-flat, fake-flake).

11. **'Walk when you hear the 2-steps'.**

    Child 'finger-walks' two steps (to a destination such as a pot of gold, or to a place on a treasure map; or up a ladder) upon hearing a consonant cluster SIWI as opposed to a singleton SIWI (e.g., the child 'walks' for 'true', but not 'two' or 'roo').

Discussion

Suggestions for multiple exemplar activities 1–11 above are provided to parents. It should be noted, however, that, for many families, the suggestions trigger their creativity and they come up with innovative and appropriate games, activities and books that are perfect for their child (and inspiring for the clinician).

Homework

Rationale

Homework administered by a parent or parents provides children with practice, reinforcement, opportunities to generalise and opportunities for discovery. It allows families to hone, generalise and enjoy the 'teaching skills' learned in therapy sessions. By engaging in activities autonomously, families can experiment, creating new opportunities for learning in natural, functional contexts. As their knowledge, skills and confidence grow, most will innovate, making up new games and fun routines, and some even instigate apposite 'next steps' in therapy. They also become more skilled in recognising 'teaching moments' weaving them seamlessly into the child's day so that they do not feel they are 'doing speech homework all the time'. Because homework suggestions are not rigid, homework is conducive to internal development and families can shape it to fit their interests, preferences and culture. Homework can assume the family 'stamp' as well as the clinician's 'style', influencing the form, content and conduct of sessions in dynamic and striking ways, letting the adults create activities a child genuinely likes and is responsive to.

Methods

Homework involves short bursts of formal home activities and the use of appropriate speech stimulation techniques (e.g., modelling corrections) when opportune. Homework comprises activities from the most recent session, delivered in 5- to 7-minute bursts once, twice, or three times daily, one-to-one with an adult in good listening conditions. Examples of 'good' and 'poor' listening conditions are discussed. Practices can be as little as 10 minutes apart (e.g., practice-craft-practice-craft-practice-craft for children who like making things; or for booklovers, practice-story-practice-story-practice-story; or practices can be alternated with playing a game: practice-game-practice-game-practice-game, or completing a puzzle: practice-puzzle-practice-puzzle-practice-puzzle), with the 50:50 split observed between listening–thinking tasks versus talking tasks. Parents are encouraged to make the homework regular, brief, naturalistic, encouraging and fun. Instructions and activities go in a homework book and are explained as often as required. If, for some reason, homework does not happen for a day or days, parents are asked not to 'compensate' by doing more than three practices in one day subsequently. It is suggested that they combine homework with activities the child likes, such as colouring and cutting, story reading or going to a park or favourite spot sometimes to do it.

Discussion

If one family member (e.g., his father in Iain's case) usually accompanies the child and participates in therapy sessions, other family members (e.g., mother and grandparents) can learn from their example during homework sessions and by watching their application of modelling, recasting and other techniques. The system will fall down if one parent does 'the bringing' to therapy and the other parent does *only* the formal homework without good communication between the two, as sometimes happens.

Younger children generally like the idea of doing 'homework' as something 'big kids' do. For some parents and older children, however, there may be interfering negative connotations and emotional baggage. In this connection, a colleague in the United States offered interesting comments on the term 'homework' which gave me pause for thought: 'I use the term 'home programming' instead of 'homework'. For me homework is something that kids might hate doing, or it may be something that children are meant to complete individually. Home programming reflects effort on the parents' part, and may not get the same negative response that 'homework' can sometimes get. It could also be called 'speech work' or such. It is just a preference based on my experience in providing after school services and working with parents. Many of my colleagues, I'm sure, use 'homework' (Mark Guiberson, personal correspondence, 2014).

Case study

Background

Josie attended a rural New South Wales Community Health Speech Pathology clinic with her mother six times between the ages of 5;2 and 5;5 for an assessment and five 'language stimulation group' sessions conducted by a locum SLP because she was a late talker and her speech was unintelligible. At 5;11, she was referred back to Community Health by a school nurse, attending an intake clinic with her father, David, for a speech assessment only. In a 20-minute session, an 88-word, 3-position screener called the *Articulation Survey* (Fisher & Atkin, 1996) was administered by a second SLP who diagnosed developmental verbal dyspraxia (DVD) and added Josie to a therapy waiting list. She had normal audiograms at 6;1 and 6;7.

Referral

A District School Counsellor (Educational Psychologist) referred Josie to me 6 months after the DVD diagnosis was made. The referral was prompted by Josie's teacher, concerned about her language development, disinterest in and difficulty with pre-reading and phonological awareness activities, and her air of unhappiness at school.

Initial presentation

Bright, bubbly and co-operative, Josie, 6;5, presented for initial consultation towards the end of her first year of school (Kindergarten in NSW). The first session involved history taking and administering a CELF-P requested by school personnel. Josie performed in the mid-average range: receptive, expressive and total language scores 103, 100 and 101, respectively. Apart from late language acquisition, poor intelligibility, and a maternal family history of speech and literacy difficulties, Josie's history was unremarkable. The conversational speech sample excerpt and the *Quick Screener* data displayed in Figures 9.6 and 9.7, respectively, were gathered at 6;6 in the second session (4 weeks after the first), and the analysis displayed in Figure 9.8 was done while her parents watched. At 6;6, her mother, Maureen, and half-sister Emma assigned Josie an intelligibility rating of (2) mostly intelligible (to them both). I gave her (3) somewhat intelligible to me; and David and Josie's teacher gave her ratings of (4) mostly unintelligible (to them both).

Screening process

Steps 1–4 were performed during the session, and Steps 5–10 were performed after it.

Single-Word sample

1. The first step in this quick screening analysis was to examine the SW sample (Figure 9.7), tally Josie's consonants correct out of approximately 100 (depending on the dialect of English), and calculate a tentative Percentage of Consonants Correct (PCC; tentative because this is a small, slightly inexact, SW *screening* sample). With scoring erring on the generous side, her SW PCC was 30%. Later it was found that both her conversational and imitated PCCs were lower than this at 27%, indicating an unusually severe SSD for a child of 6;6.
2. Using the analysis form (Figure 9.8), phonological processes with their percentages of

occurrence and other obvious errors were noted as follows: velar fronting 25% SI and SF; prevocalic voicing 57%; gliding of liquids 100%; final consonant deletion 66%; stopping of fricatives 25% SI; stopping of affricates 100% SF; and cluster reduction 100% SI and SF. Gliding of fricatives and affricates SI was prevalent, as was deletion of fricatives WF, glottal replacement, and /n/ dentalised, interdental, or produced /n^d/.

3. Counting each vowel and diphthong as one vowel, her vowels correct out of 47 were tallied and a tentative PVC calculated. With vowel errors in 12 words (*fish, kiss, bridge, wing, leaf, foot; van, crab, splash; house; stairs;* and *ear*), her PVC was about 74% (35/47). Her productions of girl and salt were not factored in because they were dialectal.

Single-word *and* conversational speech sample

4. Referring to the SW and CS sample, the vowels and consonants present were listed to record Josie's vowel and consonant inventories.
5. The marked consonants present in her SW and CS samples were circled on the form. Her marked consonants were /p t k f θ/, with /v/ and /ʃ/ considered marginal because they occurred infrequently and neither were present in both samples.
6. Any vowel and/or consonant inventory constraints were noted. Her SW consonant constraints (missing consonants) were / ŋ ð s z tʃ ʤ l/, and her CS constraints were /ŋv ð s z ʒ tʃ ʤ l ɹ/. There were no vowel inventory constraints, and one missing diphthong /ɪə/.
7. Phonotactic combinations were recorded to assess Josie's syllable/word shape inventory. She only produced one- and two-syllable combinations, and her inventory was C, V, CV, VC, CVC, CCV, CCVC, CCCV, CVCV, CCVCCV and CCVCVC.
8. Idiosyncratic or unusual features were noted. They were dentalised alveolars, glottal replacement, gliding of fricatives and

Josie:

eː ə jʌn̪ᵈ ʌn̪ᵈ mun ɒun wʌn̪ᵈ daɪd
There's a sun   and   moon   on   one   side

ʌn̪ᵈ θə daɪ ɔn̪ᵈ θi ʌdə daɪd wɪʔ ə bweɪndoʊ ‖
and   the   sky   on   the   other   side   with   a   rainbow.

θə hæudɔ ɪd bwakʌm ɒʔ
The   handle   is   broken   off,

doʊ jʌ ki jɔ pʰʌn̪ᵈ ɪn ɪt dɒn̪ᵈ jʌ ‖
so   you keep your pens   in   it,   don't   you?

weː dɪd θʌʔ kʰʌ kʌm θɒum eːbwə ‖
Where   did   the   cup   come   from,   ever?

Caroline: My friend Anna gave it to me.

Josie:

wəd ɪʔ jɔ bɜθdeɪ ‖
Was   it   your birthday?

Caroline: No, it was just for a present.

Josie:

weː ju daʔ wen θə hæju pʰʌw ɒʔ ‖
Were   you   sad   when   the   handle   fell   off?

Caroline: Actually, it didn't have a handle when she gave it to me.

Josie:

jɔ ban̪ᵈ geɪ ju ə kʰʌ wɪʔ noʊ hæudɔ ‖
Your friend   gave you   a   cup   with   no   handle.

aɪ min jaɪ hæjoʊ ‖
I   mean,   like   hello!

ʃi wədʔ ə bwi guᵈ judə ‖
She   wasn't   a   very   good   chooser.

Caroline: Do you like it?

Josie:

jet ɪtᵈ weːdi bwədi ‖
Yes.   It's   really   pretty.

Caroline: I like it too, even though it has no handle.

Josie:

bʌʔ ɪʔ wə bi betə wɪʔ ə hæudoʊ ‖
But   it   would be   better   with   a   handle.

Figure 9.6 An excerpt from Josie's conversational speech sample at 6;6

#	TARGET	TRANSCRIPTION		CC	#	TARGET	TRANSCRIPTION		CC
1	cup	ʌ	kʰʌ	1	23	jam	æ	jiæm	1
2	gone	ɒ	kʰɒn	1	24	house	aʊ	hæʊ	1
3	knife	aɪ	naɪ	1	25	path	a	pʰa	1
4	sharp	a	wjaː		26	door	ɔ	dɔ	1
5	fish	ɪ	de		27	smoke	oʊ	moʊ	1
6	kiss	ɪ	de		28	bridge	ɪ	mweʔ	
7	sock	ɒ	wjːɒk	1	29	train	eɪ	ɹeɪn	2
8	glass	a	wja		30	chair	ɛə	jɛə	
9	watch	ɒ	bwɒʔ	1	31	red	e	wjeː	
10	nose	oʊ	noʊ	1	32	spoon	u	bun	1
11	mouth	au	mau	1	33	plane	eɪ	veɪ	
12	yawn	ɔ	jɔn	2	34	fly	aɪ	fnaɪ	
13	leaf	i	wjəi		35	sky	aɪ	fnaɪ	
14	thumb	ʌ	θʌn̪ᵈ	1	36	sun	ʌ	jʌn̪ᵈ	1
15	foot	ʊ	b ɒ ʔ		37	wing	ɪ	weɪn	1
16	toe	oʊ	tʰoʊ	1	38	splash	æ	bwʌʃ	1
17	snake	eɪ	fneɪʔ	1	39	tent	e	denʔt	2
18	van	æ	bweɪn	1	40	salt	ɒ	jɒʊt	1
19	fast	a	bʰa		41	crab	æ	mbwa	
20	girl	ɜ	gwɜʊ	1	42	sweet	i	bwiʔ	1
21	stairs	eə	dʰe		43	sleeve	i	bwiʔ	
22	big	ɪ	bɪ	1	44	zipper	ɪ	wɪbə	
boy bɔɪ ear ɪə			SUBTOTAL CC:	15				TOTAL CC:	30

Figure 9.7 Josie's initial Quick Screener data at 6;6

affricates, vowel and diphthong errors, schwa insertion, final consonant deletion and no words beyond two syllables in the CS sample.

9. The data were perused for chronological mismatch, and one example was found in her correct production of /θ/ as in 'birthday' in all obligatory contexts.

10. The syllable stress inventory (assuming typical stress patterns) was recorded as S = strong and W = weak. The SW words she produced in the CS excerpt were representative of the entire CS sample (*zipper*, *better*, *other*, *handle*, *birthday*, *rainbow*, *broken*, *chooser*, *really*, and *pretty*). There were no other word stress patterns apart from one WS in 'hello' when mimicking Emma's 'cool' production with strong emphasis on the second syllable. Note that Josie spoke a non-rhotic variety of Australian English: AusE (Cox, 2012).

Velar fronting 25% SI 25% SF

#	Target SI	0 / 1	#	Target SF	0 / 1
1	cup	0	7	sock	0
6	kiss	1	17	snake	0
2	gone	0	22	big	0
20	girl	0	37	wing	1
	TOTAL	1/4		TOTAL	1/4

Palato-alveolar fronting

#	Target SI	0 / 1	#	Target SF	0 / 1
4	sharp	0	5	fish	0
30	chair	0	9	watch	0
23	jam	0	28	bridge	0
	TOTAL	/3		TOTAL	/3

Word-final devoicing

#	Target	0 / 1	#	Target	0 / 1
41	crab	0	43	sleeve	0
31	red	0	10	nose	0
22	big	0	28	bridge	0
				TOTAL	/6

Backing

#	Target SI	0 / 1	#	Target SF	0 / 1
16	toe	0	15	foot	0
39	tent	0	42	sweet	0
26	door	0	31	red	0
	TOTAL	/3		TOTAL	/3

Stopping of fricative 25% SI

#	Target SI	0 / 1	#	Target SF	0 / 1
5	fish	0	13	leaf	0
15	foot	1	11	mouth	0
14	thumb	0	6	kiss	0
7	sock	0	38	splash	0
36	sun	0	43	sleeve	0
4	sharp	0	10	nose	0
18	van	1			
44	zip(per)	0			
	TOTAL	2 /8		TOTAL	/6

Stopping of affricates 100% SF

#	Target SI	0 / 1	#	Target SF	0 / 1
30	chair	0	9	watch	1
23	jam	0	28	bridge	1
	TOTAL	/2		TOTAL	2 /2

Pre-vocalic voicing 57%

#	Target	0 / 1	#	Target	0 / 1
25	path	0	5	fish	1
16	toe	0	14	thumb	0
6	kiss	1	36	sun	1
			4	sharp	1
				TOTAL	4 /7

Liquid/glide simplification gliding 100%

#	Target	0 / 1	#	Target	0 / 1
9	watch	0	12	yawn	0
13	leaf	1	31	red	1
				TOTAL	/4

Initial consonant deletion

#	Target	0 / 1	#	Target	0 / 1
3	knife	0	7	sock	0
22	big	0	30	chair	0
18	van	0	12	yawn	0
				TOTAL	/6

Final consonant deletion 66%

#	Target SI	0 / 1	#	Target SF	0 / 1
23	jam	0	10	nose	1
44	zip	0	5	fish	1
31	red	1	28	bridge	1
				TOTAL	4/6

Initial cluster reduction 100% SI

#	Target SI	0 / 1	#	Target SI	0 / 1
33	plane	1	43	sleeve	1
8	glass	1	27	smoke	1
28	bridge	1	17	snake	1
29	train	1	32	spoon	1
41	crab	1	21	stairs	1
34	fly	1	35	sky	1
42	sweet	1	38	splash	1
				TOTAL	14 /14

Final cluster reduction 100%

#	Target	0 / 1	#	Target	0 / 1
19	fast	1	40	salt	1
39	tent	1			
				TOTAL	3/3

Figure 9.8 Josie's initial Quick Screener analysis at 6;6

11. Extensive homonymy was evident (e.g., *where*, *were*, and *red* were produced identically).
12. Her contrastive phones (phonemes) were /n m w j p b t d/, and it was interesting to see that /n m w j p b d/ were in the Early 8 and /t/ was in the Middle 8 with no Late 8 consonants functioning as phonemes. Her non-contrastive phones were /h g k f ɹ ʃ θ/.
13. Subsequent administration of the Locke Task showed that she could not reliably discriminate between the liquid /l/ from either the glide /j/ or the liquid /ɹ/.
14. Subsequent administration of the DEAP inconsistency assessment revealed predominantly *consistent* production, with only two items, *helicopter* and *vacuum cleaner*, produced inconsistently.

From this screening (1–12 above) and her performance during language testing 1 month before, it was evident that Josie had a severe phonological disorder with phonemic, perceptual and phonetic issues, and CAS was ruled out. Parental permission was obtained to share these data, including videos of therapy, for research, teaching and publication purposes. Permission to show the videos was later withdrawn.

Josie's family

The family were eager to be involved in therapy, especially if it meant the number of sessions could be reduced. They were drought affected and on a tight budget, residing 100 km (62 miles) over difficult terrain from my practice. Josie's household comprised her father (David, 52); mother (Maureen, 38); half-sister (Emma, 15), who was home-schooled by Maureen and David and who was Maureen's child; and Josie's twin brother and sister (Jasper and Ruby, 4;2). David had two sons (Ben, 16, and Aaron, 14) living overseas with their mother (Rebekah, 54). Maureen was not in paid employment, and David sent regular child support payments and school fees to Rebekah. The family was cheerful and close-knit, spending much time together and with a wide circle of friends, especially around sport, local government, community and outdoor activities. Emma assumed a 'mothering' role with Josie, Jasper and Ruby. David volunteered that he was 'Type A', 'a news junkie', and 'obsessed with finances and the price of petrol'. No one disagreed.

There was a maternal family history of speech and literacy issues, and Maureen and Emma (described as 'learning disabled' by the school psychologist who referred Josie) were poor readers and spellers. Note that in Australia the term 'learning disability' means 'specific learning difficulty' or 'specific learning disability' and not 'intellectual disability', indicating intelligence in the normal range with a difficulty in some aspect of learning such as reading. Ruby was a late talker, unintelligible at 4;2, and waiting for SLP assessment at Community Health. Ben, Aaron and Jasper were reported to have 'excellent communication skills' (like David). Maureen was a calm, competent person who had completed 4 years of high school, 2 years of a hairdressing apprenticeship and a Child Care Certificate at an NSW Technical and Further Education Commission, known as TAFE NSW, college. She was employed as a pre-school assistant prior to Josie's birth. She did not drive a car due to her epilepsy. David had a law degree and a master's degree in business and was engaged in a new venture as proprietor of a specialist book publishing company, working from home on the family farm.

Therapy planning for Josie

Although (marked) /ʃ/ appeared in Josie's CS output, she was not stimulable for it in the true sense. The (marked) affricates /tʃ/ and /dʒ/ and the (marked) fricatives /s/ and /z/ were never present in output and were also non-stimulable; so consonant inventory expansion was a priority. First, /tʃ/ was selected for stimulability training. The reasoning behind this was that there is evidence to suggest that targeting the marked voiceless affricate might: (1) evoke the emergence of *unmarked* consonants, and (2) promote generalisation to the voiced cognate, /dʒ/. A second marked consonant, /s/, was selected for stimulability training because it might help promote cluster development and generalise to /z/ and other fricatives. Consideration was given to targeting the later developing and marked /ð/, but this idea was rejected. Because Josie already had its voiceless cognate /θ/ in her repertoire, it was felt that working on /ð/ might not have as much impact on her overall system as working on /s/. On the other hand, late-developing, non-stimulable, unmarked /l/ looked like a good candidate for intervention, especially since the Locke Task revealed that Josie could not reliably discriminate/l/ from /j/. In hindsight, it *might* have been more fruitful to target /ɹ/ early on. Thinking about /l/ led naturally to deciding about her clusters. Clearly, with 100% cluster reduction in her SW sample, and only /bw/ SIWI in her CS sample, clusters were a high priority. It was decided that targeting /l/ clusters was not the best option for her. Rather, targeting the adjuncts /st/, /sp/ and /sk/, although it might not stimulate generalisation to other clusters, might give her the 'idea' of producing clusters. In hindsight, this was *not* the smartest move, and /l/ clusters might have been the better targets.

Agent, scheduling and dosage

Because of family finances and the high cost of petrol, it was decided to spread the therapy as much as was practical, with David eagerly committing to being 'very hands on'. David and Maureen were 'stuck' when it came to choosing an SLP for their daughter. They had virtually no choice with the closest SLP almost 2 hours' drive away over unsealed and mountain roads, entailing heavy petrol consumption over the round trip. They certainly did not have the luxury of questioning whether the author would be the 'best' therapist for them, whether they wanted to 'go privately', or whether the assessment administered would lead to service delivery that would fit easily with their busy family life. They did, however, consider whether the intervention offered was 'scientific' and whether the therapist was properly

credentialed and experienced, with David asking searching questions.

Their main consideration in proceeding was to minimise and 'budget' the number of appointments. In the event, Josie was seen 15 times over 12.5 face-to-face hours, spread over almost 12 months, with the support of a homework program conscientiously administered by her parents and teenage sister, Emma.

The dosage and scheduling described for Josie was mainly the result of her parents' wishes, influenced by my suggestions on how appointments could be best deployed. Aware of this, and powerless to do anything about it, they would ask periodically whether the spread-out appointment schedule might adversely affect Josie's progress, thereby pinpointing a knowledge gap. Little is known about the effects of service delivery: in terms of the primary *agent* of therapy, appropriate *dosage*, and optimal *scheduling*, and how they relate to outcomes (Dodd, 2009; Williams, 2012).

Josie's therapy

Intervention commenced in November, and the content of her 15 (out of a possible 17) therapy sessions and brief details are listed in the next section. The reader may download from www.speech-language-therapy.com many of the specific materials used in Josie's intervention.

November to December, Age 6;6–6;7: 4 sessions over 4 weeks, Session 1: 40 minutes, Present: Josie, Maureen and Emma

1. Stimulability Training (Phonetic Production Training) for /tʃ/ and /s/.
2. Sound-Picture-Symbol associations for all fricatives and affricates.
3. Auditory Discrimination Training for liquid /l/ versus the glide /j/ in CV words.
4. Auditory Discrimination Training for all fricatives and affricates in CV words.
5. Auditory Bombardment (Focused Auditory Input): /tʃ/ words SIWI (*hat shop chop*, etc.).
6. Near Minimal Pairs Games for /st/, /sp/, and /sk/ SIWI versus /t/, /p/, and /k/ SIWI.

7. Homework: 2–6 above, and Thematic Play for the voiceless affricate /tʃ/ SIWI. Thematic play was around Chinese cooking (with vocabulary like *Chinese, China, chopsticks, chicken chow mein* and *choy sum*), taking advantage of David's being an adventurous cook and the family's interest in Chinese culture and cuisine.

Session 2: 40 minutes, Present: Josie, Maureen and Emma

Josie was now stimulable for /tʃ/ SIWI in syllables and CV words *chew, chore, cha-cha-chachacha* and with intense concentration could imitate /s/ in isolation.

1. Verbal and visual imagery were introduced for /tʃ/ (the train sound), /dʒ/ (the tired train sound), and /s/ and the glides (/j/ or [ja ja] (the yes sound), and /w/ or [wa wa] (the cry-baby sound). Imagery was emphasised in sound-sorting games in which Josie had to select between glides and affricates (to target the elimination of her idiosyncratic gliding of affricates and fricatives).
2. Judgement of correctness game *chew, chore, cha-cha-cha* versus *Sue, saw, sah-sah-sah*.
3. Judgement of correctness *game chew, chore, cha-cha-cha* versus *ewe, your, ya-ya-ya*.
4. Auditory Discrimination Training for all fricatives, affricates and glides. Josie quickly learned to discriminate these, although she still had difficulty discriminating liquids from glides at word level. Emma enjoyed playing these games frequently with Josie.
5. Auditory Bombardment (Focused Auditory Input): /tʃ/ words SIWI and /s/ words SIWI
6. Production practice of 10 /tʃ/ SIWI CV and CVC words.
7. Near minimal pairs games for Final Consonant Deletion.
8. Homework: 4–7 above and practising producing /s/ in isolation.

Session 3: 40 minutes, Present: Josie and David (40 minutes)

1. Minimal triplets game with: chew, shoe, sue; chip, ship, sip; chore, shore, sore.
2. Rhyming cloze task: shoe rhymes with ch . . . , Sue rhymes with ch . . . , etc. for /tʃ/ SIWI.

3. Rhyming cloze task: ewe rhymes with ch . . . , woo rhymes with ch . . . , etc. for /tʃ/ SIWI.
4. Increased use of /ʃ/ was noted in conversation. Stimulability for /ʃ/ SIWI and SFWF was now present, so 8 production practice words for /ʃ/ SFWF were provided.
5. Production practice words for /tʃ/ SIWI were also provided.
6. 'Itchy Archie' was elicited, and Josie was promised a special sticker if she could still say it after the school holidays.
7. Games 4 and 5 from Session 2 were continued, using different words and syllables.
8. Near minimal pairs games for FCD (bee beach, cow couch, A aitch, sir search, pea peach)
9. Homework: 1–3 above.

Session 4: 1 hour, 50 minutes, Present: David, Maureen and Emma

This was a parent education session without Josie. It included PowerPoint shows on modelling, recasting and revisions and repairs. Detailed homework instructions for working with Josie in 5- to 7-minute 'bursts', once, twice or three times daily in the summer holidays were given. David kept in touch by e-mail, even attaching Josie's drawing of Itchy Archie as a Christmas card. The family's tasks were to model and reinforce /st/, /sp/ and /sk/, final consonant inclusion, and to do activities around /tʃ/, /dʒ/ and /s/, talking about the imagery and sound-letter-symbol associations, and to maintain stimulability. In this session, the difficulties both Maureen and Emma had with language processing and production, particularly the production of consonant clusters and polysyllabic words (PSWs), contrasted markedly with David's verbal abilities and quick grasp of what was needed.

Consonant clusters and multisyllabic words

During Josie's initial consultation, it emerged that there was a maternal family history of speech and literacy issues. Maureen and Emma were poor readers and spellers, and Ruby was a late talker with unintelligible speech. Maureen's conversation was characterised by many mispronunciations. For example, each time she attended with Josie, she mentioned that they would go to the village afterwards for an *advocargo sandwich*. She referred several times to a politician (The Hon Danna Vale MP) as *dallavale*, and frequently substituted *weave* for *we* (*If weave get there early . . .*), and referred repeatedly to the *ditstrict slimming carnival* (district swimming carnival), apparently without noticing. In addition, there were examples of subtle schwa insertion, especially with /pl/ and /bl/ in onset, in words like *platter, place, blister* and *blame* (/pəlætə/, /pəleɪs/, /bəlɪstə/, /bəleɪm/) and schwa deletion in words like *Malouf* and *believe* (/mluf/, /bliv/). From this speech behaviour in her mother, and the many citation-naming and spontaneous-speech consonant deletions Josie made at the outset – with words that included: *binoculars, butterfly, Beijing, carnival, computer, Dolly Magazine, Dumbledore, florist, mistake, octopus, play station, rain forest, Slim Dusty* (the family dog), *spaghetti* and *triangle* – Josie might have been expected to have particular difficulty conquering clusters and polysyllabic words, but she did not.

Dr. Debbie James is a speech pathologist and a lecturer at Southern Cross University on Australia's Gold Coast. Her expertise and research interests involve children with oral and written speech and language problems, centring on children's development of speech and language – especially their productions of polysyllabic words, language and literacy and speech improvement. Both Josie and Maureen were interesting relative to research by Dr. James into the possible clinical significance of consonant cluster errors, mispronunciation of multisyllabic words (XSWs), and consonant deletion errors, and she explores this possibility in A50.

Q50.   Deborah G. H. James: Underlying representations and surface forms of long words

An interesting feature of Josie's intelligibility rating at 6; 6 by her parents was that, even though both spent an equivalent amount of time with her, her mother who may have had 'fuzzy' underlying representations and who had many speech errors in output found her to be 'mostly intelligible', whereas her father, who was highly competent verbally, found her 'mostly unintelligible'. Can you comment on the probable relationship in individuals with persistent errors with polysyllabic words and words containing clusters, between underlying representation and surface form? In working with children who appear to have persistent errors with clusters and XSWs, what testing would you suggest, and what are the clinical implications and the directions therapy might take?

A50.   Deborah G. H. James: The relationship between the underlying representation and surface form of multisyllabic words

My interest in this relationship between children's productions of polysyllabic words and the underlying phonological representations (PRs) began with clinical observations of a mismatch between children's speech output skills whereby their performance on picture-naming tests was vastly superior to their conversational speech. This conundrum led me back to phonological theory and scrutinising the nature of words used in speech output tests. I observed that picture-naming speech tests usually comprised one- and two-syllable words but few words with three or more syllables (James, 2006), and wondered if this mattered. After completing a PhD, I decided that it *did* matter and now explain this. Concluding that clear nomenclature is important, I now use the term polysyllabic words to denote words of only three or more syllables. At times when it is expedient to group all words with *two* or more syllables, I use the term XSWs, cognisant that researchers use these terms variously. For Davis (1998) for example, PSWs have four or more syllables, whereas other scholars have applied 'PSWs' and 'XSWs' to words of two or more syllables.

Phonological representations and multisyllabic words and cluster errors

The notion that children's renditions of words provide insight into the quality of their underlying PRs is fascinating. If the idea holds, it may also have intriguing clinical implications for assessment *and* intervention. PR is the term used to describe the storage of the word's phonological information in long-term memory (Stackhouse & Wells, 1997). Accumulating evidence that accurate speech output depends on a robust PR indicates that the more accurate a person's output, the more accurate and fine-grained is the corresponding PR (Hesketh, Dima & Nelson, 2007; Sutherland & Gillon, 2005, 2007). It also implies interdependency, whereby improvement in one is associated with improvement in the other. For example, interventions designed to enhance the quality of the PR *and* output alters output (Baker, 2000; Bowen & Cupples, 1999a; Habers, Paden & Halle, 1999). Even more interesting are reports of intervention aimed only at enhancing the PRs that alter output (Moriarty & Gillon, 2006; Weiner, 1981). Moreover, studies of simultaneous treatment of PR *and* output proved more effective than treating output alone (Gillon, 2000; Hesketh et al., 2007).

An asymmetrical relationship

This PR-to-output relationship, however, appears asymmetrical, when children with typical speech have poor phonological processing. This apparent asymmetry weakens when noting syllable numbers in words used for testing speech. When speech testing relied on one- and two-syllable words, the

relationship between speech and PRs was absent or weak (Bishop & Adams, 1990; Catts, 1993). By contrast, a relationship *was* present when testing incorporated nine or more XSWs (Elbro, Borstrøm & Petersen, 1998; Larrivee & Catts, 1999; Leitão, Hogben & Fletcher, 1997; Lewis & Freebairn, 1992; Lewis, Freebairn & Taylor, 2000, 2002; Stothard, Snowling, Bishop, Chipchase & Kaplan, 1998). This suggests that XSWs provide unique information.

The uniqueness of multisyllabic words

Examining the internal structure of syllables contributes to understanding the unique information that XSWs provide. Syllable constituents include onsets, rimes, nuclei (vowels) and codas (the final consonant or consonant cluster). These constituents are modelled hierarchically, as displayed in Figure A50.1. The rime is the obligatory syllable head and its partner, the onset, is optional, allowing for words without onsets, such as *eye* and *egg*. In English, the number of consonants in the onset can vary from zero to three. The rime contains the obligatory nucleus and its optional partner, the coda, which, in English, can comprise zero to four

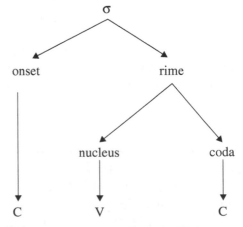

Figure A50.1 The structure of a syllable

consonants. Consequently, syllable shapes vary from one sound to eight sounds in words such as *owe* / oʊ/ and *strengths* /strɛŋkθs/.

The nucleus is the most prominent syllable constituent because it is the most sonorous (Baker, A13) resulting from an open vocal tract. Conversely, the onsets and codas at the syllable edges are relatively less prominent because the vocal tract is less open. The sonority profiles of syllables vary as their shapes and sounds within them vary, being lower at the syllable edges and peaking at the nucleus. Syllables with steeper sonority gradients are more salient than those with shallower gradients. Notably children tend to say words and/or syllables with steeper gradients more accurately than those with shallower gradients (Kehoe, 2001). For example, the word *bat* is more salient than *man* because of the greater sonority differential between its edges and nucleus than that of *man*. This is so because voiceless stops are less sonorous than nasals, giving rise to greater contrast. Similarly, syllables with onset and/or coda consonant clusters are less salient than their near minimal pair counterparts with singleton consonants because the change in sonority gradient from the syllable edge to the nucleus is more gradual. The sonority gradient in *black* is flatter than in *back*. This theory predicts children find it easier to extract sufficient details from *bat* and *back* than *man* and *black* to yield adult-like renditions, so adult-like renditions of *bat* and *back* will probably emerge before those of *man* and *black*. For all four words, the PR in young children is likely to be holistic but, possibly, the PR of *man* and *black* has to be more fine-grained than that of *bat* and *back* to yield an output of equivalent accuracy. This same logic applies to XSWs, that is, their PR may need to be even more fine-grained to yield an output of equivalent accuracy to monosyllabic words so that the additional phonological constituents are present in output. Further, some of the unique features of XSWs may strain extraction abilities more than monosyllabic words.

Another source of uniqueness of XSWs relates to the types of consonant sequences they may contain. In addition to consonant clusters, XSWs also include coda-onset sequences when codas and onsets abut at syllable edges. This generates sequences such as /k.t/, /m.b/, /ʤ.t/ /m.bj/ and /p.t/: *octopus, hamburger, vegetables, ambulance* and *helicopter*, respectively; of which none are legal onset clusters and only some are legal coda clusters (Clark & Yallop, 1995).

A third source of uniqueness is the many different levels of stress in XSWs. For example, *catamaran* with four syllables has four levels of stress, as displayed in Figure A50.2, as does, *hippopotamus* with five syllables. Your first reaction may be 'Sorry? There are only three levels of stress, primary, secondary and weak that can apply to words, and for *hippopotamus*, there are only strong and weak syllables'. This is true (Roca & Johnson, 1999). However, more levels can occur because of the metrical structure of words.

Metrical structure

Within metrical phonology (Selkirk, 1984), syllables gather into feet, and feet gather into prosodic words. As displayed in Figure A50.2 *catamaran* is one prosodic word with four syllables in 2 feet. A foot typically consists of

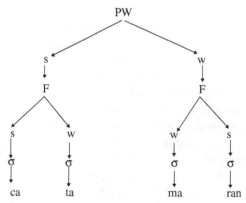

Key: PW, prosodic world; F, foot; S, stromg; W, weak; σ, syliable

Figure A50.2 The metrical structure of *catamaran*

two syllables; a head one which is strong, and second one with secondary or weak stress. A prosodic word can contain one or more feet and where there is more than 1 foot, one is more prominent than the other, giving rise to a number of different levels of stress in a word. Because the first foot in *catamaran* is the more prominent one, its strong syllable is more prominent than its counterpart in the second foot, and the same holds for the two weak syllables in both feet, resulting is four different levels of stress.

A fourth source of uniqueness of XSWs is that they contain within-word *weak* syllables, such as the two in ca*ta.ma*ran, whereas mono- and disyllabic words cannot. In these words, weak syllables be a whole word, such as *the* in a phrase *the cat*, or they can occur first or last in disyllabic words (e.g., gira*ffe* or co*la*). The importance of checking children's ability to realise within-word weak syllables, or non-final weak syllables, is underscored by the findings of Aguilar-Mediavilla, Sanz-Torrent and Serra-Raventos (2002), who reported that children with language impairment, aged 3;10 to 4;10, had more difficulty with them than their typically developing peers.

Assessment implications

Based on the above information and my findings (James, 2006), I echo Stackhouse (1985), Watts (2004) and Young (1991, 1995), who recommended that PSWs words be included routinely in child speech assessment. Importantly, their inclusion enhances *content validity* of testing because a wider array of phonological variables is sampled, including stress, non-final weak syllables and coda–onset consonant sequences. It also enhances *construct validity* because they reveal more age-related differences between groups of typically developing children than mono- and disyllabic words do (Ballard, Djaja, Arciuli, James & van Doorn, 2012; James, 2006;

James, van Doorn, McLeod & Esterman, 2008). Children are still mastering stress marking in words that begin with weak syllables such as *potato* and *tomato* between 3 and 7 years whereas it is adult-like by 3 years in words such as *butterfly* and *caterpillar* (Ballard et al., 2012). Metathesis occurred in disyllabic and PSWs but not in monosyllabic words. Also, age differences for metathesis only occurred in PSWs and not in the disyllabic words (James, 2006). They also reveal disorder-related differences, as for some children, their impairments are only apparent in PSWs (see James, 2006, for a literature review). Excluding PSWs from testing jeopardies identifying children's phonological processing and speech output difficulties that are only evident in PSWs.

Caveat

For the reasons expounded above, some PSWs are easier for children to say than others, thus it is important to use those that are clinically useful. James (2006) showed that the uniting features for clinically useful words were (a) non-final weak syllables with sonorant onsets or codas, especially the liquid /l/; (b) consonant sequences, especially those requiring an anterior/posterior articulatory movement; and (c) consonants that shared place or manner features, especially sonorants. These 10 PSWs: *ambulance, hippopotamus, computer, spaghetti, vegetables, helicopter, animals, caravan, caterpillar* and *butterfly*[1], proved to be the most clinically useful of the 39 PSWs used in the study because age differences were apparent.

Therapy

Given the evidence that working with phonological awareness brings about

---

[1] Pictures of the 10 PSWs are available from www. speech-language-therapy.com/pdf/djwordsBW1p.pdf

positive changes in the output, coupled with the assumption that accurate PSW production requires a more fine-grained PR than mono- and disyllabic words, I recommend including PSWs among the usual therapy targets and techniques. Examples include incorporating them into *focused auditory input* (Hodson, 2007, 2010 A5) and *Auditory Input Therapy* Lancaster, A24; Lancaster, Levin, Pring & Martin, 2010), *perceptually based interventions* (Rvachew, A25), and *minimal pair therapy* (Barlow & Gierut, 2002). Alternatively, one could work with families of them, such as those displayed in Table A50.1, exploring their similarities and differences.

In conclusion, by using PSWs in the management of paediatric speech impairment, several clinical efficiencies can be achieved. Clinicians can sample and expose children to a greater array of phonological variables than many mono- and disyllabic words permit. This is especially relevant for clinicians working with school-aged children because developmental changes occur more frequently in PSWs words with few, if any, in mono- and disyllabic words. It also seems that working with these variables is simultaneously enhancing the PR, thereby working on phonological awareness (for literacy) as well as speech output.

Table A50.1 Quasi minimal pairs and word families in PSWs

Root word; *ward*	Words with C+/jul/*	Words with initial weak syllable	Some quasi minimal pairs
ward	binoculars	spaghetti	reminder,
award/ing	ridiculous	zucchini	remember
reward/ing	funicular	tomato	remainder
toward	meticulous	potato	ve*randa*
forward	folliculous	banana	*Miranda*
backward	fasciculus	pyjamas	Ku*randa*
			su*rrender*

These words were listed by Gilbert and Johnson (1978).

Session 5: 1 hour, 10 minutes, Present: Josie, Maureen and David

The *Quick Screener* was administered again (Figure 9.9) with parents observing, and discussed. Josie was now stimulable for all consonants to two-syllable positions except /l/ and /f/. Her SW PCC was 65% and her Conversational PCC 50% in the clinic. There had been improvement in syllable structure with a significant reduction in final consonant deletion from 66% to zero, glottal replacement was almost eliminated, and she was attempting longer words with greater confidence, but with pervasive weak syllable deletion. Velar fronting was now confined to the velar nasal /ŋ/ only. The occurrence of prevocalic voicing, which had not been directly targeted, had dropped to 14% (previously 57%). Similarly, cluster reduction had dropped from 100% to 50% SI and 83% SF. Gliding of liquids had not changed and still stood at 100%, and stopping of fricatives (bearing in mind that she had been *gliding* fricatives) had risen to 50% SIWI and 83% SFWF. There were vowel replacements in words 13, 14, 21 and 41, and it appeared that minimal pair work for consonants, and possibly the increased attention to speech generally at home, was having a beneficial effect on vowel production also.

1. The adjuncts /st/, /sp/, and /sk/ needed more work. This was undertaken by using a multiple oppositions approach, using imagery cues, and the fixed-up-one routine for *all* s-clusters (not just the three s + voiceless stop adjuncts).
2. PSWs for production practice, focusing on weak syllable inclusion, were provided.
3. /s/ versus /ʃ/ minimal pair activities were done in the session and given for homework, along with /st/, /sp/ and /sk/ SIWI for production practice. The family were instructed to model /s/ constantly in all contexts, including polysyllables.
4. Homework: 3 and 4 above, with Josie being rewarded strongly for performing self-corrections.

Josie 6;9 PCC SW 65% CS 50%

#	TARGET	TRANSCRIPTION		CC	#	TARGET	TRANSCRIPTION		CC
1	cup	ʌ	kʌ p	2	23	jam	æ	tʃ æ m	1
2	gone	ɒ	g ɒ n	2	24	house	aʊ	h æʊ	1
3	knife	aɪ	n aɪ p	1	25	path	a	pas	1
4	sharp	a	ʃ a p	2	26	door	ɔ	d ɔ	1
5	fish	ɪ	b ɪ ʃ	1	27	smoke	oʊ	s m oʊ k	3
6	kiss	ɪ	k ɪ t	1	28	bridge	ɪ	w ɪ tʃ	0
7	sock	ɒ	ʃ ɒ k	1	29	train	eɪ	t ɹ eɪ n	3
8	glass	a	g w a tʃ	1	30	chair	ɛə	tʃ ɛə	0
9	watch	ɒ	w ɒ tʃ	2	31	red	e	w e d	1
10	nose	oʊ	n oʊ d^z	1	32	spoon	u	s b u n	2
11	mouth	aʊ	m aʊ p	1	33	plane	eɪ	p weɪ n	2
12	yawn	ɔ	j ɔ n	2	34	fly	aɪ	j aɪ	0
13	leaf*	i	j ə i p	0	35	sky	aɪ	s k aɪ	2
14	thumb	ʌ	θ ʌ m	2	36	sun	ʌ	sd ʌ n	2
15	foot*	ʊ	b ʊ t	1	37	wing	ɪ	w ɪ n	1
16	toe	oʊ	t oʊ	1	38	splash	æ	p w æ ʃ	2
17	snake	eɪ	sn eɪ k	3	39	tent	e	te n t	3
18	van	æ	b w æ n	1	40	salt	ɒ	sd ɒ t	2
19	fast	a	b a st	2	41	crab*	æ	w a b	1
20	girl	ɜ	g ɜ ʊ	1	42	sweet	i	s w i t	3
21	stairs*	eə	sd e z	2	43	sleeve	i	s w i d	1
22	big	ɪ	b ɪ g	2	44	zipper	ɪ	s ɪ p	1
boy bɔɪ ear eə		**SUBTOTAL CC:**		32		*VowelReplacement		**TOTAL CC:**	65

Figure 9.9 Josie's second Quick Screener record form at 6;9

February to April, Age 6;9–6; 11 – 5 sessions over 8 weeks (2 cancellations), Session 6 Present: Josie, Maureen, Emma and Maureen's sister

Maureen's sister, who normally minded the twins while Josie came to therapy, drove Josie, Emma and Maureen to the appointment because David was working. Josie was not well and they only stayed briefly. No homework was provided and, Josie was unable to attend her appointment the following week because she was still unwell.

Session 7: 60 minutes, Present: Josie and David

1. The whole session was devoted to clusters,' two step words' (cluster words), 'three part words' and 'four part words' (polysyllables), with 'finger walking' and *silent* tapping of syllables.
2. Using pictures from her 'speech book', Josie took great pleasure in making up her own (rather bizarre) fixed-up-one routine for clusters.
3. Homework: Reinforcement of self-corrections by David, Maureen and Emma, and Josie was

to take the speech book to school for a pat on the back from her teacher, who rose to the occasion!

Session 8: 40 minutes, Present: Josie and David

1. The velar nasal was introduced in minimal pairs (win wing, pin ping, bun bung, etc.), with multiple exemplar games and thematic play. At home, they modelled the velar nasal, modelled polysyllables (to target weak syllable deletion), and did daily production practice of polysyllables.
2. Josie was still unable to produce /f/ in CVs, but she could in VCs provided they were not real words that she knew (e.g., she could produce *uff* and *eef*, but not *if, off* and *eff*).
3. Homework: She was given a challenge to 'perfect' -iff, -off, -aff and -uff over the next week.

Session 9: 40 minutes, Present: Josie and David

1. Although clusters continued to be problematic, the velar nasal generalised within a week.
2. Playing a hunch that we could capitalise on her recent success with nasals, nasal clusters SF were emphasised for a week, particularly /-ŋk/ (sink, pink, wink, drink, link, etc.), but also /-nt/ and /-nd/.
3. Building on '–iff, -off, -aff and uff', 'iffy offy, affy and uffy' were established in the session and sent home to 'perfect'.
4. A judgement of correctness task and a fixed-up-one routine for homework, and final /-ŋk/, /-nt/ and /-nd/ words for production practice were provided (three of each).
5. Homework: 3 and 4 above.

Session 10: 40 minutes, Present: Josie, Maureen and David

The *Quick Screener* (Figure 9.10) was administered and discussed, with David doing most of the scoring! The final cluster strategy worked, and by the next session, Josie was using them inconsistently in *careful* CS.

1. Minimal pair games for stopping of fricatives were introduced.
2. Using a backward chaining technique, Josie managed at long last to produce /f/ SIWI, so: iffy-fee, offee-fee, affy-fee.
3. Homework: The family was to maintain Josie's ability to produce /f/ SIWI and to model in general. No specific homework was given, and Josie was asked to put her speech book and other materials away in a safe place and have a break. This was presented as a reward for a terrific effort on her part.

June: 3 sessions over 4 weeks, age 7;1, Session 11: 1 hour, 10 minutes, Present: Josie, Maureen and David

Josie's SW and conversational PCCs were now around about the same. Disappointingly for her, she was barely stimulable for /f/ SIWI and SFWF, and there had been no functional generalisation. She was still not stimulable for /l/, but she was now usually replacing /l/ with liquid /ɹ/ and not a glide /j/, and this replacement of a liquid with a liquid was interpreted as progress.

1. We decided to focus on /f/ and /v/ concurrently, using a combination of traditional phonetic production training and multiple exemplar activities and the aspiration trick (the f-hat, f-heat strategy; see www.speech-language-therapy.com).
2. Homework: /f/, /f/, and more /f/! And /v/!

Session 12: 40 minutes, Present: Josie, Maureen and David

1. Production practice of /f/ SIWI and /fɹ/ SIWI words.
2. Production of /ft/ using lexical innovation (laugh/laughed, cough/coughed, etc.).
3. Auditory bombardment using /f/ versus /v/ minimal pairs (fat-vat, fine-vine, fail-veil, etc.).
4. Auditory discrimination games for /ɹ/ and /l/ (lung-rung, lead-read, list-wrist, etc.).
5. Homework: 1–4 above and modelling and frequent recasting for /f/ and /v/.

#	TARGET	TRANSCRIPTION		CC	#	TARGET	TRANSCRIPTION		CC
1	cup	ʌ	k ʌ p	2	23	jam	æ	dʒ æ m	2
2	gone	ɒ	g ɒ n	2	24	house	aʊ	h æʊ s	2
3	knife	aɪ	n aɪ s	1	25	path	a	p a s	1
4	sharp	a	ʃ a p	2	26	door	ɔ	d ɔ	1
5	fish	ɪ	ʃ ɪ ʃ	1	27	smoke	oʊ	s m oʊ k	3
6	kiss	ɪ	k ɪ s	2	28	bridge	ɪ	ɹ ɪ dʒ	2
7	sock	ɒ	s ɒ k	2	29	train	eɪ	t ɹ eɪ n	3
8	glass	a	g w a s	2	30	chair	ɛə	tʃ ɛə	1
9	watch	ɒ	w ɒ tʃ	2	31	red	e	ɹ e d	2
10	nose	oʊ	n oʊ z	2	32	spoon	u	s p u n	3
11	mouth	aʊ	m aʊ θ	2	33	plane	eɪ	p w eɪ n	2
12	yawn	ɔ	j ɔ n	2	34	fly	aɪ	s w aɪ	0
13	leaf	i	j i s	0	35	sky	aɪ	s k aɪ	2
14	thumb	ʌ	θ ʌ m	2	36	sun	ʌ	s ʌ n	2
15	foot	ʊ	s ʊ t	1	37	wing	ɪ	w ɪ ŋ	2
16	toe	oʊ	t oʊ	1	38	splash	æ	s p ɹ æ ʃ	3
17	snake	eɪ	s n eɪ k	3	39	tent	e	t e n t	3
18	van	æ	b æ n	1	40	salt	ɒ	s ɒ t	2
19	fast	a	s a s t	2	41	crab*	æ	ɹ a b	2
20	girl	ɜ	g ɜ ʊ	1	42	sweet	i	s w i t	3
21	stairs*	eə	s t e z	3	43	sleeve	i	s w i z	1
22	big	ɪ	b ɪ g	2	44	zipper	ɪ	z ɪ p	2
		SUBTOTAL CC		38			**TOTAL CC**		82

Figure 9.10 Josie's third *Quick Screener* record form at 7;1

Session 13: 40 minutes, Present: Josie, David, Maureen and Emma

This was an thought-provoking session in which the family reviewed progress and future plans. Josie's name had come up on the Community Health waiting list, and they had been informed, to their surprise, that she had already been seen once at school by a newly appointed SLP. They were torn between staying with someone they knew and accessing a local service minutes by car from their home, commencing in late January. They decided to proceed with three scheduled appointments in September (2 sessions) and November (1 session) with me before chang-

ing to the new clinician. Therapy and homework were the same as for Session 12, with different vocabulary and games, plus auditory bombardment for /l/ SIWI.

September: 2 sessions over 4 weeks, age 7; 3–7;4, Session 14: 40 minutes, Present: Josie and David

1. More work on /f/ and /v/ in story retelling and narrative tasks. Both targets were beginning to show functional generalisation. This was *so* exciting for Josie, who commented, 'Ept, uh eff is my hard one, isn't it? But I can do it when I think!'

2. Homework: none, other than praising Josie (KR feedback), who was self-monitoring constantly.

Session 15: 40 minutes, Present: Josie and David

1. In the session, /l/ was elicited (in 'la') for the first time!
2. Homework: production practice: la-la-laugh, la-la-laugh, la-la-last, etc. and auditory bombardment for /l/ SIWI and SIWW.

November: 1 session, Age 7;6, Session 16: 40 minutes, Present: Josie, David, Maureen and Emma

The Screener was administered for the final time at the parent's request while the family observed (Figure 9.11). Her PCC in SW and CS was 93% or thereabouts. Josie was able to produce *laugh*, *last*, *llama*, *latte*, *Lana*, etc. perfectly, but was unable to produce /l/ preceding vowels other than /a/. Her speech was fully intelligible, and the only outstanding difficulties were with /l/ and a tendency to replace /eə/ with /e/ or /ɛ/. Josie was looking forward to seeing the Community Health SLP in the New Year. The case notes and a brief report were provided to David and Maureen for them to share with the SLP. Attempting to execute a smooth changeover, I left two telephone messages at the SLP's workplace and e-mailed her, but received no response. David also requested that the SLP speak to me and was told that Josie's speech difficulties were so mild that case discussion was unnecessary.

#	TARGET	TRANSCRIPTION		CC	#	TARGET	TRANSCRIPTION		CC
1	cup	ʌ	k ʌ p	2	23	jam	æ	dʒ æ m	2
2	gone	ɒ	g ɒ n	2	24	house	aʊ	h æʊ s	2
3	knife	aɪ	n aɪ f	2	25	path	a	p a θ	2
4	sharp	a	ʃ a p	2	26	door	ɔ	d ɔ	1
5	fish	ɪ	f ɪ ʃ	2	27	smoke	oʊ	s m oʊ k	3
6	kiss	ɪ	k ɪ s	2	28	bridge	ɪ	b ɹ ɪ dʒ	3
7	sock	ɒ	s ɒ k	2	29	train	eɪ	t ɹ eɪ n	3
8	glass	a	g w a s	2	30	chair	ɛə	tʃ ɛə	1
9	watch	ɒ	w ɒ tʃ	2	31	red	e	ɹ e d	2
10	nose	oʊ	n oʊ z	2	32	spoon	u	s p u n	3
11	mouth	aʊ	m aʊ θ	2	33	plane	eɪ	p w eɪ n	2
12	yawn	ɔ	j ɔ n	2	34	fly	aɪ	f w aɪ	1
13	leaf	i	ɹ i f	1	35	sky	aɪ	s k aɪ	2
14	thumb	ʌ	θ ʌ m	2	36	sun	ʌ	s ʌ n	2
15	foot	ʊ	f ʊ t	2	37	wing	ɪ	w ɪ ŋ	2
16	toe	oʊ	t oʊ	1	38	splash	æ	s p ɹ æ ʃ	3
17	snake	eɪ	s n eɪ k	3	39	tent	e	t e n t	3
18	van	æ	v æ n	2	40	salt	ɒ	s ɒ t	2
19	fast	a	f a s t	3	41	crab*	æ	k ɹ a b	3
20	girl	3	g 3 ʊ	1	42	sweet	i	s w i t	3
21	stairs*	eə	s t e z	3	43	sleeve	i	s w i v	2
22	big	ɪ	b ɪ g	2	44	zipper	ɪ	z ɪ p	2
		SUBTOTAL CC		44				**TOTAL CC**	93

Figure 9.11 Josie's fourth and final *Quick Screener* record form at 7;6

Epilogue

The following May, Maureen visited unexpectedly with her sister, but not Josie, to report progress. Josie, now 8;0, had been seen by her new therapist for a language assessment over 2 sessions. She had a composite language score of 100 on the CELF-4 Australian. She was grouped with two boys for weekly 30-minute sessions to work on a common target, /l/, in the lunch period at school, and a Reading Recovery teacher did individual 'l-homework' (but not Reading Recovery) with Josie and each of the boys twice weekly. No speech (or other) homework was sent home for any of the children. She had 8 group therapy sessions over 8 weeks with the SLP and 12 individual sessions with the Reading Recovery teacher, and was dismissed from therapy because she had reached the maximum allocation. Maureen was unsure, but she thought /l/ had not improved. She had not spoken to the SLP since the CELF-4 assessment. Maureen happily reported that Josie had maintained her other progress and was doing quite well academically in Year 2 (the third year of formal schooling in NSW). Plans to home-school her had been suspended for the time being because Josie was now enjoying school. Maureen said she and David might re-contact 'if the ells don't come good'.

Josie made remarkable progress with comparatively little SLP intervention in terms of therapist hours, and one has to wonder whether the outcome would have been so positive if her intervention had happened in the hands of a non-SLP within a typical (and increasingly prevalent) consultative framework or through an aide (McCartney et al., 2005).

She was on my caseload from 6;5 to 7;6. In that time, she had a language assessment (1 session), an initial speech assessment (1 session), and 15 intervention sessions, some of which incorporated ongoing assessment as required. She had two missed appointments due to illness. In all, she had 12.5 hours of in-clinic face-to-face intervention, requiring 3–4 hours of preparation for sessions by the clinician, plus the therapist's Einstein Time!

Her family's dedication to keeping scheduled appointments, participating in sessions, learning relevant skills, encouraging each other, helping Josie to maintain a positive attitude, implementing homework meticulously, and making it fun provides a wonderful example of what can be achieved even with tight limitations on the amount of intervention that can be administered. It also exemplifies the value of the SLP/SLT taking the time to plan explicitly principled therapy; the advantages of careful target selection with an eye to generalisation across a child's phonological system; the benefits of painstaking stimulability training; and the profound changes that can occur when the clinician manages every aspect of intervention him- or herself, in person, in a team effort with child and family.

Acknowledgement

Thanks are extended to Josie and her family for sharing their story; and to two of her SLPs for their willing participation in providing assessment data and other information.

References

Aguilar-Mediavilla, E. M., Sanz-Torrent, M., & Serra-Raventos, M. (2002). A comparative study of the phonology of pre-school children with specific language impairment (SLI), language delay (LD) and normal acquisition. *Clinical Linguistics and Phonetics, 16*(8), 573–596.

Baker, E. (2000). Changing nail to snail: A treatment efficacy study of phonological impairment in children. *Unpublished PhD thesis*, University of Sydney, Sydney.

Baker, E. (2010). The experience of discharging children from phonological intervention. *International Journal of Speech-Language Pathology, 12*(4), 325–328.

Ballard, K. J., Djaja, D., Arciuli, J., James, D. G. H., & van Doorn, J. (2012). Developmental trajectory for production of prosody: lexical stress contrastivity in children ages 3 to 7 years and in adults. *Journal of Speech, Language, and Hearing Research*, *55*(6), 1822–1835.

Barlow, J. A., & Gierut, J. A. (2002). Minimal pair approaches to phonological remediation. *Seminars in Speech and Language*, *2*(1), 57–67.

Bishop, D. V. M., & Adams, C. (1990). A prospective study of the relationship between specific language impairment, phonological disorders and reading retardation. *The Journal of Child Psychology and Psychiatry*, *31*(7), 1027–1050.

Bleile, K. M. (2004). *Manual of articulation and phonological disorders: Infancy through adulthood* (2nd ed.). Clifton Park, NY: Thomson Delmar Learning.

Bleile, K. M. (2013). *The late eight* (2nd ed.) San Diego, CA: Plural Publishing.

Bowen, C. (1996a). *Evaluation of a phonological therapy with treated and untreated groups of young children*. Unpublished doctoral dissertation. Macquarie University.

Bowen, C. (1996b). The quick screener. Retrieved 15 January 2014 from www.speech-language-therapy.com

Bowen, C. (1998a). *Developmental phonological disorders: A practical guide for families and teachers*. Melbourne: The Australian Council for Educational Research.

Bowen, C. (1998b). *Speech-language-therapy dot com*. Retrieved 15 January 2014 from www.speech-language-therapy.com

Bowen, C. (2007). *Les difficultés phonologiques chez l'enfant: guide à l'intention des familles, des enseignants et des intervenants en petite enfance*, Caroline Bowen; Rachel Fortin, traductrice et adaptatrice. Montréal: Chenelière-éducation.

Bowen, C. (2010). Parents and children together (PACT) intervention for children with speech sound disorders. In: A. L. Williams, S. McLeod, & R. J. McCauley (Eds.), *Interventions for speech sound disorders in children* (pp. 407–426). Baltimore, MD: Paul H. Brookes Publishing Co.

Bowen, C., & Cupples, L. (1998). A tested phonological therapy in practice. *Child Language Teaching and Therapy*, *14*(1), 29–50.

Bowen, C., & Cupples, L. (1999a). Parents and children together (PACT): A collaborative approach to phonological therapy. *International Journal of Language and Communication Disorders*, *34*(1), 35–55.

Bowen, C., & Cupples, L. (1999b). A phonological therapy in depth: a reply to commentaries. *Inter-national Journal of Language and Communication Disorders*, *34*(1), 65–83.

Bowen, C., & Cupples, L. (2004). The role of families in optimizing phonological therapy outcomes. *Child Language Teaching and Therapy*, *20*, 245–260.

Bowen, C., & Cupples, L. (2006). PACT: Parents and children together in phonological therapy. *Advances in Speech Language Pathology*, *8*(3), 282–292.

Catts, H. W. (1993). The relationship between speech-language disabilities and reading disabilities. *Journal of Speech and Hearing Research*, *36*, 948–958.

Clark, J., & Yallop, C. (1995). *An introduction to phonetics and phonology* (2nd ed.). Oxford: Basil Blackwell.

Cox, F. (2012). *Australian English: Pronunciation and transcription*. Cambridge University Press.

Crystal, D. (1996). Language play and linguistic intervention. *Child Language Teaching and Therapy*, *12*, 328–344.

Crystal, D. (1998). *Language play*. London: Penguin Books.

Day, A. (1993). *Carl goes to daycare*. New York, NY: Farrar, Straus & Giroux.

Davis, B. L. (1998). Consistency of consonant patterns by word position. *Clinical Linguistics and Phonetics*, *12*(4), 329–348.

Dean, E., & Howell, J. (1986). Developing linguistic awareness: A theoretically based approach to phonological disorders. *British Journal of Disorders of Communication*, *21*, 223–238.

Dean, E., Howell, J., Hill, A., & Waters, D. (1990). *Metaphon resource pack*. Windsor, Berks: NFER Nelson.

Dodd, B. (2009). Finding the correct dose of intervention for developmental speech impairment. In: C. Bowen (ed.), *Children's speech sound disorders* (pp. 322–327). Oxford: Wiley-Blackwell.

Dodd, B., Crosbie, S., Zhu, H., Holm, A., & Ozanne, A. (2002). *Diagnostic evaluation of articulation and phonology (DEAP)*. London: Psychological Corporation.

Elbro, C., Borstrøm, I., & Petersen, D. K. (1998). Predicting dyslexia from kindergarten: The importance of distinctness of phonological representations of lexical items. *Reading Research Quarterly*, *33*, 36–60.

Fey, M. E. (1992). Phonological assessment and treatment. Articulation and phonology: An introduction. *Language Speech and Hearing Services in Schools*, *23*, 224.

Fisher J., & Atkin, N. (1996). *Articulation survey*. Melbourne: Royal Children's Hospital.

Flynn, L., & Lancaster, G. (1996). *Children's phonology sourcebook*. Oxford: Winslow Press.

Gilbert, J. H. V., & Johnson, C. E. (1978). Temporal and sequential constraints on six-year-olds' phonological productions: Some observations on the ambliance phenomenon. *Journal of Child Language, 5*, 101–112.

Gillon, G. T. (2000). The efficacy of phonological awareness intervention for children with spoken language impairment. *Language, Speech, and Hearing Services in Schools, 31*(2), 126–141.

Grunwell, P. (1987). *Clinical phonology* (2nd ed.). Baltimore, MD: Williams & Wilkins.

Habers, H. M., Paden, E. P., & Halle, J. W. (1999). Phonological awareness and production: Changes during intervention. *Language, Speech and Hearing Services in Schools, 30*, 50–60.

Hesketh, A., Dima, E., & Nelson, V. (2007). Teaching phoneme awareness to pre-literate children with speech disorder: a randomized controlled trial. *International Journal of Language and Communication Disorders, 42*(3), 251–271.

Hodson, B. (2004). *Hodson assessment of phonological patterns* (3rd ed.). Austin, TX: Pro-Ed.

Hodson, B. (2007, 2010). *Evaluating and enhancing children's phonological systems: Research and theory to practice*. Wichita, KS: PhonoComp Publishers.

Ingram, D. (1976). *Phonological disability in children*. London: Edward Arnold.

James, D. G. H. (2006). Hippopotamus is so hard to say: Children's acquisition of polysyllabic words. *Unpublished PhD thesis*, University of Sydney, Sydney.

James, D. G. H., van Doorn, J., McLeod, S., & Esterman, A. (2008). Patterns of consonant deletion in typically developing children aged 3 to 7 years. *International Journal of Speech-Language Pathology. 10*(3), 179–192.

Johnson, C. A., Weston, A. D., & Bain, B. A. (2004). An objective and time-efficient method for determining severity of childhood speech delay. *American Journal of Speech-Language Pathology, 13*, 55–65.

Kehoe, M. (2001). Prosodic patterns in children's multisyllabic word patterns. *Language, Speech, and Hearing Services in Schools, 32*, 284–294.

Klein, E. S. (1996a). Phonological/traditional approaches to articulation therapy: A retrospective group comparison. *Language, Speech and Hearing Services in Schools, 27*, 314–323.

Klein, E. S. (1996b). *Clinical phonology: Assessment and treatment of articulation disorders in children and adults*. San Diego, CA: Singular Publishing Group, Inc.

Knowles, M. S. (1970). *The modern practise of adult education: Andragogy versus pedagogy*. New York, NY: Association Press.

Lancaster, G. S., Levin, A., Pring, T., & Martin, S. (2010). Treating children with phonological problems: Does an eclectic approach to therapy work? *International Journal of Language and Communication Disorders, 45*(2), 174–181.

Larrivee, L. S., & Catts, H. W. (1999). Early reading achievement in children with expressive phonological disorders. *American Journal of Speech-Language Pathology, 8*, 118–128.

Leitão, S., Hogben, J., & Fletcher, J. (1997). Phonological processing skills in speech and language impaired children. *European Journal of Disorders of Communication, 32*(2), 91–113.

Lewis, B. A., & Freebairn, L. (1992). Residual effects of preschool phonology disorders in grade school, adolescence and adulthood. *Journal of Speech and Hearing Research, 35*, 819–831.

Lewis, B. A., Freebairn, L., & Taylor, H. G. (2000). Follow-up of children with early expressive phonology disorders. *Journal of Learning Disabilities, 33*(5), 433–444.

Lewis, B. A., Freebairn, L. A., & Taylor, H. G. (2002). Correlates of spelling abilities in children with early speech sound disorders. *Reading and Writing: An Interdisciplinary Journal, 15*, 389–407.

Locke, J. L. (1980). The inference of speech perception in the phonologically disordered child. Part II: Some clinically novel procedures, their use, some findings. *Journal of Speech and Hearing Disorders, 45*, 445–468.

McCartney, E., Boyle, J., Bannatyne, S., Jessiman, E., Campbell, C. Kelsey, C., Smith, J., McArthur, J., & O'Hare, A. (2005). 'Thinking for two': A case study of speech and language therapists working through assistants. *International Journal of Language and Communication Disorders, 40*, 221–235.

McIntosh B., & Dodd, B. (2011). *Toddler phonology test*, London: Pearson Publishers.

McLeod, S., Verdon, S., & Bowen, C. (2013). International aspirations for speech-language pathologists' practice with multilingual children with speech sound disorders: Development of a position paper.

Journal of Communication Disorders, *46*, 375–387.

Miccio, A. W. (2005). A treatment program for enhancing stimulability. In: Kamhi, A. G., & Pollock, K. E. (Eds.), *Phonological disorders in children: Clinical decision making in assessment and intervention* (pp. 163–173). Baltimore, MD: Paul H. Brookes Publishing Co.

Moriarty, B. C., & Gillon, G. T. (2006). Phonological awareness intervention for children with childhood apraxia of speech. *International Journal of Language and Communication Disorders*, *41*, 713–734.

Ray, J. (2002). Treating phonological disorders in a multilingual child: A case study. *American Journal of Speech-Language Pathology*, *11*, 305–315.

Robey, R. R., & Schultz, M. C. (1998). A model for conducting clinical-outcome research: An adaptation of the standard protocol for use in aphasiology. *Aphasiology*, *12*, 787–810.

Roca, I., & Johnson, W. (1999). *A course in phonology*. Oxford: Blackwell Publishers.

Schmidt, R. A., & Lee, T. D. (2011). *Motor control and learning: A behavioural emphasis* (5th ed.). Champaign, IL: Human Kinetics.

Secord, W., Boyce, S. Donohue, J., Fox, R., & Shine R. (2007). *Eliciting sounds: Techniques and strategies for clinicians* (2nd ed.). Clifton Park, NY: Thompson Delmar Learning.

Selkirk, E. O. (1984). *Phonology and syntax*. Cambridge, MA: The MIT Press.

Stackhouse, J. (1985). Segmentation, speech and spelling difficulties. In: M. Snowling (Ed.), *Children's written language difficulties* (pp. 96–115). Windsor, Berkshire: The NFER-Nelson Publishing Company Ltd.

Stackhouse, J., & Wells, B. (1997). *Children's speech and literacy difficulties I: A psycholinguistic framework*. London: Whurr Publishers.

Stothard, S. E., Snowling, M. J., Bishop, D. V. M., Chipchase, B. B., & Kaplan, C. A. (1998). Language impaired preschoolers: A follow-up into adolescence. *Journal of Speech, Language and Hearing Research*, *41*, 407–418.

Strand, E., Stoeckel, R., & Baas, B. (2006). Treatment of severe childhood apraxia of speech: A treatment efficacy study. *Journal of Medical Speech Pathology*, *14*, 297–307.

Sutherland, D., & Gillon, G. T. (2005). Assessment of phonological representations in children with speech impairment. *Language, Speech and Hearing Services in Schools*, *36*, 294–307.

Sutherland, D., & Gillon, G. T. (2007). The development of phonological representations and phonological awareness in children with speech impairment. *International Journal of Language and Communication Disorders*, *42*(2), 229–250.

Unicomb, R., Hewat, S., Spencer, E., & Harrison, E. (2013). Clinicians' management of young children with co-occurring stuttering and speech sound disorder. *International Journal of Speech-Language Pathology*, *4*(15), 441–452.

Van Riper, C. (1978). *Speech correction: Principles and methods* (6th ed.), Englewood Cliffs, NJ: Prentice-Hall.

Watts, N. (2004). Assessment of vowels summary. *ACQuiring Knowledge in Speech, Language and Hearing*, Speech Pathology Australia, *6*(1), 22–25.

Watts Pappas, N., & Bowen, C. (2007). Speech acquisition and the family. In: McLeod, S. (Ed.), *The international guide to speech acquisition*. Clifton Park, NY: Thomson Delmar Learning.

Weiner, F. (1981). Treatment of phonological disability using the method of meaningful contrast: Two case studies. *Journal of Speech and Hearing Disorders*, *46*, 97–103.

Williams, A. L. (2012). Intensity in phonological intervention: Is there a prescribed amount? *International Journal of Speech-Language Pathology*, *14*(5), 456–461.

Young, E. C. (1991). An analysis of young children's ability to produce multisyllabic words. *Clinical Linguistics and Phonetics*, *5*, 297–316.

Young, E. C. (1995). An analysis of a treatment approach for phonological errors in polysyllabic words. *Clinical Linguistics and Phonetics*, *9*, 59–77.

Chapter 10
Directions and reflections

In this final chapter, Benjamin Munson, Suzanne Purdy and colleagues, Suze Leitão and Joan Rosenthal traverse a breadth of topics, including a rarely considered one in the context of child speech. It concerns sociophonetics, gender stereotyping and social indexing, and Munson (A51) approaches it with enthusiasm and empathy. Purdy, Fairgray and Asad (A52) provide an account of the important links between hearing and SSD, delivering expert guidance from an Audiology perspective. Leitão (A53) reflects on the art and science of clinical thinking, and the issues that can arise. And finally, and inspirationally, Rosenthal (A54) presents her key components of a practitioners' survival kit.

Sociophonetics

In the world of phoneticians, the burgeoning field of sociophonetics resides at the intersection of sociolinguistics and phonetics. Most of its work has involved descriptive accounts of phonetic and phonological variation within regional dialects, speech styles, or (social) speech groups and attempts to explore the relationship between phonetics and phonology (Ohala, 1990). By comparison, there has been scant exploration of the relationship between phonetic and phonological variation and how speech is perceived. Roberts (2002) provides a summary of available data, which suggest that children acquire knowledge of sociolinguistic variation from the earliest stages. Precisely *how* variation comes to be learned in the course of language acquisition is poorly understood. However, we do know that many social factors systematically shape variation in speech production, including individual differences such as age, gender, ethnicity and socio-economic status (Labov, 1994–2001), and the influence of social groups and networks with which speakers are associated (Eckert, 2000; Milroy, 1987). Sociophonetics has applications in pedagogy, foreign language teaching, forensic phonetics and multi-layered transcription (Müller, 2006). In SLP/SLT, it has undeniable implications for understanding of child-directed speech (parentese), therapy discourse, style shifting,

Children's Speech Sound Disorders, Second Edition. Caroline Bowen.
© 2015 John Wiley & Sons, Ltd. Published 2015 by John Wiley & Sons, Ltd.
Companion website: www.wiley.com/go/bowen/speechlanguagetherapy

speaker- and listener-oriented articulatory control, register, code switching and for deepening cultural and linguistic sensitivity.

Dr. Benjamin Munson is a Professor in Speech Language Hearing Sciences at the University of Minnesota, Minneapolis. His many research interests include relationships among phonology, metaphonology, and the lexicon; speech production in phonological impairment; the cognitive and linguistic bases of phonological development and disorders in children; gender typicality in children's speech, including when and how children learn to express gender through speech, with a particular focus on how this learning interacts with more general aspects of language learning; and sociophonetics.

Q51. Benjamin Munson: Sociophonetics and child speech practice

Quite inadvertently, Van Borsel, Van Rentergem and Verhaeghe (2007) pointed to the importance of SLPs/SLTs having informed views of linguistic variation, enabling them to distinguish genuine pathology from natural non-standard variation, and this is clearly an area where sociophonetics can help. What are the methods of enquiry in this non-traditional area of study? Can you explore for the interested clinician or clinical researcher the likely impact of, and clinically relevant research areas in children's SSDs for, sociophonetics as its literature base mushrooms and interfaces with clinical phonology (Müller & Ball, A3)?

A51. Benjamin Munson: Sociolinguistic variation and speech sound disorders

As practicing SLPs/SLTs know, the articulatory and perceptual characteristics of speech sounds vary from talker to talker, and within talkers, from utterance to utterance. For instance, phonetic detail can vary across talkers due to anatomic and dialectal differences; and within talkers, as a function of ambient noise (Lane & Tranel, 1971), or the presumed language abilities of the person being addressed (e.g., Bradlow, 2002).

Determining whether a variation reflects pathology, warranting treatment, or whether it is normal, is a challenge faced whenever we differentiate between language impairment and first-language interference in children from culturally and linguistically diverse backgrounds (Goldstein, A19; Zajdó, A20). Understanding of, and sensitivity to, the sources of variation simplify the task of forming these judgements.

Imagine two girls growing up in North America who demonstrate *superficially* equivalent pronunciation patterns, apparently omitting within word /ɹ/ as in *every*, substituting /f/ for /θ/ word finally as in *bath*, and omitting final /t/ and /d/ as in *hat* and *bad*, respectively. One girl has these errors because of a problem in phonological acquisition, and requires intervention. The other does not have errors *per se*, but rather, sound patterns that indicate successful acquisition of a variant of English, African American English, in which these are the speech community's pronunciations (for a review see Thomas, 2007). The second girl requires no intervention, except perhaps to say that if she were to interact with people in dialectally diverse speech communities, she might benefit from explicit instruction in appropriate code-switching.

Assessing whether variation is pathological or not can be complex, and certainly not always as straightforward, for US clinicians at least, as the comparison above would indicate. Take for example the labiodental variants of /ɹ/, transcribed as [ʋ], in some dialects of English in the United Kingdom. Superficially, they sound like /ɹ/ misarticulations that occur in typical acquisition by younger children and in older children with misarticulations. An improbable interpretation of this variant is that it represents a widespread, persistent speech error, but as Foulkes and Docherty (2000) show, rates of use of [ʊ] are highly linked to social stratification. Indeed, its use might signal, intentionally or unintentionally, membership of different social groups, rather than social-group differences in the incidence of misarticulation. SLPs/SLTs cannot determine whether a [ʊ] for /ɹ/, pattern is an error without knowing its social function in a speech community.

Sociophonetics

Sociophonetics melds methodologies and theoretical constructs from several disciplines, including experimental phonetics, psycholinguistics and sociolinguistics. Foulkes (2005) summarises how sociophoneticians catalogue variation in the sound structure of language echoing social-group membership, in production and perception, and how this interacts with other linguistically based phonetic variation: segmental and prosodic.

Perceptual studies in this sub-field reveal that listeners readily associate different pronunciation variants with social categories, often in ways contrary to the actual use of these variants in a population. Niedzielski (1999) illustrates this in an influential study of vowel perception by people in Detroit, Michigan. Participants were presented with synthesised vowels in a speaker identification task, and told that the vowels were modelled on the productions of either Detroiters, or residents of nearby Windsor, Ontario, who speak a different English dialect. Labelling of the Windsor vowels, by the Detroit participants, showed tactic knowledge of the ways that people within that dialect region speak. Interestingly, the labels listeners gave for vowels presumed to be produced by Detroiters exposed social stereotypes of the speech of Detroiters that did not match their actual vowel productions.

A qualitatively similar case comes from Mack and Munson (2012). They examined listeners' perception of men's sexual orientation according to how /s/-initial words were produced. A popular-culture stereotype in North America and in much of the Commonwealth of Nations holds that gay men lisp. Though the term 'lisp' has fallen out of scientific use among SLP/SLTs, it clearly connotes a misarticulation. Published studies on /s/ variation and sexual orientation in men show that individuals' production of /s/ is associated with both actual and perceived sexual orientation (Linville, 1998; Munson, McDonald, DeBoe & White, 2006). The distinctive /s/ associated with gay- and gay-sounding men's speech, however, is arguably a hypercorrect /s/, and not a lisp, as its acoustic characteristics serve to better differentiate it from the acoustically similar sounds /ʃ/ and /θ/ than the heterosexual and heterosexual-sounding men's /s/ (Jongman, Wayland & Wong, 2000). Munson and Zimmerman (2006) found that listeners label a talker as gayer-sounding when presented with stimuli containing a hypercorrect /s/ than when presented with stimuli containing /s/ with average acoustic characteristics. Nearly identical scores were elicited when listeners rated tokens containing a frontally misarticulated /s/, even though its acoustic characteristics differed markedly from those of hypercorrect /s/.

Other research demonstrating that listener expectations affect speech perception reinforces these findings. For example, expectations about talker gender and social class affect the categorisation of speech sounds (Hay, Warren & Drager, 2006; Munson, 2011; Strand & Johnson, 1996). Strand and Johnson, and Munson, showed that acoustically equivalent American-English lingual fricatives are labelled differently depending whether listeners believed they are listening to a man (favouring a /s/ response) or to a woman (favouring a /ʃ/ response), perhaps signifying tacit knowledge of sex differences in production of these sounds. Hay et al.

(2006) showed that listeners in New Zealand label the acoustically ambiguous diphthongs in *hair* and *here* differently depending on whether they are led to believe they are produced by a woman or a man, and by a working-class or a middle-class person.

The cases of sexual orientation and /s/, and /ɹ/ variation in the United Kingdom, are particularly interesting, illustrating that considerable variation in pronunciation can occur *within* a speech community, without appearing to be due to obvious anatomic or physiologic differences. Moreover, their origins appear to be different from those for regional dialects, the formation of which may be related to factors such as migration and language contact (Trudgill, 2004). But surely labiodental /ɹ/([ʋ]), hyperarticulated /s/ and very local phonetic variants within high school cliques (Eckert, 2000; Mendoza-Denton, 2007), cannot result from such factors. Rather, they appear to be instances of groups of individuals exploiting permissible variation in speech to convey social categories, *alongside* propositional linguistic information.

Consequences of variation

In addition to understanding the *causes* of variation, SLPs/SLTs must understand its *consequences*. Consider the fairly robust finding that: English-speaking women hyperarticulate vowels more than men (Bradlow, Torretta & Pisoni, 1996). Perceptual studies reviewed in Munson and Babel (2007) show that many listeners make tacit associations between hyperarticulation and sex typicality of speech. What if children held these stereotypes, too? If they did, they might judge less-articulate male peers as more masculine sounding, and more-articulate female peers as more feminine sounding. This in turn might promote a powerful social motivation for some children, particularly young boys, to resist speech and language therapy aimed at improving intelligibility, because 'success'

might manifest as a boy sounding less boy-like! Then again, imagine a child with a [t] for /s/ substitution being taught /s/ in therapy. One likely and reasonable instructional strategy would be for the clinician to model a hyperarticulate /s/. The social meaning associated with that phonetic variant in some English-speaking contexts might make boys in particular averse to learning it.

A child who is taught only one variant of /s/ in therapy is ill-equipped to manipulate its characteristics to convey different social registers, unless therapy promotes spontaneous learning of the full range of /s/ variants through encoding and emulation of different models in the population. To this end, peer modelling might be incorporated into therapy.

Implications for practice

When clinical SLPs/SLTs are proactive in incorporating ethnographic analysis into their practice, especially with culturally and linguistically diverse populations, they examine the range of phonetic variation throughout the communities in which a child communicates. They develop both taxonomies of phonetic variants and observations of the communicative functions of these variants, much as Eckert (2000) and Mendoza-Denton (2007) did when researching sociophonetic variation in high school students' speech. Ethnographic analysis holds promise for a rich and detailed picture, more complex, more informative and more culturally apt than traditional descriptive approaches to child speech, a suggestion that is consistent with many of the works assembled by Müller (2006).

When prescriptive standards rather than ethnographic analysis are used, the boundary between 'error' and 'normal variation' might not be clear. This is illustrated by a series of studies of the incidence of different articulations of /s/ by young adults in Belgium. Van Borsel et al. (2007)

examined an almost 23% incidence of what they characterised as dentally misarticulated /s/ in Belgian university students aged 18 to 22, reported to be 'native speakers of Dutch'. Their incidence fluctuated as a function of some variables rarely cited as being associated with misarticulation rates, such as university field of study. The lowest rates of interdental /s/ were among humanities students, with higher values for natural sciences and social sciences students, and a significant majority of those identified as lisping were unaware that they were assessed as such. Carefully indicating that their finding might not be new, they cite a palatographic study (Dart, 1991, see also Dart, 1998) that revealed dental articulation of /s/ and /z/ by French-speaking (42.1%, p. 48) and English-speaking (22.8%, p. 50) adults with no obvious speech, language or hearing impairments. Moreover, Van Borsel et al. (2007) concede that no definitive interpretation of their findings exists. They speculate, however, that they might reflect increased social tolerance to imprecision in articulation, or to the influence, on Dutch pronunciation, of English in which /θ/ and /s/ and their voiced cognates are phonemic.

How might these authors have incorporated insights from sociophonetics into their study? First, by examining more incisively the distribution of variants relative to actual or perceived social categories, especially in view of their intriguing finding that these categories differed as a function of university course. Were the students marking their affiliation to humanities or the sciences with distinctive patterns of phonetic variation? Then, analysis of listener perceptions of the participants' /s/ production might have yielded surprising insights. For example, the dental sound might have been associated more strongly with affiliation with a particular social group than with a judgement that the person produced speech less accurately. It is interesting to speculate how such a finding might help explain why the variant

is present. Consider, for example, that this research took place in Belgium, where many languages, including Belgian French and Flemish (the Belgian variant of Dutch), are spoken. As shown by Dart, French has a higher rate of dental fricative productions than English. Perhaps the higher use of dental fricative in certain groups relates to their exposure to or social identification with the French-speaking population in that country. That, of course, is mere speculation on this author's part, but it shows how sociophonetic methods could have been used to flesh out Van Borsel et al.'s findings. If, in the analysis, these variants actually indicated *pathology*, then it might be reasonable to suggest that Belgian logopedists consider treating them more aggressively in children and adolescents.

But if these are indeed normal sociophonetic variants, then they do not warrant treatment in the traditional sense, although they might legitimately be the subjects of a regimen to increase talkers' linguistic flexibility. That is, SLPs/SLTs should not be blind to the fact that non-pathological variation may be associated with negative judgements by some listeners, especially where they index membership in a group that is itself stigmatised. In this regard Van Borsel et al. (2007) cite references supporting an argument that frontal lisping can be associated with negative evaluative judgements.

An individual's communicative effectiveness, broadly speaking, resides in part on their ability to fluently switch among different phonetic variants in socially appropriate contexts, and SLPs/SLTs are best positioned, in terms of their knowledge and skill bases, to help people who find this problematic. But it must be emphasised that a population that speaks a non-standard variant is not a disordered population, and their presenting 'condition' is not a disorder. By carefully assessing whether productions are deviant, as opposed to normal, socially stratified variants, SLPs/SLTs can ensure that they do not improperly treat normal variation as pathology.

SLPs/SLTs should also be aware that a variant perceived negatively in one context or by one group might be perceived positively by another group or in another context. The association between /s/ and men's sexuality in the many English-speaking countries is a case in point. While this variant is associated with both actual and perceived sexual orientation, it is also associated with hyperarticulate speech. A man whose habitual /s/ demonstrates these characteristics would be ill-advised to change his /s/ characteristics in all communicative contexts, as doing so would prevent him from projecting the positive characteristics that are associated with clear-sounding speech.

A view from audiology

In the industrialised world at least, an Audiologist *also* assesses almost every child with SSD who is assessed by an SLP/SLT. Apart from the resultant audiogram and tympanogram being read and carefully filed, there is often little overt appreciation of this essential input. SLP/SLT clinicians who are not dually qualified in Audiology may have a poor grasp of hearing issues relative to this population. For one significant example, the high incidence of conductive hearing loss in children with cleft palate is well known, but the generalist SLP/SLT may not know how hearing acuity should be monitored.

Professor Suzanne Purdy heads Speech Science in the School of Psychology at the University of Auckland. Her clinical background is in audiology and she has received service awards from the Australian and New Zealand audiological societies. She completed her PhD in Speech Pathology and Audiology at the University of Iowa in 1990 and has published widely in the area of communication disorders, with more than 100 published articles and book chapters. She has a particular

interest in hearing loss, speech perception and auditory processing in children.

Ms. Liz Fairgray is a Speech-Language Therapist who has practised in the area of paediatric communication difficulties since 1985. Her MSc is in speech pathology and audiology. Liz has a strong interest in oral communication for children with moderate to profound hearing loss and in 2001, was the first New Zealander to become a Certified Auditory Verbal Therapist. Liz was the founding therapist for The Hearing House, a centre for oral communication for children with profound hearing loss and cochlear implants (CIs). Liz joined The University of Auckland's Listening and Language Clinic, in 2007, seeing children with a wide range of communication difficulties. She uses a family centred approach, ensuring that parents attend sessions and collaboratively develop goals and practice strategies to develop spoken communication. Liz also provides supervision to SLT students and gives lectures to masters level SLT and Audiology students.

Ms. Areej Asad is a PhD candidate in Speech Science at The University of Auckland. She previously worked as a clinician and clinical tutor in the Center for Phonetics Research, Speech and Hearing Clinic at the University of Jordan. Her research interests are in narrative language, speech outcomes of monolingual and bilingual children with hearing loss and evidence-based speech therapy.

Q52. Suzanne C. Purdy, Liz Fairgray and Areej Asad: Audiology and speech pathology

What would an Audiologist like to be able to tell SLPs/SLTs working with child speech regarding the speech spectrum and audibility of speech sounds with different types of hearing loss? Are there particular screening, referral and management consideration to be taken into account with indigenous, low SES, culturally and linguistically diverse, and other special populations; what are the research needs and directions; what communication and collaboration would you like to see between SLPs/SLTs and Audiologists; and are there any good news stories?

A52.   Suzanne C. Purdy, Liz Fairgray and Areej Asad: Hearing and children's speech sound disorders

Hearing loss degrades perceived acoustic characteristics of speech, and speech perception and speech production are closely linked. In pre-schoolers, more severe hearing loss is associated with more severe SSD (Schonweiler, Ptok & Radu, 1998). Infants with hearing loss have delayed onset of consistent canonical babbling and delayed consonant development (Moeller et al., 2007). Moeller, et al. found that infants with hearing loss, aged 10–24 months produced fewer fricatives and affricates [f, v, θ, ð, s, z, ʃ, ʒ, tʃ, ʤ] than controls. There was variability in speech development for children with similar hearing losses, so the audiogram does not completely explain speech outcomes for children with hearing loss.

Relating the acoustics of the speech signal to the audiogram

The audiogram (see Figure A52.1) plots hearing thresholds measured in *decibels hearing level* (dB HL) as a function of *speech frequency* measured in Hertz (Hz). 0 dB HL represents the softest sound heard, on average, at each frequency by young adults.

Although human hearing spans 20–20,000 Hz, audiologists routinely test hearing at 250–8000 Hz because this encompasses most of speech (see Box 10.1). For young children, frequencies tested may only include 500, 1000, 2000 and 4000 Hz. The softest and highest pitched sounds in English,

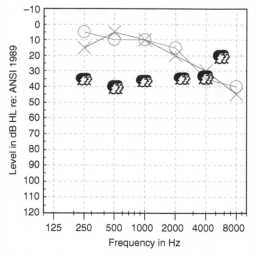

Figure A52.1 Pure tone audiogram showing mild bilateral, high-frequency hearing loss. Circles = right ear; crosses = left ear hearing thresholds. Normal hearing thresholds are in the range −10 to +15 dB HL. The dB HL scale represents hearing levels relative to hearing of young 'otologically normal' 18–30-year-olds. Face symbols on the graph represent average speech level in each frequency region for conversational speech (59 dB SPL at 1 m spoken by an adult female) (Cox & Moore, 1988). Even with mild hearing loss, high-frequency speech sounds (e.g., /s/) are close to hearing threshold, and may not be audible. The term 'speech banana' is used to refer to the speech spectrum since speech is softest for very low and high frequencies and loudest at low-mid frequencies, producing a banana shape plotted on the audiogram. Hearing thresholds of 16–25 dB HL = slight hearing loss, 26–40 dB = mild, 41–55 dB = moderate, 56–70 dB = moderate–severe, 71–90 dB = severe and >90 dB = profound (Clark, 1981).

/s/ and /ʃ/, contain significant energy above 4000 Hz, however, these frequencies may not be tested in young children. These sounds may not be audible even if the audiogram suggests normal hearing, unless the speaker is very close. Processed by hearing aids, /s/ and /ʃ/ sound very similar. Children with mild or greater hearing losses commonly misarticulate fricatives (Moeller et al., 2007).

Key aspects of speech affecting perception are intensity, frequency content and timing. Speech intensity decreases with distance; for example the speech level reduces by 6 dB when distance doubles. Speakers automatically adjust vocal effort to compensate for increased listener distance, but cannot *fully* compensate for reduced sound levels at distance. Important temporal (timing) aspects of speech include suprasegmental factors (rate, pauses between words and sentences, variations in pitch across utterances), and segmental factors, such as voice onset time (VOT, interval from plosive release to onset of voicing of vowel), and timing of vowel formant frequency transitions. Listeners with sensorineural hearing loss (SNHL) have impaired temporal processing, and may not detect short gaps or rapid sound transitions. Lane and Perkell (2005) reported a tendency for differences between voiced and voiceless VOT to be reduced in pre- and postlingually deafened speakers.

Box 10.1 Pure tone audiometry and tympanometry

Pure tone audiometry (PTA): PTA is used to measure hearing sensitivity. Tones are presented via earphones. If a loudspeaker is used with young children only the 'better' ear is tested. The softest levels at which tones are detected are hearing thresholds (measured in dB HL). In pre-schoolers, PTA is performed using conditioned play. In children 6–24 months Visual Reinforcement Audiometry (VRA) is used. Infants make a head turn response to sounds, reinforced by presenting an illuminated, moving mechanical puppet.

Tympanometry: Tympanometry is used to measure middle ear function. The tympanometer probe inserted into the ear contains a pressure pump, tone generator and microphone to measure sound levels. As ear canal pressure changes from positive to negative, the eardrum is 'clamped' by the pressure, then released, then clamped again. This causes a peak in the tympanogram near normal air pressure, as shown in Figure A52.2. The peak indicates maximum middle ear admittance (energy flow through the system); this

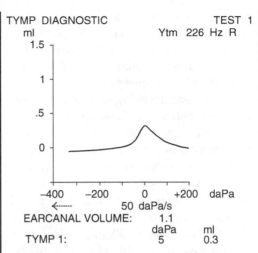

Figure A52.2 This is a normal 'Type A' tympanogram. The ear canal volume of 1.1 mL is estimated based on the admittance at +200 daPa pressure, when the eardrum is clamped with positive pressure and there is reduced energy flow through the middle ear. The peak occurs close to zero pressure, at 5 daPa, with a normal peak admittance value of 0.3 mL. 'Admittance' refers to flow of energy through a mechanical system (eardrum, middle ear space and middle ear ossicles). Peaks that occur below −100 daPa ('Type C' tympanograms) indicate negative middle ear pressure. Flat 'Type B' tympanograms indicate either a perforation in the eardrum (if volume is high) or a blocked middle ear (if volume is low), usually due to OME.

should be close to 0 decaPascals (daPa) pressure, indicating normal eustachian tube aeration of the middle ear.

Does otitis media cause SSD?

Otitis media with effusion (OME) (glue ear) is common amongst pre-schoolers (Simpson et al., 2007). OME is associated with hearing levels of about 25 dB HL and is typically worse for low frequencies. Some children with persistent OME have mild–moderate hearing loss. Treatment of OME remains controversial. A *Cochrane Review* in 2010 concluded that treatment with grommets provided some hearing improvement but found no evidence for effects on speech, language or other longer-term outcomes (Browning, Rovers, Williamson, Lous & Burton, 2010). No randomised controlled studies have investigated OME treatment effects for children with established speech and language problems. Shriberg and colleagues reviewed 27 publications (1969–1996) examining OME as a risk factor for SSD. They concluded there is 'limited evidence for a strong correlative association between early OME and [SSD]' and 'no evidence for a direct causal association between OME and speech disorder' (Shriberg et al., 2000, p. 80). Severity of hearing loss, not number of OME episodes, is a key predictor of speech and language outcomes. OME presence is commonly monitored via tympanometry (see Box 10.1, Figure A52.2), which does not test hearing sensitivity.

Young children with OME exhibit restricted phonetic inventories, a preference for bilabial stops, word initial glottal replacement, nasal deviations and limited production of velars, liquids and obstruents (Petinou, Schwartz, Mody & Gravel, 1999). Shriberg et al. (2000) reported that OME-positive Native American children had an almost fivefold increased SSD risk. OME has greater impact when risk factors co-occur, with greater hearing loss, or with earlier onset.

Intervention

Children with moderate-profound SNHL are typically fitted with hearing aids and receive SLP/SLT and other interventions once hearing loss is confirmed. Minimal hearing loss affects speech and language and hence should also be treated, but unfortunately children with mild and unilateral hearing loss may not receive any assistance, despite evidence for speech, language and school difficulties (Lieu, 2004).

CIs provide electrical auditory nerve stimulation for children with severe-profound hearing loss who do not benefit from hearing aids. Early identification of hearing loss, early age of CI, and early speech/language intervention contribute to better speech outcomes. Children with CIs show improvements in pre-first-word vocalisations (Kishon-Rabin, Taitelbaum-Swead, Ezrati-Vinacour, Kronnenberg & Hildesheimer, 2004), phonetic inventory (Blamey, Barry & Jacq, 2001), phoneme accuracy (Connor, Craig, Raudenbush, Heavner & Zwolan, 2006), phonological development (Kim & Chin, 2008), and speech intelligibility (Calmels et al., 2004). Speech is typically delayed by time without sound, and speech errors persist in some children despite early intervention. Peng, Weiss, Cheung & Lin (2004) reported that 6- to 12-year-old Mandarin-speakers with 2–6 years implant experience had fewest errors for plosives and most errors for nasals, affricates, fricatives,] and the lateral approximant /l/. Blamey et al. (2001) reported a plateau 5–6 years after implantation; eight phones failed to attain a 50% criterion in five or more of nine children (/ɔɪ, ʊə, ʒ, t, s, z, tʃ, θ/).

Early studies of children with severe-profound hearing loss using hearing aids reported sentence speech intelligibility of about 20% (Osberger, 1992). Intelligibility increases on average from 28% to 62% after 36 months CI experience in children receiving CIs before age 3 (Ertmer, 2008). Speech of children using CIs or hearing aids contains developmental and non-developmental (unusual) processes. When Flipsen Jr. and Parker (2008) examined connected speech from children implanted at age 1;8-3;0, tested over 21 months, they identified common developmental patterns such as cluster reduction, final consonant deletion, fronting, stopping, unstressed syllable deletion and liquid simplification, and non-developmental patterns, for example, vowel substitution and initial consonant deletion.

There are few studies of therapy outcomes for children with hearing loss. Auditory Verbal Therapy (AVT), a widely adopted approach for children with SNHL, emphasises listening over looking. AVT focuses on early identification, optimal amplification and good signal quality to enhance access to speech (Lim & Simser, 2005). Despite widespread practitioner support, Rhoades (2006) concluded there is little high-level evidence supporting AVT.

Paatsch, Blamey, Sarant & Bow (2006) demonstrated improvements in PCC (Flipsen Jr., A11) after computer-based speech production training for children with mild-profound hearing loss. Visual feedback is a useful component of speech therapy with individuals with hearing loss. Ultrasound and EPG (Pantelemidou, Herman & Thomas, 2003; Bacsfalvi & Bernhardt, 2011) and articulation training with a computer-animated talking head (Massaro & Light, 2004) have also been successful for hearing-impaired children and adolescents.

Communication and collaboration between SLPs/SLTs and audiologists

Audiological assessment is always recommended for children with SSD, but is particularly important for children with OME histories. Children with earlier onset of OME, more episodes, poorer hearing and other risk factors have greater SSD risk. Timely referral to otolaryngology is recommended because more aggressive medical management may eventuate if speech delay is combined with poor audiology results. For craniofacial abnormalities and/or syndromic conditions commonly associated with OME and/or SNHL (Golding-Kushner, A17; Ruscello, A48), management of speech and hearing and ear health requires a close, ongoing partnership between professionals and families.

Effective communication between SLPs/SLTs and audiologists is needed to ensure efficacious interventions for children with hearing loss. When the child has early diagnosed hearing loss, without additional complications, development of age-typical spoken language is the likely therapy goal. If there are co-existing conditions, or compromised CI electrode insertion due to cochlear calcification that can occur in meningitis, the goal may be intelligible simple spoken phrases while using signing as the primary communication and learning modality. For a goal of spoken language, interventions may include Maximal Oppositions intervention (Williams, A26), Grunwell's approach described in Chapter 4 (Grunwell, 1985, 1989, 1992), the Cycles Phonological Pattern Approach (Hodson, A5), conventional Minimal Pairs (Weiner, 1981), tactile/kinaesthetic sensory augmentation, and face and lip reading. Development of intelligible speech and language depends upon early intense, structured intervention supported by parental reinforcement of target goals.

Research needs

Prospective longitudinal studies are needed to determine the impact of OME on speech, using measures associated with longer-term outcomes. Some children with hearing loss treated at an early age have persistent speech errors. Reasons for individual variability and optimal therapy approaches children require further investigation.

Resource

An extended version of this essay is available on the *Children's Speech Sound Disorders, Second Edition* companion website.

Choices

The term 'best available evidence' is frequently taken to mean research-based knowledge, but as a process guiding intervention, E^3BP integrates a variety of data sources, including case studies by clinicians. The process also incorporates systematic on-going education of professionals and informed involvement of clients, while taking account of a mass of practical workplace issues. In the hurly burly of practice, most choices in assessment and intervention incorporate elements of clinical thinking and clinical judgement, often involving that highly prized ingredient: clinical intuition. We know these phenomena, recognising that they occur somewhere between clinical observations and clinical decision-making, but they elude precise definition and are difficult, if not impossible, to teach. As clinicians making decisions, we rely on the evidence base, solid theory and as much of 'the literature' as we can tackle in our full schedules (Highman, A41), as well as client perspectives and our own insights and experiences. This is often in situations where time is limited, access is poor, data are missing or ambiguous, and there are competing long- and short-term trade-offs to contend with.

A Fellow of Speech Pathology Australia, Dr. Suze Leitão has a long-standing clinical and research interest in children with speech and literacy difficulties. She is a senior lecturer in speech pathology in the School of Psychology & Speech Pathology at Curtin University in Western Australia. Her research interests include speech and language impairment, phonological processing and speech-literacy links. In recent years, her teaching in the areas of professional practice, ethics and clinical science has caused her to reflect on the mix of art and science involved in clinical decision-making in this age of E^3BP (Dollaghan, 2007).

Q53. Suze Leitão: Clinical thinking

In the messy real world, manualised procedures and the science of therapy often have to give way to the art of therapy. But here's the rub: the so-called art has to be consistent with our moral frameworks, ethical codes, and 'the science'. Can you reflect on these issues in relation to children's speech and literacy difficulties?

A53. Suze Leitão: Clinical decision-making: art and science

Over my years of clinical practice, I have often had to reach out for help from mentors and peers when faced with a situation where I felt doing things 'by the book' was not the right thing to do.

I have strong memories of a letter a mother sent me where she explained in great detail her anger at me for talking to her about her son's severe speech difficulties and the implications for his reading and spelling while he was in the room. As a young clinician, I had felt that describing his difficulties to Robert (aged 12) and his mother was the accurate and truthful way to give feedback and explain why I thought he needed therapy urgently at his age. I now see that, whereas the objective data may have led me to a clinical decision regarding therapy *based on evidence* (which I explained as clearly as I could), there were a number of other issues I needed to consider. Consultation with other professionals such as a psychologist and his teacher may have benefited my approach with this client, for example. Understanding the family dynamics and relationships may have influenced the way I approached the feedback session. Not only 'looking back at', but also 'reflecting on' the episode to make sense of it and try to understand it, allowed me to learn from it and incorporate this knowledge into my own developing clinical decision-making skills. Needless to say, I never saw the family again and do not know if he received treatment!

In my current role teaching clinical science to speech pathology students, I have even more cause to reflect on my own frameworks for decision-making. There is nothing better for sharpening the mind than teaching others! Unpacking the process and content of clinical decision-making in my role as a clinical educator and lecturer has opened my eyes to the complexity of what students often think we do seamlessly.

So what factors do we consider when we approach the task of making clinical decisions? How can we balance the *art* of being a clinician with clinical *science*? How can we develop a framework of proactive ethical practice? Reflecting on our own framework of morals and values and how we apply these to our own practice is one place to start. For example, most, if not all, cultures place value on telling the truth. I felt I was drawing on that principle when I explained to the young boy and his mother, the extent of his speech difficulties and the relationship of this to his spelling difficulties.

Our professional codes of ethics are another useful guide. The Speech Pathology Australia code of ethics, an aspirational framework, places strong emphasis on truth, balancing the doing of good with not causing harm, fairness and autonomy. The Code was revised in 2010 with the aim of encouraging clinicians to integrate ethical decision-making into their everyday practice. Perhaps if I had reflected in advance on the possible implications of the way I planned to run my feedback session with Robert, I could have presented my findings to his mother first, provided a clear written summary and discussed with her how best to run the session with him?

We also have the law and our legal responsibilities to our clients and our profession to provide us with another key set of principles. And this is all before we even get to the evidence base for therapy for speech, literacy and swallowing difficulties, its theoretical underpinnings, and the data we collect on therapy outcomes!

So... clinical decision-making should really be quite easy then? Giving advice to families and clients a piece of cake? Just a matter of creating some decision-making trees with yes/no junctions and procedural manuals, and always sticking to the 'truth'?

Well, no, not really.

Unfortunately the world is a messy place. To a large extent, clinical decision-making within moral, ethical, and legal frameworks is about relationships and context. Clinical decision-making requires us to analyse and interpret – to combine science with art, yet still maintain our professional integrity and do the right thing by our clients.

In one place where I used to work, children were not considered eligible for services if they were considered to have 'dyspraxia' (CAS), as the educational policy of the time was that this somewhat controversial condition did not affect language development. The term 'phonological disorder', on the other hand, or 'speech and language disorder', would allow a client to be considered eligible! So how would a diagnostic decision tree help me decide what was the 'truth' to put in my reports?

Parents of children with severe and persistent speech and literacy difficulties often contact me for advice regarding 'cures' they have read about in the papers or seen on the television or Internet. Many of these programs are expensive and involve signing a contract for a substantial fee and time frame. Some of these push a scientific or pseudoscientific approach, whereas others rely heavily on testimonials. I was recently contacted by a family who had embarked on such a program and rang me after 6 weeks to tell me that they had seen some progress but were finding the payments difficult and could not decide whether to continue or try and get their money back. What to say? There was little solid research behind the program, but the family had not seen much progress with more traditional therapy. As Powell (A39) puts it: the use of controversial treatments is not prohibited by most codes of professional ethics, but to be ethical in our practice we need to balance beneficence with non-maleficence (do good and not do harm). Like Stoeckel

(A40), I wondered how I could provide them with a variety of resources and help them evaluate the program yet remain supportive and respectful of their choices. I had to acknowledge that they had already spent a large sum of money that they would not get back and that they might be up for more payments whatever their choice, to continue or withdraw. This kind of investment does tend to bias one's evaluation of progress!

The evidence base for our profession is lacking, there is no doubt (Rosenthal, A54). But we do have a growing basis to support our clinical practice and our clinical decision-making. We must treat every client in a scientific manner: gather our data and analyse them carefully. We must, of course, draw on the evidence base for treatment approaches and the emerging number of 'manualised' procedures. But, herein lies the art – we must also take care not to lose sight of the client as an individual.

I recommend that SLPs/SLTs carefully consider the evidence you do have but interpret it within the wider context that includes client-, family-, clinician- and even wider, maybe agency- or service-related factors and frameworks. Set up hypotheses to match your clinical evidence, but do not ignore those intuitive hunches! Reflect on, and learn from, those messy real-life clinical contexts that we work in. The outcomes of our decisions may not be what we expect and this may, or may not, be a bad thing. What is important, is that we learn from them and continue to develop our clinical decision-making skills whether we are student, novice, or experienced.

To re-iterate, our clinical decision-making may well involve a mix of scientific objective facts and artistic subjective interpretations. That is the real world of decision-making. However, every decision we make will be framed by our own personal and professional moral and ethical codes and life experience and must be consistent with that.

Survival and progress

Memory is deceptive because it is coloured by today's events.

Albert Einstein

I remember the day in 2007, when my contemporary B. May Bernhardt received her question and an early draft of Chapter 5 for the first edition of this book. She was on sabbatical leave, far from her office at the University of British Columbia. Although not in work mode, she emailed almost immediately: 'Caroline – Thanks for trying with this book. I do not expect it will change the world like most books do not, but it at least gets at the knowledge translation issue … which is key if we are to advance the field a tiny centimetre before we retire'. The email was encouraging, and the word 'retire' prompted a 2002 memory of lively dinner conversation at Lasseters Casino, Alice Springs, central Australia, when she told of relishing the prospect of retirement. Among others at the table were Sharynne McLeod (A1), Peter Flipsen, Jr. (A11), John Bernthal (A16), Roslyn Neilson (A22), Nicole Watts Pappas (A30), Tom Powell (A39) and Deb James (A50). Perhaps each person thought fleetingly about retirement before the conversation changed direction, and maybe there were others at the table that thought for a moment of Joan Rosenthal and other colleagues who *had* retired.

Seven years have elapsed since our email exchange, but the retirement itch has not quite overtaken May or me. She continues in her professorial role at the University of British Columbia, and although I relinquished clinical work in September 2011, and have plans to significantly reduce my Continuing Professional Development teaching load soon, I am still absorbed with reading, thinking and writing about the interesting area that is children's speech sound disorders. Among other pleasures, it keeps me in touch with colleagues, including some I have known for a long time. As in the first edition, it seems a satisfactory and rather neat way to round off this new work by posing a question to the first person I ever consulted – with dozens of questions – for a second opinion about a child with a complex speech sound disorder.

Already a highly regarded authority in SLP/SLT clinical and academic circles when I began practice in Sydney, Australia in 1971, Joan Rosenthal was *the* person to ask for help with knotty child speech cases. She was variously referred to as a role model, an expert, the oracle and a guru – but always unassuming, she never behaved like a celebrity SLP! Theory-related and steeped in years of practical experience, her therapy approach to CAS and other developmental speech sound problems was always 'find what works with the individual child'. That was the evidence base that she trusted, stressing that 'what works' of course could change for an individual over time.

Q54. Joan Rosenthal: Resilience in the workplace

Change and progress are frequent words for clinical SLPs/SLTs in their pursuit of effective, efficient and efficacious management for each child with an SSD. All too frequently the quest takes place in work environments that are impacted by political apathy, misguided public policy, funding shortfalls, unstable levels of staffing, unmanageable waiting lists and too little time. And as you have pointed out, another sort of change that clinicians have to deal with is that children with the more severe speech problems have long-term support and intervention needs that alter, as they grow older and their conditions unfold. All this is set against the background of an information explosion in the peer-reviewed print and electronic media that leaves most of us reeling and unable to keep apace. And yet there is something that drives us to persevere: the intellectual and practical challenge, or the perceived needs of the client that require our special expertise, or the

wish to help, or our compulsion to play out the professional role. Or maybe it is to do with our personal perspective and the sheer fascination with the task at hand. What would be in your survival kit for clinicians and clinical educators as they tackle the complex working world of children's SSDs?

A54. Joan Rosenthal: Key components of a survival kit: theory, evidence and experience

Caroline, and readers,

The first point I'd like to make is that our professional evidence base is sketchy, although it's constantly developing. Still, there's not yet enough science in our knowledge of SSDs, our understanding of what is behind them, and our certainty about how we can effectively and efficaciously help children and their families through them, to rely on the published evidence base for our therapy. The same applies to knowing how and what to assess. But the limitations in our published evidence base do not mean that, as clinicians, we work in the dark in intervention. Every piece of intervention we apply is an experiment and needs to be treated as such. Do we continue? Is it working? Can we build on it? Do we need to look at the presenting problem from another angle entirely? The client's response provides the evidence. So my survival kit would contain my theoretical knowledge (continually built on by what you dramatically and accurately describe as the information explosion) hitched to my senses: what I see, hear, and intuit from my client. This indeed provides fascination with the clinical task at hand: selecting from choices about what to do, interpreting what we observe by way of response from our clients, and making further choices about what to do next.

My second point is that, not uniquely among the health professions, SLP/SLT can be beset by fads. The longer you are in this profession and working with SSD, the more you'll be exposed to our fads. They are part and parcel of the information explosion, and they are also a response to our lack of evidence-based knowledge. They come; they sweep away what has gone before; they are adopted with enthusiasm and often with expense. They spawn workshops, continuing education, even certification, sometimes research. And after a while, the next fad arrives. Experience of a succession of fads can give rise to some cynicism, but in a survival kit, I would prefer to find some healthy skepticism.

What relates these two topics: the limited evidence base and the succession of fads in intervention? There in the middle is the here-and-now: the client's behaviour and our response to it, and our behaviour and the client's response to it. Our here-and-now observation provides evidence (that can be linked to the published evidence base and that can inform our reaction to the current fad).

The third item in my survival kit would be a reminder message that flashes on an internal screen: value experience. One's individual and growing experience is a further source of evidence. I remember after my first year of practice as a speech therapist (as it was then in Australia) thinking: 'I've learned more in this year than I did in all the years of my training'. That was not an indictment of my course of study. Indeed, my course of study prepared me to be an independent learner, to be a perceptive and critical observer of my own therapy. The result was that my clinical experience provided me with a stream of evidence and a concomitant stream of questions. Look how this works! Why didn't that work? What if… ? Experience hones one's skills as a clinician, develops wisdom as well as knowledge.

The final item in my survival kit is an understanding that the development of expertise is a two-way street. There is an obligation to share such wisdom as we have acquired, and to learn from what others can contribute. Consider how you can do this. It may be by mentorship, by sharing with colleagues, by brainstorming over clinical problems, by writing, by teaching. It may also be by asking questions, by expressing ignorance, by acknowledging feelings of uncertainty and need for support. I'll confess that it was a weakness of mine, especially as a fairly recent graduate, to try to give the impression that I knew everything—doubtless from fear that someone would discover how little I did know! But it helps to realise that we have a community of wisdom. Value it and be part of it.

Two conclusions

I have thought about how to do this, and try as I might the only solution I can come up with is to give this book two conclusions, one of which is recycled. In the closing paragraph of the first edition I wrote: 'As students, clinicians, clinical educators, academics and researchers in our funny, quirky, specialised world of children with SSD, and their families, we are all workers, thinkers and life-long learners. Our work, thinking and learning with this fascinating, rewarding, challenging, engaging and sometimes frustrating population often meets the four critical criteria of all problem-based learning tasks. The problems we face are open-ended with no 'right' answers and no single route to solutions. The problems are authentic, related to real life. They are complex, involving a variety of skills, a breadth of content, and depth of thought. And they are open to self-assessment, so that we learners can determine for ourselves what work we must do in order to advance to more expert levels of performance. I hope this book will help'. The second conclusion begins with a quotation.

One does not discover new lands without consenting to lose sight of the shore for a very long time.

AndréGide

Writing this edition was an agreeable journey of discovery and re-discovery. It was made possible by the willingness and generosity of fellow travellers: the 60 contributors; the researchers who continually inspire us in their efforts to make the task of treating children with speech sound disorders more efficient, effective and efficacious; and the countless SLP/SLT and Linguist friends and colleagues from around the world who gave encouragement along the way.

References

Bacsfalvi, P., & Bernhardt, B. M. (2011). Long-term outcomes of speech therapy for seven adolescents with visual feedback technologies: ultrasound and electropalatography. *Clinical Linguistics and Phonetics*, 25(11–12), 1034–1043.

Blamey, P. J., Barry, J. G., & Jacq, P. (2001). Phonetic inventory development in young cochlear implant users 6 years postoperation. *Journal of Speech, Language, and Hearing Research*, 44, 73–79.

Bradlow, A. (2002). Confluent talker- and listener-oriented forces in clear speech production. In: Gussenhoven, C., Rietveld, T., & Warner, N. (Eds.), *Papers in Laboratory Phonology VII* (pp. 241–273). Cambridge: Cambridge University Press.

Bradlow, A., Torretta, G., & Pisoni, D. (1996). Intelligibility of normal speech I: Global and fine-grained acoustic-phonetic talker characteristics. *Speech Communication*, 20, 255–272.

Browning, G. G., Rovers, M. M., Williamson, I., Lous, J., & Burton, M. J. (2010). Grommets (ventilation tubes) for hearing loss associated with otitis media with effusion in children. *Cochrane Database of Systematic Reviews*, 6(10), CD001801.

Calmels, M. N., Saliba, I., Wanna, G., Cochard, N., Fillaux, J., Deguine, O., & Fraysse, B. (2004). Speech perception and speech intelligibility in children after cochlear implantation. *International Journal of Pediatric Otorhinolaryngology*, 68(3), 347–351.

Clark, J. G. (1981). Uses and abuses of hearing loss classification. *American Speech-Language-Hearing Association*, 23(7), 493–500.

Connor, C. M., Craig, H. K., Raudenbush, S. W., Heavner, K., & Zwolan, T. A. (2006). The age at which young deaf children receive cochlear implants and their vocabulary and speech-production growth: Is there an added value for early implantation? *Ear and Hearing*, 27(6), 628–644.

Cox, R. M., & Moore, J. N. (1988). Composite speech spectrum for hearing and gain prescriptions. *Journal of Speech & Hearing Research*, 31(1), 102–107.

Dart, S. N. (1991). articulatory and acoustic properties of apical and laminal articulations. Ph.D. Dissertation, Department of Linguistics, University of California, Los Angeles. Reprinted as *UCLA Working Papers in Phonetics*, 79, 1–155.

Dart, S. N. (1998).Comparing French and English coronal consonant articulation. *Journal of Phonetics*, 26, 71–94.

Dollaghan, C. A. (2007). *The handbook for evidence-based practice in communication disorders*. Baltimore, MD: Paul H. Brookes Publishing Co.

Eckert, P. (2000). *Linguistic variation as social practice: the construction of identity in belten high*. New York, NY: Wiley.

Ertmer, D. J. (2008). Speech intelligibility in young cochlear implant recipients: Gains during year three. *Volta Review*, 107(2), 85–99.

Flipsen, P., Jr., & Parker, R. G. (2008). Phonological patterns in the speech of children with cochlear implants. *Journal of Communication Disorders*, 41(4), 337–357.

Foulkes, P. (2005). Sociophonetics. In: Brown, K. (Ed.) *Encyclopedia of Language and Linguistics* (2nd ed., p. 495–500). Amsterdam: Elsevier.

Foulkes, P., & Docherty, G. (2000). Another chapter in the story of /r/: 'labiodental' variants in British English. *Journal of Sociolinguistics*, 4, 30–59.

Grunwell, P. (1985). Developing phonological skills. *Child Language Teaching and Therapy*, 1, 65–72.

Grunwell, P. (1989). Developmental phonological disorders and normal speech development: A review and illustration. *Child Language Teaching and Therapy*, 5, 304–319.

Grunwell, P. (1992). Process of phonological change in developmental speech disorders. *Clinical Linguistics and Phonetics*, 6, 101–122.

Hay, J., Warren, P., & Drager, K. (2006). Factors influencing speech perception in the context of merger-in-progress. *Journal of Phonetics*, 34(4), 58–84.

Jongman, A., Wayland, R., & Wong, S. (2000). Acoustic characteristics of English fricatives. *Journal of the Acoustical Society of America, 108,* 1252–1263.

Kim, J., & Chin, S. B. (2008). Fortition and lenition patterns in the acquisition of obstruents by children with cochlear implants. *Clinical Linguistics & Phonetics, 22,* 233–251.

Kishon-Rabin, L., Taitelbaum-Swead, R., Ezrati-Vinacour, R., Kronnenberg, J., & Hildesheimer, M. (2004). Pre-first word vocalizations of infants with normal hearing and cochlear implants using the PRISE. *International Congress Series. Cochlear Implants. Proceedings of the VIII International Cochlear Implant Conference, 1273,* 360–363.

Labov, W. (1994–2001). *Principles of linguistic change* (2 vols). Oxford: Blackwell.

Lane, H., & Tranel, B. (1971). The Lombard sign and the role of hearing in speech. *The Journal of Speech and Hearing Sciences, 14,* 677–709.

Lane, H., & Perkell, J. S. (2005). Control of voice-onset time in the absence of hearing: a review. *Journal of Speech Language & Hearing Research, 48*(6), 1334–1343.

Lieu, J. E. C. (2004). Speech-language and educational consequences of unilateral hearing loss in children. *Archives of Otolaryngology – Head and Neck Surgery, 130*(5), 524–530.

Lim, S. Y., & Simser, J. (2005). Auditory-verbal therapy for children with hearing impairment. *Annals, Academy of Medicine, Singapore, 34*(4), 307–312.

Linville, S. (1998). Acoustic correlates of perceived versus actual sexual orientation in men's speech. *Pholia Phoniatrica et Logopaedica, 50,* 35–48.

Mack, S., & Munson, B. (2012). The association between /s/ quality and perceived sexual orientation of men's voices: implicit and explicit measures. *Journal of Phonetics, 40,* 198–212.

Massaro, D. W., & Light, J. (2004). Using visible speech to train perception and production of speech for individuals with hearing loss. *Journal of Speech Language & Hearing Research, 47*(2), 304–320.

Mendoza-Denton, N. (2007). *Homegirls: symbolic practices in the making of latina youth styles.* Malden, MA: Blackwell.

Milroy, L. (1987). *Language and Social Networks* (2nd ed.), Oxford: Blackwell.

Moeller, M. P., Hoover, B., Putman, C., Arbataitis, K., Bohnenkamp, G., Peterson, B., Wood, S., Lewis, D., Pittman, A., & Stelmachowicz, P. (2007). Vocalizations of infants with hearing loss compared with infants with normal hearing: Part I–phonetic development. *Ear & Hearing, 28*(5), 605–627.

Müller, N. (Ed.) (2006). *Multilayered transcription.* San Diego, CA: Plural Publishing.

Munson, B. (2011). The influence of actual and imputed talker gender on fricative perception, revisited. *Journal of the Acoustical Society of America, 130,* 2631–2634.

Munson, B., & Babel, M. (2007). Loose lips and silver tongues, or, projecting sexual orientation through speech. *Language and Linguistics Compass, 1,* 416–449.

Munson, B., McDonald, E. C., DeBoe, N. L., & White, A. R. (2006). The acoustic and perceptual bases of judgments of women and men's sexual orientation from read speech. *Journal of Phonetics, 34,* 202–240.

Munson, B., & Zimmerman, L. (2006). *Perceptual Bias and the Myth of the 'Gay Lisp'.* Poster presentation at the annual meeting of the American Speech-Language-Hearing Association, Miami, FL, November 16.

Niedzielski, N. (1999). The effect of social information on the perception of sociolinguistic variables. *Journal of Language and Social Psychology, 18,* 62–85.

Ohala, J. J. (1990). 'There is no interface between phonetics and phonology: a personal view'. *Journal of Phonetics, 18,* 153–171.

Osberger, M. J. (1992). Speech intelligibility in the hearing impaired: Research and clinical implications. In: R. D. Kent (Ed.), *Intelligibility in speech disorders: Theory, measurement, and management* (pp. 233–265). Philadelphia, PA: John Benjamins Publishing.

Paatsch, L. E., Blamey, P. J., Sarant, J. Z., & Bow, C. P. (2006). The effects of speech production and vocabulary training on different components of spoken language performance. *Journal of Deaf Studies & Deaf Education, 11*(1), 39–55.

Pantelemidou, V., Herman, R., & Thomas, J. (2003). Efficacy of speech intervention using electropalatography with a cochlear implant user. *Clinical Linguistics & Phonetics, 17*(4–5), 383–392.

Peng, S. C., Weiss, A. L., Cheung, H., & Lin, Y. S. (2004). Consonant production and language skills in Mandarin-speaking children with cochlear implants. *Archives of Otolaryngology – Head & Neck Surgery, 130*(5), 592–597.

Petinou, K., Schwartz, R. G., Mody, M., & Gravel, J. S. (1999). The impact of otitis media with effusion on early phonetic inventories: A longitudinal prospective investigation. *Clinical Linguistics & Phonetics*, *13*(5), 351–367.

Rhoades, E. A. (2006). Research outcomes of auditory-verbal intervention: Is the approach justified? *Deafness & Education International*, *8*, 125–143.

Roberts, J. (2002). 'Child language variation' In: Chambers, Trudgill, & Schilling-Estes (Eds.), *The handbook of language variation and change*. (pp. 333–348). Oxford: Blackwell.

Schonweiler, R., Ptok, M., & Radu, H. J. (1998). A cross-sectional study of speech- and language-abilities of children with normal hearing, mild fluctuating conductive hearing loss, or moderate to profound sensoneurinal hearing loss. *International Journal of Pediatric Otorhinolaryngology*, *44*(3), 251–258.

Shriberg, L. D., Flipsen, P., Jr., Thielke, H., Kwiatkowski, J., Kertoy, M. K., Katcher, M. L., Nellis, R. A., & Block, M. G. (2000). Risk for speech disorder associated with early recurrent otitis media with effusion: two retrospective studies. *Journal of Speech Language & Hearing Research*, *43*(1), 79–99.

Simpson, S. A., Thomas, C. L., van der Linden, M. K., Macmillan, H., van der Wouden, J. C., & Butler, C. (2007). Identification of children in the first four years of life for early treatment for otitis media with effusion. [Update of *Cochrane Database Syst Rev.* 2003;(2):CD004163.]. *Cochrane Database of Systematic Reviews* (1), CD004163.

Strand, E., & Johnson, K. (1996). Gradient and visual speaker normalization in the perception of fricatives. In: D. Gibbon (Ed.), *Natural language processing and speech technology: Results of the 3rd Konvens conference, bielfelt, October 1996* (pp. 14–26). Berlin: Mouton de Gruyter.

Thomas, E. (2007). Phonological and phonetic characteristics of African-American English. *Language and Linguistics Compass*, *1*, 450–475.

Trudgill, P. (2004). *New-dialect formation: The inevitability of colonial Englishes*. Edinburgh: Edinburgh University Press.

Van Borsel, J., Van Rentergem, S., & Verhaeghe, L. (2007). The prevalence of lisping in young adults. *Journal of Communication Disorders*, *40*(6), 493–502.

Weiner, F. (1981). Treatment of phonological disability using the method of meaningful contrast: Two case studies. *Journal of Speech and Hearing Disorders*, *46*, 97–103.

Contributor index

Subject index

Children's Speech Sound Disorders, Second Edition. Caroline Bowen.
© 2015 John Wiley & Sons, Ltd. Published 2015 by John Wiley & Sons, Ltd.
Companion website: www.wiley.com/go/bowen/speechlanguagetherapy

CPSIA information can be obtained
at www.ICGtesting.com
Printed in the USA
LVHW051120010223
738327LV00011B/321